A Clinician's Guide to Primary Healthcare

A Clinician's Guide to Primary Healthcare

Edited by **Kelly Ward**

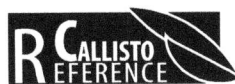

R CALLISTO
REFERENCE

New York

Published by Callisto Reference,
106 Park Avenue, Suite 200,
New York, NY 10016, USA
www.callistoreference.com

A Clinician's Guide to Primary Healthcare
Edited by Kelly Ward

International Standard Book Number: 978-1-63239-739-3 (Hardback)

Printed in the United States of America.

Contents

Preface

Every book is a source of knowledge and this one is no exception. The idea that led to the conceptualization of this book was the fact that the world is advancing rapidly; which makes it crucial to document the progress in every field. I am aware that a lot of data is already available, yet, there is a lot more to learn. Hence, I accepted the responsibility of editing this book and contributing my knowledge to the community.

The objective of primary health care is easily accessible health care facilities for all. It also tries to ensure clean and improved environment to prevent health hazards. The aim to deliver better facilities without discrimination has been prevailing ever since the dawn of globalization; but there is a vast gap between demand and supply. This book is a compilation of chapters that discuss the most vital concepts and emerging trends in this field. The readers would gain knowledge that would broaden their perspective about primary health care. Such selected concepts that redefine this field have been presented herein. Different approaches, evaluations, methodologies and advanced studies in the sector of primary healthcare have also been included in this book.

While editing this book, I had multiple visions for it. Then I finally narrowed down to make every chapter a sole standing text explaining a particular topic, so that they can be used independently. However, the umbrella subject sinews them into a common theme. This makes the book a unique platform of knowledge.

I would like to give the major credit of this book to the experts from every corner of the world, who took the time to share their expertise with us. Also, I owe the completion of this book to the never-ending support of my family, who supported me throughout the project.

Editor

Determinants of active pulmonary tuberculosis in Ambo Hospital, West Ethiopia

Authors:
Tenna Ephrem[1]
Bezatu Mengiste[2]
Frehiwot Mesfin[2]
Wanzahun Godana[3]

Affiliations:
[1]Oromia Regional Health Bureau, Addis Ababa, Ethiopia

[2]College of Health and Medical Sciences, Haramaya University, Ethiopia

[3]College of Medicine and Health Sciences, Arba Minch University, Ethiopia

Correspondence to:
Tenna Ephrem

Email:
tennnaephrem@yahoo.com

Postal address:
PO Box 24341, Addis Ababa, Ethiopia

Objectives: The aim of this study was to determine factors associated with active pulmonary tuberculosis seen in cases in Ambo Hospital, Ethiopia.

Design: A facility-based prospective case-control study.

Setting: Patients attending Ambo Hospital from 01 December 2011 to 29 March 2012.

Participants: The sample included 312 adult patients attending Ambo Hospital. The main outcome measure was presence of active pulmonary tuberculosis (TB).

Explanatory measures: Age, gender, occupation, educational status, marital status, place of residence, patient history of TB, family history of TB, human immunodeficiency virus (HIV) infection, smoking, alcohol intake, khat chewing, body mass index (BMI), employment, diabetes, history of asthma, previous history of worm infestation, history of hospitalisation, number of adults living in the household (HH), person per room, housing condition.

Results: A total of 312 study participants, including 104 active pulmonary tuberculosis (PTB) cases (cases) and 208 non-active PTB cases (controls), were recruited for the present study. Having one or more family member with a history of TB (OR = 4.4; 95% CI: 1.50–12.90), marital status (OR = 7.6; 95% CI: 2.2–12.6), male gender (OR = 3.2; 95% CI: 1.4–7), rural residence (OR = 3.3; P = 0.012), being a current or past smoker (OR = 2.8; 95% CI: 1.1–7.2), BMI < 18.5 (OR = 2.1; 95% CI: 1.03–4.2), HIV infection (OR = 8.8; 95% CI: 2.4–23.8) and a history of worm infestation (OR = 6.4; 95% CI: 2.6–15.4) remained significant independent host-related factors for active PTB.

Conclusion: Patients who came from a compound with more than two HHs were more likely to develop active PTB than those who came from a compound with only one HH. Those who lived in houses with no windows were more likely to develop active PTB than those who lived in houses with one or more windows, had a family history of TB, lived in rural areas. Sex of the patient was a predicting factor. Not being the owner of the house was significantly more associated with active PTB. Measures taken to reduce the prevalence and burden of active PTB should consider these determinant factors.

Les déterminants de tuberculose pulmonaire active à l'hôpital d'Ambo, en Ethiopie occidentale.

Objectifs: Le but de cette étude était de déterminer les Facteurs associés de Tuberculose pulmonaire active à l'Hôpital d'Ambo.

Conception: Une étude cas-témoins prospective au sein d'un établissement.

Cadre: les patients qui sont venus à l'hôpital d'Ambo du 15 décembre 2011 au 29 mars 2012.

Participants: 312 patients adultes sont venus à l'hôpital d'Ambo. Résultats principaux: présence de Tuberculose pulmonaire active.

Mesures explicatives: Age, Sexe, Profession, niveau d'études, état civil, lieu de résidence, état tuberculeux du patient, antécédents de Tuberculose, infection VIH, tabagisme, consommation d'alcool, mastication de khât, BMI, emploi, diabète, antécédents d'asthme, antécédents d'infection par des vers, hospitalisations passées, nombre d'adultes vivant au HH, nombre de personnes par chambre, conditions de logement.

Résultats: On a recruté 312 participants pour cette étude, 104 cas de Tuberculose pulmonaire active (PTB) et 208 cas de PTB non active (Contrôles). Les patients ayant un membre ou plus de leur famille atteint de Tuberculose (OR = 4.4, 95% CI : 1.50–12.90), les célibataires (OR 7.6, 95% CI : 2.2–12.6), les personnes de sexe masculin (OR 3.2, 95% CI : 1.4–7), les personnes des régions rurales (OR 3.3, p = 0.012), les fumeurs ou anciens fumeurs (OR 2.8, 95% CI : 1.1–7.2), la sous-alimentation (BMI < 18.5) (OR 2.1 et 95% CI : 1.03–4.2), l'Infection VIH (OR 8.8 et 95% CI : de 2.4–23.8), les antécédents d'infection de vers (OR 6.4 et 95% CI : 2.6–15.4) sont indépendamment des facteurs importants propres aux personnes atteintes de Tuberculose pulmonaire active.

Conclusions: les patients provenant d'un composé de plus de deux HH étaient plus susceptibles de développer la Tuberculose pulmonaire active que ceux qui provenaient d'un composé avec un seul HH. Ceux qui vivent dans des maisons sans fenêtres étaient plus susceptibles de développer la Tuberculose pulmonaire active que ceux qui vivent dans des maisons à une fenêtre ou plus. Ceux qui n'étaient pas propriétaire de la maison étaient beaucoup plus susceptibles d'être atteint de Tuberculose pulmonaire active. Les mesures prises pour diminuer la prévalence et le fardeau de la Tuberculose pulmonaire active devraient considérer ces facteurs décisifs.

Introduction

Tuberculosis (TB) is an airborne bacterial disease. The causal agent is the tubercle bacillus *Mycobacterium tuberculosis*, and sometimes *Mycobacterium bovis* or *Mycobacterium africanum*.[1,2] The most common form of disease, caused by *M. tuberculosis*, is pulmonary tuberculosis (PTB). In the lungs, the bacterium is taken up and if it is not contained by the immune system, it is able to grow uncontrollably, resulting in the subsequent development of TB. The pulmonary form of TB is infectious because it is transmitted through aerosol whenever individuals with active PTB cough, sneeze, talk or laugh, and droplets in the air are inhaled by those who are in close contact with the infectious case.[3,4,5,6]

Globally, TB represents one third of the world's health problems; roughly two billion people are affected.[7,8] Annually, an estimated eight to ten million people develop TB owing to primary infection, reactivation or re-infection.[8] In 2009, there were an estimated 9.4 million new cases, 14 million existing cases and 1.68 million deaths from TB. Most cases were in the South-East Asia, African and Western Pacific regions (35%, 30% and 20%, respectively).[7,9] Ninety-five per cent of TB cases in low-income countries are amongst people between 15 and 50 years old.[10,11]

TB is still the leading cause of infection in some tropical countries. In some countries, overcrowding in urban slums further aggravates the situation. The co-existence of human immunodeficiency virus (HIV) infection and TB worsen the health of the population.[4,8,12]

Ethiopia is amongst the world's 22 high-burden TB countries. An overall incidence rate (people acquiring PTB) increases from time to time. The trend of increment in incidence rate rose from 331 per 100 000 in 2000 to 378 per 100 000 in 2007.[1,13]

TB is a multifactorial disease in which environmental and individual factors contribute to the disease process.[5,14] An individual with acquired immune deficiency syndrome (AIDS) is 110–170 times more likely to develop TB than a person with no known risk factors, and an individual with HIV has a risk of 50–110 times greater than a person with no known risk factors.[3] Individuals with HIV have deficient immune systems for immunologic containment. Globally, TB is the leading cause of mortality of people with HIV.[15]

Many factors are related to TB, such as smoking,[16,17] and rates of TB infection, disease and mortality are significantly higher amongst smokers.[18,19,20] Another factor that is related to TB is diabetes mellitus (DM)[2,13] and a recent meta-analysis found that patients with DM were three times more likely to have TB than controls.[21] Drinking alcohol excessively also increases the likelihood of developing TB by three times more than in those who do not. Generally, there are different explanations for this scenario.[22]

Relatively little data are available concerning the association between nutrition or low body mass index (BMI) and TB.

One recent review on TB and low BMI indicated a strong dose–response relationship with TB incidence; in the six summarised studies, TB increased exponentially as BMI decreased.[23] Owing to the widespread global prevalence of under-nutrition, on a population level, the effect of this risk factor has been predicted to be substantial.[24] Deficiencies for protein and micronutrients such as vitamin D, arginine and zinc[3] increase the risk of TB. There is a documented inverse relationship between BMI and risk of progression from TB infection to TB disease.[25]

Concerning individual host factors, results from multivariate analyses from three West African countries (Guinea, Guinea-Bissau and The Gambia) identified TB to be related to male gender, a family history of TB, absence of a Bacillus Calmette–Guérin (BCG) scar, smoking, alcohol use, anaemia, seropositive HIV status, and history of and treatment for worm infestation.[14]

A study conducted in Gonder, Ethiopia on TB risk factors for PTB found that there is a strong relationship between TB and HIV status (7.8 times higher in cases) and between TB and intestinal helminth infestation (4.2 times higher in cases).[26]

TB burden follows a socio-economic gradient; therefore, poverty and its related conditions are strong social and environmental determinants of TB.[24] Studies from Russia, The Gambia and south-west Ethiopia revealed that family history of TB was independently related to active PTB.[26,27,28] Furthermore, there was some evidence that this effect was higher when the previous or former TB case was in close family, as compared with unrelated household members. The clustering of TB within families could reflect not only the place of transmission within the family, but also a genetic contribution to the susceptibility to active PTB.[29]

Efforts to decrease the rates of TB must focus on controlling transmission and identifying associated factors as a means of reducing the overall burden of the disease. It has been observed that not all patients who have PTB transmit the disease; therefore, research must include an examination of specific determinant factors to show which influence and result in development of the disease without difference in the infection status. The present research focused on PTB patients to identify the factors related to developing active PTB in comparison with people without TB.

Research methods and design
Study area and period

The study was conducted in Ambo Hospital, the zonal referral hospital of the West Shoa zone of Oromia Regional State, from 15 December 2011 to 29 March 2012. The town Ambo is located 115 km away from Addis Ababa in the western part of Ethiopia. It is the only governmental institution in the zone that has a functional X-ray machine for chest radiography to detect smear-negative TB cases. The hospital serves the population of the zone and neighbouring districts as a referral hospital.

Study design

A facility-based prospective case-control study was conducted amongst patients visiting the adult outpatient department (OPD) of Ambo Hospital.

Active PTB patients (smear-positive and smear-negative TB cases) diagnosed in the OPD of the hospital during the study period were included in the study. Active PTB was defined as bacteriologically, radiologically or clinically detected TB. A smear-positive or smear-negative TB case was defined as one for which chest radiography findings were consistent with TB, there was a lack of response to a trial of broad-spectrum antimicrobial agents (excluding anti-TB drugs and fluoroquinolones) and a physician's judgement on detecting a case as TB. The TB screening and diagnosis protocol of the World Health Organization (WHO) was used.

Controls were OPD patients who were free of active PTB and TB screening signs and symptoms during the study period. According to the WHO standards, individuals who are free of these constitutional symptoms are declared free of active TB although they may be infected with the TB bacterium.

Study population

The study population included all patients aged 15 years and older who attended the OPD of Ambo Hospital during the study period. On average, there were 73 OPD patients per day.

Sample size

Sample size was estimated using the Open-Epi sample size calculator software (CDC, Atlanta) according to the following factors:

- power: 80%
- confidence interval (CI): 95%
- sample ratio of controls to cases: 2:1
- proportion of family history of PTB amongst controls: 17%
- odds ratio (OR) of family history of TB from previous studies[14] (in three West African countries): 2.38

With the Fleiss continuity correction, the sample size was set at 95 cases and 189 controls, and with a 10% non-respondent rate the sample size became 104 cases and 208 controls. The total sample size was therefore 312.

Sampling procedure

All active PTB patients (smear-positive and smear-negative TB cases) aged 15 years and older at the OPD of the hospital during the study period were included. The first OPD attendee who was free of active PTB and aged 15 years or older following each case was approached to serve as a control in the study. If these individuals refused participation, the next eligible OPD attendee was approached.

Study design

The outcome variable of the study was active PTB status. Independent variables included the following host-related variables: age, gender, occupation, educational status, marital status, place of residence, patient history of TB, family history of TB, HIV status, smoking history, alcohol intake, khat chewing, BMI, employment, diabetes status, history of asthma, previous history of worm infestation, history of hospitalisation, and history of incarceration. Environment-related variables were as follows: number of households (HHs) in the compound, number of adults in the HH, number of people per room, wall type, floor type, type of roof and/or ceiling, number of windows, availability of electricity, separate kitchen, latrine, ownership of the house, and type of cooking fuel.

Data collection

A pre-tested structured questionnaire was used to collect all data on the study variables, a beam balance scale was used to measure weight, and a tape measure to measure the height of the respondents. All OPD patients were interviewed by data collectors for their cases at exit to identify PTB cases and consult with the OPD physician to confirm the case. Study participants answered a structured questionnaire that was conducted in their own language by trained diploma nurses. Information was collected on a wide range of potential host-related and environment-related risk factors for active PTB. Host information included basic demographic data (age, gender and ethnicity), past medical history of asthma and diabetes, history of smoking and alcohol consumption, schooling and category of occupation, and previous history of TB. The environmental factors included the type of cooking fuel used, building structure and materials of the house, housing conditions, whether there was another member of the HH with TB disease, and a crowding index (such as number of adults living in the HH, number of HHs in the compound and people per room). All HIV test results of the cases and controls were recorded, the height and weight of the respondents were measured, and BMI was calculated.

Data analysis

The data were entered into a pre-drafted coding sheet on Epi Info software (version 3.5.3) by two different data clerks. A binary logistic analysis with conditional method was used to measure the association between the dependent variable and independent variables using an OR and 95% CI. Statistical significance was set at $\alpha \leq 0.05$. In an attempt to identify the relative effects of explanatory variables on the outcome variable, hierarchical multivariate analyses were applied. Independent predictor variables with a P-value < 0.25 were entered into the final regression model, based on the likelihood ratio for further analyses in different models.

A backward stepwise entry method was used for the logistic regression for each model. Finally, a combined multivariate model was constructed from the individual host- and environment-related risk factors for analysis.

Data quality control

A properly designed and pre-tested questionnaire was used. Training, close supervision during data collection and double data entry were implemented as quality control measures.

Ethical considerations

Ethical approval and clearance for this study were obtained from the Institutional Research Ethics Review Committee of the College of Health and Medical Sciences, Haramaya University. At all levels, officials were contacted and permission from administrators was secured. All the necessary explanation about the purpose of the study and its procedures was explained with the assurance of confidentiality. Written and verbal consent from the study participants were also secured.

Result and discussion

Results

A total of 312 study participants (104 active PTB cases [cases] and 208 non-active PTB cases [controls]) were recruited. The median age of cases and controls was 32 and 30, respectively. The majority of the study participants (93.9%) were of the Oromo ethnic group. More than half (58.3%) of the respondents were orthodox in their religion (Table 1).

Host-related factors

There were more male patients amongst the cases (74; 71.2%) than amongst the controls (94; 45.2%). The majority of the cases (64; 61.5%) and controls (141; 67.8%) were married; more widowed or divorced patients were part of the cases group (14; 13.5%) than the control group (9; 4.3%). A total of 66 case patients (63.5%) and 109 of the controls (52.4%) were from rural areas. Patient history of TB was higher amongst cases (15; 14.4%) than amongst controls (12; 5.8%). Family history of TB was also higher in cases (20; 19.2%) than in controls (12; 5.8%). Current or past history of smoking was more common amongst cases (24; 23.1%) than amongst controls (15; 7.2%). Khat was more commonly chewed in cases (13; 12.5%) than

TABLE 1: Demographic characteristics of pulmonary tuberculosis cases and controls in Ambo Hospital, Western Ethiopia, 2011 and 2012.

Variables	Cases *n* (%)	Controls *n* (%)	Total *n* (%)
Age			
Mean(standard deviation)	35 (13.4)	35.7(16.1)	35.5 (15.1)
Median (Range)	32 (64)	30 (58)	31 (66)
Religion (%)			
Orthodox	66 (63.5)	116 (55.8)	182 (58.3)
Protestant	33 (31.7)	83 (39.8)	116 (37.2)
Muslim	3 (2.9)	7 (3.4)	10 (3.2)
Other	2 (1.9)	2 (1.0)	4 (1.3)
Ethnicity (%)			
Oromo	94 (90.4)	199 (95.7)	293 (93.9)
Amhara	5 (4.8)	8 (3.8)	13 (4.2)
Other	5 (4.8)	1 (0.5)	6 (1.9)

TABLE 2: Bivariate analysis of host-related factors associated with active pulmonary tuberculosis in Ambo Hospital, Western Ethiopia, 2011 and 2012.

Variables	Cases (%)	Controls (%)	COR (95% CI)	P-value
Age†				
15–24	28 (26.9)	56 (26.9)	1.00	
25–34	22 (21.2)	64 (30.8)	0.68 (0.35, 1.34)	0.27
35–44	25 (24)	43 (20.7)	1.16 (0.60, 2.27)	0.66
> 44	29 (27.9)	45 (21.6)	1.29 (0.67, 2.47)	0.45
Gender†				
Female	30 (28.8)	114 (54.8)	1.00	
Male‡	74 (71.2)	94 (45.2)	3.0 (1.8, 5.0)	0.000
Educational status				
No formal education	42 (40.4)	90 (43.3)	0.89 (0.55, 1.43)	0.63
Formal education	62 (59.6)	118 (65.7)	1.00	
Marital status†				
Married	64 (61.5)	141 (67.8)	1.00	
Single	26 (25)	58 (27.9)	1.0 (0.57, 1.7)	0.988
Widowed/divorced‡	14 (13.5)	9 (4.3)	3.4 (1.4, 8.3)	0.007
Residence†				
Urban	38 (36.8)	99 (46.7)	1.00	
Rural	66 (63.5)	109 (52.4)	1.6 (0.97, 2.56)	0.064
Occupation†				
Civil/public servant	17 (16.3)	46 (22.1)	1.00	
Farmer	45 (43.3)	87 (41.8)	1.4 (0.72, 2.7)	0.32
Merchant	9 (8.7)	12 (5.8)	2.0 (0.73, 5.7)	0.18
Student	12 (11.5)	43 (20.7)	0.76 (0.32, 1.76)	0.52
Daily labour‡	14 (13.5)	11 (5.3)	3.4 (1.3, 9.)	0.012
Other	7 (6.7)	9 (4.3)	2.1 (0.77, 6.54)	0.20
Patient history of TB†				
No	89 (85.6)	169 (94.2)	1.00	-
Yes‡	15 (14.4)	12 (5.8)	2.8 (1.24, 6.12)	0.013
Family history of TB†				
No	84 (80.8)	196 (94.2)	1.00	-
Yes‡	20 (19.2)	12 (5.8)	3.9.0 (1.82, 8.3)	0.000
Smoking†				
Never	80 (76.9)	193 (92.8)	1.00	-
Current/past‡	24 (23.1)	15 (7.2)	3.9 (1.9, 7.6)	0.000
Khat chewing†				
Never	91 (87.5)	197 (94.7)	1.00	-
Current/past‡	13 (12.5)	11 (5.3)	2.6(1.1, 5.9)	0.029
BMI†				
< 18.5‡	66 (63.5)	87 (41.8)	2.4 (1.5, 3.9)	0.000
≥ 18.5	41 (36.5)	121 (58.2)	1.00	-
Employment				
Employed	22 (21.2)	48 (23.1)	1.00	-
Unemployed	82 (78.8)	160 (78.8)	1.12 (0.63, 2.0)	0.70
HIV status‡				
Negative	83 (79.8)	202 (97.1)	1.00	-
Positive‡	21 (20.2)	6 (2.9)	8.5 (3.32, 21.9)	0.000
History of worm infestation‡				
No	65 (62.5)	185 (88.9)	1.00	-
Yes‡	39 (37.5)	23 (11.1)	4.8 (2.7, 8.7)	0.000
Incarceration in last 2 years				
No	98 (94.2)	201 (96.6)	1.00	-
Yes	6 (5.8)	7 (3.4)	1.8 (0.58, 5.37)	0.32

†, Variables with at least one category significant at 25% for further analysis; ‡, Significant at 5%.
BMI, body mass index; COR, crude odd ratio; HIV, human immunodeficiency virus.

in controls (11; 5.3%). Under-nutrition (BMI < 18.5) was higher amongst cases (66; 63.5%) than amongst controls (87; 41.8%). HIV infection was higher in cases (21; 20.2%) than in controls (6; 2.9%) (Table 2).

TABLE 3: Environmental factors related to active pulmonary tuberculosis in Ambo Hospital, Western Ethiopia, 2011 and 2012.

Variables	Cases (%)	Controls (%)	Cr OR (95% CI)	Cr P-value
HHs in the compound†				
1	67 (64.4)	168 (80.8)	1.00	-
>1	37 (35.6)	40 (19.2)	2.32 (1.4, 4)	0.002
Adults living in the HH				
1–5	63 (61.8)	120 (58.5)	1.00	-
>5	39 (38.2)	85 (41.5)	0.9 (0.54, 1.4)	0.56
Persons per room†				
≤2	23 (22.1)	64 (30.8)	1.00	-
>2	81 (77.9)	144 (69.2)	1.57 (0.9, 2.7)	0.104
Wall type				
Cement	7 (6.7)	17 (8.2)	1.00	-
Mud	97 (93.3)	191 (91.8)	1.2 (0.5, 3.1)	0.65
Floor type†				
Cement	9 (8.7)	36 (17.3)	1.00	-
Earth/other	95 (91.3)	172 (82.7)	2.2 (1.0, 4.8)	0.044
Roof type†				
Corrugated iron sheet	83 (79.8)	188 (90.4)	1.00	-
Thatch	21 (20.2)	20 (9.6)	2.4 (1.2, 4.6)	0.011
Ceiling				
Yes	50 (48.1)	93 (44.7)	1.00	-
No	54 (51.9)	115 (55.3)	0.87 (0.55, 1.4)	0.57
Windows†				
Present	79 (76)	188 (90.4)	1.00	-
Absent	25 (24)	20 (9.6)	3.0 (1.56, 5.66)	0.001
Electricity				
Yes	54 (51.9)	98 (47.1)	1.00	-
No	50 (48.1)	110(52.9)	0.83 (0.83, 1.3)	0.42
Electric cooker				
Present	10 (6.9)	14 (6.7)	1.00	-
Absent	94 (90.4)	194 (93.3)	0.68 (0.3, 1.6)	0.37
Separate kitchen				
Yes	82 (78.8)	154 (74)	1.00	-
No	22 (21.2)	54 (26.0)	0.77 (0.44, 1.3)	0.35
Ownership of house†				
Yes	66 (63.5)	180 (86.5)	1.00	-
No	38 (36.5)	28 (13.5)	3.7 (2.1, 6.5)	0.000

†, Significant at 25% level of significance.
CI, confidence interval; Cr, crude; HH, household

In the multivariate analysis, male patients were 3.2 times more likely (95% CI: 1.4–7.0) to develop active PTB than female patients. Patients who were from rural areas were 3.3 times more likely to develop active PTB than those who were from urban areas ($P = 0.012$). Family history of TB had a significant association with active PTB (Table 2). Under-nutrition (BMI < 18.5) was significantly associated with the development of active PTB, with an adjusted OR of 2.1 and 95% CI of 1.03–4.2. HIV infection was found to have a high association with active PTB, with an adjusted OR of 8.8 and 95% CI of 2.4–23.8. A history of worm infestation was also significantly associated with active PTB, with an adjusted OR of 6.4 and 95% CI of 2.6–15.4 (Table 3).

Environment-related factors

In the bivariate analysis of environmental factors for active PTB, the number of HHs in the compound, number of persons per room, type of house floor, type of house roof, number of windows and ownership of the house were all found to be associated with active PTB. Of the 12 variables entered into the bivariate analysis, only six predictor variables were significantly associated with active PTB cases (see Table 3). These variables were included for further analyses in multivariate models.

In the combined multivariate analysis of host- and environment-related factors, patients who lived in houses with more than one HH in the compound were significantly more likely to develop active PTB than with those who lived in HHs with only one house in the compound (adjusted OR: 2.2; 95% CI: 1.02–4.8). Patients who lived in houses with no windows were more likely to develop active PTB than those who lived in houses with one or more windows (OR: 4.3; 95% CI: 1.7–11.0). Not being the owner of the house was found to have an association with active PTB, with an adjusted OR of 10.8 and 95% CI of 3.85–13.3 (Table 4).

Discussion

In the present study, the risk factors for active PTB amongst patients at Ambo Hospital were as follows: being male, being single, living in a rural area, having a history of household exposure to a known TB case, smoking, a BMI < 18, HIV infection and a history of worm infestation. These were independent predictors of active PTB. It was also found that having more than one HH in the compound, more than two people living per room, an absence of windows and not being the owner of the house were factors independently associated with active PTB.

Cigarette smoking was independently associated with active PTB, with a clear effect from duration of smoking. This finding is in line with previous studies elsewhere (West African countries, Spain and India), in which a similar association between tobacco smoking and PTB was reported.[14,29,30] Similarly, several systematic reviews have found that rates of TB infection, disease and mortality are significantly higher amongst smokers.[18,19,20] It is reported that smoking results in histological changes in the lower respiratory tract, including bronchial inflammation, fibrosis, vascular intimal thickening and destruction of alveoli.[16] These changes affect epithelial function (e.g. reduced ciliary activity, difficulty in clearance of inhaled substances and altered vascular and epithelial permeability). The results of the current study therefore supports the hypothesis that there is an increased risk of smokers developing active PTB, which is commonly attributed to physiological changes in the lungs caused by long-time smoking.[16,30] As smoking is becoming an increasing public health problem in low-income countries, especially amongst younger age groups, these results reinforce the need for appropriate public health interventions, as recommended by the WHO Framework Convention on Tobacco Control, which is aimed at helping younger individuals not to develop active PTB.[31] This issue can be adequately addressed in TB control programme policies. In the meantime, TB-control personnel should have counselling skills to advise TB-infected individuals and their relatives about the advantages of stopping smoking.

TABLE 4: Combined environmental- and host-related factors for active pulmonary tuberculosis: multivariate analysis (n = 312) in Ambo Hospital, Western Ethiopia, 2011 and 2012.

Variables	Cases	Controls	Adj OR (95% CI)	Adj P-value
Gender				
Female	30	114	1.00	-
Male	74	94	3.16 (1.4, 7.0)	0.005
Marital status				
Married	64	141	1.00	-
Single	26	58	7.6 (2.2, 12.6)	0.001
Widowed/divorced	14	9	3.3 (0.7, 8.5)	0.12
Residence				
Urban	38	99	1.00	-
Rural	66	109	3.3 (1.3, 8.6)	0.012
Patient history of TB				
No	89	169	1.00	-
Yes	15	12	2.7 (0.8, 8.7)	0.09
Family history of TB				
No	84	196	1.00	-
Yes	20	12	4.4 (1.5, 12.9)	0.008
Smoking				
Never	86	193	1.00	-
Current/past	18	15	2.8 (1.1, 7.2)	0.034
BMI				
< 18.5	66	87	2.1 (1.03, 4.2)	0.042
≥ 18.5	38	121	1.00	-
HIV status				
Negative	83	202	1.00	-
Positive	21	6	8.8 (2.4, 23.8)	0.001
History of worm infestation				
No	65	185	1.00	-
Yes	39	23	6.4 (2.6, 15.4)	0.001
No of HHs in the compound				
1	67	168	1.00	-
> 1	37	40	2.2 (1.02, 4.8)	0.046
Persons per room				
≤ 2	23	64	1.00	-
> 2	81	144	4.1 (1.7, 9.7)	0.001
Floor type				
Cement	9	36	1.00	-
Earth/other	95	172	4.5 (1.3, 15.7)	0.018
Window				
Present	79	188	1.00	-
Absent	25	20	4.3 (1.7, 11.0)	0.003
Ownership of house				
Yes	66	180	1.00	-
No	38	28	10.8 (3.85, 13.3)	0.001

Adj, adjusted; BMI, body mass index; HH, household; OR, odds ratio.

HIV infection is amongst the determinants that have measurably increased the risk for active TB and has had a substantial effect on altering TB incidence rates over the past few decades. At a population level, rising HIV prevalence is strongly associated with dramatic increases in PTB notification rates. This is especially so in sub-Saharan Africa, where there are high HIV infection and prevalence rates, and new TB infections are three to five times higher than in 1980.[2]

In the present study, HIV infection was a significant independent risk factor for active PTB, which is consistent with previous studies conducted in African countries.[14] According to the WHO, 30% of TB cases amongst 15- to 49-year-old adults in sub-Saharan Africa are commonly because of HIV,[13] and every year nearly a 10% continuous increase in TB is expected in countries with high HIV infection rates. The major factors contributing to the increased number of HIV-associated TB cases in Africa are the increased risk of reactivation of latent TB infection in HIV-infected persons because of decreased immunity, and the increased risk of progression of TB disease because of HIV infection, which will, in turn, result in increased TB transmission rates in the community.

The present study showed that under-nutrition (BMI < 18.5) was an independent determinant factor for active PTB, which is in agreement with previous studies.[24,26] There are relatively little data on the relationship between BMI and TB, which may be due to the complexity of mechanisms linking nutrition, the immune system and TB, and the difficulties in identifying the relevant biologic markers. One recent review on TB and low BMI indicated that a strong dose–response relationship with TB incidence increases exponentially as BMI decreases.[23] At a population level, the effect of this risk factor has been predicted to be substantial owing to the widespread global prevalence of under-nutrition.[24]

A history of worm infestation has also been shown to have a significant independent association with active PTB (prevalence of 37.5% amongst cases compared with 11.1% amongst controls; adjusted OR: 11.3; P < 0.001). This finding is consistent with a previous case-control study conducted in northern Ethiopia, which included 230 TB cases and 510 controls. In that study, the prevalence of intestinal helminths was 71% in cases compared with 36% in controls, with an OR of 4.2 (P < 0.001).[25] A case-control study conducted in south-western Ethiopia on people living with HIV and/or AIDS also showed that a history of worm infestation is significantly associated with active PTB.[26] It is suggested that infection with helminths can lead to the development of active TB through enhancing the helper T-cell type 2 (Th-2) immune responses.[32]

Another determinant factor of active TB in the present study was exposure to a family member with known TB infection. This is also consistent with findings from a study conducted in The Gambia, where 45% of PTB cases had a family history of TB compared with 11% of the controls (OR: 7.55; P < 0.001). In the present study, 19% of cases reported household exposure to a known TB case, compared with 5.8% of controls (OR: 4.4; P = 0.008). Other studies have reported similar findings. In addition, the risk appears to increase when the contact is with a close family member as the primary TB case, compared with unrelated household members.[27,33]

Data on income were difficult to obtain, as income-generating activities were commonly carried out in the 'informal' economic sector. In addition, it was difficult to assess whether the income of the individual reflects the overall income of the household; however, ownership of the house remained a consistent marker of socio-economic status throughout the study and showed a statistically significant association with active PTB.

Being single was another determinant factor for development of active TB. By virtue of their marital status, single people have a different lifestyle to those who are married. This is especially the case for male patients, who often migrate to different towns in search of jobs, where they frequently live alone or with peers;[24] therefore, in the present study, being single was independently associated with active PTB. However, further study is needed to explore the factors underlying marital status as being a determinant to active TB.

The present study also revealed that place of residence has a significant independent association with active PTB, with rural residents being at higher risk than those from urban areas. This factor has not been previously addressed by other studies and may be due to the differences in lifestyle or differences in standard of living or socio-economic status. Further study is needed to explore this association.

Limitations

Social desirability bias in the community associated with questions about history of worm infestation can be seen as a weakness in the study design, as mild forms of infestation may have gone undiagnosed and the variable was therefore assessed based purely on personal history. In addition, selection of clinic controls is reasonable when the source population is difficult to define, but bias can be introduced during selection and the effect of the variables under study may be underestimated. Another problem is that recall bias is inherent to case-control studies. In this study, recall bias might have led to the underestimation of the effect; a short recall duration was used to limit the effect.

Another concern in this study was its failure to identify the temporal relationships between exposure factors and the result (reverse causality). This could be the situation with smoking and khat chewing, as health workers may advise newly diagnosed TB cases and their family to give up this habit.[34] For that reason, we collected information on the duration of smoking to differentiate past from current smoking, so that reverse causality was unlikely to explain the findings.

Conclusion

The present study highlighted many host-related and environment-related factors that contribute to the development of active PTB in humans. In this study, the most important contributing factors to developing active PTB included being single, widowed or divorced, living in rural areas, having a family member with a history of TB, smoking, being under-nourished or having a BMI of less than 18.5, being infected with HIV, and having a history of worm infestation. Furthermore, not being the owner of a house is a powerful predictor of active PTB. Measures taken to reduce the prevalence and burden of active PTB should consider these factors.

Based on our findings, the following recommendations are made to curbing TB infection and the associated burden of the disease:

- Reducing or ceasing smoking should be actively encouraged through measures such as working on long-term behavioural changes and health education.
- Efforts to stop the pandemic effect of HIV should be strengthened.
- Measures to tackle the prevalence of worm infestation in the community through different approaches should be strengthened.
- New PTB patients should be educated on how to protect their family and community. To reduce the transfer of disease, health extension workers should also provide health education regarding the care of any family members who have developed active PTB to reduce the risk of exposure in other family members.
- Further prospective cohort studies should be conducted to clearly identify other determinant factors, as the current study could not identify the temporal relationships between predictor variables and outcome variables.

Acknowledgements

The authors wish to thank and acknowledge the Federal Ministry of Education of Ethiopia for providing the opportunity to conduct the study. We also thank the data collectors and supervisors, hospital staff and the study community. The *African Journal of Primary Health Care and Family Medicine* is thanked for covering article processing charges. The reviewers' comments and suggestions for improving the article are appreciated.

Competing interests

The authors declare that they have no financial or personal relationship(s) that may have inappropriately influenced them in writing this article.

Authors' contributions

T.E. (Oromia Regional Health Bureau) conceived and designed the study, supervised data collection, analysed the data, drafted the manuscript and approved the final version. B.M. and F.M. (both Haramaya University) contributed to the conception and design of the study, data analysis, and drafting and approval of the manuscript. W.G. (Arba Minch University) participated in interpretation of the findings, contributed to the drafting and writing of the manuscript, critical writing and revision of the manuscript and updated the manuscript to this version. All authors read and approved the manuscript.

References

1. Ait-Khaled N, Enarson DA. Tuberculosis: a manual for medical students. Geneva: World Health Organization; 2003.

2. Harries AD, Dye C. Tuberculosis. Ann Trop Med Parasitol. 2006;100:415–431.

3. Menzies D, Khan K. Diagnosis of tuberculosis infection and disease. In: Long R, Ellis E, editors. Canadian Tuberculosis Standards. 6th ed. Ottowa: Public Health Agency of Canada, 2007; 53–91.

4. Gryzbowski S. Tuberculosis and its prevention. Missouri, USA: Warren H. Green, 1983; p. 3–10.

5. Flynn J. Lessons from experimental *Mycobacterium tuberculosis* infections. Microbes Infect. 2006;8(4):1179–1188. http://dx.doi.org/10.1016/j.micinf.2005. 10.033

6. Daschuk J, Hackett P, MacNeil S. Treaties and tuberculosis. First Nations people in late 19th-century western Canada, a political and economic transformation. Can Bull Med Hist. 2006;23(2):307–330.

7. Coberly JS, Chaisson RE. Tuberculosis. In: Nelson KE, Williams CM, editors. Infectious disease epidemiology. 2nd ed. London; 2007.

8. Lucas AO, Gilles HM. Short textbook of public health medicine for the tropics. 4th ed. London: Jones & Bartlett; 2003.

9. World Health Organization (WHO). WHO global tuberculosis control report, 2010. Geneva: World Health Organization, 2010; p. 5–8.

10. Knight L. Tuberculosis and sustainable development. Geneva: World Health Organization; 2005. (Document WHO/CDS/STB/2000.4; Stop TB Initiative Series.)

11. World Bank. Global TB control program. World Bank 2006. Accessed July 30, 2011

12. Dye C, Watt CJ, Bleed DM, Hosseini SM, Raviglione MC. Evolution of tuberculosis control and prospects for reducing tuberculosis incidence, prevalence and deaths globally. JAMA 2005;293:2767–2775. http://dx.doi.org/10.1001/jama.293.22.2767

13. World Health Organization. WHO diabetes factsheet (no 312). Geneva: World Health Organization; c n.d. [cited 2011, July 28]. Available from http://www.who.int/mediacentre/

14. Lienhardt C, Fielding K, Sillah JS, et al. Sequence of *Mycobacterium tuberculosis* H37RV. Microbiology 148(1), 2967-2973.

15. Houston S, Brassard P, FitzGerald M, Wobeser W. Tuberculosis and Human Immunodeficiency Virus. In: Long R, Ellis E, editors. Canadian Tuberculosis Standards, 6th ed. Ottawa: Public Health Agency of Canada, 2007; p. 37–53.

16. Aubry MC, Wright JL, Myers JL. The pathology of smoking-related lung diseases. Clin Chest Med 2000;21:11–35. http://dx.doi.org/10.1016/S0272-5231(05)70005-8

17. World Health Organization. Russian oblast is model in fight against TB. Bull World Health Organ 2007;85(5): 331–332.

18. Bates MN, Khalakdina A, Pai M, Chang L, Lessa F, Smith KR. Risk of tuberculosis from exposure to tobacco smoke: a systematic review and meta-analysis. Arch Intern Med. 2007;167:335–342. http://dx.doi.org/10.1001/archinte.167.4.335

19. Lin HH, Ezzati M, Murray M. Tobacco smoke, indoor air pollution and tuberculosis: a systematic review and meta-analysis. PLoS Med. 2007;4:e20. http://dx.doi.org/10.1371/journal.pmed.0040020

20. Slama K. Tobacco and tuberculosis: a qualitative systematic review and meta-analysis. Int J Tuberc Lung Dis. 2007;11:1049–1061.

21. Jeon CY, Murray MB. Diabetes mellitus increases the risk of active tuberculosis: a systematic review of 13 observational studies. PLoS Med. 2008;5:e152. http://dx.doi.org/10.1371/journal.pmed.0050152

22. Lönnroth K, Williams BG, Stadlin S, Jaramillo E, Dye C. Alcohol use as a risk factor for tuberculosis: a systematic review. BMC Public Health. 2008;8:289. http://dx.doi.org/10.1186/1471-2458-8-289

23. Lönnroth K, Williams BG, Cegielski P, Dye C. A consistent log-linear relationship between tuberculosis incidence and body mass index. Int J Epidemiol. 2007;39:149–155. http://dx.doi.org/10.1093/ije/dyp308

24. Lönnroth K, Jaramillo E, Williams BG, Dye C, Raviglione M. Drivers of tuberculosis epidemics: the role of risk factors and social determinants. Soc Sci Med. 2009;68:2240–2246. http://dx.doi.org/10.1016/j.socscimed.2009.03.041

25. Elias D, Mengistu G, Akuffo H, Britton S. Are intestinal helminths risk factors for developing active tuberculosis? Trop Med Int Health. 2006;11(4):551–558. http://dx.doi.org/10.1111/j.1365-3156.2006.01578.x

26. Mohammed T, Amare D, Fasil T, Sahilu A, Duchateau L, Colebunders R. Risk factors of active tuberculosis. Ethiop J Health Sci. 2011;21(2).

27. Singh M, Balamurugan A, Katoch K, Sharma SK, Mehra NK. Immunogenetics of mycobacterial infections in the North Indian population. Tissue Antigens. 2007;69(Suppl 1):228–230. http://dx.doi.org/10.1111/j.1399-0039.2006.77311.x

28. Hill PC, Jackson-Sillah D, Donkor SA, Otu J, Adegbola RA, Lienhardt C. Risk factors for pulmonary tuberculosis: a clinic-based case control study in The Gambia. BMC Public Health. 2006;6:156. http://dx.doi.org/10.1186/1471-2458-6-156

29. Kolappan C, Gopi PG. Tobacco smoking and pulmonary tuberculosis. Thorax. 2002;57:964–966. http://dx.doi.org/10.1136/thorax.57.11.964

30. Alcaide J, Altet MN, Plans P et al. Cigarette smoking as a risk factor for tuberculosis in young adults: a case-control study. Tuber Lung Dis 1996;77:112–116. http://dx.doi.org/10.1016/S0962-8479(96)90024-6

31. World Health Organization. WHO Framework Convention on Tobacco Control. Geneva: World Health Organization; 2003.

32. Fine PE. Immunogenetics of susceptibility to leprosy, tuberculosis, and leishmaniasis. An epidemiological perspective. Int J Lepr Other Mycobact Dis. 1981;49(4):437–454.

33. Zerihun Z, Girmay M, Adane W, Gobena A. Prevalence of Pulmonary Tuberculosis and Associated Risk Factors in Prisons of Gamo Goffa Zone, South Ethiopia: A Cross-Sectional Study. American Journal of Health Research. Vol. 2, No. 5, 2014, pp. 291-297. http://dx.doi.org/10.11648/j.ajhr.20140205.21

34. Gustafson P, Gomes V, Vieira CS et al. Tuberculosis in Bissau: incidence and risk factors in an urban community in sub-Saharan Africa. Int J Epidemiol. 2004;33:163–72. http://dx.doi.org/10.1093/ije/dyh026

Prevalence and causes of visual impairment in patients seen at Nkhensani Hospital Eye Clinic, South Africa

Authors:
Modjadji M. Maake[1]
Olalekan A. Oduntan[2]

Affiliations:
[1]Department of Public Health, School of Health Sciences, University of Limpopo, South Africa

[2]Department of Optometry, School of Health Sciences, University of Kwazulu-Natal, South Africa

Correspondence to:
Modjadji Maake

Email:
mjajimus@yahoo.com

Postal address:
Private Bag X1106, Sovenga 0727, South Africa

Background: Knowledge of the prevalence and causes of visual impairment (VI) amongst hospital patients is useful in planning preventive programmes and provision of eye-care services for residents in the surrounding communities.

Aim: The aim of this study was to determine the prevalence and causes of VI amongst eye clinic patients at Nkhensani Hospital. The relationship between VI and age was also investigated.

Setting: Nkhensani Hospital in the Greater Giyani subdistrict municipality, Mopani district, Limpopo Province, South Africa.

Methods: Four hundred participants aged 6–92 years were selected for the study using a convenient sampling method. Presenting and best corrected visual acuities (VA) were measured with a LogMAR E chart. Presenting VA (PVA) in the right and left eyes and in the better eye of the patients was used to determine the prevalence of VI, low vision (LV) and blindness. Ophthalmoscope was used to diagnose the eye conditions causing VI amongst participants.

Results: The prevalence of VI based on the PVA in the right eye was 34.8% and in the left eye, the prevalence was 35.8%. There was a significant association between age of the participants and VI in the right and left eyes ($p = 0.00$) in each case, respectively. Based on the vision in the better eye of each patient, the prevalence of VI was 28.0% and there was a significant association between VI and age of the participants ($p = 0.00$). The main causes of VI were uncorrected refractive errors, cataract and glaucoma.

Conclusion: Findings in this study indicate that a large proportion of VI is preventable. Focusing on refractive error correction and surgical intervention for cataract would significantly reduce the burden of VI amongst patients utilising this hospital.

Fréquence et causes de déficience visuelle chez les patients examinés à la Clinique phtalmologique de l'Hôpital Nkhensani, Afrique du Sud.

Contexte: Une connaissance de la fréquence et des causes de déficience visuelle (VI) chez les patients des hôpitaux est utile pour mettre en œuvre des programmes de prévention et des services de soins oculaires pour les habitants des communautés avoisinantes.

Objectif: Le but de cette étude était de déterminer la fréquence et les causes de VI chez les patients de la clinique ophtalmologique de l'Hôpital Nkhensani. On a aussi examiné la relation entre la déficience visuelle et l'âge.

Cadre: L'hôpital Nkhensani dans la municipalité du sous-district du Greater Giyani, district de Mopani, province du Limpopo, Afrique du Sud.

Méthodes: Pour l'étude on a sélectionné quatre cent participants âgés de 6 à 92 ans et utilisé une méthode pratique d'échantillonnage. On a mesuré les acuités visuelles présentes et la meilleure acuité visuelle corrigée (VA) au moyen d'un tableau LogMAR E. On s'est servi de la (PVA) dans l'œil droit et l'œil gauche et dans le meilleur œil des patients pour déterminer la fréquence de VI, la vision basse (LV) et la cécité. On a utilisé un ophtalmoscope pour diagnostiquer les conditions oculaires causant la VI chez les participants.

Résultats: La fréquence de VI basée sur la PVA dans l'œil droit était de 34.8% et dans l'œil gauche elle était de 35.8%. Il y avait une relation significative entre l'âge des participants et la VI dans l'œil droit et gauche ($p = 0.00$) dans tous les cas, respectivement. En se basant sur la vision du meilleur œil de chaque patient, la fréquence de VI était de 28.0% et il y avait une relation significative entre la VI et l'âge des participants ($p = 0.00$). Les causes principales de VI étaient des erreurs de réfraction non corrigées, la cataracte et le glaucome.

Conclusion: les résultats de cette enquête montrent qu'une grande proportion de VI peut être évitée. En mettant l'accent sur la correction des erreurs de réfraction et les interventions chirurgicales pour la cataracte, on réduirait beaucoup le fardeau de la déficience visuelle chez les patients de cet hôpital.

Introduction

According to the World Health Organization (WHO),[1] there are four levels of visual function, namely: normal vision; moderate visual impairment (VI); severe VI; and blindness. Moderate combined with severe VI are grouped together under the term 'low vision'; and low vision (LV) taken together with blindness represents total visual impairment.[1] Visual acuity (VA) of less than 6/18 constitutes VI, acuity less than 6/18 to 3/60 constitutes LV and visual acuity less than 3/60 is blindness.[1,2] From a global perspective, 'uncorrected refractive errors are the main causes of moderate and severe visual impairment and cataract remains the leading cause of blindness in middle and low income' countries.[1] In the past, VI estimates have been based on corrected vision, but in order to assess the magnitude of VI caused by uncorrected refractive errors (URE), estimates need to be based on presenting VA.[2] In 2010, it was estimated that 285 million people of all age groups were visually impaired, of whom 39 million were blind; the major causes were UREs (43.0%) and cataracts that had not been operated on (33.0%).[3] The majority of the impairments were correctable, hence preventable.[3]

The prevalence of VI has been reported amongst different populations, with cataracts and refractive errors (RE) being reported as common causes. For example, in a population-based study amongst subjects aged 1–91 years of age in Botucatu, Brazil, Schellini et al.[4] reported a prevalence of presenting LV (5.2%) and blindness (2.2%) and the main causes were UREs, cataracts and retinal disease. Ramke et al.[5] found that amongst the people aged ≥ 40 years of age in Timor-Leste, the age, gender and domicile-adjusted prevalence of functional blindness (presenting VA of 6/60 in the better eye) was 7.4% and blindness (≥ 3/60) was 4.1%. The adjusted prevalence of LV (< 6/18 – 6/60) was 17.7%. Cataract was responsible for 72.9% of the cases of blindness and 17.8% of those involving LV. Haq et al.[6] reported that the prevalence of VI, LV and blindness amongst those members of the population aged 20 years or older in Aligarh, India, based on presenting VA were 13.0%, 7.8% and 5.3%, respectively, whilst the main causes of VI were cataract, RE, glaucoma and corneal opacities. In Tehran, Iran, Fotouhi et al.[7] found the prevalence of VI to be 2.52% for presenting VA and 1.39% for corrected VA amongst participants aged one year and older. The most frequent cause of VI was UREs (33.6%), followed by cataract (25.4%), macular degeneration (12.7%) and amblyopia (8.2%). Based on the best corrected vision, common causes were cataract (36.0%), macular degeneration (20.0%) and amblyopia (10.7%).[7]

In Nigeria, amongst adults aged ≥ 40 years, Abdull et al.[8] found that UREs were responsible for 57.1% of moderate VI (< 6/18 – 6/60) and cataract (43.0%) was the most common cause of blindness (VA < 3/60). Cataract-related blindness had a prevalence of 1.8% and glaucoma-related blindness, 0.7%.

In a study of RE and VI amongst school-aged children aged 5–15 years in Durban, South Africa, Naidoo et al.[9] found that VA of 6/12 or worse in the better eye had a prevalence of 1.4% (uncorrected), 1.2% (presenting) and 0.32% (best-corrected). Refractive errors (63.0%) were the main causes of VI, whilst amblyopia (7.3%), retinal disorders (9.9%), corneal opacities (3.7%), other causes (3.1%) and unexplained causes (12.0%) were responsible for the rest. The main causes of blindness and LV were cataract, posterior segment diseases, glaucoma, uncorrected aphakia and globe abnormalities. Refractive errors (22.0%) were reported as being the cause of LV in their sample population.[9]

Age and gender have an influence on visual impairment and it has been reported that, in all age groups, prevalence increases with age and women have a significantly higher risk of developing VI than men in every region of the world.[3] This was consistent with the reports by Abdull et al.,[8] Zainal et al.,[10] Resnikoff et al.[11] and Shahriari et al.[12]

Visual impairment has significant socioeconomic implications. Resnikoff et al.[2] indicated that VI resulting from UREs has both immediate and long term consequences 'such as lost educational and employment opportunities, lost economic gain for individuals, families and societies, and impaired quality of life'.[2] In children, poor vision as a result of uncorrected or under-corrected myopia can lead to an inability to read information written on the blackboard and can thus have a serious impact on a child's participation in learning.[13] This results in poor school performance which will adversely affect a child's educational, occupational and socioeconomic status in life. Visual impairment has also been associated with decreased quality of life (QoL) in persons aged 40 years or older;[14] correction of RE amongst older people improved their vision-specific QoL.[15]

In a national guideline for the prevention of blindness in South Africa, the Department of Health[16] reported a 0.75% prevalence of blindness in the country; 80.0% of these cases of blindness were reportedly avoidable. The Department of Health[17] has also reported a severe lack of epidemiological data on the magnitude of URE in the country. Considering the burden and impact of visually-disabling anomalies on the society and economy, data on their prevalence would be a valuable tool for appropriate planning and resource allocation in the country.

Aim and objectives

Data on the prevalence and causes of VI in South Africa are few and no studies have been conducted specifically in the Mopani district of Limpopo Province. Hospital data have been used by several authors[18,19,20] to report eye problems in various populations worldwide, but such a report for South Africa could not be found in the literature. The purpose of this study was to determine the prevalence and causes of VI amongst patients presenting to the eye clinic at Nkhensani Hospital, Limpopo Province. The relationship of VI with age was also examined. Findings reported in this article will provide an insight into the causes of VI amongst patients using the hospital for eye-care services and will be useful for both prevention and intervention planning.

Research methods and design

Study setting

Nkhensani Hospital is a level 1 district hospital situated in the Greater Giyani subdistrict municipality, Mopani district, Limpopo Province, South Africa. Most people using Nkhensani Hospital are from the rural areas of the Greater Giyani subdistrict municipality. Eye-care services at the hospital are provided by both optometrists and ophthalmic nurses. Patients who needs specialist care are referred to the ophthalmologist at Elim Hospital or Mankweng Hospital who provides subsequent management and feedback. Where necessary, the diagnosis of the ophthalmologist was used to confirm any ocular diagnosis reported in this study.

Study population and sampling strategy

The study population was the patients attending the Nkhensani Hospital Eye Clinic in Giyani, Limpopo Province, South Africa between August 2012 and March 2013 – an estimated total population of about 3400 patients. Based on this population size, using the Krejcie and Morgan Table,[21] a sample of 400 participants was considered adequate for this study. The table provides appropriate sample sizes for listed population sizes, which can be read directly from the table. Resnikoff et al.[11] found visual impairment to be uniquely distributed across age groups, therefore participants in this study were stratified by age in order to determine the distribution of VI across age strata. Participants were stratified by age (6–18; 19–35; 36–59; ≥ 60 years) and 100 participants were included in each age stratum. All patients six years and older presenting at eye clinic for the first time for eye-care services during the study period were included in the study by the convenient sampling method until the desired number of participants in each age stratum was reached. All those who were recruited agreed to participate in the study. Children below the age of six (possible poor comprehension of instructions) and follow-up patients (to avoid duplication of data) were excluded.

Data collection

A LogMAR (log of the minimal angle of resolution) illiterate E acuity chart was used to measure presenting (habitual), pinhole and best corrected VA. A pinhole disc was used to detect if reduced VA was a result of RE or eye disease or another anomaly. Where reduced VA resulted from REs, subjective refraction (lenses providing the best vision were determined by the choice made by the patient, when difference lenses were placed in front of their eyes) was done and the REs and corrected vision value recorded. Direct ophthalmoscope examination was used to examine the external and internal structures of the eye. A digital hand-held tonometer was used to measure the intraocular pressure. A confrontation test was performed to estimate the extent of visual field. Those with eye diseases were referred to the ophthalmic nurse and/or

TABLE 1: Visual acuity ranges, categories and classification of visual impairment according to the World Health Organization classification.

Snellen VA	VA (LogMAR)	Category	Classification
≥ 6/18	0.0 – 0.50	0	Mild or no VI
< 6/18 – 6/60	0.52 – 1.0	1	Moderate VI
< 6/60 – 3/60 (6/120)	1.02 – 1.30	2	Severe VI
< 3/60 – 1/60	1.32 – 1.80	3	Blindness
< 1/60 – LP[†]	1.82 – 3.0	4	Blindness
NLP[†]	4.0	5	Blindness

Note: Moderate and severe visual impairment constitute low vision.
VA, visual acuity; LogMAR, logarithm of the minimum angle of resolution, VI, visual impairment; †, LP is light perception and NLP is no light perception.

ophthalmologist for further management. In cases where the researcher had doubts regarding diagnoses – such as differential diagnoses of the retinopathies – the diagnosis of the ophthalmologist was used to confirm diagnosis. Visual impairment was based on presenting VA and the WHO classification,[2] modified for LogMAR values using the Holladay[22] and Johnson[23] tables. Table 1 below shows the categories and classification of VI used in the study.

Data analysis

Data were analysed using the descriptive and inferential statistics of the Statistical Package for Social Sciences (SPSS) version 21 (IBM Corp., Armonk, NY 2012). Descriptive statistics (range, mean and standard deviation) were used to describe the cohort and the visual values. The relationship between VI and age was tested for significance using the Chi-squared test; a p-value of < 0.05 was considered to be significant at 95% confidence interval.

Ethical consideration

Approval to conduct the study was obtained from the University of Limpopo Ethics Committee (MEDUNSA), approval number MREC/HS/63/2012:PG. Permission was obtained from the Limpopo provincial department of health, Mopani district Health Office and the Chief Executive Officer of Nkhensani Hospital. Informed consent was obtained from the participants and parents of the children included in the study after they had been provided with appropriate information regarding the purpose and method of the study.

Results

A total of 400 participants was included in the study, all attending the Nkhensani Hospital Eye Clinic for eye-care services during the period of the study. Their ages ranged from 6 to 92 years, with a mean of 39.5 ± 23.5 years. They comprised 161 (40.3%) men and 239 (59.7%) women.

Prevalence of visual impairment

The prevalence of VI (combined LV and blindness) based on presenting VA in the right and left eyes ($N = 400$) were 34.8% and 35.8%, respectively (Tables 2 and 3). In the right eye, the prevalence of LV and blindness were 16.3% and 18.5%, respectively; and in the left eye, the prevalence of LV and blindness were 17.5% and 18.3%, respectively. The distribution of the various categories of VI in the right

TABLE 2: Ages and percentages of participants with various levels of visual status in the right eye based on presenting visual acuity.

Ages (years)	Mild/NVI	Low vision		Blindness			Total VI (%)
	0	1	2	3	4	5	
6–18	22.0	1.5	0.3	0.3	1.0	0.0	3.0
19–35	19.5	2.8	0.0	0.3	1.5	1.0	5.5
36–59	15.0	4.3	0.0	1.5	2.8	1.5	10.1
≥ 60	8.8	7.3	0.3	1.5	6.8	0.5	16.3
Total	**65.3**	**15.8**	**0.5**	**3.5**	**12.0**	**3.0**	**34.8**

Note: Mild and no visual impairment (NVI) (category 0), moderate and severe visual impairment (VI) (categories 1 and 2) constituting low vision and blindness (categories 3–5) are shown in the Table. The total percentage of VI participants is shown in the last column.

TABLE 3: Ages and percentages of participants with various levels of visual status in the left eye based on presenting visual acuity.

Ages (years)	Mild/NVI	Low vision		Blindness			Total VI (%)
	0	1	2	3	4	5	
6–18	20.8	1.8	0.3	0.8)	1.5	0.0	4.3
19–35	18.8	2.5	0.0	0.8)	1.3	1.8	6.3
36–59	15.5	5.0	0.0	1.0)	2.5	1.0	9.5
≥ 60	9.3	7.8	0.3	1.8)	4.3	1.8	15.8
Total	**64.3**	**17.0**	**0.5**	**4.3**	**9.5**	**4.5**	**35.8**

Note: Mild and no visual impairment (NVI) (category 0), moderate and severe visual impairment (VI) (categories 1 and 2) constituting low vision and blindness (categories 3–5) are shown in the Table. The total percentage of VI participants is shown in the last column.

TABLE 4: Ages of the participants and percentage distribution of low vision, blindness and visual impairment (VI) based on the visual acuity in the better eye.

Age (years)	Low vision	Blindness	Total VI
6–18	1.5	1.0	2.5
19–35	2.8	1.8	4.6
36–59	4.5	2.8	7.3
≥ 60	8.3	5.3	13.6
Total	**17.1**	**10.9**	**28.0**

and left eye in relation to the age of the participants is shown in Tables 2 and 3.

There was a significant association between age of the participants and VI in the right and left eye ($p = 0.00$). Based on the presenting VA in the better eyes of the patients, the prevalence of VI was 28.0% (LV = 17.1%; blindness = 10.9%) (Table 4). There was a significant association between VI and the age of the participants ($p = 0.00$).

Causes of visual impairment

The main causes of VI were UREs, cataract and glaucoma (Figure 1) accounting for 38.0%, 25.9% and 17.6%, respectively. The main causes of LV were UREs (56.7%) and cataract (20.9%), whereas the main causes of blindness were cataract, glaucoma and corneal anomalies (accounting for 34.1%, 31.7% and 17.1%, respectively).

Discussion

Visual impairment is an important public health issue since it impairs the QoL and limits the career choices/job opportunities of those affected, thus constituting a socioeconomic burden on society.[13,14] It is, therefore, important that the prevalence and causes of the conditions be investigated so that health authorities may have relevant values that can help them in making informed decisions with regard to prevention and management programmes. Population-based studies are the most appropriate method of establishing the prevalence and causes of VI, however, such methods are expensive and

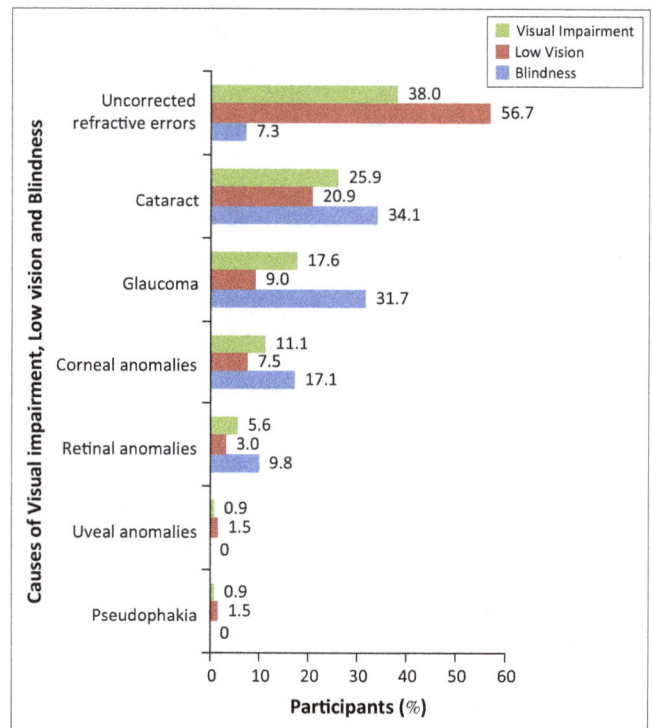

FIGURE 1: The percentage distributions of causes of visual impairment amongst participants ($N = 400$). Uncorrected refractive errors (UREs) were the most common causes of visual impairment and low vision. Cataract was the main cause of blindness.

time consuming. Hospital-based studies are less expensive and provide useful information that can be used to plan eye-care services in the particular hospital as well as preventive programmes in the surrounding communities. Therefore, this study is of significance in providing data that could be used to improve eye-care services at the Nkhensani Hospital Eye Clinic and may serve as a comparative tool for similar hospital studies in South Africa and other parts of the world.

Prevalence and causes of visual impairment

The prevalence of VI, LV and blindness were 28.0%, 17.1% and 10.9%, respectively. The main causes of VI were

UREs (38.0%), cataract (25.9%) and glaucoma (17.6%). A comparable hospital-based retrospective study[24] in which the records of all new eye-care patients seen at Adoose Specialist Hospital, Jos, North Central Nigeria were reviewed, found bilateral blindness of 11.0% and LV prevalence of 9.2% in the patients; blindness as well as VI increased significantly with age. Although the prevalence values of LV in that study were lower than found in this study (Tables 2 and 3), the prevalence of bilateral blindness is similar to the 10.9% reported in the present study (Table 4). Refractive errors (33.3%), cataract (28.3%) and glaucoma (13.3%) were also the common causes of VI in that study and their percentages are similar to those found in this study (Figure 1). This similarity reflects the reports in previous population-based studies that REs and cataract,[3,4,5,6,7,8,9] as well as glaucoma,[8,9] are common causes of VI. The findings of UREs and cataract as the main causes of VI in this study are consistent with those in many population-based studies[4,6,7] and can be attributed to age-related cataracts and to the fact that occurrence of REs is common to all age groups.

Although REs can simply be corrected with a pair of spectacles, the majority of people in South Africa remain visually impaired because of URE. This may be because of an absence of eye-care personnel, poor accessibility to the services or inability to afford the service cost, especially amongst those living in rural and remote areas.

Relationship between age and visual impairment

The significant association between age and VI ($p = 0.00$) in this study is consistent with that found in various population-based studies.[4,7,8,11,25,26] The reason for increase in VI with increasing age, especially amongst the elderly, is a common occurrence in age-related eye conditions such as cataract and glaucoma.

Limitations

A major limitation of hospital-based studies, including this study, is that they are biased toward those seeking (in this case) eye-care services, hence findings may be higher than would be seen in the population at large. For this reason, the VI prevalence of 28.0% and causes reported here cannot be generalised to the entire district, province or national population. Also, findings should be compared with those in the literature with caution because VI reports in the literature could vary as a result of differences in the ages, study sites or ethnicity of participants as well as the socioeconomic status of the participants. Findings in this study could not be directly compared to the majority of those of the previous prevalence and VI studies because of various factors such as differences in methodology and ages of participants. Also, reports here are based only on presenting, not corrected, VA. Most previous studies on prevalence and causes of VI were population based.[4,5,7,8,9,10,11,12] Hospital-based studies were few and some of them concentrated only on REs[18,19] or eye diseases.[20,27] Furthermore, age differences preclude direct

comparison with those studies on REs. For example, the age range of those in the Qureshi et al. study[18] was 15 to 35 years, hence cannot be compared to the present study where the age range was six to 92 years. Socioeconomic differences may also influence prevalence and causes of VI,[28] hence should be taken into consideration when comparing these data with other studies.

Although a previous hospital-based study on VI in South Africa could not be found in the literature, findings in this study reflect the views of previous population-based studies in the country which found that cataract[25,29,30] and REs[9] are the leading causes of blindness in the country. According to Lecuona and Cook,[29] 'human resources available for eye-care and cataract surgery in 2006 in the indigent population are far below the number recommended for the public sector', hence 'additional posts for ophthalmologists, optometrists and ophthalmic nurses should be provided and more medical officers trained for cataract surgeries'.[30] We agree with this recommendation because, if implemented, it has the potential to drastically improve eye-care services, reducing the prevalence of cataract and REs and, hence, VI at district, provincial and national levels in South Africa.

Recommendations

It is recommended that the Department of Health prioritise the elimination of REs and cataract if the prevalence of VI is to be reduced in the country. Sustainable programmes toward correction of REs and cataract surgery are needed in Nkhensani Hospital in order to reduce the burden of VI amongst patients receiving eye-care services in the hospital. As glaucoma is the third most common cause of VI in this study, appropriate programmes should be put in place to detect and manage glaucoma cases before they result in visual impairment. Strengthening awareness programmes and screening campaigns (with appropriate screening equipment) in the Giyani subdistrict where this hospital is located will provide an opportunity for identifying potentially blinding conditions before they cause visual loss.

Conclusion

This study indicates that the overall prevalence of VI in this hospital sample is high (28.0%), as is shown in Table 4. As the main causes of LV and blindness, based on PVA amongst patients, were UREs and cataract, respectively, VI is preventable as these conditions are correctable. A focus on the optical correction of REs and surgical intervention in the case of cataract would lead to a significant reduction in the burden of VI amongst patients who utilise Nkhensani Hospital for eye-care services.

Acknowledgements

This article was adapted from a Master of Public Health project by M.M. Maake, University of Limpopo, supervised by O.A. Oduntan.

Competing interests

The authors declare that they have no financial or personal relationship(s) that may have inappropriately influenced them in writing this article.

Authors' contributions

M.M.M. (University of Limpopo) was responsible for the project design, data collection and analysis, in addition to contributing to the writing of the article. O.A.O. (University of KwaZulu-Natal) supervised the project and contributed to the writing of the article.

References

1. World Health Organization (WHO). Visual impairment and blindness. Fact Sheet No. 282, updated August 2014 [page on the Internet]. c2014 [cited 2014 Aug 18]. Available from: http://www.who.int/mediacentre/factsheets/fs282/en/

2. Resnikoff S, Pascolini D, Mariotti SP, et al. Global magnitude of visual impairment caused by uncorrected refractive errors in 2004. Bull World Health Organ. 2008;86(1):63–70. http://dx.doi.org/10.2471/BLT.07.041210

3. Pascolini D, Mariotti SP. Global estimates of visual impairment: 2010. Brit J Ophthalmol. 2012;96(5):614–618. http://dx.doi.org/10.1136/bjophthalmol-2011-300539

4. Schellini SA, Durkin SR, Hoyama E, et al. Prevalence and causes of visual impairment in a Brazilian population: The Botucatu Eye Study. BMC Ophthalmol. 2009;9:8. http://dx.doi.org/10.1186/1471-2415-9-8

5. Ramke J, Palagyi A, Naduvilath T, et al. Prevalence and causes of blindness and low vision in Timor-Leste. Br J Ophthalmol. 2007;91(9):1117–1121. http://dx.doi.org/10.1136/bjo.2006.106559

6. Haq I, Khan Z, Khalique N, et al. Prevalence of common ocular morbidities in adult population of Aligarh. Indian J Community Med. 2009;34(3):195–201. http://dx.doi.org/10.4103/0970-0218.55283

7. Fotouhi A, Hashemi H, Mohammad K, et al. The prevalence and causes of visual impairment in Tehran: The Tehran Eye Study. Br J Ophthalmol. 2004;88(6):740–745. http://dx.doi.org/10.1136/bjo.2003.031153

8. Abdull MM, Sivasubramaniam S, Murthy GV, et al. Causes of blindness and visual impairment in Nigeria: The Nigeria national blindness and visual impairment survey. Invest Ophthalmol Vis Sci. 2009;50(9):4114–4120. http://dx.doi.org/10.1167/iovs.09-3507

9. Naidoo KS, Raghunandan, Mashige KP, et al. Refractive error and visual impairment in African children in South Africa. Invest Ophthalmol Vis Sci. 2003;44(9):3764–3770. http://dx.doi.org/10.1167/iovs.03-0283

10. Zainal M, Ismail SM, Ropilah AR, et al. Prevalence of blindness and low vision in the Malaysian population: Results from the National Eye Survey 1996. Br J Ophthalmol. 2002;86(9):951–956. http://dx.doi.org/10.1136/bjo.86.9.951

11. Resnikoff S, Pascolini D, Eya'ale D, et al. Global data on visual impairment in the year 2002. Policy and Practice. Bull World Health Organ. 2004;82:844–851.

12. Shahriari H, Izadi S, Rouhani M, et al. Prevalence and causes of visual impairment and blindness in Sistan-va-Baluchestan Province, Iran: Zahedan Eye Study. Br J Ophthalmol. 2007; 91(5):579–584. http://dx.doi.org/10.1136/bjo.2006.105734

13. Taylor HR. 2000. Refractive errors: Magnitude of the need. Community Eye Health. 2000;13(33):1–2.

14. Broman AT, Muñoz B, Rodriquez J, et al. The impact of visual impairment and eye disease on vision-related quality of life in a Mexican-American population: Proyecto VER. Invest Ophthalmol Vis Sci. 2002;43(11):3393–3398.

15. Coleman AL, Yu F, Keeler E, et al. Treatment of uncorrected refractive error improves vision-specific quality of life. J Am Geriatr Soc. 2006;54(6):883–890. http://dx.doi.org/10.1111/j.1532-5415.2006.00817.x

16. Department of Health. National guideline: prevention of blindness in South Africa [document on the Internet]. c2002 [cited 2014 Sep 05]. Available from: http://www.westerncape.gov.za/text/2003/blindness.pdf

17. Department of Health. National guideline: Refractive errors screening for persons 60 years and older. Pretoria; 2004.

18. Qureshi N, Ahmed T, Ghaffar Z, et al. Clinical study of types of 'refractive errors' at a tertiary care hospital. Pak J Surg. 2012;28(3):226–228.

19. Ayoob M, Dawood Z, Mirza SA, et al. Refractive errors and their relation to age and sex. Med Channel. 2011;17(2):28–31.

20. Adenuga OO, Samuel OJ. Pattern of eye diseases in an air force hospital in Nigeria. Pak J Ophthalmol. 2012;28(3):144–148.

21. Krejcie RV, Morgan DW. Determining sample size for research activities. Educ Psychol Meas. 1970;30:607–610.

22. Holladay JT. Proper method for calculating average visual acuity. J Ref Surg. 1997;13:388–391.

23. Johnson GJ, Minassian DC, Weale RA, et al. 2003. The epidemiology of eye disease. 2nd ed. London: Imperial College Press.

24. Malu KN. Blindness and visual impairment in north central Nigeria: A hospital based study. Niger Postgrad Med J. 2013;20(2):98–103.

25. Cook L, Kluever H, Mabena L, et al. Rapid assessment of cataract at pay points in South Africa. Br J Ophthalmol. 2007;91(7):867–868. http://dx.doi.org/10.1136/bjo.2006.108910

26. Fegghi M, Khataminia G, Ziaei H, et al. Prevalence and causes of blindness and low vision in Khuzestan Province, Iran. J Ophthalmic Vis Res. 2009;4(1):29–34.

27. Al-Akily SA, Bamashmus MA, Gunaid AA. Causes of visual impairment among Yemenis with diabetes: A hospital-based study. East Mediterr Health J. 2011;17(11):831–837.

28. Cockburn N, Steven D, Lecuona K, et al. Prevalence, causes and socio-economic determinants of vision loss in Cape Town, South Africa. PLoS ONE. 7(2):e30718. http://dx.doi.org/10.1371/journal.pone.0030718

29. Van Dijk KM, Cook CD, Razum O. Rapid assessment of cataract in a rural health district. Mingaphi Iminwe, Gogo? S Afr Med J. 2000;90(10):991–993.

30. Lecuona, K, Cook C. South African cataract surgery rates: Why are we not meeting our targets? S Afr Med J. 2011;101(8):510–512.

3

'If you have a problem with your heart, you have a problem with your life': Self-perception and behaviour in relation to the risk of ischaemic heart disease in people living with HIV

Authors:
Ronel Roos[1]
Hellen Myezwa[1]
Helena van Aswegen[1]

Affiliations:
[1]Department of
Physiotherapy, University
of the Witwatersrand,
South Africa

Correspondence to:
Ronel Roos

Email:
ronel.roos@wits.ac.za

Postal address:
0 7 York Road, Park Town
2193, South Africa

Background: Ischaemic heart disease (IHD) is a global health problem and specifically relevant in the African context, as the presence of risk factors for IHD is increasing. People living with the human immunodeficiency virus (HIV)/acquired immune deficiency syndrome (AIDS) (PLWHA) are at increased risk for IHD due to increased longevity, treatment-specific causes and viral effects.

Aim: To determine the self-perception and behaviour in relation to risk for IHD in a cohort of South African PLWHA.

Methods: A qualitative study using semi-structured interviews with a card-sort technique was used to gather data from 30 individuals at an HIV clinic in Johannesburg. Descriptive analysis and conventional content analysis were done to generate the findings.

Results: The median age of the cohort was 36.5 (31.8–45.0) years and they were mostly women (*n* = 25; 83.3%) who were employed (*n* = 17; 56.7%) and supporting dependents (*n* = 26; 86.7%). Fifteen (50%) participants did not perceive themselves at risk of IHD and reported having adequate coping behaviour, living a healthy lifestyle and being healthy since initiating therapy. Twelve (40%) did feel at risk because they experienced physical symptoms and had poor behaviour. Knowledge and understanding related to IHD, insight into own risk for IHD and health character in a context of HIV infection were three themes.

Conclusion: This study highlights that participants did not perceive themselves to be at risk of IHD due to their HIV status or antiretroviral management. Education strategies are required in PLWHA to inform their personal risk perception for IHD.

'Si vous avez un problème cardiaque, vous avez un problème de vie': La perception de soi et le comportement par rapport au risque de maladie cardiaque ischémique chez les patients atteints du VIH.

Contexte: Les maladies cardiaques ischémiques (IHD) sont un problème de santé mondial particulièrement pertinent dans le contexte africain étant donné que la présence de facteurs de risques d'IHD augmente en raison de la présence élevée du virus humain de déficience immunitaire (HIV). Les personnes vivant avec le VIH ont un risqué accru de IHD dû à l'augmentation de la longévité, à des causes spécifiques du traitement et à des effets viraux. Cette étude a déterminé la perception de soi et le comportement par rapport au risque d'IHD chez un groupe de Sud-africains atteints du VIH. Un plan d'étude qualitatif par le biais d'entrevues semi-structurées avec une technique de sélection des cartes a été utilisé pour collecter les données de trente individus à une clinique VIH à Johannesburg, en Afrique du Sud. Une analyse descriptive et une approche inductive avec une analyse conventionnelle du contenu ont été utilisées pour obtenir les résultats.

Résultats: L'âge moyen du groupe était de 36.5 (31.8–45.0) ans et comprenait surtout de femmes (*n* = 25; 83.3%) qui avaient un emploi (*n* = 17; 56.7%) et des personnes à charge (*n* = 26; 86.7%). Quinze des participants (50%) ne se considéraient pas exposés au risque d'IHD car ils savaient faire face à la situation, en vivant sainement et en étant en bonne santé depuis qu'ils avaient commencé une thérapie antirétrovirale très active. Douze des participants (40%) se sentaient vulnérables car ils avaient ressenti des symptômes physiques et avaient un mauvais comportement dû à un mauvais régime alimentaire, des taux élevés de stress et le manque d'exercice. Trois des participants (10%) n'étaient pas sûrs de leur risque d'IHD. Les connaissances et la compréhension concernant l'IHD, la conscience de leurs propres risques d'IHD et le caractère sanitaire dans le contexte du VIH ont été identifiés comme les trois thèmes principaux se dégageant des données.

Conclusion: Cette étude montre que les participants ne se considèrent pas en danger d'IHD en raison de leur statut VIH ou de leur traitement antirétroviral. Il faut éduquer les gens atteints du VIH pour influencer leur perception personnelle de risque d'IHD ce qui en retour pourrait amener des changements de comportement et la prévention d'IHD.

Introduction

Ischaemic heart disease (IHD) is a global health concern, and this condition combined with stroke accounted for 12.9 million deaths globally in 2010.[1] The greatest burden associated with IHD occurs in developing countries due to epidemiological transition: increased longevity of individuals, urbanisation and lifestyle changes.[2,3] In sub-Saharan Africa IHD is a concern due to risk factors for IHD such as hypertension, diabetes, overweight and obesity, physical inactivity and dyslipidaemia.[4,5,6] Additionally, the high prevalence of infection with the human immunodeficiency virus (HIV) augments the potential burden of IHD into the future.

Studies have shown that people living with HIV/acquired immune deficiency syndrome (AIDS) (PLWHA) are at an increased risk for developing IHD compared to non-infected individuals.[7,8] Increased risk can be attributed to the presence of traditional risk factors, for example, smoking prevalence,[8] metabolic effects of highly active antiretroviral therapy (HAART)[9,10] and specific viral effects (e.g. increased inflammation[11,12]). Little research has been published regarding PLWHA's perception of IHD risk. Cioe, Crawford and Stein[13] indicated that knowledge of IHD risk factors was fairly high, but not predictive of individuals' perceived risk for IHD in the United States of America (USA). Additionally, the authors found that individuals' risk perception was inaccurate when compared to their actual risk as determined by the Framingham Risk Score.

Aim and objective

The aim of this study was to determine self-perception and behaviour in relation to the risk of IHD in a cohort of South African PLWHA. Considering the potential burden of IHD in sub-Saharan Africa, it is prudent to determine if PLWHA in Africa perceive themselves as at risk for IHD. This information may inform clinical practice and enable tailored education programmes.

Research methods and design

Study design

A qualitative study design was chosen to achieve the aims of the study. Qualitative inquiry provides the ideal means to describe the complex nature of humans and how individuals perceive their own experiences within a specific social context.[14]

Study population

Participants were purposefully sampled according to the following inclusion criteria: 20–65 years of age, on HAART treatment for 6–12 months and ambulatory without an assistive device. Participants with a past medical history of cardiovascular disease, complaints of difficulty walking at the time of recruitment, pregnancy, complaints of acute illness or active opportunistic infection were excluded. The sample size was dependent upon information gathered during the interview process, until the point of saturation was reached.

Assessment procedure

Participants completed a demographic questionnaire to capture their social and HIV background. Pharmacological treatment and details of specific HAART medication were collected from the clinic files. Participants' latest CD4 count and viral load values were collected from the clinic laboratory database and clinic files.

Interviews were conducted in a private room using a semi-structured interview questionnaire. Open-ended questions related to living a healthy lifestyle and IHD were asked, with secondary prompting questions added. The card-sort technique was used to assist in generating information; this is associated with a constructivist approach, specifically Kelly's Personal Construct Theory: 'they assume that people make sense of the world by categorising it, and that people can describe their own categorisation of the world with reasonable validity and reliability'.[15] Card sort elicits individual understanding about topics and their relationships with each other. It is systematic and easy to use for both respondents and researchers.[15,16]

For the purposes of this study, a closed card-sort technique was used. Twenty three cards consisting of key phrases (English and isiZulu translation) with supporting pictures related to components of living a healthy lifestyle were utilised. An additional blank card was included that enabled each participant an opportunity to add an aspect of living a healthy lifestyle that was not presented on the other cards. Participants were asked to review the cards and sort them, from most important to least important on a continuum according to hierarchy of living a healthy lifestyle. Participants had freedom to overlap cards into piles on the line if the cards had similar importance. Their card selections were discussed and led to the open-ended questions related to IHD. All interviews were tape-recorded to allow for verbatim transcription at a later stage.

Data analysis

An inductive approach to data analysis was followed using conventional content analysis.[17] As stated by Thomas[18]: 'inductive analysis refers to approaches that primarily use detailed readings of raw data to derive concepts, themes or a model through interpretation made from the raw data by an evaluator or researcher'. All interviews were transcribed verbatim from beginning to end in Microsoft Word. Codes and keywords were identified vertically and then for each question horizontally in all transcribed documentation. The frequencies on how often codes appeared were analysed question by question as a means of highlighting their importance. The frequency of similar codes contributed to data saturation. This was supported by the percentage of participants who had concepts in similar categories.

To reduce the data, the codes were collapsed into subcategories, then categories and lastly themes.[19] Explanatory qualitative quotations provide descriptive data as per participants' contextual explanations. Demographic information was analysed using SPSS IBM 21. Categorical data are presented as frequencies and percentages. Numerical data are expressed as medians (interquartile range).

Ethical considerations

The study was approved by the University of the Witwatersrand Human Research Ethics Committee, permission was received from the clinic where the study was undertaken, and participants provided informed consent.

Triangulation strategies to improve trustworthiness of research findings included member checks of transcribed interviews by a senior qualitative researcher; a second researcher analysed 20% of transcribed interviews; 20% of study participants returned for a second appointment to review transcribed interviews and clarify key findings; and two focus group discussions with the researcher and three senior qualitative researchers were held to assist in identifying themes. A transparent coding process and inter-coder verification added to dependability of the research findings.

Results

Demographic characteristics

The median age of participants was 36.5 (31.8–45.0) years with 10.5 (7.0–12.0) months being the median time spent on HAART (Table 1). Most participants were diagnosed as having HIV infection between 2009 and 2010 (n = 21; 70%), and they were on the HAART regimen consisting of lamivudine, efavirenz and stavudine (n = 13; 43.3%) (Table1). The majority of participants were female (n = 25; 83.3%), employed (n = 17; 56.7%), with a secondary school education (n = 16; 53.3%), and were supporting dependents (n = 26; 86.7%) (Table 1). Most perceived their health status as good (n = 17; 56.7%).

Self-perception and behaviour in relation to the risk of Ischaemic heart disease

Fifty percent of the participants (n = 15) did not perceive themselves as at risk for IHD; 12 (40%) did and three (10%) were unsure. Twenty six individuals (87%) thought one can prevent IHD from occurring in one's life. Two (6.6%) said it was unavoidable and two (6.6%) additional individuals were unsure if it was preventable.

Three prominent themes were identified during the data analysis: knowledge and understanding related to IHD, insight into their own risk, and health character in a context of HIV.

Knowledge and understanding related to Ischaemic heart disease

Participants demonstrated knowledge and understanding related to the causes of IHD. Psychological factors such as

TABLE 1: Demographic characteristics of study participants (N = 30).

Variable	N	Median (interquartile range)	Variable	
			n	%
Age (years)	30	36.5 (31.8–45.0)	-	-
Gender	30	-		
Male	-	-	5	16.7
Female	-	-	25	83.3
Time on HAART (months)	30	10.5 (7.0–12.0)	-	-
CD4 count (cells/mm³)	30	282 (211.0–357.5)	-	-
Viral load (copies/mL)	28*	22.5 (0.0–51.3)	-	-
Diagnosed with HIV infection				
Prior to 2005	-	-	3	10.0
Between 2005 to 2008	-	-	6	20.0
Between 2009 to 2010	-	-	21	70.0
HAART categories				
Lamivudine, efavirenz, tenofovir	-	-	10	33.3
Lamivudine, efavirenz, stavudine	-	-	13	43.3
Other	-	-	7	23.3
Educational level				
No education	-	-	1	3.3
Primary school education	-	-	5	16.7
Secondary school education	-	-	16	53.3
Post-secondary school education	-	-	8	26.7
Employment status				
Unemployed	-	-	12	40.0
Employed	-	-	17	56.7
Self-employed	-	-	1	3.3
Participants who had dependents				
No	-	-	4	13.3
Yes	-	-	26	86.7
Perception of health status				
Average	-	-	8	26.7
Good	-	-	17	56.7
Excellent	-	-	5	16.7

*, Viral load findings only available for 28 participants.
N = 30.

stress and thinking too much were codes that presented often (n = 20; 66%). One participant stated this as follows:

> 'Sometimes I wonder if it is not due to stress overload. The heart is always pumping fast and it can't relax.' (Participant 21, female, 49 years, no education and employed)

Not accepting one's HIV status (n = 1; 3%) and keeping problems to themselves (n = 3; 10%) to a lesser extent were noted to add to the risk for IHD:

> 'When one has a lot of problems that you can't solve on your own, that you keep on yourself inside, that can cause heart disease.' (Participant 6, female, 39 years, secondary school education and employed)

The second most prominent cause of IHD reported by participants was related to nutrition, as reflected by specifics on diet (n = 16; 53%). This was voiced as follows:

> 'I think eating habits, you need to feed your body just like you feed your mind, and you need to select what you eat.' (Participant 1, female, 36 years, post-secondary school education and employed)

Thirdly, participants explained the cause of IHD in relation to impaired structure and function of the heart. Understanding regarding the link between diet and altered function of the heart was also demonstrated:

> 'When you are eating too much fat, the fat clots the heart. Pumping of the heart is not good. When it is very bad your heart can fail.' (Participant 11, male, 25 years, secondary school education and employed)

Smoking (n = 4; 13%) and not being active (n = 2; 7%) as causative factors for IHD were codes but did not appear often. Participants demonstrated knowledge and understanding related to the consequences of IHD by highlighting signs and symptoms, morbidity and mortality aspects related to IHD. Chest pain (n = 13; 43%) and breathing difficulties (n = 11; 37%) were issues most often highlighted. Illustrative quotes of signs and symptoms of IHD were:

> 'I think swelling because the circulation is not well. Sweating and breathing problems and chest pains most of the time.' (Participant 8, female, 28 years, post-secondary school education and employed)

Participants knew that an increased risk for mortality was linked with IHD (n = 8; 27%):

> 'If someone is having heart disease they can die from heart disease or if they take care of themselves they can live long.' (Participant 29, female, 32 years, secondary school education and employed)

Lastly, knowledge and understanding regarding prevention strategies for IHD in the form of lifestyle change, coping behaviour, health-seeking behaviour and medical management were reported. These facets were explained:

> 'Yes, if you do all the right things like not eating fatty food, not using cooking oil, if you don't smoke, if you do your exercises and eat your vegetables and fruit. Healthy balanced life; drink enough water, sleep enough and don't stress too much. You always make sure that you are in the middle and level.' (Participant 29, female, 32 years, secondary school education and employed)

Some participants stated that outside assistance was needed to prevent IHD:

> 'Yes, they must come to the clinic at the hospital to get treatment. Only the hospital can make the heart disease right ... A person can't help themselves; they can't do something, the hospital must help.' (Participant 26, female, 45 years, primary school education and employed)

Another reported:

> 'Yes you can ... like an operation to your heart. I don't know anything else that will help.' (Participant 10, female, 26 years, secondary school education and unemployed)

Insight into own risk for Ischaemic heart disease

Participants who perceived themselves not at risk for IHD explained that this was due to following a healthy lifestyle, specific coping behaviours and maintaining

health since using HAART. One participant voiced it as follows:

> 'No, at the moment with HIV and the life I have been leading before, it has been a healthy life throughout and I have never thought that I could get heart disease. But in the course of time you are no longer as young and fit as you used to be, you can come across a lot of problems and could get heart disease, but at the moment I don't think so.' (Participant 28, male, 49 years, secondary school education and employed)

Another stated:

> 'No because something that can cause a painful heart I try and take away or leave alone.' (Participant 21, female, 49 years, no education and employed)

Antiretroviral therapy was seen as a protective factor against IHD:

> 'No since I am taking ARVs I am healthy.' (Participant 14, female, 32 years, secondary school education and unemployed)

In contrast, participants who perceived themselves to be at an increased risk for IHD explained that it was due to their behaviour and/or experiencing physical symptoms:

> 'Sometimes, because of the stress and unhealthy diet and not exercising. I think sometimes I can feel my heart tension that is not normal. Maybe you feel that you are stressed and angry. Anger causes your high blood to go higher and you can even feel that your heart is not "*klopping*" [*beating*] normal. You feel that it is beating faster. It feels like you can hold it, then you feel the short breath and everything.' (Participant 3, female, 36 years, secondary school education and employed)

Another stated:

> 'I think so because when I am worried there is pain straight in the heart. Sometimes I feel weak and the pain goes to my back.' (Participant 7, male, 45 years, post-secondary school education and unemployed)

Health character in a context of HIV infection

Participants demonstrated knowledge and understanding regarding why it is important to adhere to HAART. One participant stated:

> 'To live longer, that is why I am taking ARVs so that I live longer for my children. I know that the ARVs are helping me to keep the sickness down ...' (Participant 6, female, 39 years, secondary school education and employed)

Participants had knowledge of comorbidities that might develop during the course of their illness:

> 'TB, losing weight, skin can change, some people gets a rash or get sores in the mouth.' (Participant 22, male, age 34 years, primary school education and unemployed)

Coping was deemed an important facet that influenced participants' health character and coping beliefs. Certain coping behaviours were identified as ways in which participants attempted to improve their lives. One participant explained:

'It is important to have support from my family especially my mother, because in many ways she supported me in my life; if I am sick, she was there for me.' (Participant 10, 26 years, secondary school education and unemployed)

Being able to live a healthy life was often hindered by environmental factors such as unemployment. One participant explained:

'To get a job, that is what makes me stressed. Not having a job.' (Participant 19, female, 48 years, post-secondary school education and unemployed)

The importance of having employment to ensure an adequate diet was emphasised:

'Yes, it is important to have a job so that you will be able to buy food to be able to take your medication.' (Participant 25, female, 31 years, primary school education and unemployed)

Taking responsibility for health and self-regulating behaviour even in challenging circumstances were important components for functioning with HIV infection. This self-regulation was especially noted when participants' discussed how they used HAART ($n = 17$; 56.7%):

'I think to take my medication at the right time. Not to take my medication at any time. If I take my medication at eight o'clock I need to take my medication at the same time. It is very important and healthy.' (Participant 14, female, 32 years, secondary school education and unemployed)

Another said:

'You must eat first then take your medication like ARVs. You can't drink it on an empty stomach.' (Participant 10, female, 26 years, secondary school education and unemployed)

Discussion

In a South African context prevalence of HIV infection remains disproportionally high in females in comparison to males.[20] More women access HAART in sub-Saharan Africa[21] and in South Africa.[22] The international literature suggests that individuals often underestimate their risk for IHD,[23,24] and this is identified more often in women.[25,26] So it was important to evaluate self-perception and behaviour in relation to the risk of IHD in a South African cohort of PLWHA.

Participants had some knowledge and understanding of IHD, and the majority of participants had a secondary educational level. These two factors might explain why 12 participants (40%) perceived themselves at risk for IHD. The literature suggests that one's knowledge of risk factors for IHD influences one's self-perception.[23] Potvin, Richard and Edwards[27] report that individuals are more likely to know behavioural compared to physiological risk factors of IHD. Out of a sample of 23 129 Canadian participants, 60% reported fat in food, 52% smoking, and 41% lack of exercise as risk factors for IHD. Only 32% reported excess weight, 27% elevated cholesterol and 22% high blood pressure. The education level of participants was strongly associated with participants' ability to recall risk factors of IHD.[27]

Ansa, Oyo-Ita and Essien,[28] who investigated knowledge of risk factors for IHD in university staff in Nigeria, reported smoking (70.6%), use of alcohol (52.8%), obesity (41.6%), sedentary lifestyle (16.6%) and oral contraceptive use (6.4%) as risk factors named. Senior staff with more education were more likely than junior staff to report all of the risk factors. Pace et al.[29] reported an interesting finding regarding education and IHD, in that individuals with a secondary school education or less were likely to report that they know about heart disease but that it was not a concern to them.

In contrast Cioe et al.[13] found a low, non-significant relationship between risk factor knowledge (Heart Disease Fact Questionnaire) and perceived risk (Perception of Risk of Heart Disease Scale) ($r = 0.13$; $p > 0.05$). Cioe et al.'s study was conducted in PLWHA in Rhode Island, USA and consisted mostly of men (62.3%), whilst our study primarily includes women. Even though the authors found a low, non-significant relationship, 97% of their population knew that smoking and being overweight were risk factors for cardiovascular disease.

In our study smoking as a risk factor for IHD was voiced by four individuals (13%), but none voiced overweight or obesity as a risk factor for IHD. This is of concern, considering that obesity in PLWHA is becoming more prevalent.[30] Hurley et al.[31] found that when individuals are on a regimen containing stavudine a significant change ($p < 0.001$) in body mass index of 2.2 kg/m^2 (95% CI 1.5–2.9) in women and 2.4 kg/m^2 (95% CI 1.7–3.1) in men occurs during the first year following initiation. Ninety per cent of participants in Cioe et al.'s study[13] also knew that a high cholesterol, high fat diet and lack of exercise contribute to an increased risk for IHD. Similarities exist between Cioe et al.'s and our study with regard to dietary contribution and lack of exercise as risk factors for IHD. Our study therefore highlights that education strategies are necessary to enlighten PLWHA living in South Africa about the impact of smoking and obesity on their potential future risk for IHD.

Participants in this study who perceived an increased risk for IHD explained that it was due to lifestyle risk factors such as stress and poor diet. The general public in South Africa are known to have higher levels of stress[32] compared to individuals living in the USA.[33] Participants in our study also had to cope with the stigma that surrounds HIV infection and the difficulties associated with employment and participation in the wider community. This risk factor was therefore highlighted as an important factor to address when implementing management strategies for IHD in PLWHA in South Africa.

Individual participants experienced symptoms such as chest pain, especially when they were under a lot of stress. A number of factors contribute to reasons why participants did not address their symptoms. Bodily sensations provide information to an individual, and depending on one's past experiences a person might or might not act on these experiences.[34] Corbin[34] states that individuals are likely to wait and see what happens, and if the sensations become more frightening they will seek medical advice.

The Shifting Perspectives Model of chronic illness described by Paterson[35] could also be used to explain why participants did not seek medical advice. The Shifting Perspectives Model demonstrates that individuals living with chronic illness (e.g. PLWHA) continually shift between two states: illness-in-the-foreground or wellness-in-the-foreground. Wellness is determined by comparing the experience (e.g. chest pain) to what is known and understood about illness, and vice versa. Paterson[35] explains that a perception of losing control is the major factor that will move an individual from a state of wellness-in-the-foreground to illness-in-the-foreground. It is therefore important to monitor subjective symptoms of IHD closely in PLWHA to identify individuals who require further investigations, as they might not see their symptoms as problematic when compared to previous illness experiences.

It was encouraging to note that participants understood the importance of adhering to their HAART regimens and followed advice given by the clinic on how to take their medication on a daily basis. Reda and Biadgilign[36] reported that lack of adherence to HAART in Africa is due to financial constraints and poor food security. Individuals in our study voiced that being unemployed influenced their diet and created significant amounts of stress. Educational strategies would therefore not completely address individuals' stress levels and dietary choices. Part of the wider response addressing social problems facing South Africa should include addressing unemployment and livelihood.

The following limitations should be acknowledged when interpreting the findings from the current study. This study used a qualitative approach and consisted of 30 individuals from one HIV clinic in an urban setting, which limits generalisation of findings to the larger South African and African HIV community. In addition, statistical conclusions from the quantitative data presented here can only be related to the current study population. Data saturation occurred in that the same codes did occur more frequently; however, those that did not were interpreted as knowledge gaps, as this was directed content analysis and participants gave information they knew about within the conceptual framework used. It should also be noted that self-perception and behaviour of participants were influenced by participants' knowledge and understanding of IHD.

Conclusion

Our study supports the need to develop educational programmes to improve IHD risk perception in PLWHA in Johannesburg, South Africa. Programmes are needed to educate and focus on the impact of advancing age, obesity,

physical inactivity, HIV and HAART sequelae on risk for IHD.

Stress was highlighted as a significant risk factor for IHD by participants and often given as a reason why they perceived themselves to be at risk. Intervention strategies to assist individuals on how to manage their stress levels, such as exercise programmes, is key to reduce risk factors for IHD.

As the roll-out of HAART to PLWHA increases in South Africa, morbidity associated with non-communicable diseases such as IHD could increase, as has been shown internationally. Educating PLWHA about risk factors for IHD, screening for risk factors and implementing intervention strategies to change behaviour are important means to lessen the potential burden of IHD in PLWHA.

Acknowledgements

This study was possible due to support from Themba Lethu HIV clinic, Clinical HIV Research Unit, Right to Care and the Department of Medicine at Helen Joseph Hospital in Gauteng, South Africa.

This work was supported by the National Research Foundation Thuthuka Programme (Grant number: 76280); National Research Foundation Sabbatical Grant to Complete Doctoral Degrees (Grant number: 86485); University of the Witwatersrand, Faculty Research Committee Grants (Grant number: 4759); Medical Research Council Self-Initiated Research Grant (Grant number: MZWA012); and South African Society of Physiotherapy, Research Foundation Grant.

Any opinion, findings and conclusions or recommendations expressed in this material are those of the author(s) and therefore the NRF and MRC do not accept any liability in regard thereto.

Competing interests

The authors declare that they have no financial or personal relationship(s) that may have inappropriately influenced them in writing this article.

Authors' contributions

R.R. (University of the Witwatersrand) was responsible for design of the study, data collection and analysis and write-up. H.M. (University of the Witwatersrand) made conceptual contributions, especially towards experimental and study design, and assisted with data analysis and write-up. H.vA. (University of the Witwatersrand) made conceptual contributions and assisted with manuscript write-up.

References

1. Lozano R, Naghavi M, Foreman K, et al. Global and regional mortality from 235 causes of death for 20 age groups in 1990 and 2010: A systematic analysis for the Global Burden of Disease Study. Lancet. 2010;380(9859):2095–2128. http://dx.doi.org/10.1016/S0140-6736(12)61728-0

2. Mensah GA. Ischaemic heart disease in Africa. Heart. 2008; 94(7):836–843. http://dx.doi.org/10.1136/hrt.2007.136523

3. Gaziano TA. Cardiovascular disease in the developing world and its cost-effective management. Circulation. 2005;112(23):3547–3553. http://dx.doi.org/10.1161/CIRCULATIONAHA.105.591792

4. Onen CL. Epidemiology of ischaemic heart disease in sub-Saharan Africa. Cardiovasc J Afr. 2013; 24(2):34–42. http://dx.doi.org/10.5830/CVJA-2012-071

5. Danaei G, Finucane MM, Lin JK, et al. National, regional, and global trends in systolic blood pressure since 1980: Systematic analysis of health examination surveys and epidemiological studies with 786 country-years and 5.4 million participants. Lancet. 2011;377:568–577. http://dx.doi.org/10.1016/S0140-6736(10)62036-3

6. Finucane MM, Stevens GA, Cowan MJ, et al. National, regional, and global trends in body-mass index since 1980: Systematic analysis of health examination surveys and epidemiological studies with 960 country-years and 9.1 million participants. Lancet. 2011;377:557–567. http://dx.doi.org/10.1016/S0140-6736(10)62037-5

7. Triant VA, Lee H, Hadigan C, Grinspoon SK. Increased acute myocardial infarction rates and cardiovascular risk factors among patients with human immunodeficiency virus disease. J Clin Endocrinol Metab. 2007;92(7):2506–2512. http://dx.doi.org/10.1210/jc.2006-2190

8. Saves M, Chene G, Ducimetiere P, et al. Risk factors for coronary heart disease in patients treated for human immunodeficiency virus infection compared with the general population. HIV/AIDS. 2003;37:292–298. http://dx.doi.org/10.1086/375844

9. De Wit S, Sabin CA, Weber R, et al. Incidence and risk factors for new-onset diabetes in HIV-infected patients: The DATA Collection on Adverse Events of Anti-HIV Drugs (D:A:D) Study. Diabetes Care. 2008;31:1224–1229. http://dx.doi.org/10.2337/dc07-2013

10. Friis-Møller N, Weber R, Reiss P, et al. Cardiovascular disease risk factors in HIV patients – association with antiretroviral therapy. Results from the DAD study. AIDS. 2003;17(8):1179–1193. http://dx.doi.org/10.1097/00002030-200305230-00010

11. De Luca A, De Gaetano Donati K, Colafigli M, et al. The association of high-sensitivity C-reactive protein and other biomarkers with cardiovascular disease in patients treated for HIV: A nested case-control study. BMC Infect Dis. 2013;13(414):1–12. http://dx.doi.org/10.1186/1471-2334-13-414

12. Triant VA, Meigs JB, Grinspoon SK. Association of C-Reactive protein and HIV infection with acute myocardial infarction. J AIDS. 2009;51(3):268–273. http://dx.doi.org/10.1097/QAI.0b013e3181a9992c

13. Cioe PA, Crawford SL, Stein MD. Cardiovascular risk-factor knowledge and risk perception among HIV-infected adults. JANAC. 2013;25(1):60–69.

14. Portney LG, Watkins MP. Qualitative Research. In: Cohen M, editor. Foundations of Clinical Research; applications to practice, 3rd ed. Pearson Education, Inc., New Jersey: Upper Saddle River, 2009; pp. 306–313.

15. Rugg G, McGeorge P. The sorting techniques: A tutorial paper on card sorts, picture sorts and item sorts. Expert Systems. 1997;14(2):80–93. http://dx.doi.org/10.1111/1468-0394.00045

16. Fincher S, Tenenberg J. Making sense of card sorting data. Expert Systems. 2005;22(3): 89–93. http://dx.doi.org/10.1111/j.1468-0394.2005.00299.x

17. Hsieh HF, Shannon SE. Three approaches to qualitative content analysis. Qual Health Res. 2005;15(9):1277–1288. http://dx.doi.org/10.1177/1049732305276687

18. Thomas DR. A general inductive approach for analysing qualitative evaluation data. Am J Eval. 2006;27(2):237–246. http://dx.doi.org/10.1177/1098214005283748

19. Smith CP. Content analysis and narrative analysis. In: Reis T, Judd C, editors. Handbook of research methods in social and personality psychology. New York: Cambridge University Press, 2000; pp. 313–326.

20. Statistics South Africa. Mid-year population release, 2013. Pretoria: Government of South Africa: 2013.

21. Braitstein P, Boulle A, Nash D, et al. Gender and the use of antiretroviral treatment in resource-constraint settings: Findings from a multicentre collaboration. J Womens Health. 2008;17(1):47–55. http://dx.doi.org/10.1089/jwh.2007.0353

22. Cornell M, Schomaker M, Garone DB, et al. Gender differences in survival among adult patients starting antiretroviral therapy in South Africa: A multicentre cohort study. PLOS Med. 2012;9(9):e1001304. http://dx.doi.org/10.1371/journal.pmed.1001304

23. Meischke H, Sellers DE, Goff DC, et al. Factors that influence personal perceptions of the risk of an acute myocardial infarction. Behav Med. 2000;26(1):4–13. http://dx.doi.org/10.1080/08964280009595748

24. Avis NE, Smith KW, McKinlay JB. Accuracy of perceptions of heart attack risk: What influences perceptions and can they be changed? AJPH. 1998;79(12):1608–1612. http://dx.doi.org/10.2105/AJPH.79.12.1608

25. Hart PL. Women's perceptions of coronary heart disease: An integrative review. J Cardiovasc Nurs. 2005;20(3):170–176. http://dx.doi.org/10.1097/00005082-200505000-00008

26. Legato MJ, Padus EP, Slaughter E. Women's perceptions of their general health, with special reference to their risk of coronary artery disease: Results of a national telephone survey. J Womens Health. 1997;6(2):189–198. http://dx.doi.org/10.1089/jwh.1997.6.189

27. Potvin L, Richard L, Edwards AC. Knowledge of cardiovascular disease risk factors among the Canadian population: Relationships with indicators of socioeconomic status. CMAJ. 2000;162(9):S5–S11.

28. Ansa VO, Oyo-Ita A, Essien OE. Perception of ischaemic heart disease, knowledge of and attitude to reduction of its risk factors. EAMJ. 2007;84(7):318–323.

29. Pace R, Dawkins N, Wang B, et al. Rural African Americans' dietary knowledge, perceptions, and behaviour in relation to cardiovascular disease. Ethn Dis. 2008;18:6–12.

30. Crum-Cianflone N, Roediger MP, Eberly L, et al. Increasing rates of obesity among HIV-infected persons during the HIV epidemic. PLOS One. 2010;5(4):e10106. http://dx.doi.org/10.1371/journal.pone.0010106

31. Hurley E, Coutsoudis A, Giddy J, Knight SE, Loots E, Esterhuizen TM. Weight evolution and perceptions of adults living with HIV following initiation of antiretroviral therapy in a South African urban setting. SAMJ. 2011;101(9):645–650.

32. Hamad R, Fernald LCH, Karlan DS, Zinman J. Social and economic correlates of depressive symptoms and perceived stress in South African adults. JECH. 2008;62:538–544. http://dx.doi.org/10.1136/jech.2007.066191

33. Cohen S, Janicki-Deverts D. Who's stressed? Distributions of psychological stress in the United States in probability samples from 1983, 2006 and 2009. J Applied Soc Psychol. 2012;42(6):1320–1334. http://dx.doi.org/10.1111/j.1559-1816.2012.00900.x

34. Corbin JM. The body in health and illness. Qual Health Res. 2003;13(2):256–267. http://dx.doi.org/10.1177/1049732302239603

35. Paterson BL. The Shifting Perspectives Model of chronic illness. J Nurs Scholarsh. 2001;33(1):21–26. http://dx.doi.org/10.1111/j.1547-5069.2001.00021.x

36. Reda AA, Biadgilign S. Determinants of adherence to antiretroviral therapy among HIV-infected patients in Africa. AIDS Res Treat. 2012:574656. http://dx.doi.org/10.1155/2012/574656

4

Evaluation of universal newborn hearing screening in South African primary care

Authors:
Katijah Khoza-Shangase[1]
Shannon Harbinson[1]

Affiliations:
[1]Faculty of Humanities, Department of Audiology, University of the Witwatersrand, South Africa

Correspondence to:
Katijah Khoza-Shangase

Email:
katijah.khoza@wits.ac.za

Postal address:
PO Box 57, Wits 2050, South Africa

Background: Universal Newborn Hearing Screening (UNHC) is the gold standard toward early hearing detection and intervention, hence the importance of its deliberation within the South African context.

Aim: To determine the feasibility of screening in low-risk neonates, using Otoacoustic Emissions (OAEs), within the Midwife Obstetric Unit (MOU) three-day assessment clinic at a Community Health Centre (CHC), at various test times following birth.

Method: Within a quantitative, prospective design, 272 neonates were included. Case history interviews, otoscopic examinations and Distortion Product OAEs (DPOAEs) screening were conducted at two sessions (within six hours and approximately three days after birth). Data were analysed via descriptive statistics.

Results: Based on current staffing profile and practice, efficient and comprehensive screening is not successful within hours of birth, but is more so at the MOU three-day assessment clinic. Significantly higher numbers of infants were screened at session 2, with significantly less false-positive results. At session 1, only 38.1% of the neonates were screened, as opposed to more than 100% at session 2. Session 1 yielded an 82.1% rate of false positive findings, a rate that not only has important implications for the emotional well-being of the parents; but also for resource-stricken environments where expenditure has to be accounted for carefully.

Conclusion: Current findings highlight the importance of studying methodologies to ensure effective reach for hearing screening within the South African context. These findings argue for UNHS initiatives to include the MOU three-day assessment to ensure that a higher number of neonates are reached and confounding variables such as vernix have been eliminated.

Evaluation du test universel de dépistage auditif chez les nouveau-nés dans les soins primaires sud-africains.

Contexte: Le Test universel de Dépistage auditif chez les Nouveau-nés (UNHC) est la norme d'excellence pour le dépistage et le traitement précoces de la surdité ; il est donc important d'en discuter dans le contexte sud-africain.

Objectif: Déterminer la faisabilité du dépistage chez les nouveau-nés à faible risque, au moyen d'Emissions otoacoustiques (OAE), au sein de la clinique d'évaluation de trois jours de l'Unité d'Obstétrique des Sages-femmes (MOU) dans un Centre de Santé communautaire (CHC), à différentes périodes d'essais après la naissance.

Méthode: On a inclus 272 nouveau-nés au sein d'une conception prospective et quantitative. On a effectué des entrevues sur les antécédents médicaux, des examens otoscopiques et des dépistages de produits de distorsion d'émissions otoacoustiques (DPOAEs) au cours de deux sessions (dans les six heures et environ trois jours après la naissance). Les données ont été analysées par satistiques descriptives.

Résultats: Selon le profil actuel et les pratiques du personnel, le dépistage complet et efficace n'est pas performant dans les heures suivant la naissance, mais il a plus de succès dans les cliniques d'évaluation de trois jours du MOU. Un plus grand nombre de bébés a été dépisté à la session 2, avec beaucoup moins de résultats faussement positifs. A la session 1, seuls 38.1% des nouveau-nés ont été dépistés, contre plus de 100% à la session 2. La session 1 a donné un taux de 82.1% de résultats faussement positifs, ce qui a des conséquences importantes pour le bien-être émotionnel des parents; mais aussi pour les environnements à ressources limitées où il faut rendre compte soigneusement des dépenses.

Conclusion: Les résultats actuels soulignent l'importance de l'étude des méthodologies pour assurer la portée efficace du dépistage de la surdité dans le contexte sud-africain. Ces résultats plaident pour que les initiatives de l'UNHS incluent l'évaluation de trois jours du MOU pour pouvoir inclure un plus grand nombre de nouveau-nés et que les facteurs de confusion comme le vernix soient éliminés.

Introduction

The profession of audiology has focused on childhood hearing screening for several years and the screening for paediatric hearing impairment has subsequently become an important component of neonatal care. The Health Professions Council of South Africa (HPCSA) and the Joint Committee on Infant Hearing (JCIH) endorse, advocate and stipulate the early identification of hearing loss through the employment of objective physiological screening measures, so that the timely diagnosis and treatment for congenital auditory impairment may occur.[1,2] This, therefore, highlights the intention of neonatal hearing screening, which is to ensure the early identification of congenital hearing impairment as well as the early intervention for those identified with a hearing loss.[3] Screening for hearing impairment is viewed as a method of prevention and is mandated in several developed countries. Screening has also been deemed as an attainable public health programme in developing countries.[4]

The aim of neonatal hearing screening may be achievable through the appropriate screening of all infants,[5] otherwise called universal newborn hearing screening (UNHS). UNHS refers to a prevention programme in which all newborns are screened for hearing impairment, after birth, prior to discharge from the newborn nursery.[6] In contrast to UNHS, targeted hearing screening denotes a selective screening method based on the presence of established risk factors. According to Flynn et al.[7] a comparison between UNHS and targeted hearing screening procedures has indicated that universal hearing screening measures are generally preferred.

There is evidence to suggest that the lack of UNHS programmes may be detrimental to several hearing-impaired children. These newborn hearing screening programmes are considered to be valid and are thus likely to result in the timeous identification of, and intervention for, congenital hearing loss.[3] The primary rationale underlying UNHS and the early detection of hearing impairment is that hearing-impaired children who are provided with suitable intervention services within the first six months of life, present with considerably better language skills when compared to children who receive this intervention at a later stage.[8] Considering the age at which the detection of, and intervention for, hearing impairment occurs, a properly implemented neonatal hearing screening programme is able to offer acceptable outcomes in terms of language and emotional development, as well as educational and vocational outcomes.[9] However, in the absence of an appropriate hearing screening programme, a hearing-impaired child may only be identified once the child is of school-going age.[3] UNHS has therefore been proposed as a means to speeding up the identification, diagnostic and intervention process for hearing-impaired children.[10] Neonatal hearing screening programmes are deemed as advantageous and are, therefore, accepted in many developed countries.[11] These early hearing detection programmes have been implemented as components of the public health system in many countries[12] and the establishment of UNHS programmes has been on the increase internationally.[3]

The increase in UNHS programmes may be a result of the existing evidence that UNHS is a cost-effective approach for the timeous and effective detection of congenital hearing impairment;[13] and may also be attributed to reports of feasibility and value of such programmes.[4] Neonatal hearing screening is gradually becoming a standard procedure internationally.[14] However, it is of great concern that the implementation of extensive neonatal audiological screening drives has mainly been limited to the developed world. This implementation has not yet been intensified in the developing world, namely, the developing countries of Asia, Latin America, the Caribbean and Africa (and 80% of the world's population).[15]

If UNHS is valid, then it must also be established as effective and viable across geographically-varied hospital collections, with differing staffing attitudes and resources.[16] This implies that UNHS needs to be embraced in the developing world, considering that most children with a hearing impairment are reported to live in third-world countries.[17]

According to Olusanya, Luxon and Wirz,[17] the feasibility of newborn hearing screening programmes for developing countries seems inadequate in view of the diversities in the socioeconomic and health standing of these countries. This may be because of the perception of hearing impairment that, although hearing loss is debilitating, it is not life-threatening when compared to various fatal childhood diseases. In spite of this, a great number of developing countries are exploring practical and culturally-appropriate options for early hearing screening.

Whilst the available technology for newborn hearing screening is appropriate for employment in developing countries, the advantages and benefits of early detection and early intervention services for infants with a hearing impairment are not always available and easily reachable. Moreover, administrative systematisation for UNHS has not been established in several of these countries.[11] Findings from ongoing infant hearing screening programmes in South Africa and in Nigeria have even proposed that hearing screening programmes be integrated into early childhood immunisation programmes in developing countries, especially where a number of births occur outside regular hospitals and clinic settings.[18] However, regardless of the numerous recommendations,[19] researchers have acknowledged that the establishment of a UNHS programme in settings with such limitations may be a challenging task.

Notwithstanding the challenges associated with the establishment and implementation of these UNHS programmes in developing countries such as South Africa, there are accessible structures that need to be explored and considered as potential platforms from which these programmes can be realised.[20] In South Africa, the professional board for speech, language and hearing professionals has suggested that community-based developmental hearing screening programmes be put into operation at the primary healthcare level within the district health services model.[1] Structures that may be explored include the community health centres (CHCs), where babies are followed up after being discharged from the hospital, hence the current study.

According to the JCIH,[2] the establishment of suitable practices is a necessary part of the foundation for newborn hearing screening programmes. Intensified research and the development of appropriate screening programmes for the detection of, and intervention for, hearing impairment in the newborn population are required. There is a pressing call for further research comparing hearing screening programmes in various contexts; that is, research is required that aims to establish whether the programme, equipment and protocols are designed to meet the specific objectives according to the context.[21] This is particularly true for developing countries, where resources are scarce and decisions are mostly financially driven.

Olusanya and Okolo[18] have highlighted South Africa's means to realise valuable and feasible neonatal audiological screening programmes. However, in order to guide the implementation process of neonatal hearing screening programmes in South Africa, research to collate evidence concerning the efficacy and practicability of these screening programmes is required,[1] hence the current study.

The primary aim of the study was to determine the feasibility of otoacoustic emissions (OAE) screening in low-risk neonates at different times and places following birth in a primary care setting. Specific objectives of the study were:

- To investigate the practicability and efficiency when OAE screening takes place within six hours after birth, prior to discharge from the newborn nursery.
- To investigate the practicability and efficiency when OAE screening takes place at three days after birth at the Midwife Obstetric Unit (MOU) three-day assessment clinic.
- To compare the findings of the OAE screening obtained across the two differing test times.

Research methods and design
Study design

This study employed a quantitative research design. Quantitative research designs entail the utilisation of standardised measures, with fixed categories, to which numbers are assigned. For the purposes of this study, the standardised measures were the audiological screening measures (otoscopic examinations and OAEs) and the fixed categories were the screening results obtained (*pass/refer*).[22]

Within the quantitative research design application for this study, a longitudinal approach was adopted. A longitudinal design, or within-subject design, involves the collection of data from the same sample of participants at two or more points in time.[22] For the purpose of this study, two data collection sessions – one on the day of birth and then one at the Midwife Obstetric Unit (MOU) three-day assessment clinic, with approximately three days between the sessions – were adopted. All testing was conducted by a qualified registered audiologist.

Setting

The study was conducted at a Community Health Centre's MOU department in Gauteng, South Africa. The CHC is run daily by midwives, with a majority of babies born there being discharged within six hours of birth, with a clinic follow up appointment for the MOU three-day assessment clinic. The CHC has an audiologist in its staff establishment who keeps 08:00–16:30 working hours on weekdays and attends every scheduled MOU assessment clinic. Dippenaar[23] has described the South African context where midwives care for 77% of pregnant women and are, therefore, an integral part of the healthcare system. These midwives manage low-risk pregnancies, with high-risk pregnancy being referred to the hospital system. Hence, all the neonates attended to at the research site are considered to be low risk.[24]

Study population

The target population for the current study was the low-risk neonatal population in Gauteng, whilst the accessible population was all neonates at the CHC where data were collected. All neonates during a one-month period were potentially included in the study (from 30 August to 30 September 2009), which had the following inclusion and exclusion criteria.[25]

Participants were required to be well, full-term neonates and to be born by normal vaginal delivery. A full-term neonate is one that is born at 38–42 weeks' gestation.[26] Participants were required to present with an unremarkable prenatal and perinatal history, as reported in the participant's clinic file.

Newborns older than seven days at session 2 were not included in this study. The rationale for this is that the aim of UNHS is to identify congenital hearing loss, a hearing loss present at birth.[27] A postnatal hearing loss is a hearing loss which is acquired after the perinatal period,[28] where the perinatal period refers to the period from 28 weeks' complete gestation to day 7 after delivery.[29] Based on this, the seven-day cut-off was applied in an attempt to differentiate postnatal hearing loss from congenital hearing loss.

Of the 272 participants, 149 (54.8%) were boys and 123 (45.2%) were girls. The mean age (SD) at session 1 was 4.2 (1.3) hours and at session 2 was 3.9 (1.1) days.

The sample for this study (N = 272) was further divided into three distinct groups: the first group (n = 99) comprised the neonates tested at session 1, the second group (n = 173) comprised newborns tested only at session 2 and the third group (n = 95) comprised neonates tested at both session 1 and session 2.

Instrumentation and materials

The materials which were employed included a case history checklist form and a data collection form, a Heine mini 2000 otoscope and a GSI AUDIOscreener, as well as a sound level meter to monitor noise levels during the hearing screening. The GSI AUDIOscreener is a portable, hand-held screener with automatic operations for quick and simple screening and is designed for universal newborn hearing screening (UNHS) purposes.

Details pertaining to the pregnancy were included in the case history interview and were aimed at determining whether the pregnancy was a healthy one and whether any complications existed, as well as to determine the age of the mother, with younger than 15 years and older than 35 years being regarded as the limits for maternal age.[30] Details regarding the birth, postnatal conditions and a family history of hearing impairment were also included in the case history, with the aim of establishing whether any risk factors were present. Although it did not form part of the set objectives of the current study, it was important to identify and document any possible risk factors for congenital hearing impairment which the participants presented with, as part of ensuring context-specific and context-relevant evidence.

Ethical considerations

The current study was examined and approved by the appropriate ethics committee and has therefore been performed in accordance with the ethical standards laid down in the 2012–2013 World Medical Association's Declaration of Helsinki. Permission to conduct the study was also obtained from hospital management at the research site and the Head of Department of Speech Therapy and Audiology. Data collection only began following permission from the Human Research Ethics Committee (Medical) at the University of the Witwatersrand (Ethical Clearance Number: M090836).

Test procedures
The collection of case history information

Following the attainment of informed consent for participation in the study, a case history was obtained. The case history information was drawn from the participant's clinic file and from interviews with the participant's mother. In the presence of a language barrier, the services of a trained interpreter were employed in order to ensure the gathering of adequate case history details and to facilitate clear communication between the researcher and the mothers of the participants.[31]

Audiological screening

Two newborn hearing screening test sessions occurred. The initial screening session (session 1) took place at the CHC in the MOU department's newborn nursery, within six hours of the participant's birth, before discharge from the birth facility. The second screening session (session 2) also took place at the CHC but as part of the scheduled MOU three-day assessment clinic, approximately three days after the participant's birth.

Tattersall and Young[32] have suggested that, in the case of a healthy infant obtaining a *pass* result during the initial screening process, no additional testing is necessary. Despite this suggestion, for the purposes of this study, irrespective of the result obtained at the initial screening session, all neonates were booked for re-screening at the MOU three-day assessment clinic.

At each audiological screening session, an otoscopic examination was carried out in both ears on each participant. An otoscopic examination is a subjective procedure deemed to be useful in the assessment for the presence or absence of middle ear effusion and is used to examine the external auditory meatus in order to assist with the selection of an appropriate probe tip for further tests.[33] In the past, specialists have purposely highlighted the diagnostic worth of the otoscopic examination, claiming that the appropriate utilisation of this procedure may lead to improved diagnosis of middle ear pathology.[34] Although the otoscopic examination is a subjective measure, it is also a cost-effective and highly-rated diagnostic tool.[35] The otoscopic examination, therefore, ought to form part of standard paediatric audiological evaluations.[36]

For the otoscopic examination, a *pass* result represented a clear external auditory meatus with no foreign bodies or debris in the external auditory canal, no obvious middle ear pathology and a visibly intact and healthy tympanic membrane. The otoscopic examination is a key stage in the newborn hearing screening process, as middle ear pathology and/or obstruction has a documented adverse effect on the detectability of OAE responses; and the presence of cerumen or vernix in the external auditory meatus is implicated frequently in failed hearing screenings.[37]

Following the otoscopic examination, a distortion product otoacoustic emissions (DPOAE) screening was conducted. In order to obtain a DPOAE response, a small probe is inserted into the participant's external auditory meatus.[32] To enhance the probe fitting, the tester may remove and clean the probe tip and then re-test immediately[38] and this was done from time to time in the current study.

The GSI AUDIOscreener was employed to obtain the DPOAE measures. This screener incorporates calibration within the test ear, which promotes total screening accuracy.[39] The test parameters were set according to the default screening protocol setting – 'Quick DPOAE' – and three frequencies (2000 Hz, 3000 Hz and 4000 Hz) were assessed for each ear per participant. The criteria for an overall *pass* result were based on passing at least two of the three frequencies tested.

The hearing screening test results can be obtained in only a few seconds as DPOAE screening devices conveniently feature pass-fail algorithms.[3] Screening methodologies that include automated response detection are preferable to the screening methodologies that require operator interpretation. Therefore, to decrease tester error, a programmed OAE machine with pass or fail criteria is recommended[40] and was employed for the purposes of the current study. The audiological screening results obtained, per participant, across the two screening sessions, were recorded using the data collection form. The screening results were recorded across the *pass/refer* category. The term *refer* was used in place of the term *fail*, with the aim of emphasising that not passing the screening session indicates necessity for follow-up testing to confirm or exclude the presence of a hearing impairment.[41]

The overall *pass* criteria for the purposes of this research project were a normal otoscopic examination in both ears, as well as a bilateral *pass* result for the DPOAE screening. It has been suggested that newborns that do not pass the initial hearing screening session can be re-tested prior to hospital discharge.[42] It has been implied that test repetition may result in a reduction in the high *refer* rates from UNHS.[13] The overall specificity of a screening protocol can thus be increased by testing infants twice.[42] In line with this, for the purposes of this study, participants not obtaining a *pass* result were re-screened immediately.

All neonates who do not pass the birth admission audiological screening session and any follow-up screening sessions are to undergo thorough audiologic and medical examinations in order to verify the presence of a hearing impairment before the infant is three months of age.[43] Therefore, for the purposes of the current study, in the case of a neonate not passing the second screening session, the neonate was referred for a full audiological assessment.

OAE responses can be obtained in a non-soundproofed environment.[44] Therefore, for the initial testing session, within six hours of birth, audiological screening took place in the post-delivery room, in the MOU department at the CHC. Screening was conducted whilst the neonate was lying in an open crib. The participants need not be asleep for the OAE testing, as an OAE can be obtained in various states of arousal.[45] Screening during the second test session took place in the Rehabilitation department at the CHC, which is off the same corridor as the MOU department.

Validity and reliability

A trained interpreter was employed when indicated in order to obtain an accurate case history for each participant. To ensure that an accurate case history was obtained, information obtained during the interview was cross-checked with the details recorded in the participant's clinic file. In terms of test procedures, the employment of an otoscopic examination, conducted prior to the OAE screening, ensured an accurate interpretation of the OAE result obtained and thus added to the aspects of validity and reliability. The OAE screening measure contributed to reliability and validity, as these screening measures are reportedly both reliable and sensitive.[46] The appropriate screening equipment was utilised and protocol strictly adhered to across all participants. Protocols also remained constant between participants and calibration of the OAE machine was ensured. Furthermore, it has been suggested that, in order for OAE measures to be reliable, ambient noise levels should not exceed 50 to 55 dB A of noise.[47] Noise levels in both of the test environments were measured using a sound level meter to ensure that the environment remained appropriate for audiological screening, that is between 50 to 55 dB A of noise.

Data analysis and statistical procedures

This study entailed the collection of categorical data, used for classification purposes, where categorical data can be defined as the frequency of observations falling into various categories.[48] The categories pertaining to this project were those of *pass* and *refer*.

In order to determine the feasibility of audiological screening in low-risk neonates, using OAEs, at different times following birth, various statistical tests were conducted. These included cross-tabulations and the matched pairs *t*-test.[49]

The number of neonates presenting with *refer* findings were analysed both unilaterally and bilaterally using descriptive statistics. After tabulation and coding of the data, followed by frequency distribution, measures of central tendency, variability, relative position and measures of relationship were adopted.

In terms of practicability, aspects taken into account included the availability of participants. Asma et al.[50] defines the coverage rate, which encompasses components of practicability, as the percentage born during the study that were tested, available resources in the form of staffing, the working hours of the audiologist and the time-frames of discharge from the newborn nursery, as well as the test equipment. In terms of efficiency, aspects taken into consideration included the results obtained for the otoscopic examination and for the otoacoustic emission, as well as the referral rate. The time taken per screening measure also forms part of the evaluation of the efficiency of OAE screening within six hours after birth; but this aspect was not measured in the current study. According to Hall,[51] the OAE, when used as part of a UNHS programme, has a fairly short test time. The time taken to conduct the hearing screening on each participant is recognised as an aspect in the evaluation of the efficiency of OAE screening within six hours after birth, prior to discharge from the newborn nursery. However, this aspect was not formally measured as part of the current study, although it was noted from clinical experience on the part of the researcher audiologist that it was not problematic, so the time taken with each neonate was deemed appropriate for a screening session.

Results

A sample of 272 low-risk neonates was screened for hearing impairment during the current study, across the two screening sessions. This sample comprised 149 male participants and 123 female participants.

The practicability and efficiency of screening within six hours of birth

During the time of the current study, 260 neonates were born at the research site. However, only 99 (38.1%) of these newborns were screened at session 1. The 99 newborns screened at session 1 were available for screening at session 1; that is, the time period between the neonate's birth and discharge from the newborn nursery fell within normal working hours, when the audiologist was on duty to perform the screening. It is notable that the 99 newborns screened at session 1 comprised all the participants approached to participate in the study, as no participants declined the screening services as part of the current study. A total of 161 newborns were missed at the first screening session, as these neonates were born over weekends or during the night. The time period between these neonates' births and their discharge from the newborn nursery did not fall within normal working hours when the audiologist was on duty to perform the screening.

In evaluating the efficiency of OAE screening at session 1; the screening results obtained have been taken into account. Of the 99 participants screened at session 1, 16 newborns obtained an overall *pass* result for the audiological screening and the remaining 83 participants obtained an overall *refer* result; which equates to an 83.8% refer rate. With the overall *pass* criteria for the purposes of the current study being a normal otoscopic examination bilaterally as well as a bilateral *pass* result for the DPOAE screening, the results for both the otoscopic examination as well as for the DPOAE screening at session 1 are detailed in Table 1 below.

As depicted in Table 1, of the 99 participants screened at the first session; a small minority presented with *pass* findings, depicted by only 17 neonates presenting with a bilateral *pass* result for the otoscopic examination and 16 with a bilateral *pass* result for the DPOAE screening measure. A large majority presented with *refer* findings for both of these measures. Two newborns obtained a bilateral *pass* result for the otoscopic examination, yet obtained a unilateral *refer* result for the DPOAE screening. No neonates obtained a *refer* otoscopic examination result and a *pass* DPOAE screening result. These data are detailed in Table 2 below.

TABLE 1: Summary of the screening results obtained during session 1 of the current study (*n* = 99 participants, 198 ears).

Procedure and result obtained	Unilateral	Bilateral
Otoscopic examination – *Pass*	7	17
Otoscopic examination – *Refer*	7	75
DPOAE – *Pass*	9	16
DPOAE – *Refer*	9	74
Total Participants examined	**99**	

DPOAE, Distortion Product Otoacoustic Emissions.

TABLE 2: Breakdown of screening results obtained during session 1 (*n* = 99).

Detailed results obtained	Number of participants
Number of bilateral *refer* results for Otoscopic examination and DPOAE screening.	74
Number of bilateral *pass* results for Otoscopic examination and DPOAE screening.	16
Number of unilateral *pass* results for Otoscopic examination and DPOAE screening on the left ear.	4
Number of unilateral *pass* results for Otoscopic examination and DPOAE screening on the right ear.	3
Number of bilateral *pass* results for Otoscopic examination, unilateral *refer* results for DPOAE screening.	2
Total number of newborns screened at session 1.	**99**

DPOAE, Distortion Product Otoacoustic Emissions.

The practicability and efficiency of screening three days after birth

During the time of the current study, 260 neonates were born at the research site. It is noteworthy that a total of 268 neonates, 147 boys and 121 girls, were screened at the second screening session – 173 more than at session 1. This indicates that eight newborns not born at the CHC were also captured at the second screening session.

For session 2, there was still only one audiologist on duty from 08:00 to 16:30 on weekdays. As screening was conducted as part of the MOU three-day assessment programme, during scheduled times daily, no newborns were missed because of discharge time-frames or the audiologist's working hours.

In the evaluation of the efficiency of audiological screening at session 2, of the 268 participants screened at session 2, 266 participants obtained an overall *pass* result. Two participants obtained an overall *refer* result, which equates to an overall *refer* rate of 0.7% for the audiological screening results obtained during session 2. The audiological screening results obtained during the second screening session are detailed in Table 3 below.

There were no neonates that presented with bilateral *refer* results for both the otoscopic examination and the DPOAE screening measure during session 2. There was one participant that presented with a unilateral *pass* result for both the otoscopic examination and the DPOAE screening measure. In this case, the laterality of the ear in which the *pass* result for the otoscopic examination as well as the DPOAE result were obtained correlated. There was one newborn that obtained a bilateral *pass* result for the otoscopic examination, yet obtained a unilateral *refer* result for the DPOAE screening. It is worth noting that both the DPOAE *refer* results obtained were unilateral. There were no neonates that obtained *refer*

TABLE 3: Summary of the screening results obtained during session 2 (n = 268).

Procedure and result obtained	Unilateral	Bilateral	Total participants examined
Otoscopic Examination – *Pass*	1	267	268
Otoscopic Examination – *Refer*	1	0	268
DPOAE – *Pass*	2	266	268
DPOAE – *Refer*	2	0	268

DPOAE, Distortion Product Otoacoustic Emissions.

TABLE 4: Breakdown of screening results obtained during session 2 (n = 268).

Detailed results obtained	Number of participants
Bilateral *refer* results for Otoscopic examination and DPOAE screening.	0
Bilateral *pass* results for Otoscopic examination and DPOAE screening.	266
Unilateral *pass* results for Otoscopic examination and DPOAE on the left ear.	0
Unilateral *pass* results for Otoscopic examination and DPOAE on the right ear.	1
Bilateral *pass* results for otoscopic examination, unilateral *refer* results for DPOAE.	1
Total newborns screened at session 2.	**268**

DPOAE, Distortion Product Otoacoustic Emissions.

otoscopic examination results and *pass* DPOAE screening results. This information is detailed in Table 4.

In terms of efficiency, the follow-up rate is to be taken into account. In the current study, of the 99 newborns that were screened at session 1, 95 participants returned for follow-up screening at session 2, as part of the MOU three-day assessment clinic. This equates to a follow-up return rate of 96%.

Comparison of findings across the two screening sessions

During the time of the current study, 260 newborns were born at the research site. During session 1, only 99 newborns were screened, but 268 newborns were screened at session 2. The eight additional newborns who were screened at session 2 comprised babies born at home and not at the CHC during the same period, but whose parents still utilise the MOU three-day clinic for neonatal assessments and follow up, which is standard practice in the area.

A total of 161 neonates were missed at the first screening session as these neonates were born over weekends or during the night and, because of the discharge time-frames, the audiologist was not on duty to perform the screening. There were 268 newborns tested at session 2 as screening at session 2 was not affected by time of birth and discharge being outside of working hours. Audiological screening at session 2, as part of the MOU three-day assessment clinic, was the final screening session where referrals for diagnostic assessments were made.

In the current study, a total of 95 participants underwent screening at both sessions. The screening results for each of these participants has been captured across the two screening sessions and compared. It is notable that the majority of these participants (73.7%) obtained bilateral

refer results at session 1 and then obtained bilateral *pass* results at session 2. There was one participant who obtained an overall *refer* result at both sessions and 16 participants who obtained an overall *pass* result at both sessions. A total of 78 participants obtained a *refer* result at session 1 and a *pass* result at session 2. It is notable that there were no participants that obtained a *pass* result at session 1 and a *refer* result at session 2.

It is also notable that there were no participants that obtained a *pass* result at session 1 that did not present for screening at session 2, but there were three participants with bilateral *refer* results at session 1 that did not present for re-screening at session 2.

In comparing the feasibility and efficiency of audiological screening at various times following birth, the number of *refer* results obtained across the two sessions has been taken into account. With regard to the otoscopic examination results, of the total *refer* results obtained, 99.4% of these were obtained during session 1; whilst only 0.6% were obtained at session 2. This indicates a considerably higher *refer* rate for otoscopic examinations at session 1 compared with session 2, approximately three days later.

In comparing the feasibility and efficiency of audiological screening at various times following birth, the number of DPOAE *refer* results obtained across the two sessions has been taken into account. Of the total *refer* results obtained; 98.8% of these were obtained during session 1, whilst only 1.2 % were obtained at session 2. The *refer* rate for DPOAE screening at session 1 is thus notably increased when compared with the rate at session 2.

It is notable that $p < 0.0001$, which indicates a very small chance that the differences are a result of variables other than group membership, where group membership refers to whether or not newborns were tested at session 2. The matched pairs t-test indicated statistically-significant differences between session 1 and session 2 *pass/refer* findings ($p < 0.0001$).[52]

Discussion

The current study focused on low-risk newborns, as the newborns enrolled in the clinic system are considered to be low risk. Any newborns presenting with prenatal or perinatal conditions are referred to the hospital setting and would thus not be available for testing at the clinic or for participation in the current study. In light of this, noted risk factors for hearing impairment that were identified during the current study were collated and documented so that data could be analysed accordingly. In the current study, one newborn was identified as having a positive family history for permanent childhood hearing loss. Lahr and Rosenberg[53] have listed this as a risk factor for hearing impairment. It is noteworthy that no other risk factors for hearing impairment were identified during the data collection of the current study. This is consistent with what would be considered appropriate in

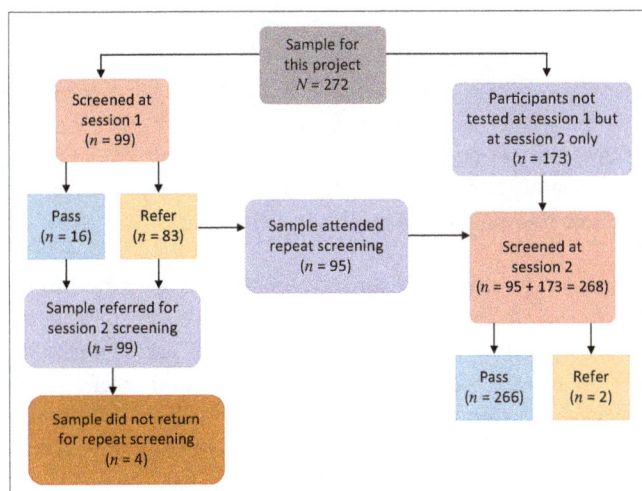

FIGURE 1: Summary of screening outcomes in the current study.

low-risk neonates and indicates that the current sample is representative of the general low-risk neonatal population.

During the time of the current study, 260 neonates were born at the CHC, yet only 99 of newborns underwent screening at session 1 – a mere 38.07%. There were no newborns whose parents refused screening at session 1; yet 161 newborns were missed at the first screening session.

Factors contributing to the reduced number of participants at session 1 may include the time of birth, as the audiological screening at session 1 only took place at the centre during normal working hours, being on a Monday to Friday (08:00 to 16:30). Many newborns were born outside this time frame or were discharged within six hours of birth and were thus not screened. The findings from the current study are consistent with reports by Ng et al.,[54] where neonates were discharged without screening because of the time of birth and discharge outside of normal working hours. Another study by Abdullah et al.[55] reported that 10.8% of newborns were missed at the session 1 screening whilst, in the current study, 61.92% were missed at session 1. This number is significantly higher and has serious implications for the current context. The reasons for this, as documented by Abdullah et al.,[55] included discharge during weekends, absent screening personnel and neonates that were overlooked unintentionally. Although this is similar to the findings from the current study, a marked difference between the study by Abdullah et al.[55] and the current study exists. In the current study, newborns were discharged within six hours of birth; in the study by Abdullah et al.,[55] neonatal screening at session 1 took place within 24 hours of birth. The longer hospital stay meant that fewer newborns were missed because of working hour limitations in the study by Abdullah et al.[55] when compared with the current study. In spite of these findings, it is notable that Lim and Daniel[56] have reported that screening prior to discharge after birth offers the greatest coverage. Nonetheless, this is a significant factor which reduces practicability of neonatal audiological screening using OAEs within six hours of birth in the context of the current study.

Adelola et al.[57] refer to a newborn hearing screening programme where the screening takes place in the maternity ward within 48 hours of birth from Monday through Friday. In their programme, the missed babies are sent for session 2 screening at the outpatient department. In a private healthcare setting, the minimal period for hospital stay post-birth is 24 hours and this is sufficient time to allow for universal newborn hearing screening to be conducted.[12] In addition to this, it is possible for screening to be conducted from Monday through to Saturday in these contexts; again because of the availability of resources.[12] This scenario is different to that in a government clinic where newborns are discharged from the clinic six hours post-birth and where the audiologist is only available to conduct the screening during normal working hours. This implies that the practicability for session 1 in this context is compromised. This has significant implications for implementing UNHS in CHC settings across South Africa, where similar protocols are followed in terms of discharge times and the availability of audiologists or other screening staff.

Early hearing detection and intervention (EHDI) coordinators are to be attentive to circumstances under which infants may be lost to the UNHS system. These may include home/out-of-hospital births and hospital missed screenings when infants are discharged prior to the hearing screening being conducted.[2] This is especially significant for efficiency of screening at session 1 in the current study, where newborns are discharged within six hours of birth and where the audiologist conducting the screening is only available during normal working hours. Spivak[58] has emphasised that a course for managing home births, early hospital discharge as well as private births needs to be instituted so that high coverage and consistent services can be delivered; and it is the opinion of the current researcher that this is crucial in a developing country such as South Africa.

In terms of resources related to staffing, there was only one audiologist on site to conduct the neonatal audiological screening. The audiologist adhered to normal working hours and this resulted in several newborns being missed at the initial screening session. This was proven to have a negative impact on the practicability of neonatal audiological screening at session 1. Theunissen and Swanepoel[59] have stated that the most commonly reported grounds for the lack of neonatal screening programmes are the shortage of suitable screening equipment, as well as personnel shortages. Widen et al.[41] have also explained that trained nursing staff and volunteers are able to conduct newborn hearing screening tests, which is consistent with the statement made by Hayes[60] that newborn hearing screening can be conducted by trained volunteers. Hayes[60] has, however, stipulated that an audiologist's supervision is required in this event. The notion of newborn hearing screening being conducted by non-audiological staff is supported by the study conducted by Ferro et al.,[61] where Newborn Hearing Screening programmes in Illinois were compared. In their study, hearing screening was conducted most commonly by the nursing staff.

Throughout areas such as Latin America, the availability of hearing healthcare professionals is limited, especially in rural communities.[62] In the study by Chan and Leung,[63] the screening was conducted by enrolled nurses who had received training on OAE testing. These nurses conducted automated OAE screening and performed standard nursing duties as well. In contrast to this, in the current study, screening was only carried out by a qualified audiologist. This is the standard protocol in South Africa, for the most part; and it was also a result of time and resource limitations. Chan and Leung[63] report that UNHS programmes, where screening is conducted by nurses, is a practical option; with concentrated and direct training. In the current study, in the event of the audiologist being ill for a day, the programme would be gravely affected as no other screening staff were available; a finding that can be generalised to a majority of clinics in South Africa as similar staffing and scope of practice conditions apply.

Hall[51] has stated that universal newborn hearing screening through the use of OAE measures can be recorded dependably by non-audiologic personnel. In the current study, if screening was conducted by trained nursing staff, this would have meant that screening could have been conducted seven days a week and 24 hours a day. Thus the number of newborns missed at session 1 would have been greatly reduced.

In determining the efficiency of screening at session 1 for the current study, the audiological screening results, an overall *refer* rate of 83.83% was obtained. In light of such a high *refer* rate, it is essential to consider the possibility of false-positive results where a neonate does not pass the hearing screening but does not truly present with a hearing impairment.[64] In the case of neonatal audiological screening, false-positive screening results have been reported as being a major concern.[16] False-positive results may be obtained when the transmission of sound from the earphone to the cochlea and back to the recording microphone is interrupted.[65] Screening newborns on the day of birth is of particular concern because of the presence of vernix in the external auditory meatus.[65] Based on this fact, the high *refer* rate at this screening session is not unexpected. Albuquerque and Kemp[66] have stated that, when newborns are discharged from the birthing facility within six hours of birth, OAEs will render an unacceptably high false-positive rate; a finding supported by the results of the current study. Hall[51] has stated that the higher the *refer* rate is, the lower the OAE specificity is; and this, therefore, has a negative impact on the efficiency of screening at session 1 for the current study. This does highlight the pitfalls of screening at this time and reduces the efficiency of screening at this session. These findings are not consistent with the American Academy of Paediatrics,[67] where it has been stated that OAEs render a 5% – 20% *refer* rate in the first 24 hours post-birth. The findings in the current study are also not consistent with the results reported by Abdullah et al.,[55] where, at session 1 within 24 hours of birth, a *refer* rate of 19.7% was obtained. The reason for this inconsistency may be attributable to the time difference, namely, six hours

for the current study and the 24 hour discharge time-frame for the study by Abdullah et al.[55] Current study findings provide evidence that, within the South African context, screening prior to discharge (which is often within six hours of birth) might not be the best time and might also be more detrimental than beneficial because of the impact of false-positive findings on the mother's well-being.

The second objective of the current study was to determine the practicability and efficiency when OAE screening takes place approximately three days after birth as part of the MOU three-day assessment clinic. The larger number of infants covered in session 2 implies that newborns born outside the CHC presented to the clinic and were included at the second screening session. Place of birth may influence the outcomes of a UNHS programme as this has an impact on the number of newborns that cannot be tested at session 1 – purely because they may not have been born at the CHC. Olusanya and Somefun[68] have emphasised that a sizeable percentage of neonates with hearing impairment in numerous developing countries are born outside hospital settings. This accentuates the necessity for community-oriented UNHS, which will lead to early detection and intervention. In terms of coverage, Akhtar et al.[69] have stated that, in order to identify all newborns with a hearing loss, all newborns need to be screened. In developing countries, many newborns with sensorineural hearing loss are born at home and, therefore, session 2 testing may be more practical as these newborns can then be included in the screen as well.[68] Based hereon, it is evident that screening newborns for hearing loss at the MOU three-day assessment clinic is practicable, as more newborns can be tested during this time-frame.

For the purposes of the current study, only one hearing healthcare professional was on duty at CHC. However, the impact of this staffing limitation was less influential at the second screening session as newborn screening was only conducted during scheduled times of the day and there was thus no impact resulting from discharge time and birth times. The MOU three-day assessment clinic is where medical check-ups on both the mother and baby take place, so the attendance is higher since the neonate will be undergoing a medical examination as well as a hearing screening. This highlights the importance of scheduling a hearing screening at the same time as a routine medical check-up. This will ensure that attendance is less costly for the parents in that it is cost effective to come for a single appointment to see several professionals than to present for appointments on different days. Ng et al.[54] have stated that the ideal time for screening would be when the neonate and mother present for a routine medical check-up. The findings of the current study support this, which again highlights the value of the MOU three-day assessment clinic, where both the mother and child present for a post-birth medical check-up.

Bartley and Digby[70] have reported that OAEs stabilise after day 2 post-birth and this may explain the decrease in the number of *refer* results obtained at the second screening session in the current study. In a study conducted by Vaid et al.,[71] 1238 well newborns were screened. In their study, a *refer* rate of 11.14% was reported when newborn hearing screening was conducted at three days post-birth. This finding is consistent with the results reported by Doyle et al.,[72] where 200 well newborns were tested at five to 120 hours post-birth. These authors have reported that the OAE *pass* rate increases in infants older than 24 hours. The findings of the current study are consistent with this as a *refer* rate of 0.74% was obtained at session 2. The high *refer* rate at session one reduces the efficiency of session 1 as a platform for UNHS. The JCIH[2] has stated that less than 4% of newborns should fail audiological screening at session 1 and at session 2 before being referred for diagnostic tests. The HPCSA stipulates that a referral rate of less than 5% should be achieved.

In the current study, session 1 does not meet the stipulated criteria and this implies that session 1 may not be a feasible test time; and might actually be a costly exercise in an already resource-stricken environment.

In terms of efficiency, the follow-up return rate was taken into account. In the current study, 95 of the 99 neonates screened at session 1, returned for follow-up screening at session 2. This equates to a follow-up return rate of 95.95% and indicates that session 2 is efficient as a platform for UNHS. This return rate is significantly better than the HPCSA benchmark of a minimum rate of 95%. The HPCSA stipulates that a 70% or greater follow-up return rate of infants and their caregivers is ideal.

Abdullah et al.[55] highlights the fact that audiological screening before 24 hours of age does result in a high false-positive rate. Consistent with the findings obtained in the current study, Stevens and Parker[73] have outlined how the *pass* rate for OAE neonatal screening is reduced in the first 24 hours after birth. It has also been stipulated by Wada et al.[11] that the accuracy of newborn hearing screening seems to improve with time. This highlights the value and reliability of screening at a time outside the first 48 hours post-birth, when vernix no longer has an impact on the findings and at a time when parents are still eager to return to the clinic for follow-up visits.

In agreement with this, Torrico et al.[74] have suggested that screening should not take place within the first 24 hours of birth. Sun et al.[75] conducted a study in which various time intervals for in-patient UNHS were compared and results have indicated that testing on day 3 was more effective than screening on the first or second day post-birth. These findings and notions are in line with the findings of the current study.

The results of the current study are similar to the results obtained from the research conducted in Sweden by Hergils.[76] In that study, 14 287 newborns at two maternity wards were screened over two sessions. Session 1 took place on the day of birth and session 2 took place at three days post-birth. The results of their study indicate that screening

on the day of birth is less effective than screening on day 2 or 3 after birth.[76] This is consistent with Gabbard, Northern and Yoshinaga-Itano,[77] who have also reported a significant difference in OAE screening within the first 24 hours after birth and thereafter.

Conclusion

Research strives to contribute to a scientific body of knowledge and aims to enhance health services and health outcomes. In the current study, a community-based newborn hearing screening programme has been considered in terms of efficacy and practicability. Research in this field is important as the drive behind the execution of extensive neonatal hearing screening programmes has not yet reached developing countries where more than half of the world's hearing impaired children reside. Current findings indicate that a need exists for the establishment of community-oriented primary ear care services in the developing world.

The current research project has addressed one of the many barriers regarding newborn hearing screening – that of the timing of neonatal OAE audiological screening, relative to post-birth discharge. The researcher has thus strived to ascertain the impact that time frames for neonatal audiological screening may have on the dependability of these programmes in primary healthcare settings in South Africa. Through the current study, the practicability and efficiency of an audiological screening programme within the MOU three-day assessment clinic has been positively proven.

The HPCSA[1] position statement on hearing screening has referred to three hearing screening contexts: the well-baby nursery, on discharge from the neonatal intensive care unit, as well as Mother Child Health Clinics at the six-week immunisation clinic. The current study has rendered results that suggest an additional screening platform not previously considered or recommended. Whilst the HPCSA has made bold and positive recommendations and has proposed guidelines regarding EHDI, contextualising such recommendations remains crucial. Current findings have verified that the MOU three-day assessment clinic could be one of the most appropriate test times and may present as a suitable platform to roll out neonatal audiological screening in South Africa. This platform would ensure wide coverage, whilst keeping the rate of false-positive test results at a minimum.

Current findings have also emphasised the importance of having personnel other than an audiologist conducting the hearing screening. This would ensure that, if UNHS had to be conducted before discharge, personnel such as nurses or midwives who are available 24 hours every day could conduct the screening.

The outcomes of the current study add to the development of methodologies for the early identification of hearing impairment within the South African neonatal population.

Acknowledgements

Competing interests

The authors declare that they have no financial or personal relationship(s) that may have inappropriately influenced them in writing this article.

Authors' contributions

K.K.-S. (University of the Witswatersrand) was the postgraduate research project supervisor and co-conceptualised the research idea, wrote the first draft of the manuscript and provided editorial input. S.H. (University of the Witswatersrand) co-conceptualised the research idea and performed all data collection and analysis as part of her postgraduate research project.

References

1. Health Professions Council of South Africa (HPCSA). Professional board for speech, language and hearing professions: Early hearing detection and intervention programmes in South Africa. Position statement: year 2007. Pretoria: HPCSA; 2007.

2. Joint Committee on Infant Hearing. Year 2007 position statement: Principles and guidelines for early hearing detection and intervention programs. Pediatrics. 2007;120(4):898–921. http://dx.doi.org/10.1542/peds.2007-2333

3. Hyde ML. Newborn hearing screening programs: overview. J Otolaryngol. 2005;34(Suppl. 2):S70–S78.

4. Olusanya BO, Swanepoel D, Chapchap MJ, et al. Progress towards early detection services for infants with hearing loss in developing countries. BMC Health Serv Res. 2007;7:14. http://dx.doi.org/10.1186/1472-6963-7-14

5. Rouev P, Mumdzhiev H, Spiridonova J, et al. Universal newborn hearing screening program in Bulgaria. Int J Pediatr Otorhinolaryngol. 2004;68(6):805–810. http://dx.doi.org/10.1016/j.ijporl.2004.01.013

6. Windmill S, Windmill IM. The status of diagnostic testing following referral from universal newborn hearing screening. J Am Acad Audiol. 2006;17(5):367–378. http://dx.doi.org/10.3766/jaaa.17.5.6

7. Flynn M, Austin N, Schmidtke-Flynn T, et al. Universal newborn hearing screening introduced to NICU infants in Canterbury Province, New Zealand. N Z Med J. 2004;117(1206):U1183.

8. Kennedy C, McCann D, Campbell MJ, et al. Universal newborn screening for permanent childhood hearing impairment: An 8-year follow-up of a controlled trial. Lancet. 2005;366(9486):660–662. http://dx.doi.org/10.1016/S0140-6736(05)67138-3

9. Uus K, Bamford J. Effectiveness of population-based newborn hearing screening in England: Ages of interventions and profile of cases. Pediatrics. 2006;117(5):e887–e893. http://dx.doi.org/10.1542/peds.2005-1064

10. Grill E, Uus K, Hessel F, et al. Neonatal hearing screening: Modelling cost and effectiveness of hospital- and community-based screening. BMC Health Serv Res. 2006;6:14. http://dx.doi.org/10.1186/1472-6963-6-14

11. Wada T, Kubo T, Aiba T, et al. Further examination of infants referred from newborn hearing screening. Acta Otolaryngol Suppl. 2004; 554:17–25. http://dx.doi.org/10.1080/03655230410018435

12. Swanepoel D, Ebrahim S, Joseph A, et al. Newborn hearing screening in a South African private health care hospital. Int J Pediatr Otorhinolaryngol. 2007;71(6):881–887. http://dx.doi.org/10.1016/j.ijporl.2007.02.009

13. Korres SG, Balatsouras DG, Nikolopoulos T, et al. Making universal newborn hearing screening a success. Int J Pediatr Otorhinolaryngol. 2006;70(2):241–246. http://dx.doi.org/10.1016/j.ijporl.2005.06.010

14. Boone RT, Bower CM, Martin PF. Failed newborn hearing screens as presentation for otitis media with effusion in the newborn population. Int J Pediatr Otorhinolaryngol. 2005;69(3):393–397. http://dx.doi.org/10.1016/j.ijporl.2004.11.006

15. Population Reference Bureau. 2008 World population data sheet. Washington, DC; 2008.

16. Lam BCC. Newborn hearing screening in Hong Kong. Hong Kong Med J. 2006;12(3):212–218.

17. Olusanya BO, Luxon LM, Wirz SL. Ethical issues in screening for hearing impairment in newborns in developing countries. J Med Ethics. 2006;32(10):588–591. http://dx.doi.org/10.1136/jme.2005.014720

18. Olusanya B, Okolo A. Early hearing detection at immunization clinics in developing countries. Int J Pediatr Otorhinolaryngol. 2006;70(8):1495–1498. http://dx.doi.org/10.1016/j.ijporl.2006.04.002

19. Llanes EG, Chiong CM. Evoked otoacoustic emissions and auditory brainstem responses: Concordance in hearing screening among high-risk children. Acta Otolaryngol. 2004;124(4):387–390. http://dx.doi.org/10.1080/00016480410017305

20. Swanepoel DW, Hugo R, Louw B. Infant hearing screening at immunization clinics in South Africa. Int J Pediatr Otorhinolaryngol. 2006;70(7):1241–1249. http://dx.doi.org/10.1016/j.ijporl.2006.01.002

21. Johnson JL, White KR, Widen JE, et al. A multicenter evaluation of how many infants with permanent hearing loss pass a two-stage otoacoustic emissions/automated auditory brainstem response newborn hearing screening protocol. Pediatrics. 2005;116(3):663–672. http://dx.doi.org/10.1542/peds.2004-1688

22. Breakwell GM, Rose D. Theory, method and research design. In: Breakwell GM, Hammond S, Fife-Schaw C, et al., editors. Research methods in psychology. 3rd ed. London, UK: Sage Publications Ltd, 2006; p. 2–23.

23. Dippenaar J. Assessment and risk screening. In: de Kock J, van der Walt C, Jones CM, editors. Maternal and newborn care: A complete guide for midwives and other health professionals. Lansdowne, Cape Town: Juta & Company (Pty) Ltd, 2004; p. 18.3–18.8.

24. Department of Health. A district hospital service package for South Africa: A set of norms and standards. [document on the Internet]. c2002 [cited 2013 Mar 23]. Available from http://www.ruralrehab.co.za/uploads/3/0/9/0/3090989/norms_and_standards_district_hospital.pdf

25. Rubin A, Babbie E. Research methods for social work. 4th ed. Pacific Grove, CA: Brooks/Cole Publishing Company; 2004.

26. Harrison V. The newborn baby. 5th ed. Cape Town, South Africa: Juta & Company (Pty) Ltd; 2008.

27. Madell JR, Flexer C. Hearing test protocols for children. In: Madell JR, Flexer C, editors. Pediatric audiology: Diagnosis, technology, and management. New York, NY: Thieme Medical Publishers, Inc, 2008; p. 45–53.

28. Weichbold V, Nekahm-Heis D, Welzl-Mueller K. Universal newborn hearing screening and postnatal hearing loss. Pediatrics. 2006;117(4):e631–e636. http://dx.doi.org/10.1542/peds.2005-1455

29. Mangate HL. Maternal and infant health profiles. In: van der Walt C, de Kock J, Jones CM, editors. Maternal and newborn care: A complete guide for midwives and other health professionals. Lansdowne, Cape Town: Juta & Company (Pty) Ltd, 2004; p. 4.1–4.8.

30. Norwitz ER, Schorge JO. Obstetrics and gynecology at a glance. 2nd ed. Malden, MA: Blackwell Publishing Limited; 2006.

31. Schenker Y, Wang F, Selig SJ, et al. The impact of language barriers on documentation of informed consent at a hospital with on-site interpreter services. J Gen Intern Med. 2007;22(Suppl. 2):294–299. http://dx.doi.org/10.1007/s11606-007-0359-1

32. Tattersall H, Young A. Deaf children identified through newborn hearing screening: Parents' experiences of the diagnostic process. Child Care Health Dev. 2006;32(1):33–45. http://dx.doi.org/10.1111/j.1365-2214.2006.00596.x

33. Jones WS, Kaleida PH. How helpful is pneumatic otoscopy in improving diagnostic accuracy? Pediatrics. 2003;112(3 Pt 1):510–513. http://dx.doi.org/10.1542/peds.112.3.510

34. Orji FT, Mgbor NC. Otoscopy compared with tympanometry: An evaluation of the accuracy of simple otoscopy. Niger J Med. 2007;16(1):57–60. http://dx.doi.org/10.4314/njm.v16i1.37282

35. Olusanya BO, Okolo AA, Aderemi AA. Predictors of hearing loss in school entrants in a developing country. J Postgrad Med. 2004;50(3):173–179.

36. Psarommatis I, Valsamakis T, Raptaki M, et al. Audiologic evaluation of infants and preschoolers: A practical approach. Am J Otolaryngol. 2007;28(6):392–396. http://dx.doi.org/10.1016/j.amjoto.2006.11.011

37. Hof JR, Anteunis LJC, Chenault MN, et al. Otoacoustic emissions at compensated middle ear pressure in children. Int J Audiol. 2005;44(6):317–320. http://dx.doi.org/10.1080/14992020500057822

38. Nicholson N, Widen JE. Evoked otoacoustic emissions in the evaluation of children. In: Robinette MS, Glattke TJ, editors. Otoacoustic emissions: Clinical applications. 3rd ed. New York, NY: Thieme Medical Publishers, Inc, 2007; p. 385–402.

39. Viasys Healthcare. GSI AUDIOscreener: OAE and ABR hearing screening [document on the Internet]. c2009 [cited 2015 Mar 16]. Available from: http://www.audiomed.com/Audiomed.com/SchoolPDFs/Entries/2008/11/3_OAEs_Grason_Stadler_files/GSI-AUDIO_Screener.pdf.

40. Coates H, Gifkins K. Diagnostic tests: Newborn hearing screening. Austr Prescriber. 2003;26(4):82–84.

41. Widen JE, Bull RW, Folsom RC. Newborn hearing screening: What it means for providers of early intervention services. Infants and Young Children. 2003;16(3):249–257. http://dx.doi.org/10.1097/00001163-200307000-00007

42. Shoup AG, Owen KE, Jackson G, et al. The Parkland Memorial Hospital experience in ensuring compliance with Universal Newborn Hearing Screening follow-up. J Pediatr. 2005;146(1):66–72. http://dx.doi.org/10.1016/j.jpeds.2004.08.052

43. Prieve BA. Otoacoustic emissions in neonatal hearing screening. In: Robinette MS, Glattke TJ, editors. Otoacoustic emissions: Clinical applications. 3rd ed. New York, NY: Thieme Medical Publishers, Inc, 2007; p. 343–364.

44. Durante AS, Carvallo RMM, da Costa FS, et al. [Characteristics of transient evoked otoacoustic emissions in newborn hearing screening program]. Portugese. Pro Fono. 2005;17(2):133–140. http://dx.doi.org/10.1590/S0104-56872005000200002

45. Lustig LR, Niparko JK, Minor LB, et al. Clinical neurotology: Diagnosing and managing disorders of hearing, balance and the facial nerve. London, UK: Martin Dunitz Ltd; 2003.

46. Kemp DT. The basics, the science, and the future potential of otoacoustic emissions. In: Robinette MS, Glattke TJ, editors. Otoacoustic emissions: clinical applications. 3rd ed. New York, NY: Thieme Medical Publishers, Inc, 2007; p. 7–42.

47. Rhoades K, McPherson B, Smyth V, et al. Effects of background noise on click-evoked otoacoustic emissions. Ear Hear. 1998;19(6):450–462. http://dx.doi.org/10.1097/00003446-199812000-00006

48. Howell DC. Fundamental statistics for the behavioral sciences. 5th ed. Belmont, CA: Thomson-Brookes/Cole; 2004.

49. Cramer D. Introducing statistics for social research: Step-by-step calculations and computer techniques using SPSS. London, UK: Routledge; 1994.

50. Asma A, Wan Fazlina WH, Almyzan A, et al. Benefit and pitfalls of newborn hearing screening. Med J Malaysia. 2008;63(4):293–297.

51. Hall JW. Handbook of otoacoustic emissions. San Diego, CA: Singular Thomson Learning; 2000.

52. Stevens J, Parker G. Screening and surveillance. In: Newton VE, editor. Paediatric audiological medicine. 2nd ed. West Sussex, UK: John Wiley & Sons Ltd, 2009; p. 29–51.

53. Lahr MB, Rosenberg KD. Oregon's early hearing detection and intervention program (EHDI): The first fifteen years (1989–2004). Calif J Health Promot. 2004;2:59–66.

54. Ng PK, Hui Y, Lam BCC, et al. Feasibility of implementing a universal neonatal hearing screening programme using distortion product otoacoustic emission detection at a university hospital in Hong Kong. Hong Kong Med J. 2004;10(1):6–13.

55. Abdullah A, Hazim MYS, Almyzan A, et al. Newborn hearing screening: Experience in a Malaysian hospital. Singapore Med J. 2006;47(1):60–64.

56. Lim S, Daniel LM. Establishing a universal newborn hearing screening programme. Ann Acad Med Singapore. 2008;37(12 Suppl):63–65.

57. Adelola OA, Papanikolaou V, Gormley P, et al. Newborn hearing screening: A regional example for national care. Ir Med J. 2010;103(5):146–149.

58. Spivak LG. Universal newborn hearing screening. New York, NY: Thieme Medical Publishers, Inc; 1998.

59. Theunissen M, Swanepoel D. Early hearing detection and intervention services in the public health sector in South Africa. Int J Audiol. 2008;47(Suppl. 1):S23–S29. http://dx.doi.org/10.1080/14992020802294032

60. Hayes D. Screening methods: current status. Ment Retard Dev Disabil Res Rev. 2003;9(2):65–72. http://dx.doi.org/10.1002/mrdd.10061

61. Ferro LM, Tanner G, Erler SF, et al. Comparison of universal newborn hearing screening programs in Illinois hospitals. Int J Pediatr Otorhinolaryngol. 2007;71(2):217–230. http://dx.doi.org/10.1016/j.ijporl.2006.10.004

62. Gerner de Garcia B, Gaffney C, Chacon S, et al. Overview of newbornhearing screening activities in Latin America. Rev Panam Salud Publica. 2011;29(3):145–152.

63. Chan KY, Leung SSL. Infant hearing screening in maternal and child health centres using automated otoacoustic emission screening machines: A one-year pilot project. HK J Paediatr (New Series). 2004;9:118–125.

64. Herrero C, Moreno-Ternero JD. Hospital costs and social costs: A case study of newborn hearing screening. Investigaciones Económicas. 2005;29(1):203–216.

65. Korres S, Nikolopoulos T, Ferekidis E, et al. Otoacoustic emissions in universal hearing screening: Which day after birth should we examine the newborns? J Otorhinolaryngol Relat Spec. 2003;65(4):199–201. http://dx.doi.org/10.1159/000073114

66. Albuquerque W, Kemp DT. The feasibility of hospital-based universal newborn hearing screening in the United Kingdom. Scand Audiol Suppl. 2001;30(2): 22–28. http://dx.doi.org/10.1080/010503901750166565

67. Erenberg A, Lemons J, Sia C, et al. Newborn and infant hearing loss: detection and intervention. Pediatrics. 1999;103(2):527–530. http://dx.doi.org/10.1542/peds.103.2.527

68. Olusanya BO, Somefun AO. Place of birth and characteristics of infants with congenital and early-onset hearing loss in a developing country. Int J Pediatr Otorhinolaryngol. 2009;73(9):1263–1269. http://dx.doi.org/10.1016/j.ijporl.2009.05.018

69. Akhtar N, Datta PG, Alauddin M, et al. Neonatal hearing screening. Bangladesh J Otorhinolaryngol. 2010;16(1):54–59. http://dx.doi.org/10.3329/bjo.v16i1.5782

70. Bartley J, Digby J. Universal screening of newborns for hearing impairment in New Zealand. N Z Fam Physician. 2005;32(1):46–49.

71. Vaid N, Shanbhag J, Nikam R, et al. Neonatal hearing screening – The Indian experience. Cochlear Implants Int. 2009;10(Suppl. 1):111–114. http://dx.doi.org/10.1179/cim.2009.10.Supplement-1.111

72. Doyle KJ, Burggraaff B, Fujikawa S, et al. Newborn hearing screening by otoacoustic emissions and automated auditory brainstem response. Int J Pediatr Otorhinolaryngol. 1997;41(2):111–119. http://dx.doi.org/10.1016/S0165-5876(97)00066-9

73. Stevens J. Intermediate statistics: A modern approach. 2nd ed. Mahwah, NJ: Lawrence Erlbaum Associates, Inc; 1999.

74. Torrico P, Gómez C, López-Ríos J, De Cáceres MC, Trinidad G, Serrano M. [Age influence in otoacoustic emissions for hearing loss screening in infants]. Spanish. Acta Otorrinolaringol Esp. 2004;55(4):153–159. http://dx.doi.org/10.1016/S0001-6519(04)78500-3

75. Sun X, Shen X, Zakus D, et al. Development of an effective public health screening program to assess hearing disabilities among newborns in Shanghai: A prospective cohort study. World Health Popul. 2009;11(1):14–23.

76. Hergils L. Analysis of measurements from the first Swedish universal neonatal hearing screening program. Int J Audiol. 2007;46(11):680–685. http://dx.doi.org/10.1080/14992020701459868

77. Gabbard SA, Northern JR, Yoshinaga-Itano C. Hearing screening in newborns under 24 hours of age. Semin Hear. 1999;20(4):291–304. http://dx.doi.org/10.1055/s-0028-1082945

5

A situational analysis of training for behaviour change counselling for primary care providers, South Africa

Authors:
Zelra Malan[1]
Bob Mash[1]
Katherine Everett-Murphy[2]

Affiliations:
[1]Family Medicine and Primary Care, Stellenbosch University, South Africa

[2]Chronic Diseases Initiative in Africa (CDIA), Faculty of Health Sciences, University of Cape Town, South Africa

Correspondence to:
Zelra Malan

Email:
zmalan@sun.ac.za

Postal address:
PO Box 19063, Tygerberg 7505, South Africa

Background: Non-communicable diseases and associated risk factors (smoking, alcohol abuse, physical inactivity and unhealthy diet) are a major contributor to primary care morbidity and the burden of disease. The need for healthcare-provider training in evidence-based lifestyle interventions has been acknowledged by the National Department of Health. However, local studies suggest that counselling on lifestyle modification from healthcare providers is inadequate and this may, in part, be attributable to a lack of training.

Aim: This study aimed to assess the current training courses for primary healthcare providers in the Western Cape.

Setting: Stellenbosch University and University of Cape Town.

Methods: Qualitative interviews were conducted with six key informants (trainers of primary care nurses and registrars in family medicine) and two focus groups (nine nurses and eight doctors) from both Stellenbosch University and the University of Cape Town.

Results: Trainers lack confidence in the effectiveness of behaviour change counselling and in current approaches to training. Current training is limited by time constraints and is not integrated throughout the curriculum – there is a focus on theory rather than modelling and practice, as well as a lack of both formative and summative assessment. Implementation of training is limited by a lack of patient education materials, poor continuity of care and record keeping, conflicting lifestyle messages and an unsupportive organisational culture.

Conclusion: Revising the approach to current training is necessary in order to improve primary care providers' behaviour change counselling skills. Primary care facilities need to create a more conducive environment that is supportive of behaviour change counselling.

Analyse situationnelle de la formation à donner aux fournisseurs de soins primaires en Afrique du Sud pour leur permettre de faire changer les comportements.

Contexte: Les maladies non contagieuses et les facteurs de risques associés (la cigarette, l'abus d'alcool, l'inactivité physique et un régime malsain) contribuent fortement à la morbidité des soins primaires et au fardeau de la maladie. Le Département de la Santé national reconnaît le besoin de former des prestataires de soins pour modifier les modes de vie. Cependant, les études locales suggèrent que les conseils donnés par les prestataires pour changer les modes de vie sont insuffisants ce qui peut être attribué en partie à un manque de formation.

Objectif: Cette étude avait pour but d'évaluer les formations actuelles pour les prestataires de soins primaires dans la province du Western Cape.

Cadre: Université de Stellenbosch et Université de Cape Town.

Méthodes: Des entrevues qualitatives ont eu lieu avec six informateurs importants (formateurs d'infirmières en soins primaires et secrétaires généraux de médecine familiale) et deux groupes de consultation (neuf infirmières et huit médecins) des Universités de Stellenbosch et de Cape Town.

Résultats: Les formateurs manquaient de confiance dans l'efficacité des conseils à donner pour effectuer un changement de comportement et dans l'approche actuelle à la formation. La formation actuelle est limitée par des contraintes de temps et n'est pas intégrée dans tout le programme - l'accent est plutôt mis sur la théorie que sur le modèle et la pratique, et il y a un manque d'évaluation formatrice et globale. La mise en pratique de la formation est limitée par le manque de matériel éducatif pour les patients, la continuité des soins et la mauvaise tenue des dossiers, des conseils de mode de vie contradictoires et une absence de culture d'organisation.

Conclusion: Il faut réviser la démarche actuelle de formation pour améliorer les compétences des prestataires de soins primaires qui aideront à faire changer les comportements. Les établissements de soins primaires doivent créer un environnement plus adapté qui soutient les services de conseils pour changer les comportements.

Introduction

The burden of non-communicable diseases (NCD) is predicted to increase worldwide due to the ageing of populations, urbanisation and the globalisation of underlying risk factors. The rising morbidity and mortality related to NCDs has major implications for the delivery of acute and chronic healthcare services.[1]

The risk factors associated with NCDs have been clearly identified through international research and have been confirmed locally.[2,3] Smoking, excessive alcohol consumption, physical inactivity and unhealthy diet are the key modifiable factors contributing to morbidity and mortality from NCDs.[4] In South Africa, the burden of NCDs disproportionately affects the socio-economically disadvantaged and places increased demands on the public sector primary care services.[3] Improving risky lifestyle behaviours is an important approach to decreasing health disparities and for more cost-effective utilisation of scarce resources in the public health sector.

Healthcare providers can play an important role in counselling and supporting patients with lifestyle risk factors or an established NCD.[3] Patients have frequent contact with healthcare professionals, who are well positioned to provide counselling and who are also viewed by patients as being reliable sources of information. The best interface for this counselling in South Africa would be within public-sector, primary healthcare (PHC) services, as this is where the majority of the population encounters the healthcare system on a regular basis.[5]

Health services in low-/middle-income countries, such as South Africa, are based on a model of treating acute episodic illness and are not well organised for the prevention and management of NCDs. Counselling and education about risky lifestyle factors is usually inadequate.[1] Until recently, the prevention of these lifestyle risk factors received little attention in South Africa's health-related priorities.[6]

Recently, however, the need for healthcare-provider training in evidence-based lifestyle interventions, both at an undergraduate level and as part of continuing professional development, has been acknowledged by the National Department of Health in their strategic plan for NCDs.[7] In line with World Health Organization recommendations, the strategic plan prioritises cost-effective and feasible interventions to address the NCD epidemic.[8] Brief behaviour change counselling in primary care is recommended for all four risk factors.[7,8] Training healthcare providers in effective communication skills is seen as necessary and is particularly important, given the potential for prevention and control of NCDs at primary care level.[8] A patient-centred approach , which actively engages the patient in decision making about their health, is seen as an objective in 're-orienting' the PHC system to effectively address NCDs.[7,8]

To date, there has been very little research assessing the capacity of healthcare providers in South Africa to deliver behaviour change counselling, however these few studies suggest that counselling is inadequate.[5,9] Although it is primarily nurses who provide behaviour change counselling in the public sector, nurses were found to have limited knowledge of how to counsel patients on NCD risk factors.[5] Private general practitioners have also been found to struggle with documenting and counselling overweight or obese patients.[9] Two other local studies, which investigated the knowledge, attitudes and practices of obstetricians and midwives respectively, around the delivery of smoking-cessation counselling to pregnant smokers, showed very low levels of counselling practice and knowledge of best-practice methods amongst both categories of healthcare providers.[10,11] This poor performance amongst practitioners may reflect a lack of training in behaviour change counselling skills.

Brief behaviour change counselling is the ability to skilfully help patients change risky lifestyle behaviours. This study forms the first part of a larger research project, which aims to develop and implement a training intervention for PHC providers on brief behaviour change counselling, as well as to assess the provider's competency in delivering this counselling intervention. The aim of this study was to analyse the factors which were important for the design of a behaviour change counselling training programme in our setting.

The ADDIE (Analysis, Design, Development, Implementation and Evaluation) model provides a systematic approach to the creation of new educational programmes.[12] This study reports on the analysis step of the ADDIE model, which helped the researchers to understand the current situation with regard to behaviour change counselling in our primary care context and the learning needs of primary care providers. The aim of this study, therefore, was to conduct a situational analysis of the current training courses and practice of primary care providers in the Western Cape with regard to brief behaviour change counselling. The specific objectives were:

- To explore the perceived effectiveness of current counselling and the factors that influence this.
- To explore the perceived effectiveness of current and prior training courses and the factors that influenced this.

Research methods and design
Study design

This was a qualitative situational analysis that made use of both individual in-depth and focus group interviews to explore the perceptions of primary care nurses and doctors as well as training programme coordinators. This situational analysis subsequently informed the design, development and evaluation of a new approach to training (using the ADDIE model), which will be reported on in future articles.[12]

Setting

In the Western Cape Province, doctors are trained at Stellenbosch University and the University of Cape Town. After undergraduate studies, internship and community service, doctors can choose further postgraduate training. Postgraduate training for primary care is via a four-year Masters of Medicine degree in family medicine. Basic training for nurses is offered by universities (such as the University of Western Cape) and nursing colleges. After basic training, nurses can qualify as a clinical nurse practitioner through a one-year Higher Diploma course, which is offered by Stellenbosch University and the Western Cape College of Nursing.

Primary care services are offered via a network of fixed and mobile clinics as well as community health centres throughout all the health districts in the Province. Patients with NCDs are mostly managed in these facilities. At clinics, the service is offered by a nurse with periodic support from a doctor. At health centres, service is also offered mainly by nurses, but with more involvement from doctors as well as a broader multidisciplinary team that might include health promoters, occupational therapists, physiotherapists and pharmacists.

In qualitative research, the degree of objectivity of the researcher can partly be judged by their own self-awareness and relationship to the topic. The researcher in this study is a qualified family physician and spent many years working in private general practice. She developed an interest in behaviour change counselling through previous research on general practitioners counselling overweight and obese patients,[9] which prompted her to think about possible training interventions that could improve the counselling skills of PHC providers.[9]

Study population and selection of participants

Key informants were selected on the basis that they coordinated postgraduate training for either primary care nurses or registrars in family medicine in the Western Cape. Interviews were conducted with the two programme managers involved in the training of nurses for the Diploma in Clinical Nursing Science, Health Assessment, Treatment and Care at Stellenbosch University (this course is not offered at the University of Cape Town) as well as three programme managers involved with the training of registrars in Family Medicine at Stellenbosch and Cape Town Universities. An additional family physician working at a public PHC facility in the Western Cape, who supervises registrars and is actively involved in research on teaching and assessment of registrars, was interviewed to gain a complete picture of current training in behaviour change counselling in the clinical training environment.

Focus group interviews were conducted with nurses and doctors currently working in primary care and who had experience of these training programmes. Nine nurses working at a primary care clinic, situated in a low socioeconomic area of the Cape Winelands, were selected. The researcher was familiar with the nursing staff at this clinic, as she has been involved with the training of undergraduate medical students at this facility on a weekly basis, for the last few years. The nurses were established primary care

providers and were trained in the Western Cape. They were familiar with the community and had been working at their facility for more than a year. All nurses were interviewed to get an overall view from each level of trained nurse. Four of the nurses were clinical nurse practitioners, four were staff nurses and one was an assistant nurse.

The second focus group interview was with a group of eight registrars in family medicine at the University of Cape Town. The registrars ranged from first- to third-year students, had previously been working as junior doctors and had received their undergraduate training at a variety of different universities. At the time of the research it was logistically difficult to conduct a focus group interview with Stellenbosch registrars.

The design allowed for further interviews to be conducted if the analysis and triangulation of these initial interviews suggested the need to identify and explore additional issues.

Data collection

The researcher performed and audio-taped in-depth interviews with all the key informants listed above. Interviews were conducted in the key informant's choice of language, either Afrikaans or English. The researcher used an interview guide and skills such as open-ended questions, reflective listening, summarising and elaboration to conduct the interview. Topics discussed were: the current teaching modules, if any, on behaviour change counselling; prior experiences and beliefs about the effectiveness of such training; attitude toward the introduction of a new training module; and their beliefs about the long-term effect of current training in clinical practice.

The focus group interviews were also conducted by the researcher and audio-taped. The interview with the nurses took place at the clinic and the interview with the registrars at the university campus. The nurses preferred to be interviewed in Afrikaans and the registrars in English. During these interviews the researcher used an interview guide to explore their successes and failures with counselling, their perceptions of factors that enabled or obstructed counselling and their perceived effectiveness/competency in delivering counselling. Participants were also asked about prior formal training received and perception of their knowledge on NCDs.

Data analysis

All interviews were transcribed verbatim and analysed using Atlas.ti software (v. 6.2.15 2011) using the framework approach.[13] The framework approach to content analysis involves the following steps:

- Familiarisation: The researcher listened to the tapes, read the transcripts and listed recurrent issues or ideas that emerged from the data.
- Construction of thematic framework: The researcher organised these issues and ideas into a framework that was aligned with the interview guide and objectives of the

study. In Atlas.ti, this related to a list of codes organised into families.

- Coding: The researcher applied the thematic framework systematically to all the data by annotating the transcripts with the codes using Atlas.ti.
- Charting: All the data from the specific codes included in a family in Atlas-ti were brought together in one document or chart.
- Mapping and interpretation: The researcher used the charts to interpret the data for themes and look for any associations or relationships between themes.

All three researchers were involved in this process: familiarisation, coding, construction of the thematic framework, charting and interpretation of the charts.

Ethical considerations

This study was approved by the Health Research Ethics Committees (HREC) at Stellenbosch University (Reference number: N11/11/321). Key informants and focus group participants gave written consent. The confidentiality and privacy of all interviewees and participants were respected in data analysis and reporting.

Results

Overall, 23 people were interviewed, comprising six key informants, nine nurses working in primary care and eight doctors training in family medicine and primary care, as described in the methods. Fifteen of the respondents were women and eight were men, with ages ranging from 24 to 56 years.

Both doctors and nurses believed that healthcare providers (HCPs) should be skilful in their ability to help patients make difficult decisions about changing risky lifestyle behaviours:

'Everybody needs to be able to do it and do it effectively.' (Nurse programme manager)

'I think it is a crucial part of the skills set that any family physician should have.' (Family medicine programme manager)

'We can't just waste it, in the sense of giving more medication, but the cause of the problem is not addressed [*through counselling*].' (Nurse)

Although it was seen as an integral and important part of an HCP's competencies, nobody expressed confidence in the current training or its impact on practice in the clinical setting:

'So we haven't found a form of behaviour change counselling that really works and can work at scale in the context of our primary care scenario, where things are very pressurised, you know, and with nurses it is a huge challenge.' (Family medicine programme manager)

'The current training programmes do not meet the needs of the country.' (Nurse programme manager)

'We have not gone as far as changing the clinical picture.' (Family physician)

The current training of registrars was seen as being mainly theoretical and did not enable the development of practical skills. Time constraints, as a result of other competing issues in the curriculum, resulted in a lack of continuity throughout the curriculum and made it difficult for HCPs to fully integrate new skills into clinical practice. Registrars felt that the limited time spent on training in behaviour change counselling led to the impression that it is of lesser importance:

'So I am very concerned about how little time they actually have and you know, what they are picking up and then even more concerned about whether they will practise in any of that skills, in a way that will encourage you know their on-going learning.'(Family medicine programme manager)

'We just had one session which makes it feel almost as if it's of lesser importance. It's *ja*, so and we're always told you know, you need to counsel your patients its important and I don't think we get taught enough about it undergrad and postgrad.' (Registrar).

Nurses on the one-year diploma course had only seven contact sessions of two hours allocated to the module, Principles and Processes of Primary Care; and the training in this module focused on breaking bad news, substance abuse and intimate partner violence. During this module there was virtually no training or assessment of behaviour change counselling skills. They did role play and audio-taped a normal consultation with a patient, then received feedback from the lecturer on general communication skills. Final assessment of their communication skills involved a single role play that did not necessarily focus on counselling. Nurses were thought to be starting at a much lower level in terms of their prior communication skills because less focus was placed on these skills in their basic training and they had less experience of consulting in their work environment prior to training as primary care nurses. Typically, the nursing consultation tended to be more task oriented, which made it difficult for them to adopt a holistic patient-centred approach. During their training they were not taught knowledge related to risky lifestyle behaviours for NCDs, but rather a general approach to communication. It was apparent that lecturers did not expect nurses to be competent after the training and also that there was no follow up after completion of the training programme:

'What tends to happen is that because it is so short and because some of them start with a very low baseline, it is difficult to get them to significance.' (Nurse programme manager)

'Remember our students have only seven contact sessions in which we need to teach them everything. You must understand that everybody wants their specific thing to be concentrated on and we only have seven lectures.' (Nurse programme manager)

'I don't teach them to become professional counsellors at all, it's teaching for concepts.' (Nurse programme manager)

Family medicine lecturers commented on an organisational culture in the health services whose values were often incongruent with the style required for behaviour change counselling, namely, one that is respectful, empathic and collaborative. Lack of support from clinic managers for behaviour change counselling and modelling of an authoritarian and directive style of communication, made it challenging for HCPs to implement any training they received:

> 'How do you get a health worker to behave in a guiding style, in an organisation that manifests values almost directly opposite to those values you know?' (Family medicine programme manager)

Registrars at both universities were exposed to communication skills training, including motivational interviewing, early in their four-year programme. The training was over a three-month period in first year, as part of a consultation module. This actually involved a 1–2 week section where they studied basic motivational interviewing (MI). This involved several readings, watching a video that modelled the counselling approach and a written assignment that reflected on attempts to counsel behaviour change at the end of the module. During the second year, registrars at Stellenbosch attended a one-day workshop on brief MI. The registrars at Cape Town developed and practised consultation skills by using audio-taped role plays with no specific focus on counselling. After the more formal teaching in the first and second years there was no specific requirement for these counselling skills to be observed or reinforced as part of their work-based training and portfolio assessment, although the portfolio does require observation and feedback on consultation skills in general.

Registrars at both universities were assessed in fourth year on their ability to perform behaviour change counselling in a simulated consultation, which is one out of four such consultations in the final examination, all of which focus on communication skills. In the new national exit exam for family medicine, organised by the College of Family Physicians, candidates are required to perform three observed consultations and the assessment tool includes an assessment of their general counselling skills. This section of the tool, however, defines counselling more in terms of general health education than behaviour change counselling:

> 'So what they really have taken out, and what is actually incorporated into their consultation, is not known.' (Family medicine programme manager)

> 'We have not gotten [sic] as far as saying we want to be absolutely sure that every registrar is competent in that skill.' (Family medicine programme manager)

> 'It's really difficult to assess.' (Family physician)

Although feedback is considered an important factor in developing and maintaining a new skill, once registrars and nurses were in actual clinical training practice, no feedback on their skills was available, mainly because most supervisors had not received training in specific counselling skills:

> 'How confident are you at using it and if you don't get feedback on your success at using it, it is very difficult to develop enough

confidence to carry on trying to use that skill.' (Family medicine programme manager)

> 'They're from all over the country and so we don't know, they pass the programme, they get their diploma and they're out of here.' (Nurse programme manager)

> 'It is one thing to be taught how to do it, it is another thing actually changing your practice to actually doing that. It is much easier probably for people to just go back to doing things the way they have always done them.' (Family medicine programme manager)

> 'In terms of the registrar's supervision, absolutely no idea if any of the supervisors do any teaching around brief motivational interviewing at the training sites.' (Family medicine programme manager)

Doctors expressed the need for feedback in future training:

> 'I think it will be a big help if we have to counsel someone with a supervisor or somebody or a lecturer watching us and giving feedback.' (Registrar)

> 'When you are trying to use a new technique which you have admittedly only had six hours training in, how confident are you at using it and if you don't get feedback on your success at using it, it is very difficult to develop enough confidence to carry on trying to use that new skill.' (Family medicine programme manager)

As a result, doctors and nurses lacked confidence in their counselling skills and did not feel equipped to counsel effectively:

> 'So it is not an easy procedure to verbally tell someone you must stop smoking.' (Nurse)

> 'I cannot just tell a person to quit smoking; there is no way that you can just quit smoking.' (Nurse)

> 'The only counselling skills that I know is like HIV counselling skills or the counselling of the dying patient, but not really the steps of making someone stop smoking.' (Registrar)

> 'We have been taught but you don't actually, I don't think I'm confident enough to do it in the right way, I'm doing it in the way that I feel is best.' (Registrar)

Nurses did not recall being trained to counsel a patient to change risky behaviour, thus basing their current counselling methods on their own past experiences. Counselling was viewed as part of the consultation and not a specific technique. Nurses used a more directive style, where asking and informing patients about the risk factor seem to be the dominant skills used. There was a perception that one had to use a direct style if you had limited time. Most of the knowledge used during this counselling was reportedly obtained from magazines, the radio and newspapers:

> 'We have taught ourselves with experience.' (Nurse)

> 'It's part of how we anyway see a patient.' (Nurse programme manager)

> 'There is no specific technique, actually we just talk.' (Nurse)

> 'I ask are you smoking, are you drinking, then I try to convince them that it is not good.' (Nurse)

'I ask them a question and I inform them what the risks are towards that. For example, I ask "do you smoke?"' (Nurse)

'To do it all in five minutes you have to be direct.' (Nurse)

Registrars tried to involve the patient in decision making, but still relied on information giving when counselling, using a brief 1–2 minute intervention as part of the consultation. Interestingly, both nurses and doctors felt more comfortable with regard to counselling a patient on diet and exercise than with regard to advising them to stop or reduce smoking tobacco or drinking alcohol. There was a perception that you would be wasting your time trying to counsel someone on tobacco smoking or alcohol use:

'I make them aware of what I think needs attention and we have learnt with, like, getting the patient to participate in the decision making and sometimes I will ask, "so what do you think you can do differently?"' (Registrar)

'So it's easier to tell someone to eat salad, he will more willingly eat salads and tomatoes and stuff like that, than you telling him to quit smoking.' (Nurse)

'I feel sometimes diet, people can change and exercise, but smoking sometimes I just feel like someone's going to smoke anyway.' (Registrar)

Nurses felt overwhelmed in a situation where they were expected to counsel, lacked practical skills, had time constraints and pressure of workload, lacked appropriate support materials and felt that patients were likely to be irresponsible anyway, despite knowing the risks:

'They have the information but they are still smoking. They see it on television, they see it on the cigarette packet, they see it in the newspaper, in a book they are reading and we tell them. They still smoke.' (Nurse)

'It will be much easier with what you say to have colourful pictures, because there are people who can't read.' (Nurse)

'So you need to give them something to read about the danger of smoking and all that stuff, it would be much better.' (Nurse)

'How can we do all of this in five minutes?' (Nurse)

Despite these barriers, registrars remained sympathetic toward patients' circumstances, but also felt that poverty made it difficult to adopt a healthier lifestyle:

'A lot of times our patients' lives are just so miserable, like they are just so poor and so like the areas they live are such bad areas and, for example, if someone smokes then sometimes I feel like *ag* shame just let them smoke, like, it's their only little pleasure.' (Registrar)

'You can't tell a diabetic that doesn't have an income and three children with only child support grants they must have a low GI [*glycaemic index*] diet. I mean they eat what they can to stay alive.' (Registrar)

Doctors reported poor continuity of care, poor record keeping, lack of a standardised approach, language and cultural issues as being additional difficulties. Both doctors and nurses expressed difficulties in counselling a patient when they themselves were smokers or overweight. Doctors felt that nurses had a better understanding of the patient's language and culture because they often stay in the community, but sometimes lacked the knowledge on risk factors and NCDs when counselling. This also led to the problem of HCPs giving conflicting or contradictory messages:

'Continuity of care, we never see the patient twice so you can't really say let's talk a little bit today and then next week we will continue ...' (Registrar)

'You don't always see the notes, or recordings about previous brief things are not always in the notes.' (Registrar)

'They understand a person's culture better and when you work with them although sometimes a problem is also that sometimes their knowledge might not be adequate enough and then we get a problem where they say one thing, you say another.' (Registrar)

Doctors did not think counselling alone would be sufficient to change a patient's behaviour and that it needed to be combined with giving printed patient information material. They also felt that patients preferred to see a doctor and trusted their advice more than the nurses, although it was not clear if this was because of the counselling style, higher professional status of doctors in the patient's perspective or for some other reason:

'If it comes from the doctor's mouth then it's like, no, this is definitely the correct thing I'm not listening to the nurse. Unless they've actually bonded with the nurse or they have had a good experience or with someone that's very patient-centred, but from my experience patients tend to prefer doctors.' (Registrar)

'I think they remember more if you actually tell them rather than say here's the pamphlet, go read up on hypertension and diet or something.' (Registrar)

Nurses felt that they should target young people in future because old people are set in their ways and less likely to change. They reported that counselling for smoking-cessation in future could be more successful if the patients are prescribed medication to assist them in changing their behaviour, but unfortunately not many could afford it:

'Our major problem is that we don't start with the right people. We must start with the children.' (Nurse)

'So you must start from where you started smoking, people from 20 or between 25 or wherever. If you are 14 you smoke because it is fun, your friends are smoking, but if you are smoking at the age of 20, you smoke because you smoke.' (Nurse)

'Patients that really want to stop ask the doctor to write a prescription that they get at the private chemists and it is a bit expensive but those that are given prescriptions, were successful and they wanted to stop.' (Nurse)

The nurse programme managers felt that counselling skills need to be integrated into current nursing practice in order to make the time available for counselling more skilful and effective. Trying to implement counselling as an additional task would not be successful:

'You have to incorporate whatever you are doing into what the nurses are already doing, because you're not going to get it done separately. They don't have the time or the interest, and how

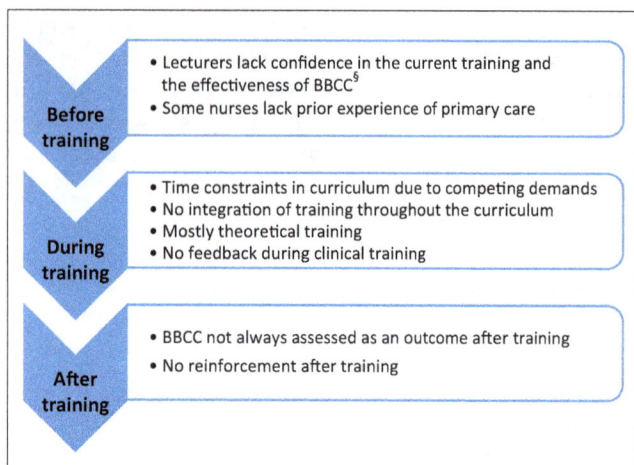

BBCC, brief behaviour change counselling.
FIGURE 1: Current training difficulties.

to, and you know every time you add something to a nurse's workload they tell you, okay so where am I going to fit this into my day?' (Nurse programme manager)

A simple unified structured approach based on the best evidence available should be adapted and implemented in the primary care system. Future training should be aimed at improving supervisors and other HCPs counselling skills at undergraduate and postgraduate levels. Competence after training should be assessed and the importance of brief behaviour change counselling (BBCC) needed to be stressed by both policy makers and managers at the clinic level:

'We must seriously look at integrating some of these things that only happen at the end and at the very beginning, integrate that far more into a form of a workplace based assessment throughout the four years.' (Family medicine programme manager)

'We need much more regular training and much more regular assessment.' (Family medicine programme manager)

'So having a simple structure that people can remember and apply almost generically to behaviour change issues that, could actually be highly beneficial in getting people to do this.' (Family physician)

Discussion

Training of primary care nurses and family physicians in BBCC is not designed to really build competency. Training programmes seem to be promoting the theory of lifestyle modification, but are not delivering on the practical skills. The opportunity to practise key skills and to receive constructive feedback on performance is largely missing, thus HCPs do not transfer these skills to clinical practice. As a result, HCPs lack confidence in their ability to counsel patients effectively. The current difficulties with training are summarised in Figure 1.

The Department of Health's recommendations to revitalise PHC focuses on improving PHC providers' capacity to counsel effectively, by teaching HCPs to deliver personalised, patient-centred behaviour change counselling.[7] Traditionally, HCPs rely mostly on the directive style when counselling patients on behaviour

change, resulting in resistance from the patient and frustration for the HCP.[5,14,15] A patient-centred approach to counselling patients on lifestyle change outperforms a directive, advice-giving approach in 80% of studies.[16] Involving the patient in decision making is essential in order to create a collaborative, culturally relevant and efficient interaction, especially in our diverse context.

Brief behaviour change counselling is built on the foundation of a patient-centred style and incorporates a guiding style derived from MI.[17] It is designed for use in PHC settings, with brief interactions in mind.[4,17] This study echoed other research, which showed that many programme managers and HCPs are unaware of the evidence in support of BBCC and are sceptical about its effectiveness.[5,18,19,20] International evidence exists to show that BBCC can be delivered by a range of healthcare providers with minimum investment of time, in a variety of settings, for patients of different ages, genders and ethnicities.[21,22] Healthcare providers from different training backgrounds, working in different settings, devoting a small amount of extra time with their patients and building a patient-centred relationship, can expect 10% – 15% additional improvement in patients across a wide variety of behaviours.[21,22] This evidence can possibly be used to increase HCPs' awareness of their potential role and to build their confidence as well as to sensitise programme managers and decision makers to the potential value of BBCC.

The relevance and applicability of BBCC has not been widely assessed in low- and middle-income country settings. The first attempt to apply BBCC skills in a primary care setting in a developing country such as South Africa in 2004, demonstrated that it has great potential for general practitioners.[17] They felt less frustrated with behaviour change consultations and reported having more skills in counselling for behaviour change.[17] During 2008, 38 lay- and nurse counsellors were trained to counsel pregnant mothers about behaviour changes related to the prevention of mother to child transmission of HIV in sub-Saharan Africa.[23] This research developed recommendations to guide the development of future training programmes in this setting. One of the key messages was to tailor-make the training according to the HCP's baseline communication skills. Other recommendations included avoiding reinforcing problems, deficiencies and failures of the counsellors, but rather focusing on successes and aiming to build self-confidence.[23]

Healthcare providers in practice reported a number of barriers to the delivery of BBCC, such as a lack of time, lack of confidence in their ability to counsel and a lack of supportive materials for patients (see Figure 2). There was a perception that counselling was ineffective, with poor patient adherence; and language barriers were also amongst the main difficulties in counselling. These same barriers have been reported in similar studies from the same setting.[5,20]

Even if current training programmes are adapted and optimised, we are still faced with numerous challenges in our

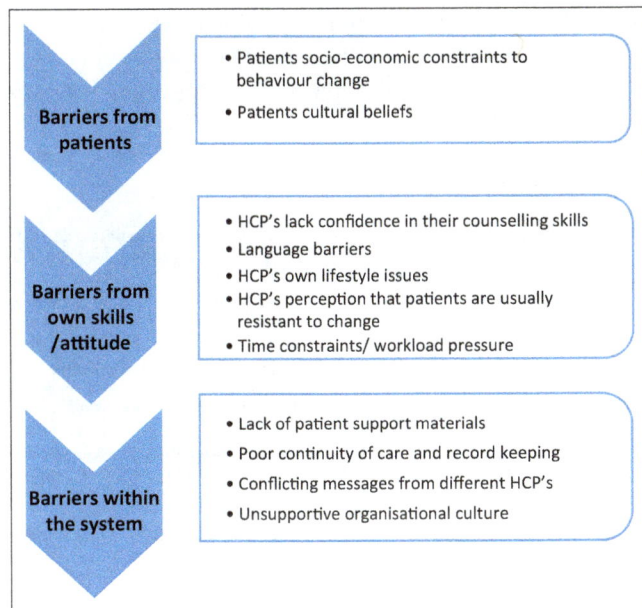

HCPs, Healthcare providers.

FIGURE 2: HCPs'[§] barriers to behaviour change counselling in clinical practice.

public, PHC system that may be a barrier to HCPs' ability to engage in patient-centred counselling. A recent study in the Western Cape reported that three-quarters of junior doctors working in community-level PHC facilities, are suffering from clinically-significant burnout.[24] Emotional exhaustion and depersonalisation may diminish HCPs' commitment to engage patients in patient-centred counselling.[24]

Future training could optimise training outcomes by targeting HCPs with the most potential to provide successful BBCC. Empathy has been identified as one of the essential skills valued most by patients, in communicating with a healthcare provider who uses a patient-centred approach.[25,26] Healthcare providers who are low in empathy show indifference or active dismissal of the patient's perspective, whereas those high in empathy are curious and spend the time required to explore the patient's story. Patients experience this attitude as positive: they feel listened to, which then leads to an increased possibility of change.[26] Recent international research suggested that training can make a significant difference in PHC providers' empathic expression during patient interactions.[25] Screening before training, as well as offering additional input as required, may be necessary in order to optimise gains in patient-centred communication skills training for counsellors with lower baseline empathy.[25]

The development of future training programmes should take note of current counselling barriers and aim to reduce those barriers that can be addressed through training skills. Training can teach communication skills and can change the HCP's attitude about the effectiveness of counselling.[15,25,27,28] Doctors with good communication skills identify patients' problems more accurately.[27] In addition, they have greater job satisfaction and less work stress.[27] The inclusion of training modules on communication skills for primary HCPs is therefore essential.[6,15,18]

Group education could also be explored as a possibility to deal with some of the barriers in PHC settings with limited resources. Health professionals regard group interactions as the most practical approach to counselling in our demanding primary care clinic setting. The first trial in an African context, on the effectiveness of a group diabetes education programme in the Western Cape, demonstrated that healthcare promoters have the potential to deliver effective group diabetes education.[16] A combination of both structured and systematic group education, together with more ad hoc individual BBCC, could be a model to explore further.

Training has very limited impact on practice if there is no follow-up support and feedback.[23,29,30] Offering feedback on real consultations could ensure more effective transfer of skills after initial training.[27] Formative feedback is an essential part of a supervisor's role and including observation of BBCC in the registrar's portfolio of learning (the portfolio is now a national requirement in South Africa, for entry to the college exams) could strengthen the training in this area. The portfolio requires direct observation of consultations with feedback and could require that some of these focus more on BBCC. However, supervisors should also be trained on the best evidence-based methods for BBCC. In-service training and ongoing support can be effective in overcoming some of the barriers and improving clinician's provision of behaviour change counselling.[18,23]

Limitations of the study

Interviews were conducted by the researcher, who is a family physician at the Division of Family Medicine and Primary Care at Stellenbosch University. Previous research conducted by the researcher on general practitioners' management of overweight and/or obese patients, could have had a negative influence on her perception of the primary HCP's efficacy in counselling. The researcher has been involved primarily as the interviewer in all the interviews undertaken for this study, as well as the analysis and interpretation of the findings. The interview process, analysis and interpretation were, however, supervised by the other co-authors.

The researcher triangulated data from different types of respondents (trainers, nurses and doctors), from different genders, ages, institutions and with different levels of expertise and qualifications. However, a broader selection of study participants could have added to the credibility of the results. For example, focus group interviews with nurses from other clinics or with other primary care doctors outside of the training programme might have revealed additional themes.

Recommendations

Based on the current training challenges identified by this study, future BBCC training programmes should aim to:

- Raise awareness of the evidence on the benefits of BBCC amongst primary care providers and decision makers.
- Include the evidence base for BBCC in the training.

- Focus on the development of competency in BBCC, rather than the theories of behaviour change, or general communication skills. Include time to both model and practise skills in the training.
- Reinforce the initial training provided throughout the rest of the programme.
- Ongoing, on-site feedback and supervision should be provided in the clinical training setting.
- Competency in BBCC should be assessed summatively as part of the programme.
- Based on the barriers to BBCC in clinical practice, the following recommendations can support the implementation in primary care:
  - Provide patient education materials to reinforce and supplement BBCC on risk factors and key behaviours.
  - Encourage record keeping and continuity of care to enable follow up of BBCC interventions.
  - Ensure that all relevant health workers are trained in BBCC and share the same understanding of lifestyle modification messages.
  - Develop an organisational culture that is patient-centred and which encourages learning and innovation so that BBCC is congruent with this culture.

Future research in our setting will focus on the development and implementation of a training intervention for primary HCPs on BBCC, based on the findings of this study and best-practice models.

Conclusion

Current training on behaviour change counselling for primary care providers in the Western Cape is viewed as insufficient to achieve competence in clinical practice. Primary care providers' current experience of counselling in practice tends to be discouraging and challenging, in view of the numerous barriers that they face. Revising the approach to current training is necessary in order to ensure that skills can be learnt and transferred to the clinical setting.

Acknowledgements

This research was supported by a grant from the CDIA (Chronic Disease Initiative for Africa) via the Division of Family Medicine and Primary Care, Stellenbosch University. We would like to acknowledge the Cancer Association of South Africa for their funding contribution to the project as part of CDIA's programme of work.

Competing interests

The authors declare that they have no financial or personal relationship(s) that may have inappropriately influenced them in writing this article.

Authors' contributions

Z.M. (Stellenbosch University) interviewed participants, then analysed and interpreted the qualitative data. B.M. (Stellenbosch University) and K.E.-M. (University of Cape Town) conceptualised the study and supervised the research process. All of the authors approved the final manuscript.

References

1. Mayosi BM, Flisher AJ, Lalloo UG, et al. The burden of non-communicable diseases in South Africa. Lancet. 2009;374(9693):934–947. http://dx.doi.org/10.1016/S0140-6736(09)61087-4

2. Whitlock EP, Orleans CT, Pender N, et al. Evaluating primary care behavioral counseling interventions: An evidence-based approach. Am J Prev Med. 2002;22(4):267–284. http://dx.doi.org/10.1016/S0749-3797(02)00415-4

3. Beaglehole R, Epping-Jordan J, Patel V, et al. Improving the prevention and management of chronic disease in low-income and middle-income countries: A priority for primary health care. Lancet. 2008; 372(9642):940–949. http://dx.doi.org/10.1016/S0140-6736(08)61404-X

4. Spanou C, Simpson SA, Hood K, et al. Preventing disease through opportunistic, rapid engagement by primary care teams using behaviour change counselling (PRE-EMPT): Protocol for a general practice-based cluster randomised trial. BMC Fam Pract. 2010;11:69. http://dx.doi.org/10.1186/1471-2296-11-69

5. Parker WA, Steyn NP, Levitt NS, et al. They think they know but do they? Misalignment of perceptions of lifestyle modification knowledge among health professionals. Public Health Nutr. 2011;14(8):1429–1438. http://dx.doi.org/10.1017/S1368980009993272

6. Kautzky K, Tollman SM. A perspective on primary health care in South Africa. In: Barron P, Roma-Reardon J, editors. South African Health Review 2008. Durban: health Systems Trust, 2008; pp. 17–30.

7. Health Systems Trust. Green paper: National health insurance in South Africa [page on the Internet]. c2011 [cited 2015 Jan 14]. Available from: http://www.hst.org.za/publications/green-paper-national-health-insurance-south-africa

8. World Health Organization. Global status report on non-communicable diseases [page on the Internet]. c2010 [cited 2015 Feb 15]. Available from: http://www.who.int/nmh/publications/ncd_report2010

9. Malan JE. The influence of information given on general practitioners' management of overweight patients. Masters thesis. Department of Family Medicine. University of Pretoria; 2008.

10. Everett-Murphy K, Paijmans J, Steyn K, et al. Scolders, carers or friends: South African midwives' contrasting styles of communication when discussing smoking cessation with pregnant women. Midwifery. 2011;27(4):517–524. http://dx.doi.org/10.1016/j.midw.2010.04.003

11. De Feijter EM. Smoking: Our care! A quantitative study among South African midwives, focussing on the determinants of their educational behaviour in relation to smoking cessation of disadvantaged coloured women. Masters thesis. Health Education & Health Promotion. Maastricht, The Netherlands: University of Maastricht; 2003.

12. Allen WC. Overview and evolution of the ADDIE Training System. Advances in Developing Human Resources. 2006;8(4):430–441. http://dx.doi.org/10.1177/1523422306292942

13. Richie J, Spencer L. Qualitative data analysis for applied policy research. In: Bryman A, Burgess R, editors. Analyzing qualitative data. London: Routledge, 1994; pp. 173–194. http://dx.doi.org/10.4324/9780203413081_chapter_9

14. Green LA, Cifuentes M, Glascow RE, et al. Redesigning primary care practice to incorporate health behaviour change. Am J Prev Med. 2008;35(5 Suppl): S347–S349. http://dx.doi.org/10.1016/j.amepre.2008.08.013

15. Emmons KM, Rollnick S. Motivational interviewing in health care settings. Opportunities and limitations. Am J Prev Med.2001;20(1):68–74. http://dx.doi.org/10.1016/S0749-3797(00)00254-3

16. Botes AS, MajikelaDlangamandla B, Mash R. The ability of health promoters to deliver group diabetes education in South African primary care. Afr J Prm Health Care Fam Med. 2013;5(1), Art. #484, 8 pages.

17. Mash RJ, Allen S. Managing chronic conditions in a South African primary care context: Exploring the applicability of Brief Motivational Interviewing. SAMJ. 2004;46(9):21–26.

18. Achhra A. Health promotion in Australian general practice: A gap in GP training. Aust Fam Physician. 2009;38(8):605–608.

19. Sim MG, Wain T, Khong E. Influencing behaviour change in general practice – Part 1 – brief intervention and motivational interviewing. Aust Fam Physician. 2009;38(11):885–888.

20. Van der Does AM, Mash R. Evaluation of the 'Take Five School': An education programme for people with Type 2 Diabetes in the Western Cape, South Africa. Prim Care Diabetes 2013;7(4):289–295.

21. Artinian N, Fletcher G, Mozaffarian D, et al. Interventions to promote physical activity and dietary lifestyle changes for cardiovascular risk factor reduction in adults: A scientific statement from the American Heart Association. Circulation. 2010; 122(4):406–441.

22. Lundahl B, Moleni T, Burke L, et al. Motivational interviewing in medical settings: A systematic review and meta-analysis of randomized controlled trials. Patient Educ Couns. 2013;93(2):157–168.

23. Mash R, Baldassini G, Mkhatshwa H, et al. Reflections on the training of counsellors in motivational interviewing for programmes for the prevention of mother to child transmission of HIV in sub-Saharan Africa. SA Fam Pract. 2008;50(2):53–59.

24. Rossouw L. The prevalence of burnout and depression among medical doctors working in the Cape Town metropole community health care clinics and district hospitals of the provincial government of the Western Cape: a cross-sectional study. Masters thesis. Division of Family Medicine and Primary Care. University of Stellenbosch. Cape Town; 2011.

25. Bonvicini KA, Perlin MJ, Bylund CL, et al. Impact of communication training on physician expression of empathy in patient encounters. Patient Educ Couns. 2009;75(1):3–10.

26. Miller WR, Rollnick S. Motivational interviewing: Helping people change. 3d ed. New York, NY: The Guildford Press; 2013.

27. Maguire P, Pitceathly C. Key communication skills and how to acquire them. BMJ.2002; 325(7366):697–700.

28. Everett-Murphy K., Steyn K., Matthews C. et al The effectiveness of adapted, best practice guidelines for smoking cessation counseling with disadvantaged, pregnant smokers attending public sector antenatal clinics in Cape Town, South Africa. Acta Obstet Gynecol Scand.2010;89(4): 478-489.

29. Kinect Australia, for the Lifescripts Consortium. Lifescripts practice manual: Supporting lifestyle risk factor management in general practice [document on the Internet]. c2005 [cited 2015 Feb 15]. Available from: www.pnml.com.au/home/doc_download/149-lifescripts-manual

30. The Royal College of General Practitioners. SNAP: A population health guide to behavioural risk factors in general practice. College House, Melbourne, Australia: RACGP; 2004.

Utilisation of a community-based health facility in a low-income urban community in Ibadan, Nigeria

Authors:
Ayodeji M. Adebayo[1]
Michael C. Asuzu[1]

Affiliations:
[1]Department of Preventive Medicine and Primary Care, College of Medicine, University of Ibadan, Ibadan

Correspondence to:
Ayodeji Adebayo

Email:
davidsonone@yahoo.com

Postal address:
PO Box 1517, UI Post Office, Ibadan

Background: Primary healthcare is established to ensure that people have access to health services through facilities located in their community. However, utilisation of health facilities in Nigeria remains low in many communities.

Aim: To assess the utilisation of community-based health facility (CBHF) amongst adults in Ibadan, Nigeria

Settings: A low-income community in Ibadan North West Local Government Area of Oyo State.

Methods: A cross-sectional survey was conducted using a simple random sampling technique to select one adult per household in all 586 houses in the community. A semi-structured interviewer-administered questionnaire was used to collect information on respondents' sociodemographic characteristics, knowledge and utilisation of the CBHF. Data analysis included descriptive statistics and association testing using the Chi-square test at $p = 0.05$.

Results: The mean age of the respondents was 46.5 ± 16.0 years; 46.0% were men and 81.0% married; 26% had no formal education and 38.0% had secondary-level education and above; traders constituted 52.0% of the sample; and 85.2% were of low socioeconomic standing; 90% had patronised the CBHF. The main reasons for non-utilisation were preference for general hospitals (13.8%) and self-medication (12.1%). Respondents who had secondary education and above, were in a higher socioeconomic class, who had good knowledge of the facility and were satisfied with care, utilised the CBHF three months significantly more than their counterparts prior to the study ($p < 0.05$). However, only satisfaction with care was found to be a significant predictor of utilisation of the CBHF.

Conclusion: The utilisation of the CBHF amongst adults in the study setting is high, driven mostly by satisfaction with the care received previously. Self-medication, promoted by uncontrolled access to drugs through pharmacies and patent medicine stores, threatens this high utilisation.

Utilisation d'un établissement communautaire de santé dans un quartier urbain à faibles revenus d'Ibadan, Nigéria.

Contexte: Les soins de santé primaire ont été établis pour permettre aux gens d'avoir accès aux services de santé dans des établissements installés dans leur communauté. Cependant, l'utilisation des équipements sanitaires au Nigeria est faible dans de nombreuses communautés.

Objectif: Evaluer l'utilisation d'un établissement communautaire de santé (CBHF) par les adultes à Ibadan, Nigéria

Situation: Une communauté à faibles revenues dans la Zone de Gouvernement local d'Ibadan Nord Ouest (IBNWLGA) de l'état d'Oyo.

Méthodes: On a effectué une enquête transversale au moyen d'une technique d' échantillonnage simple au hasard pour sélectionner un adulte par ménage dans les 586 maisons de la communauté. On s'est servi d'un questionnaire semi-structuré administré par l'interviewer pour collecter les informations sur les caractéristiques sociodémographiques, les connaissances et l'utilisation du CBHF par les personnes interrogées. L'analyse des données comprenait des statistiques descriptives et des tests d'association au moyen du test de Chi-carré à $p = 0.05$.

Résultats: L'âge moyen des personnes interrogées était de 46.5 ± 16.0 ans; 46.0% étaient des hommes et 81.0% étaient mariés. Vingt-six pour cent n'avaient pas d'éducation formelle; et 38.0% avaient fait des études secondaires et plus. Les commerçants constituaient 52.0% de l'échantillon; et 85.2% avaient un statut socioéconomique modeste. Quatre-vingt-dix pour cent avaient fréquenté le CBHF. Les raisons principales pour la non utilisation de l'établissement étaient une préférence pour les hôpitaux généraux (13.8%) et l'automédication (12.1%). Les personnes interrogées qui avaient fait des études secondaires et plus, appartenaient à une classe sociale supérieure; ils connaissaient bien l'établissement et étaient satisfaits des soins, et ils avaient considérablement utilisé le CBHF trois mois avant l'enquête par rapport à leurs homologues ($p < 0.05$). Cependant, seule la satisfaction des soins était un indice significatif de l'utilisation du CBHF.

Conclusion: L'utilisation du CBHF par les adultes de l'étude est élevée, et liée essentiellement à la satisfaction des soins reçus au paravent. L'automédication, encouragée par l'accès incontrôlé aux médicaments des pharmacies et des magasins qui vendent des médicaments brevetés, menace l'utilisation élevée de l'établissement.

Introduction

Primary healthcare (PHC) is defined as:

> essential healthcare based on practical, scientifically-sound and socially-acceptable methods and technology made universally accessible to individuals and families in the community by means acceptable to them at a cost that the community and country can afford to maintain at every stage of their development in a spirit of self-reliance and self-determination.[1]

It forms an integral part of both the countries' health system of which it is the central function and the main focus of the overall social and economic development of the community. It is also the first level of contact of individuals, families and communities with the national health system, bringing healthcare as close as possible to where people live and work and constitutes the first element of continuing health care process.[1]

Emphasis in healthcare has changed from healthcare *for* the people to healthcare *by* the people. Health is meant to be earned and maintained by the individuals.[2] However, despite the fact that it is a fundamental human right, the community also has a role to play in contributing to the health of its members and the community as a whole. Apart from contributing toward the planning and implementation of planned programmes aimed at developing the community, the community also needs to utilise relevant health facilities in an appropriate manner.

The inception of PHC has facilitated some communities to have at least one health care facility sited as close as possible to where they live or work in all the districts or local government areas of many of the states in Nigeria. However, siting of health care facility does not necessarily translate to its utilisation; more so, that one of the major factors maintaining high mortality rate in Nigeria is poor access to and utilisation of health services.[3,4] Several other factors, such as availability and cost of services, location of facility from clients/patients, competencies and attitudes of service providers, the peculiarity of patients' need and adequacy of resources can affect effective healthcare delivery. In a literature review of the situation of health-seeking behaviour in developing countries, by Shaikh and Hatcher in Pakistan,[5] physical, socioeconomic, cultural and political contexts were documented as being the factors responsible for utilisation of a healthcare system, whether public or private, formal or informal.[5] Details of these factors may include sociodemographics, social structures, educational status, gender discrimination, cultural beliefs and practices, employment status, women status, political will, the disease pattern, environmental conditions and healthcare system itself.[5]

Primary healthcare is established to ensure that people have access to health services through health facilities located in their community. However, utilisation of health facilities in Nigeria remains unacceptably low in many communities. A household survey amongst 630 respondents in Northern Nigeria showed that the majority preferred to use patent medicine stores (53.63%) compared with only 7.6% who utilised the PHC services.[6] In another study to assess the utilisation of PHC facilities in a rural community in south-western Nigeria, 44% of the respondents who were ill in the three months preceding the survey had used the health facility.[7] In many, if not all countries in Africa, as well as in other developing countries worldwide, most morbidities are treated at home and are never reported to the formal healthcare system.[8] Clinical problems that present to the formal healthcare facilities are, therefore, only the tip of the iceberg. For example, for every case of febrile illness attended to in the formal healthcare facilities, approximately 4–5 more existed in the community in resource-poor countries.[8]

Studies on health services utilisation often seek to understand both the frequency and trends in the use of health services, as well as the possible mechanisms that may be associated with the pattern of use.[9] Good knowledge and understanding of utilisation also help health providers and health systems managers to plan and improve on health services. However, it has been observed that such studies have been neglected, especially since the early 1990s. Given that most PHC facilities in Nigeria were established without an evaluation of their accessibility to the communities they are meant to serve, gaining an understanding of how people use health facilities cannot be over-emphasised. This is even more so in developing countries, including Nigeria, where people's knowledge of and attitude toward health services and the use of these services are still poor.[4,10,11,12]

Aims and objectives

Given that the utilisation of the CBHF by the community members at Idikan, Ibadan, Nigeria has hitherto not been assessed since its advent, the current study aimed to assess the utilisation of the facility within the three months preceding the study and to identify reasons for any lack of utilisation. It is hoped that the findings of this study will inform interventions for the improvement of PHC services in the community, hence the need for this study. Achieving this will enable better decisions to be made, which should result in better, more effective primary care for the people of the area in the long run. Therefore, the objective of this study was to assess the utilisation of the facility within the three months preceding the interview as well as to assess any reasons for any lack of utilisation of the facility, so that these can be corrected, if possible, for the improvement of PHC in the area.

Research methods and design
Study design

This was a community-based descriptive cross-sectional survey.

Research setting

The study was conducted in Idikan, a low-income urban community located in Ibadan North West Local Government

Area of Oyo State, South-western Nigeria. The community has an estimated population of 13 902 based on the 2006 population census.[13] The majority of the inhabitants are petty traders, artisans and farmers – the men are mostly artisans and farmers whilst the women are traders. Almost everybody in the community is from the Yoruba tribe – the dominant ethnic group in the south-western part of Nigeria. A great majority of the inhabitants have no formal education and belong to a low socioeconomic class. Idikan, as with other traditional areas of Ibadan, is grossly unplanned and has limited access to pipe-borne water and an irregular electricity supply. The CBHF was established in 1963 to serve the urban Idikan community. The programme was designed to promote health and to provide basic medical services to the community members as well as to provide an avenue for teaching urban community healthcare to the students of the Ibadan Medical School. With the advent of PHC in 1978, the service was expected to provide as much of all community/PHC services to the community as possible. The services are run from Monday to Friday for six hours per day by community health nurses and resident doctors, supervised by consultant community physicians from the Department of Community Medicine, University College Hospital, Ibadan. Two members of the community (community health assistance) provide assistance in the running of services at the facility. Currently, the clinic attends to an average 15–20 adults per day. There is a community health committee meant to ensure community participation in sustaining the services provided at this facility. The members of the committee contribute to the planning and implementation of programmes for their development through provision of funds, logistic and human resources; and in the utilisation of this facility.

Study population

The study population consisted of male and female adults residing in selected households.

Sample size calculation

The sample size was calculated using Leslie Kish's formula for descriptive surveys.[14] A minimum sample size of 398 respondents was estimated, taking into consideration the prevalence of utilisation of health facilities of 44% from a previous study,[15] with a critical ratio of 1.96, a level of precision of 5% and a non-response rate of 5%.

Sampling methods

There were a total of 586 houses in Idikan community with an average of 3–4 households per dwelling. All 586 houses were visited. In places where there were more than one household per house, one household was selected randomly by balloting. In the selected household, one adult was selected by a simple random sampling technique by balloting.

Research instrument and data collection

The study was conducted using a semi-structured interviewer-administered questionnaire. Five research assistants were recruited from the community and trained in order to administer the questionnaire. The interview was conducted mostly in the evening, which is when most of the community members were around. The questionnaire covered: sociodemographic characteristics; perception of community health services by adult members in the community; pattern of presentation in the three months preceding the interview; the utilisation of the CBHF for common illnesses in the three months preceding the interview; and obstacles against use of the community health services.

The questionnaire was standardised after it had been critiqued during a departmental proposal presentation with consultants, senior registrars and registrars present. Through constructive criticism, any possible shortcomings which could affect the quality and feasibility of the study were identified and rectified. The questionnaire was translated into Yoruba for the benefit of the majority who were predominantly Yoruba speaking, then translated back to formal English by a different translator from the first to ensure that there was no error in translation and that the original meaning was retained.

Pretesting was carried out on 15 subjects in Abebi, an adjoining community in the area which was not part of the study area but has similar characteristics. The pre-test was found necessary in order to ensure clarity of interpretation, ease of completion, reduce respondents' bias and generate useful questions not initially conceived but very germane to the quality of the study and to correct any ambiguity whatsoever detected. Corrections and relevant restructuring were made in places of ambiguity.

Data collation and analysis

The data obtained were sorted out, edited and manually cleaned and recoded where necessary. Data were entered into the computer and analysed with SPSS software v 16.0 (SPSS Inc., Chicago, IL 2007). Data analysis was done with the assistance of a statistician using both descriptive and inferential statistics. Descriptive statistics such as percentages or proportions were used to describe the qualitative or categorical variables. The Chi-square test was used to examine the relationship between two categorical variables. The test was carried out at 5% level of significance.

Responses to questions on knowledge of the CBHF were converted to a 40-point score by coding a correct answer as '1' and a wrong answer as '0'. The knowledge scores were generated giving minimum and maximum obtainable scores of 0 and 40 respectively. Respondents were categorised into having good, fair and poor knowledge using 75% and above, 50% – 74% and 49% and below of the maximum obtainable scores, respectively. Seventy-five per cent was used as the lowest limit for good knowledge because the CBHF had been in Idikan community for more than two decades before this assessment. It was located both centrally and within 1 km of all the community members for easy accessibility. Hence, respondents with a knowledge score of 30 and above were reported as having good knowledge, fair (20–29) and poor (< 20). Similarly, responses to perception questions were converted to a 60-point score. Perception scores were generated with minimum and maximum obtainable scores of 12 and 60 respectively. Respondents were classified into having poor, fair and good perception of some characteristics of the CBHF using 75% and above, 50% – 74% and 49% and below of the total obtainable scores, respectively. Hence, those with scores of 36 or less were regarded as having poor perception, 37–49 fair and ≥ 50 good perception. Satisfaction with the services at the CBHF was assessed by asking if respondents were satisfied with the services received at the facility, generating a 'yes' or 'no' response.

Multivariate analysis using binary logistic regression[16] was used to identify predictors of utilisation of the CBHF. The independent variables entered into the logistic regression model were those that were significant at 10% ($p < 0.1$) on bivariate analysis.

The occupation of respondents was classified into high and low occupational class for ease of bivariate analysis, in some instances by modifying the social class based on occupation alone, as adopted from Rose and Pevalin (2001).[17] Those classified as high occupational class were those in social class I and II (including professionals, senior civil servants and those in managerial occupations), whilst the low occupational class consisted of those in social class III, IV and V (including traders, artisans, farmers, drivers, etc.). Socioeconomic status was classified into high and low using the educational level and occupation of respondents. Those in the high occupational class with tertiary education were classified as the high socioeconomic class whilst those in the low occupational class with secondary education and below were classified as the low socioeconomic class.

Ethical considerations

Ethical approval was obtained from Oyo State Ethical Review Committee, State Ministry of Health (reference number AD/13/479/146). Permission and cooperation were sought from the High Chief of Idikan Community. Verbal informed consent was also ensured from all the participants. No names were recorded on the questionnaire so as to ensure confidentiality; and codes were used for identification of respondents instead of names.

Results

A total of 586 households were visited, from which 554 respondents consented – a response rate of 95%. The respondents' sociodemographic characteristics are shown in Table 1. The mean age was 46.5 ± 16 years with the highest proportion ($n = 237$, 42.6%) being in the 30–49 year age group. Most were women ($n = 300$, 54%) and from a monogamous family setting ($n = 352$, 63.5%). Traders comprised 52.2% ($n = 289$) of the sample, 173 (31.2%) had secondary education and 347 (62.2%) were of the Islamic religion. Most of the respondents were married ($n = 447$, 80.7%), of the Yoruba

TABLE 1: Sociodemographic characteristics of respondents.

Variables ($N = 554$)	Frequency	Percentage
Gender		
Male	254	46
Female	300	54
Age group		
< 20	4	0.7
20–29	78	14.1
30–39	121	21.8
40–49	116	20.8
50–59	87	15.7
60–69	74	13.4
> 70	57	10.3
No response	17	3.1
Ethnicity		
Yoruba	507	91.5
Igbo	43	7.8
Hausa	4	0.7
Marital status		
Single	29	5.2
Married	447	80.7
Separated	13	2.3
Divorced	13	2.3
Widowed	52	9.4
Religion		
Islam	347	62.6
Christianity	205	37
Traditional	2	0.4
Type of marriage		
Monogamous	352	63.5
Polygamous	202	36.5
Level of education		
No formal education	143	25.8
Quranic	49	8.8
Primary	153	27.6
Secondary	173	31.2
Tertiary	36	6.5
Occupation		
Professional†	24	4.3
Civil servant	25	4.5
Artisan	90	16.2
Trading	289	52.2
Unemployed	56	10.1
Other‡	70	12.6
Monthly income[Naira]		
< 5000	241	43.5
5000–9999	79	14.3
> 10 000	124	22.3
No response	110	19.9
Socioeconomic status		
Low (1–5)	472	85.2
High (6–9)	82	14.8
Distance of respondents house from health facility		
≤ 5 km	434	78.3
> 5 km	120	21.7

†, Engineers, teachers; ‡, Clergy, students, drivers, farmers.

tribe ($n = 507$, 91.5%) and within the low socioeconomic status ($n = 472$, 85.2%).

The majority ($n = 484$, 82.5%) of the respondents felt that the best place to seek help when sick is the CBHF. Regarding the service components of PHC available at the CBHF, 211

(42.5%) knew about health education and 183 (36.9%) were aware of referral services. This was followed by knowledge of antenatal services (n = 169, 34.1%) and immunisation (n = 118, 23.8%). Questions were asked to test the respondents' knowledge about some of the characteristics of the services provided at the CBHF, for example: if they were provided free; rendered 24 hours daily; availability of a community health committee; and if members of the community are part of the working staff. In each of the first three knowledge questions, well above 50% (n = 336, 67.7%; n = 361, 72.8%; and n = 310, 62.5%, respectively) answered correctly, except for the last question (if members of the community are part of the working staff), where only 47.6% were correct. Just over half of the respondents (n = 284, 57.3%) had good knowledge of the administrative structure and functions of the CBHF as well as the services there (Table 2).

Most the respondents (n = 496, 89.5%) had patronised the CBHF. Of the 554 respondents, 369 (76.1%) reported that they were satisfied with the care received at the CBHF. Amongst those that had ever received treatment in the facility, the perceived reasons for seeking care include good services (89.5%), nearness to the house (84.1%), prompt attention (69.2%) and available of essential drugs (68.5%) (Figure 1). Amongst those that had never utilised the CBHF, 21 (36.2%)

proffered reasons for non-patronage as preference for general hospital (13.8%), self-medication (12.1%) and one person (1.7%) reported a preference for traditional practitioners.

Amongst those that sought medical care outside the home in the three months preceding the interview, 212 (93.8%) specified their sources of care. One hundred and fifty-one respondents (66.8%) reported the CBHF as their source of medical care three months prior to interview, 34 (15.0%) a private hospital, 16 (7.1%) government-owned hospitals and 11 (4.9%) a faith-based organisation.

Results of the bivariate analysis are shown in Table 3, indicating that the higher occupational class (p = 0.013), higher socioeconomic class (p = 0.01), having secondary education and above (p = 0.023), being unmarried (p = 0.002), satisfaction with previous care (p < 0.001) and having good attitude, perceptions and knowledge (p < 0.001) were all associated with having received treatment from the CBHF in the preceding three months.

In the multivariate logistic regression analysis (Table 4), only satisfaction with care received was a significant predictor of utilisation of services at the CBHF. Respondents that were not satisfied with care were less likely (OR = 0.378; 95% CI = 0.144–0.994; p = 0.049) to use the CBHF.

Discussion

This study was carried out to assess the utilisation of the CBHF by adult members in a low-income urban community in Ibadan for the purpose of promoting/optimising and upgrading PHC in the area. The majority of the respondents (89.5%) had utilised the CBHF at one time or the other and utilisation of services in the preceding three months was equally high (89%). Utilisation in the preceding three months was in relation to treatment of injuries and ailments, whether acute or chronic. However, the respondents' awareness of the service components of PHC provided at the CBHF was low. Less than half knew about health education, 36.9% were aware of referral services, followed by antenatal services (34.1%) and immunisation (23.8%). This means that respondents were not aware of the full range of the services provided at the CBHF based on the PHC service components. Utilisation of services in the preceding three months showed that they were more familiar with use of the facility for treatment of disease conditions such as malaria, hypertension and diabetes. The low awareness of the service components of PHC amongst respondents in this study may be a result of poor enlightenment of the public regarding the component services available at the centre with health workers, provision of services for only six hours without admission; non-provision of delivery services, in addition to antenatal care, which would have encouraged patients and relatives to stay for a longer period in the facility and provide opportunities for exposure to the other services being offered at the centre. The poor awareness reported in our study is in contrast to a community-based study in India where awareness of services was high but utilisation was relatively

TABLE 2: Distribution of respondents regarding knowledge of the community-based health facility.

Knowledge areas (N = 496)	Correct n (%)	Incorrect n (%)
Owner of the facility	373 (75.2)	123 (24.8)
Types of services provided		
Antenatal care	327 (65.9)	169 (34.1)
Immunisation	378 (68.2)	118 (23.8)
Family planning	454 (91.5)	42 (8.5)
Treatment of common ailments	389 (78.4)	107 (21.6)
Health education	285 (57.5)	211 (42.5)
Referral	313 (61.3)	183 (36.9)
Ultra Sound Scan	298 (60.1)	198 (39.9)
Characteristics of services provided		
Free	336 (67.7)	160 (32.3)
24 hours	361 (72.8)	135 (27.2)
Availability of community health committee	310 (62.5)	186 (37.5)
Members of the community provide assistance at the facility	236 (47.6)	260 (52.4)
Overall knowledge rating regarding the community-based health facility		
Good (30 and above)	284	57.3
Fair (20-29)	116	23.4
Poor (19 and below)	96	19.3

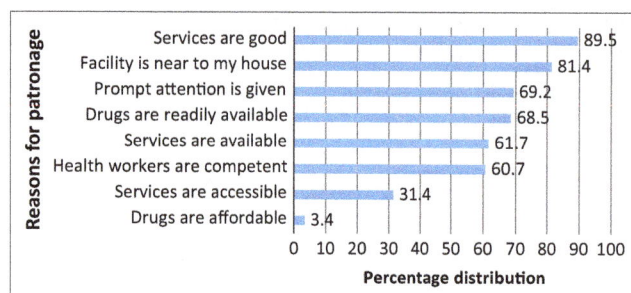

FIGURE 1: Percentage distribution of respondents by reasons for utilising the community-based health facility.

TABLE 3: Association between utilisation of services at the community-based health facility for three months before survey and respondents' characteristics.

Variables	Received treatment in last 3 months		X^2	p-value
	Yes n (%)	No n (%)		
Age group (yrs)				
< 30	21 (25.6)	61 (74.4)		
30–59	96 (29.6)	228 (70.4)	3.938	0.140
60 and above	27 (20.6)	104 (79.4)		
Gender				
Male	72 (28.2)	183 (71.8)		
Female	79 (26.4)	220 (73.6)	0.228	0.633
Occupational class				
High	18 (43.9)	23 (56.1)		
Low	133 (25.9)	380 (74.1)	6.188	0.013*
Educational level				
No formal	41 (21.4)	151 (78.6)		
Primary	40 (26.1)	113 (73.9)	7.569	0.023*
Secondary and above	70 (33.5)	139 (66.5)		
Socioeconomic status				
Low	119 (25.2)	353 (74.8)		
High	32 (39.0)	50 (61.0)	6.722	0.010*
Occupation of head of household				
Professional	13 (43.3)	17 (56.7)		
Civil servant	9 (28.1)	23 (71.9)		
Artisan	24 (23.3)	79 (76.7)	5.130	0.275
Traders	69 (28.0)	177 (72.0)		
Other	36 (25.2)	107 (74.8)		
Marital status				
Never	15 (51.7)	14 (48.3)		
Ever	136 (25.9)	389 (74.1)	9.24	0.002*
Ethnicity				
Yoruba	139 (27.4)	368 (72.6)		
Other	12 (25.5)	35 (74.5)	0.077	0.781
Religion				
Christianity	62 (30.2)	143 (69.8)		
Islam	89 (25.5)	260 (74.5)	1.465	0.226
Family type				
Polygamous	92 (26.1)	260 (73.9)		
Monogamous	59 (29.2)	143 (70.8)	0.611	0.435
Household income				
< 5000	71 (31.4)	157 (68.6)		
5000–9000	23 (25.3)	68 (74.7)	1.424	0.491
10 000 and above	34 (27.4)	90 (72.6)		
Satisfaction				
Yes	136 (36.9)	233 (63.1)		
No	8 (6.9)	108 (93.1)	37.948	<0.001*
Distance				
≤ 5	113 (26.0)	321 (74.0)		
> 5	38 (31.7)	82 (68.3)	1.503	0.220
No of days sickness lasted				
≤ 14 days	136 (30.8)	306 (69.2)		
> 14 days	15 (30.6)	34 (69.4)	0.001	0.982
Severity				
Mild	104 (31.1)	230 (68.9)		
Severe	47 (30.3)	108 (69.7)	0.033	0.856
Knowledge				
Poor (< 20)	6 (6.3)	90 (93.8)		
Fair (21–29)	26 (22.4)	90 (77.6)	43.269	< 0.001*
Good (30 and above)	114 (40.1)	170 (59.9)		
Perception				
Poor	5 (5.3)	90 (94.7)		
Fair	12 (40.0)	18 (60.0)	33.421	< 0.001*
Good	129 (34.8)	242 (65.2)		

*p-values < 0.05

TABLE 4: Adjusted odds ratio of predictors of utilisation of the community-based health facility.

Variables	Odds ratio	95% CI	p-value
Occupational class			
High	1.000		
Low	0.594	0.203–1.737	0.342
Level of education			
No formal	1.000		
Primary	0.904	0.520–1.571	0.719
Secondary	0.913	0.514–1.621	0.756
Socioeconomic status			
Low	1.000		
High	1.437	0.615–3.353	0.402
Marital status			
Never	1.000		
Ever	0.409	0.138–1.213	0.107
Satisfaction			
Yes	1.000		
No	0.378	0.144–0.984	0.049*
Knowledge			
Poor	1.000		
Fair	0.831	0.132–5.249	0.844
Good	1.711	0.276–10.618	0.564
Perception			
Poor	1.000		
Fair	4.278	0.495–36.982	0.187
Good	3.326	0.448–24.682	0.240

*p-value < 0.05

low (54.9%).[12] Whilst our study assessed the various service components of PHC, the Indian study only inquired whether respondents were aware of the availability of PHC without exploring awareness of the various service components on offer. The relatively low awareness of the various services available at the CBHF, as documented by this study, will cause under-utilisation of the available services. Efforts at creating awareness of the available component services of PHC and promoting community mobilisation with the support of the community members will further benefit the community members by enhancing their use of the available promotive and preventive services at this facility.

The reasons adduced for utilisation of the CBHF were that services were good and readily available, health facility was nearer to their homes, drugs were readily available and attention was prompt. Reasons for non-utilisation in this study included preference for general hospitals, self-medication, private hospitals and traditional healers. In a study to determine utilisation of approved health facilities for delivery in Ile-Ife, the reasons given for non-utilisation of the health facilities at hand were time of onset of labour, problems with transport, fear of surgery, husband and/or family influence and the fact that delivery was assisted by Traditional Birth Attendants (TBAs) and relatives.[15] Even though our study assessed services in relation to various service components of PHC compared with the Ile-Ife study, which was specifically in facilities for delivery services, the different hours of service are not comparable: six hours in our facility as opposed to 24 hours in Ile-Ife. Reasons for non-utilisation in India were 'faith in quacks, inconvenient timing of the primary health centre, long queues, non-availability of drugs, and investigations'.[12] Interventions to address these factors will improve the current utilisation rate.

The practice of self-medication amongst 12.1% of the respondents is worthy of mention. Considering the fact less than a third reported that the services at the CBHF were not readily accessible may be explained by the fact that services are only accessible in this facility for a maximum of six hours per day. This may force community members to become more dependent on self-medication and traditional healers because drugs are not available at all hours. This automatically makes the services of 'quacks' and patent medicine merchants readily available. However, there is also the possibility that their low level of education and strong cultural beliefs could contribute equally to this. However, a survey in Kathmandu, Nepal, showed that individuals turned to modern health sector 'because they are dissatisfied with the previous folk or traditional professional consultation or because or traditional practitioners had advised them to seek modern hospital services'.[18] Another study in South Africa on community knowledge and perception of malaria reported that 66.9% of the respondents would seek treatment at the hospital when symptoms are severe.[19] From a study conducted in the former Soviet Union on health service utilisation, the main reason for not seeking care was lack of funds to pay for treatment (42.5%), self-treatment with home remedies (32.9%) and purchase of non-prescription medication.[20] An extension of the hours of services at the CBHF may reduce clients' exposure to use of self-medication and traditional healers. This will prevent the clinical and policy implications of buying over-the-canter drugs which may generate drug resistance, increased morbidity and mortality through incompletely-treated cases, use of wrong medication, sub-normal doses and the adverse effects of drugs and herbal medications.

The findings of this research on bivariate analysis indicated that utilisation patterns can be explained, to a large extent, by factors relating to occupational class, socioeconomic status, level of education and level of satisfaction, as well as knowledge of and perception of respondents toward the services. However, it was only the level of satisfaction that was a significant predictor on logistic regression. These findings are consistent with findings from prior research: a bivariate analysis in determinants of utilisation of health services in the western states of Nigeria revealed age, level of education, type of education, place of work and attitudes toward services as being significant factors.[21] A similar study in the determinants of maternal services in a rural Nigeria city showed that the mother's education and occupation of, as well as the husband's religion and occupation were associated significantly with delivery at a health facility on logistic regression analysis. This study showed a higher likelihood of utilisation of health services amongst post-primary education mothers than those with no occupation; and in Christian mothers versus their counterparts.[22] 'The woman's educational level and total number of living children were the most significant predictors of prenatal care utilization' in Vietman.[23] In another study on utilisation

of an approved health facility for delivery in Ile-Ife, south west Nigeria, 'educational status of the mother, religious beliefs, distance from approved health facilities more than 5 km and attitude of health workers were amongst the factors significantly influencing choice of place of delivery' by the mother.[15] This shows that promoting most of these factors through female education and positive attitudes of health workers toward work will further enhance the patronage of the CBHF. The results from both bivariate and multivariate analyses confirmed the importance of a mother's education in explaining the utilisation of maternal health services in a study to determine the use of such services in rural Bangladesh. The Bangladesh study also reported the significant effect of severity of disease condition in predicting the utilisation of maternal health care. Multivariate analysis indicated that women having had a life-threatening condition were more likely to seek care from a health facility.[24]

'The distance patients must travel in order to obtain treatment has long been recognized as a primary determinant of the utilization of health care facilities'.[25] However, it was not found to be a significant factor in this study, contrary to the findings of Esimai et al.[15] and Chakraborty et al.[24] The distance is especially significant in:

> [the] Third World settings where the density of Western type health facilities is often low, where the majority of patients are likely to make the journey for treatment as pedestrians and where there are viable and usually more accessible alternate sources of medicine.[25]

Conclusion

The utilisation of the CBHF at Idikan was high but the awareness of the various service components of PHC was low. Higher occupational and socioeconomic status, higher level of education, satisfaction with previous care, good awareness and perception of the CBHF were factors associated with utilisation of CBHF, although only satisfaction with previous care predicted utilisation on logistic regression.

Implications or recommendations

Information on healthcare utilisation has important policy implications in health systems development. Public awareness programmes that mobilise the community to participate in the design and running of the CBHF need to be developed in order to increase awareness and sustain utilisation of the services at the CBHF. Issues surrounding waiting time, availability of drugs and accessibility should also be addressed by the institution in order to sustain the current level of utilisation. The stakeholders should review the hours of service from the current maximum of six hours to 24 hours; this might require scaling up of resources.

Acknowledgements

The authors would like to acknowledge the contributions of the research assistants, data entry clerk and analyst, the nursing officers at the community-based health facility and the community leaders and members for their cooperation and support.

Competing interests

The authors declare that they have no financial or personal relationship(s) that may have inappropriately influenced them in writing this article.

Authors' contributions

A.M.A. (University of Ibadan) was responsible for the conceptualisation of the study, supervision of the process of data collection, entry and analysis; and the writing of the manuscript. M.C.A. (University of Ibadan) was involved in the conceptualisation and supervision of the manuscript writing.

References

1. Lucas AO, Gilles HM. Organization of health services. In: Short textbook of public health medicine for the tropics. 4th ed. London: Arnold Publishers, 2003; p. 303.

2. Singh AR, Singh SA. The goal: Health for all. The commitment: All for health. Mens Sana Monogr. 2004; 2(1):97–110.

3. Mojekwu JN, Ibekwe U. Maternal mortality in Nigeria: Examination of intervention methods. International Journal of Humanities and Social Science 2012;2(20):135–149.

4. OlayinkaOA, Achi OS, Amos AO, et al. Awareness and barriers to utilization of maternal health care services among reproductive women in Amassoma community, Bayelsa State. Int J Nurs Midwifery. 2014 6(1):10–15. http://dx.doi.org/10.5897/IJNM2013.0108

5. Shaikh BT, Hatcher J. Health seeking behavior and health service utilisation in Pakistan: Challenging the policy makers. J Public Health (Oxf). 2004;27(1):49–54. http://dx.doi.org/10.1093/pubmed/fdh207

6. Muhammed KA, Umeh KN, Nasir SM, et al. Understanding the barriers to the utilization of primary health care in a low-income setting: implications for health policy and planning. J Public Health Africa. 2013;4(2):64–67. http://dx.doi.org/10.4081/jphia.2013.e13

7. Sule SS, Ijadunola KT, Onayade AA, et al. Utilization of primary health care facilities: Lessons from a rural community in southwest Nigeria. Niger J Med. 2008;17(1):98–106. http://dx.doi.org/10.4314/njm.v17i1.37366

8. Agyepong IA, Kangeya-Kayonda J. Providing practical estimates of malaria burden for health planners in resource-poor countries. Am J Trop Med Hyg. 2004;71 (2 Suppl):162–167.

9. Habib OS, Vaughan JP. The determinants of health services utilization in Southern Iraq: A household interview survey. Int J Epidemiol. 1986;15(3):395–403. http://dx.doi.org/10.1093/ije/15.3.395

10. Streefland PH. Public doubts about vaccination safety and resistance against vaccination. Health Policy. 2001;55(3):159–172. http://dx.doi.org/10.1016/S0168-8510(00)00132-9

11. Houweling TA, Ronsmans C, Campbell OM, et al. Huge poor–rich inequalities in maternity care: An international comparative study of maternity and child care in developing countries. Bull World Health Organ. 2007;85(10): 745–754. http://dx.doi.org/10.2471/BLT.06.038588

12. Chandwani H, Jivajarani P, Jivarajani H. Community perception and client satisfaction about the primary health care services in a tribal setting of Gujarat – India. The Internet Journal of Health. 2009;9(2):7.

13. National Population Commission (NPC). Nigerian population facts and figures [page on the Internet]. No date [cited 2014 Mar 16]. Accessed from: http://www.population.gov.ng/factsandfigures.htm [URL no longer valid]

14. Abbo C, Ekblad S, Waako W, et al. The prevalence and severity of mental illnesses handled by traditional healers in two districts in Uganda. Afr Health Sci. 2009;9(Suppl 1):S16–S22.

15. Esimai OA, Ojo OS, Fasubaa OB. Utilization of approved health facilities for delivery in Ile-Ife, Osun State, Nigeria. Nig J Med. 2002;11(4):177–179.

16. Allison PD. Multiple regression: A primer. Thousand Oaks, CA: Pine Forge Press; 1999.

17. Rose D, Pevalin DJ. The national statistics socio-economic classification: Unifying official and sociological approaches to the conceptualisation and measurement of social class. ISER working paper 2001-4. Institute for Social and Economic Research, University of Essex, Colchester.

18. Subedi J. Modern health services and health care behaviour: A survey in Kathmandu, Nepal. J Health Soc Behav. 1989;30(4):412–420. http://dx.doi.org/10.2307/2136989

19. Govere J, Durrheim D, La Grange K, et al. Community knowledge and perception about malaria and practices influencing malaria control in Mpumalanga province, South Africa. S Afr Med J. 2000;90(6):611-616.

20. Balabanova D, McKee M, Pomerleau J, et al. Health service utilisation in the former Soviet Union: Evidence from eight countries. Health Serv Res. 2004;39(6 pt 2):1927–1950. http://dx.doi.org/10.1111/j.1475-6773.2004.00326.x

21. Ademuwagun ZA. Determinants of pattern and degree of utilization of health services in Western State, Nigeria. Isr J Med Sci. 1997;13(9):896–907.

22. Nwakoby BN. Use of obstetric services in rural Nigeria. J R Soc Health. 1994;114(3):132–136. http://dx.doi.org/10.1177/146642409411400304

23. Swenson IE, Thang NM, Nhan VQ, et al. Factors related to the utilization of prenatal care in Vietnam. J Trop Med Hyg. 1993;96(2):76–85.

24. Chakraborty N, Islam MA, Chowdhury RI, et al. Determinants of the use of maternal health services in rural Bangladesh. Health Promot Int. 2003;18(4): 327–337. http://dx.doi.org/10.1093/heapro/dag414

25. Stock R. Distance and the utilization of health facilities in rural Nigeria. Soc Sci Med. 1983;17(9):563–570. http://dx.doi.org/10.1016/0277-9536(83)90298-8

7

Development of Family Medicine training in Botswana: Views of key stakeholders in Ngamiland

Authors:
Radiance M. Ogundipe[1]
Robert Mash[1]

Affiliations:
[1]Division of Family Medicine and Primary Care, Faculty of Medicine and Health Sciences, Stellenbosch University, Tygerberg, South Africa

Correspondence to:
Radiance Ogundipe

Email:
radiance.ogundipe@mopipi.ub.bw

Postal address:
PO Box 80903, Gaborone, Botswana

Background: Family Medicine training commenced in Botswana in 2011, and Maun was one of the two sites chosen as a training complex. If it is to be successful there has to be investment in the training programme by all stakeholders in healthcare delivery in the district.

Aim: The aim of the study was to explore the attitudes of stakeholders to initiation of Family Medicine training and their perspectives on the future roles of family physicians in Ngami district, Botswana.

Setting: Maun and the surrounding Ngami subdistrict of Botswana.

Methods: Thirteen in-depth interviews were conducted with purposively selected key stakeholders in the district health services. Data were recorded, transcribed and analysed using the framework method.

Results: Participants welcomed the development of Family Medicine training in Maun and expect that this will result in improved quality of primary care. Participants expect the registrars and family physicians to provide holistic health care that is of higher quality and expertise than currently experienced, relevant research into the health needs of the community, and reduced need for referrals. Inadequate personal welfare facilities, erratic ancillary support services and an inadequate complement of mentors and supervisors for the programme were some of the gaps and challenges highlighted by participants.

Conclusion: Family Medicine training is welcomed by stakeholders in Ngamiland. With proper planning introduction of the family physician in the district is expected to result in improvement of primary care.

Lancement d'une Formation en Médecine familiale au Botswana: Points de vue des principales parties prenantes au Ngamiland.

Contexte: On a commencé la Formation en Médecine familiale au Botswana en 2011, et Maun était l'un des deux sites choisis comme centre de formation. Pour que le projet réussisse il faut que tous les acteurs des prestations de soins de santé de la région s'investissent dans le programme de formation.

Objectif: L'étude avait pour but d'examiner les attitudes des parties prenantes envers le lancement d'une formation en médecine familiale et leurs points de vue concernant le futur rôle des médecins de famille dans le district de Ngami, au Botswana.

Lieu: Maun et le sous-district avoisinant de Ngami au Botswana.

Méthodes: On a effectué des entrevues avec des intervenants clé expressément sélectionnés parmi les services de santé du district. On a enregistré, transcrit et analysé les données suivant la méthodologie du cadre.

Résultats: Les participants ont bien accueilli le développement d'une Formation en Médecine familiale à Maun et espèrent que cela amènera une amélioration de la qualité des soins primaires. Les participants désirent que les directeurs et les médecins de famille offrent des soins de santé holistiques et une expertise de meilleure qualité que celle fournie à l'heure actuelle, fassent des recherches appropriées sur les besoins en santé de la communauté, et réduisent le besoin de référence. Les participants ont souligné certaines lacunes et défis tels que les services insuffisants de bien-être personnel, les services auxiliaires de soutien irréguliers et une équipe insuffisante de mentors et de surveillants pour le programme.

Conclusion: Les acteurs du Ngamiland ont bien accueilli la formation en médecine familiale. Avec une bonne planification, la mise en place d'un médecin de famille dans le district devrait améliorer les soins primaires.

Introduction

In response to the Alma-Ata Declaration of 1978, many developing countries embraced primary health care (PHC) as the most cost-effective approach to providing accessible and affordable health care for their people.[1] However, the benefits of this comprehensive and equitable approach to health care were not achieved in most countries of sub-Saharan Africa due to failure to address the socio-economic determinants of health problems, the introduction of vertical and disease-orientated health programmes in a selective PHC system, a short-term focus and a *laissez faire* approach to the emergence of unregulated commercialisation in health provision.[2,3] The World Health Report 2008, however, reiterates the need to strengthen PHC as the cornerstone of health systems.[3] The report recommends transformation from a focus on specific diseases and vertical programmes to PHC that comprehensively responds to all of the people's health needs. Furthermore, the report argues that countries with successful PHC systems have included doctors with postgraduate training in Family Medicine or general practice.[3]

Like many other African countries, Botswana adopted PHC as their strategy to improve healthcare delivery. To this end, the Government made organisational changes at both national and local levels. A department of Primary Health Care was established at national level to coordinate preventive, promotive, curative and rehabilitative health services. Prior to 2010 PHC was managed separately by the Ministry of Local Government, but it was subsequently transferred to the Ministry of Health.

District health teams were established to oversee implementation of the Government health policies at local level and to encourage community participation in healthcare delivery. The PHC approach in Botswana has been largely nurse-driven, with various different cadres of nurses providing the interventions. PHC is supported by a network of primary hospitals, which are currently functioning poorly with many gaps in service provision. A number of new and well-equipped district hospitals have been built, with posts for general specialists such as obstetricians, paediatricians and surgeons.

Botswana established its first medical school in 2008 and has just graduated its first fully home-trained medical graduates. There has been high attrition amongst the medical workforce over the years, with recruitment skewed in favour of secondary and tertiary care settings. In 2012 the density of doctors and nurses per 10 000 population was 3.4 and 31.4 respectively, and significantly lower in rural districts than in urban districts.[4] This has made it difficult to achieve the goal of accessible, high-quality PHC services at community level.[4] Access to specialist care is also difficult, and leads to significant mortality and complications as a result of referring patients over long distances.[4] Many of the medical officers in the district are currently foreign graduates with little understanding of local language and culture, a wide range of competencies, and no postgraduate education in Family Medicine.

In the light of these shortcomings in healthcare provision, Botswana has realised that introducing family physicians as expert generalists into its district healthcare system may help to solve some of these problems. Family Medicine was one of the initial postgraduate programmes introduced at the School of Medicine at the University of Botswana, and two training complexes were created in Maun and Mahalapye. The Botswana Health Professions Council has created a register for family physicians and the Ministry of Health appears committed to creating posts for the first cohort of locally trained family physicians in 2016. Recent policy documents suggest that family physicians will initially be placed at primary hospitals with outreach to the PHC platform.[4]

Although the core values and principles of Family Medicine are shared globally, the specific competencies and organisational principles that define the role of Family Medicine need to be explored in each region where the specialty is introduced.[5] The training programme for family physicians in Botswana has been significantly influenced by the established programme in South Africa.[6] The Botswana family physician is expected to have competencies appropriate to the District Health Services in the following clinical areas: Cardiology, Neurology, Nephrology, Gastro-enterology, Haematology, Oncology, Respiratory medicine, Endocrinology and Musculoskeletal, Dermatology, Ophthalmology and Ear-Nose-Throat (ENT); Consultation Skills; Women's Health; Internal Medicine; Surgery; Infectious diseases, HIV and/or AIDS, Tuberculosis (TB) and sexually transmitted diseases, and Emergency Medicine.[7]

It is expected that the family physician in Botswana will play the following roles in the health system:

- Practitioners with thorough knowledge, professionalism and requisite skills in Family Medicine, particularly those critical to the local environment;
- communicators and collaborators;
- managers capable of providing evidence-based, cost-effective patient care;
- advocates able to identify important social determinants of health affecting their patients and to advocate for their resolution;
- scholars committed to lifelong learning and clinical governance, and
- teachers educating and mentoring students and junior colleagues in the discipline of Family Medicine.[7]

These roles for the family physician in the district need to be explored with all stakeholders, taking into cognisance the district health needs, availability of other specialists, and cultural and socio-economic factors affecting the community.[8]

This study therefore sought to explore the perspective of key stakeholders in Maun and the surrounding Ngami subdistrict of Botswana on the new Family Medicine training programme and the future role of the family physician in the district health system.

Research methods and design

Study design

The study design was qualitative, utilising in-depth recorded interviews with each of the relevant stakeholders.

Setting

Ngami subdistrict is the southern half of the North West District of Botswana. The entire district, also known as Ngamiland, is made up of two subdistricts: Ngami and Okavango. The entire Ngamiland has a population estimated at 133 000.[9] Ngami subdistrict has a population estimated at 56 865,[9] and consists of Maun, a rural town with a population estimated at 48 000. It is divided into eight wards, each with a clinic or health post. There are 23 surrounding villages with a total estimated population of 8865.[9]

Health care in Ngami subdistrict is coordinated by a District Health Management Team consisting of the hospital arm and the PHC arm. Ngami subdistrict is served by 68 mobile clinic stops, 17 health posts, and five clinics with maternity units, three other clinics, and a district hospital. The district hospital, Letsholathebe II Memorial Hospital, is located in Maun and serves as a referral centre for all the facilities in Ngamiland. Although called a district hospital, it has separate specialist departments such as Medicine, Surgery, Obstetrics and gynaecology and Paediatrics.

The PHC clinics are run by PHC doctors, without postgraduate training, who consult patients, carry out minor procedures like suturing of lacerations, and refer patients that need admission. There is usually one doctor assigned to a clinic as well as general or family nurse practitioners, who also consult. The doctors in charge of the clinics regularly consult on a weekly outreach basis at other health facilities in the district to conduct health programmes on issues such as antiretroviral therapy or TB clinics. The nurses rely on the doctors for guidance whenever they are available at their clinic, and consult with them when they have patients with conditions beyond their capability. Although usually administered by the nurses, the district health programmes are also supervised and at times run by the clinic doctors.

The Family Medicine training programme in Botswana seeks to provide family physicians with enhanced competence and professionalism to support and strengthen healthcare delivery at the primary care clinics and primary hospitals. The training is a four-year programme entailing core modules and clinical rotations. The core modules include Communication, Ethics and Professionalism; Clinical research and Medical Literature; Principles and Techniques of Medical Education; Public Health Principles and International Health; Human Growth, Development and Family-orientated Primary Care; and Health Care Management and Administration. The clinical rotations are in the disciplines of Internal Medicine; Cardiology; Nephrology; Neurology; Endocrinology; Haematology; Musculoskeletal and Respiratory Medicine; Oncology; Women's Health; Infectious diseases – HIV and/or AIDS, TB, STDs; Surgery; Emergency Medicine; Dermatology; ENT; and Ophthalmology.[7]

During the rotations the registrars' learning is supervised by consultants at the district hospitals to which they are attached as well as family physicians who oversee their learning outcomes. The family physicians are responsible for supervising the primary care exposure of the registrars to ensure their grasp of the essential concepts of Family Medicine. There are eight registrars in the programme presently. At the end of the clinical rotations registrars are assessed for their ability to apply clinical knowledge, communication and clinical skills, judgement and decisiveness, and professional attributes and values.

Selection of key stakeholders

Purposeful sampling was used to select the interviewees who were key managers within the local district health system, and who had control over the training environment and service delivery platform, as well as senior clinicians. Fifteen key stakeholders were defined as follows: the coordinator of the district health management team, the managers of the district hospital (three people), the managers of PHC (three people), a principal medical officer from the hospital and PHC (two people), three doctors in charge of clinics, and three nurses in charge of clinics.

Data collection

Interviews were conducted over a six-week period in 2012, lasted between 30 and 45 minutes each, and were conducted in English by the researcher at a place convenient for the interviewees. An interview guide, shown in Box 1, was used to conduct the in-depth interviews, but respondents were allowed to express themselves freely in answering.

The opening question was: 'How do you feel about having these new Family Medicine registrars in the district?' Subsequent questions explored attitudes towards the training programme, perspectives on the future roles of family physicians, and issues that needed to be addressed by the health services. The interviews were audio-recorded, backed up by field notes, transcribed verbatim by a research assistant and checked in comparison to the recording by the researcher.

Data analysis

The transcribed data were analysed using the framework method.[10] After thorough familiarisation with the data a thematic index was developed by coding the data and organising the codes into categories using the Atlas-ti qualitative analysis software. The transcripts were indexed by systematically applying the codes in the thematic index to all the data. Charting was done to bring all data with the same codes together. These were then interpreted by the researcher to identify the range and depth of different themes and any relationships between themes.

BOX 1: Interview guide.

Opening question: 'How do you feel about having these new Family Medicine registrars in the district?'

Further questions were then used to explore the respondent's attitude towards the development of a Family Medicine training complex:

- How important is the development of the Family Medicine training complex for you?
- What do you think are some of the benefits of developing a Family Medicine training complex?
- What do you look forward to as the Family Medicine training complex develops?
- What are some of the difficulties that you anticipate in the development of a Family Medicine training complex?
- Do you have any concerns regarding the development of a Family Medicine training complex?

These questions were used to explore their perspective on the future role of family physicians and Family Medicine registrars in the district health care delivery system:

- Once these registrars graduate and become specialist family physicians, what role do you see them fulfilling in the district health system?
- What concerns do you have about having these specialist family physicians in the future?
- Do you anticipate any other difficulties?
- What do you think are the pros and cons of having specialist family physicians in the district health system?
- What impact or effect do you think these specialist family physicians will have on the district health system?

These questions were used to identify gaps in the training opportunities and facilities that need to be addressed to meet the standards of Family Medicine in sub-Saharan Africa:

- What changes do you think are necessary to your facility to make it suitable for training of Family Medicine?
- What are the main training opportunities that your facility can offer to registrars in Family Medicine?
- What essential training opportunities do you think the district will struggle to provide?
- Do you anticipate any issues with the supervision of these registrars?

HCW, healthcare workers.

Ethical considerations

The research was approved by the Health Research Ethics Committee at Stellenbosch University (Reference Number N/11/06/187) and the Ministry of Health Botswana Research and Ethics Board. The study was conducted according to the ethical guidelines and principles of the International Declaration of Helsinki, South African Guidelines for Good Clinical Practice and the Medical Research Council Ethical Guidelines for Research.

Results

Thirteen interviews were conducted, as the head of the district health management team had resigned and one principal medical officer refused consent. Interviews were conducted with the district chief public health officer, two senior managers at the hospital, the principal medical officer in charge of the clinics, doctors in charge of four clinics, and nurses in charge of five clinics. One audiotape of an interview with a doctor in charge of a clinic was discarded due to poor quality. The key themes that emerged from the interviews are described below.

Advent of Family Medicine training complex welcome

Most respondents were excited about the development of the Family Medicine training complex:

'The coming of the Family Medicine training especially in Maun is really welcomed. It has offered to us as a nation, a background where we can have the knowledge and skills. It has brought to us a forum to discuss from time to time as doctors and be closely guided.' (Doctor in charge of a clinic in Maun)

The training was expected to increase knowledge and information sharing through interactions between the registrars and other healthcare workers in the district. This was expected to facilitate upgrading of their skills and performance with improved health delivery to the community:

'It is important. Like I said, it is going to benefit the community and the health workers, not only the community but also health workers. They can get more information and new ideas from doctors who are doing Family Medicine.' (Nurse in charge of a clinic in Maun)

Some respondents felt the training would lead to better interaction between healthcare workers and the community, encouraging better understanding of community health needs whilst facilitating the appreciation of health services provided to the community. Others felt that the training will attract and enhance the retention of Batswana medical doctors who would have better understanding of the local culture and no language barrier. This, they felt, would improve patient-doctor interaction, and lead to better diagnosis and more holistic health provision at individual, family and community levels. Some felt that developing Maun into a Family Medicine training complex would offer the registrars an opportunity to experience life in a remote rural setting and encourage them to remain after graduation:

'By training here also, they will know it's a nice place and whenever they are posted here they will not hesitate to come. I think it's a good thing.' (Senior district administrator)

The Family Medicine training complex was seen as reducing inequity and bringing significant benefit to the community because of the remote location of Maun, far away from other urban centres where most of the specialists are usually based:

'So, bringing the training this side is a good thing because it will help us to develop this area at this level of health care and training people this side directly will also increase the number of healthcare providers that you can have who can work directly here.' (Principal medical officer)

Other benefits expressed as expectations of Family Medicine training in Maun were improved economic and social growth. The perceived benefits of the training complex are summarised in Figure 1.

Roles and expectations of Family Medicine registrars and family physicians

Family Medicine was expected to foster community engagement and champion community-oriented primary

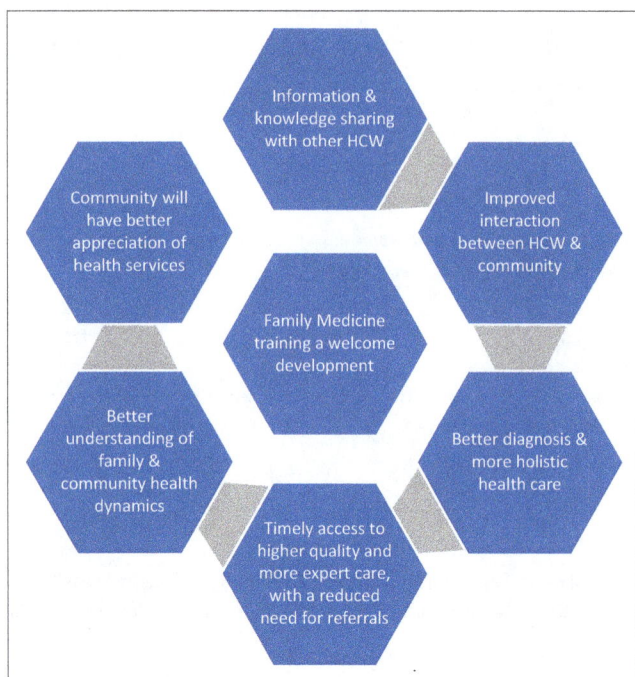

HCW, healthcare workers.

FIGURE 1: Expected benefits from the advent of Family Medicine training in Maun.

care. It was suggested that exposure of Family Medicine registrars and family physicians to the community would lead to a community diagnosis, with a better understanding of the causes of diseases and health conditions. Community identification with, acceptance of and participation in healthcare provision was also expected to result in greater benefits from the health services for the community:

'I think they will be better prepared in the sense that they will be managing the cases and the conditions of the people who surround them. So, I see them as having been better prepared unlike studying in a different place and sending them to another place to go and serve, [*then you*] meet more challenges unlike when you started, knowing exactly the type of community you are serving.' (Senior district nursing administrator)

Added one principal medical officer: 'The most important activity to embark on is to understand exactly the community and how they function; what are their needs?'

The Family Medicine registrars and physicians were also expected to understand family dynamics and their role in the disease processes, which should lead to more holistic patient care.

Other roles expected of the registrars and family physicians as a result of their closer interaction with the community included primary care research into the health needs and burden of disease in the community, stated by a nurse in charge of a clinic in Maun as follows: 'Family medicine being a specialty course on its own will enable further research and contribution into [*solving*] the problems patients are bringing forth.'

This primary care research, arising from issues identified within the community or at the primary care facility, was expected to yield findings that would be more acceptable

to the community and to bring about more effective interventions.

Another role expected of the registrars and family physicians was provision of high-quality health care and mentoring of other healthcare providers. The family physicians are expected to provide guidance and avail current evidence-based ways of caring for patients. Respondents felt that the family physicians will provide a critical mass of skilled and capable practitioners that will support high-quality healthcare at the community level:

'With this development, we can have people at hand and with proper organisation of specialist clinics regarding to health care in this district, we shall be able to have quite a number of skilled practitioners.' (Doctor in charge of a clinic in Maun)

Timely access to expert generalist care and reduced referrals to other specialists was another benefit expected from the presence of the registrars and family physicians. Expert generalist care of commonly presenting and locally prevalent conditions across many fields of health care was expected to be provided by the family physicians, although this was conceptualised as a combination of skills from other specialties:

'Family Medicine, as it incorporates all those specialities: obstetrics, gynaecology and what ... I think the whole community will benefit because, now it will be a doctor who has done Family Medicine who will be able to do all those ... in one person. So, you will be looking at the client holistically.' (Nurse in charge of a peripheral clinic)

Development of other healthcare workers through information sharing and clinical mentoring was another role expected of the registrars and family physicians, as stated by this nurse in charge of a clinic in Maun: 'So, they give information to staff members. So, the staff members benefit from the new information which they didn't know. Thus, those working are being empowered.'

However, one participant felt the advent of Family Medicine registrars and family physicians was a threat to other medical practitioners. He explained further that this threat to the job security of other generalist medical officers could materialise after some years:

'Those who are trained in family medicine, for them to work, they have to replace the doctors who were not trained then, that's ... that's where I can see some kind of friction coming there because it means, getting jobs, losing your job to somebody else.' (Doctor in charge of a clinic in Maun)

Participants did not anticipate problems with integration of the Family Medicine specialty into the district health system. Their views on the different roles of the registrars and family physicians are summarised in Figure 2.

Gaps in training opportunities and challenges of developing Family Medicine training

A number of personal lifestyle challenges and expectations of the registrars in this rural area were discussed. Personal

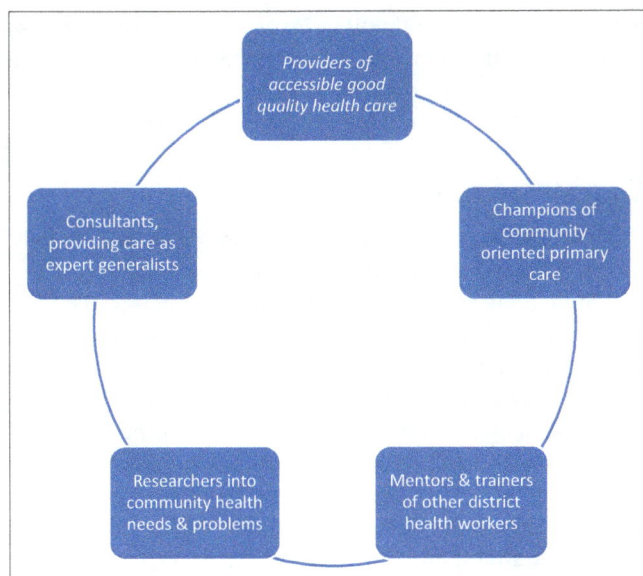

FIGURE 2: Summary of the roles expected from family physicians in Maun.

issues raised by participants included concerns about accommodation, transport, electricity, potable safe water and access to good-quality food. Although most respondents agreed that there is a need for the registrars to be trained at community level, they anticipated that this would be a challenge in terms of these personal issues:

'They can, they have to be accommodated so we have to find a place for that in Maun. I mean if this accommodation can be found and then when you go to places where water … running water is the problem, or electricity is not provided.' (Doctor in charge of a clinic in Maun)

Transport to 'hard to reach' areas such as the communities in the swamps of the Okavango Delta was viewed as particularly challenging. One participant actually felt that these personal issues may hinder recruitment for the programme, but others suggested starting with an initial low number of registrars and providing a retention allowance to compensate for the personal challenges involved in compulsory short- term rotations to rural facilities:

'But I feel if we have to retain them in this area, we need to change the issues around accommodation and to place a specific retention allowance for such people who accept to do service to people in the remote [areas].' (Senior health administrator in Maun)

Participants were concerned about the scale of the training programme and whether there would be sufficient infrastructure to accommodate a large number of registrars, even in the town of Maun. However, the general consensus was that the anticipated personal lifestyle challenges could be overcome by proper planning and resource allocation.

The general staff complement in the district health team was considered inadequate to provide a conducive learning environment to support the training of family physicians in Maun:

'If you place a family physician in a facility that is understaffed, he might end up doing a job of a simple nurse who has just

graduated and therefore dilute the whole reason why we place a family physician there.' (Senior district health administrator)

They also expressed concern that there may not be an adequate complement of family physicians and other specialists to supervise and mentor the registrars and ensure good-quality professional exposure and training in Maun:

'I think for a good training in Family Medicine, we would have loved to have all these specialists well represented here so that when the new physician is graduating, he or she becomes a rounded up somebody who has a hint of everything up to scratch.' (Senior district health administrator)

The reason for the dearth of specialists was attributed to the remoteness of Maun, and there were suggestions that the Government should consider providing incentives to attract specialists to assist with the training. Participants also felt that there could be financial challenges to the development of Maun into a Family Medicine training complex. They were concerned that the present Government budgetary constraints may impact adversely on the training:

'We need a budget which has been allocated to do those kinds of things to train the doctors. … even the people who train, maybe those professionals, who come from outside; the Government has to look into how the, the package … the remuneration for those kind of people, maybe it can be a challenge, a problem for the training to go on.' (Nurse in charge of a peripheral clinic)

One participant felt that the Government ought to see the financial commitment to the training as an investment which would have considerable future benefits. Another felt that if the Government prioritised the training, it would be feasible. A further participant believed that coping with deficiencies and learning to improvise were characteristics of working in remote areas, and should be an essential aspect of the training:

'I believe that is part of the training, to be able to work in any type of environment even if it is under a tent.' (Doctor in charge of a clinic in Maun)

Another issue that participants felt could affect learning opportunities for the Family Medicine training in Maun was substandard ancillary facilities:

'They will have loved to have all the right investigation support here, equipment like scan, sophisticated laboratories and X-ray facility. But what we have currently in Maun are just the basic things, and that might be a challenge to their learning process, it will limit them.' (Senior district health administrator)

The inadequate support facilities were also perceived as a limitation to the effective performance of the family physicians after they qualify. Inadequate drug supply was also expressed as a concern that could limit learning opportunities for the registrars and affect their future role as family physicians in the district:

'When they come here, do they have adequate drugs to use because that come from the central medical stores, and how regular[ly] are we going to receive our supplies?' (Senior district nursing administrator)

Supervision and mentoring of Family Medicine registrars

Participants felt that this was a crucial challenge to overcome for successful Family Medicine training. The need for adequate numbers of family physician trainers that have in-depth knowledge of Family Medicine and would be able to give the necessary hands-on training to the registrars was expressed:

> 'We need people that are qualified enough to supervise and monitor the students. Students come to provide services but they need to be guided, oriented and monitored and supervised in what they are doing. So, it will take someone who is qualified to know the needs of the students of the Family Medicine programme to be able to offer the right supervision.' (Principal medical officer in charge of clinics)

The need for specialists in other clinical specialties was also emphasised as a necessary prerequisite for the successful training of registrars, as the presently available family physicians will be inadequate to meet all aspects of their learning needs in other disciplines:

> 'We need doctors, specialised doctors ... who will be directly linked to the academics of these students, but who will be working in these hospitals where they will be attached to.' (Senior district health administrator)

There was also concern about the lack of a local benchmark for the quality of the training programme, especially considering the need for adherence to international standards whilst training with a locally relevant curriculum:

> 'Do we have the correct curriculum? That is going to determine the quality of doctors that we will, we are producing. ... But if we don't plan, again we don't plan well in teaching of these students concerned, we will have so many graduates ... but we will have mediocre type[s] of specialist[s].' (Senior district health administrator)

The possibility that the textbooks recommended for training may not be locally relevant was expressed as a concern. It was suggested that having a formalised training institute for Family Medicine may be a better approach for planning and developing the training complex. It was also felt that the present clinics and hospital may be substandard in design and thus not meet the prerequisites for acceptable Family Medicine training:

> 'The institutions in terms of infrastructure, for example, hospitals and clinics and other health facilities, were not constructed primarily for training. So they might not meet the prerequisites for training.' (Principal medical officer in charge of clinics)

Need for community awareness of Family Medicine

Some participants felt that a general lack of awareness of the nature and importance of Family Medicine by the community in Maun could be a challenge to the learning opportunities for the registrars and their future role as family physicians. The need to educate the community on the nature and importance of Family Medicine was seen as very important

to the success of the training in Maun. It was considered that community education and mobilisation will help prepare the way for the training complex and facilitate the integration of the family physician into the district health system.

Discussion

The participants welcomed the development of a Family Medicine training complex and anticipated better-quality and more holistic care, a reduced need for referral to higher levels of care, and more exploration of the social and family dynamics involved in health and disease. These expectations from key health stakeholders in the district suggest that they recognise many deficiencies in PHC and saw the advent of Family Medicine as part of a solution.

However, for respondents to see the introduction of Family Medicine training and later family physicians in the health system as a panacea for all the problems or deficiencies in primary care may also be unrealistic and create expectations that cannot be fulfilled. As the impact of Family Medicine was still largely aspirational, it was probably difficult for respondents to clearly identify the limits of the likely impact. Overall respondents were hopeful and expressed the need for the necessary budgetary allocation and incentives to ensure the successful development of the discipline and its integration into the health system of the country.

In a recent study exploring the views of key academic and government leaders in some African countries on Family Medicine, the respondents similarly expressed their expectation that Family Medicine will lead to improved quality and more comprehensive health care, and reduce referrals to the overburdened higher level of health care.[11] This expectation was reported to be a reality in the Western Cape, South Africa, when the impact of Family Medicine on district healthcare delivery was evaluated.[12]

In another evaluation, also in the Western Cape, family physicians and registrars were perceived by the district health managers to have made positive impacts on the clinical processes of key medical conditions like trauma, HIV and/or AIDS care, TB and chronic non-communicable diseases.[13] However, this impact was not uniform across the province, depending on the number of family physicians available and their differing abilities to function optimally. Although the impact was perceived to be in the early stages of development, participants in the study remarked that this positive impact had increased the acceptance of the specialty and the demand by junior doctors for training as family physicians. Other aspects of the district health system perceived to have been impacted positively by the family physicians and registrars included access to health care, coordination of health services, comprehensiveness of health service provision and efficiency of health delivery.[13]

The roles of family physicians in South Africa have been described as care provider, consultant to the PHC team, capacity builder and mentor to other healthcare workers;

supervisors of junior doctors and medical students, and champion of clinical governance and community-orientated primary care.[12] These were similar to the roles expected of family physicians and registrars by key health stakeholders in Maun, although they expressed a greater interest in research at community level. The roles identified in the study are also consistent with those agreed to in the regional consensus statement on Family Medicine.[8]

Challenges to the development of Maun as a Family Medicine training complex expressed by the stakeholders are indeed genuine concerns. The performance of the first cohort of family physicians trained will influence others who may consider training in the future. It will also influence the credibility and recognition of the discipline by specialists in other clinical domains.[12,13]

Inadequacies of training facilities, mentors and supervisors can be detrimental to the quality of the family physicians produced. Training programmes also tend to undergo a development journey, as has been seen in South Africa. Initial training was strongly based in the regional hospitals under the supervision of other specialists. This was because there were insufficient family physicians in the district platform and facilities were poorly developed to train on all the skills required. This initial model was also necessary to get buy-in from the other specialists on the training of family physicians. However, registrars often felt orphaned in specialist departments and were not trained in the correct context. Subsequently, however, training has largely shifted into the district under the direct supervision of family physicians.[12] One can anticipate a similar shift over time in the Botswana context.

Poor working conditions may also discourage further intake of registrars into the training programme. A suggestion to donor organisations to commit 15% of their budgets to the strengthening of PHC systems in developing countries rather than vertical disease-orientated programmes may be an avenue to explore for financial leverage to address the working conditions and some of the infrastructural inadequacies that will be a challenge to the success of the programme.[14]

At the recent First Botswana Family Medicine Conference, held in May 2013 in Gaborone, the collaborative support of Stellenbosch University for the University of Botswana in the development of Family Medicine was acknowledged. This collaboration may help to build capacity amongst the new academic staff and faculty members.

There is a need in Botswana for family physicians to be employed in the health services as role models and mentors and not just as academics. There is also a need to decide whether they will be employed at the primary care level or at primary hospitals. If, as seems likely, they will initially be employed at primary hospitals to meet a critical skills gap, this will follow the pattern seen in South Africa, but differ considerably from the role of the frontline general

practitioner in Europe and America. In South Africa the family physician as a well-trained scarce resource is now focusing more on the subdistrict as a whole, and whilst based at a hospital would provide extensive outreach to the primary care services.[15] Botswana, with its relatively small population and middle-income status, seems more able to employ doctors at all the clinics, and could in future move towards ensuring they have postgraduate training. It was also proposed at the conference that the support of the private health sector should be explored in developing the Family Medicine programme.

Opinions of the key health stakeholders interviewed in this study seem strongly in favour of retaining Maun as a training location, rather than shifting the training closer to Gaborone, as suggested by some participants at the conference. This is supported by findings in the Western Cape and Gelukspan health ward in South Africa, where training of the registrars in rural communities enhanced their understanding of the health issues and increased the chance that they would remain in those communities after graduation.[12,14,16] Relocating the training closer to an urban setting may also further perpetuate inequitable distribution of healthcare provision.[17]

Limitations

A few participants might have expressed themselves more fully if the interview had been conducted in Setswana. The researcher (R.M.O.) was a Family Medicine registrar at the time this study was done, and has a deep desire for the successful integration of the specialty into the health system in Botswana. Although he did his level best to remain neutral whilst conducting the interviews, this interest could have affected his perception of the views expressed by the respondents. R.M.O. has worked as a senior level officer in the health team in Maun for more than six years, in both the clinics and the hospital. Most of the respondents are known to him and some have worked with him. This fact may also have affected the way they expressed their views, despite assurances of confidentiality. The Principal Medical Officer who declined to participate in the study for undisclosed reasons could have provided an alternative viewpoint, but his reason for declining is not known. Similarly, the audio file of one of the clinic doctors that was discarded owing to poor audio quality could have provided additional information. However, by continuous familiarisation with the data during the interviewing phase, it was concluded that no new themes were emerging after the eleventh interview.

Implications and recommendations

The following recommendations can be made on the basis of this study:

- There is an urgent need to improve working conditions and develop incentive packages to attract and retain health workers in the rural areas of Botswana.
- Maun should be retained as a rural training complex within the Family Medicine training programme.

- The University of Botswana will need to explore ways of incorporating family physicians in clinical practice into the programme.
- The supply of resources to district level medical facilities should be improved so as to create a better training environment.
- Maun as a training complex will need to develop measures for evaluating the impact of the registrars and Family Medicine on PHC in the district.
- Research to evaluate the cost-effectiveness and impact of the introduction of family physicians in similar districts in sub-Saharan Africa will be useful to demonstrate objectively the benefits of Family Medicine.

Conclusion

Key health stakeholders in Ngamiland support the need for the training of Family Medicine registrars and placement of family physicians in the district health services in Maun. The roles described for the family physicians by the stakeholders are consistent with the roles identified in South Africa and the broader region.

Gaps in facility infrastructure, resources and learning opportunities may be a challenge to the development of the training complex.

There was a generally optimistic outlook by the stakeholders that with proper planning the challenges would be overcome, and PHC in the district would benefit from the introduction of Family Medicine registrars and family physicians.

Acknowledgements

I am grateful to the University of Botswana Family Medicine Department and Medical Education Partnership Initiative (MEPI) for allowing me to use the department's digital audio recorder for my interviews, and for the initial take-off grant. I am also grateful to Stellenbosch University Rural Medical Education Partnership Initiative (SURMEPI) for the grant awarded to me that facilitated my completion of the research and also enabled me to attend the first Botswana Family Medicine conference. I am deeply appreciative of my supervisor, Prof. Bob Mash, for his dedicated supervision and encouraging corrections, which made this research a reality. I appreciate Dr Luise Parsons, formerly acting coordinator for Family Medicine training in Maun (now running her own private facility), for her encouragement and for allowing me to include her for my pilot interview. I appreciate the assistance of every one of the key health stakeholders in Ngami who consented to be interviewed for this study.

Competing interests

The authors declare that they have no financial or personal relationship(s) that may have inappropriately influenced them in writing this article.

Authors' contributions

R.M.O. (Stellenbosch University) was the primary researcher as a registrar in Family Medicine with Stellenbosch University. Under the supervision of R.M. (Stellenbosch University), R.M.O. conducted the interviews, analysed the data and wrote the draft of the article. The draft article was reviewed with corrections and suggestions by R.M., and he also approved the final manuscript.

References

1. International Conference on Primary Health Care, Alma-Ata, USSR, 6–12 September 1978, Declaration of Alma-Ata [document online]. Sept 1978 [cited 2015 Mar 25]. Available from: www.who.int/publications/almaata_declaration_en.pdf

2. Werner D, Sanders D. Questioning the solution: The politics of primary health care and child survival. Palo Alto: Healthwrights; 1997.

3. World Health Organization. The World Health Report 2008: Primary Health Care now more than ever [book on the Internet]. c2008 [cited 2013 Jul 13]. Available from: www.who.int/whr/2008/en/

4. Nkomazana O, Peersman W, Wilcox M, Mash R, Phaladze N. Human resources for health in Botswana: The result of in-country database and reports analysis. Afr J Prim Health Care Fam Med. 2014;6(1), Art # 716 dx. doi:10.4102/phcfm.v6:1.716

5. Mash B. The definition of family medicine in sub-Saharan Africa. S Afr Fam Pract J. 2008;50(3):58–59. http://dx.doi.org/10.1080/20786204.2008.10873719

6. Couper I, Mash B, Smith S, Shweitzer B. Outcomes for family medicine postgraduate training in South Africa. S Afr Fam Pract J. 2012;54(6):501–506. http://dx.doi.org/10.1080/20786204.2012.10874283

7. University of Botswana. Course outline for the MMED in Family Medicine. Gaborone: University of Botswana; 2011.

8. Mash R, Reid S. Statement of consensus on Family Medicine in Africa. Afr J Prim Health Care Fam Med. 2010;2(1). doi:10.4102/phcfm.V2i 1.151

9. Central Statistics Office. Population census. Gaborone: Central Statistics Office; 2011 [cited online 2013 Jul 17]. Available from: www.cso.gov.bw

10. Ritchie J, Spencer L. Qualitative data analysis for applied policy research. In: Bryman A, Burgess RG, editors. Analysing qualitative data. London: Routledge, 1994; p. 173–194. http://dx.doi.org/10.4324/9780203413081_chapter_9

11. Moosa S, Downing R, Mash R, Reid S, Essuman A. Understanding of family medicine in Africa: A qualitative study of leaders' views. Br J Gen Pract. 2013. doi:10.3399/bjgp13x664261

12. Mash B. Reflection on the development of family medicine in Western Cape: A 15-year review. S Afr Fam Pract J. 2011;53(6):557–562. http://dx.doi.org/10.1080/20786204.2011.10874152

13. Swanepoel M, Mash B, Naledi T. Assessment of the impact of family medicine in the district health system of Western Cape, South Africa. Afr J Prim Health Care Fam Med. 2014;6(1). Art. #695, 8 pages. http://dx.doi.org/10.4102/phcfm.v6i1.695

14. Mash R. Family medicine is coming of age in sub-Saharan Africa. S Afr Fam Pract J. 2008;50(6):50–51.

15. Mash B. The contribution of family physicians to district health services: A position paper for the National Department of Health [document on Internet]. 2014 [cited 2015 Jun 24]. Available from: www.saafp.org/index.php/news/48-national-position-paper-on-familymedicine

16. De Jonge M. Sound primary health care demands a strong role for family medicine. S Afr Fam Pract J. 1995;16:161–171.

17. Boelen C, Haq C, Hunt V, Rivo M, Shahady E. Improving health systems: The contribution of family medicine. A guidebook. Singapore: Wonca, 2002; p. 140–143.

8

Knowledge and practices about multidrug-resistant tuberculosis amongst healthcare workers in Maseru

Authors:
Ntambwe Malangu[1]
Omotayo D. Adebanjo[1]

Affiliations:
[1]Department of Epidemiology & Biostatistics, University of Limpopo, Medunsa Campus, South Africa

Correspondence to:
Ntambwe Malangu

Email:
gustavmalangu@gmail.com

Postal address:
PO Box 215, Medunsa 0204, South Africa

Background: To date, no study has been found that described the knowledge and practices of healthcare workers surrounding multidrug-resistant tuberculosis (MDR-TB) in Lesotho.

Aim and setting: This study was conducted to fill this gap by investigating the knowledge level and practices surrounding MDR-TB amongst healthcare workers at Botsabelo Hospital in Maseru, Lesotho.

Method: This was a cross-sectional survey conducted by means of a questionnaire designed specifically for this study. Data collected included sociodemographic and professional details; and responses to questions about knowledge and practices regarding MDR-TB. The questions ranged from the definition of MDR-TB to its treatment. Respondents' practices such as the use of masks, guidelines and patient education were also assessed.

Results: A response rate of 84.6% (110 out of 130) was achieved. The majority of participants were women (60%), married (71.8%) and nursing staff (74.5%). Overall, less than half (47.3%) of the participants had a good level of knowledge about MDR-TB. With regard to practice, about 83% of participants stated that they used protective masks whilst attending to MDR-TB patients. About two-thirds (66.4%) reported being personally involved in educating patients about MDR-TB; whilst about 55% stated that they referred to these guidelines.

Conclusion: The level of knowledge about MDR-TB amongst healthcare workers at the study site was not at an acceptable level. Unsafe practices, such as not wearing protective masks and not referring to the MDR-TB treatment guidelines, were found to be associated with an insufficient level of knowledge about MDR-TB. An educational intervention is recommended for all healthcare providers at this facility.

Connaissances et pratiques du personnel de santé de Maseru au sujet de la tuberculose multi-résistante.

Contexte: A ce jour, on n'a pas trouvé d'étude qui décrive les connaissances et pratiques des professionnels de la santé sur la tuberculose multi-résistante (MDR-TB) au Lesotho.

Objectif et cadre: Cette étude a été menée pour combler cette lacune en étudiant le niveau des connaissances et les pratiques relatives à la MDR-TB parmi le personnel de santé à l'Hôpital Botsabelo de Maseru, Lesotho.

Méthode: Cette étude transversale a été effectuée au moyen d'un questionnaire conçu spécifiquement pour cette étude. Les données collectées comprennent des informations sociodémographiques et professionnelles; et des réponses à des questions sur les connaissances et pratiques relatives à la MDR-TB. Les questions allaient de la définition de la MDR-TB à son traitement. Les pratiques des personnes interrogées telles que l'utilisation de masques, les directives et l'éducation des patients ont aussi été évaluées.

Résultats: On a obtenu un taux de réponse de 84.6% (110 sur 130). La majorité des participants étaient des femmes (60%), mariées (71.8%) et des infirmières (74.5%). En tout, moins de la moitié (47.3%) des participants avait un bon niveau de connaissances sur la MDR-TB. En ce qui concerne la pratique, environ 83% des participants ont déclaré qu'ils utilisaient des masques protecteurs pendant qu'ils s'occupaient des patients souffrant de MDR-TB. Environ les deux tiers (66.4%) ont déclaré qu'ils s'occupaient personnellement d'éduquer les patients sur la MDR-TB; alors que 55% ont dit qu'ils se référaient à ces directives.

Conclusion: Le niveau des connaissances sur la MDR-TB parmi le personnel de santé sur le lieu de l'étude n'était pas à un niveau acceptable. Des pratiques dangereuses, comme de ne pas porter de masque protecteur et de ne pas se référer aux directives de traitement pour la MDR-TB, étaient associées à un niveau de connaissances insuffisant sur la MDR-TB. Il est donc recommandé d'organiser une formation éducative pour tous les professionnels de santé de cet établissement.

Introduction

Lesotho is one of the countries with the highest *per capita* incidence of tuberculosis (TB) in the world. With 637 incident cases of TB per 100 000 people, it was the fifth most affected country by 2006.[1] Despite having achieved a high detection rate of 84% and adopted the directly observed therapy short-course (DOTS) strategy, several cases of multidrug-resistant tuberculosis (MDR-TB) had been reported since 2005. By 2009, a least 259 cases of MDR-TB had been identified in a total population of about 1.8 million people.[2,3] Given this alarming figure, it is imperative that healthcare providers in Lesotho be knowledgeable about MDR-TB and be able to adopt practices to curb further transmission of this serious condition.

Although it is generally assumed that healthcare service workers (HCWs) know about MDR-TB and its implications, the evidence from several studies worldwide have found that HCWs do not always have sufficient knowledge or the correct positive attitude; and do not exhibit acceptable practices regarding prevention and treatment of MDR-TB.[4,5,6,7,8] To date, no study has been found describing the knowledge and practices of HCWs with regard to MDR-TB at Botsabelo Hospital in Maseru, Lesotho.

This study was conducted to fill this gap by investigating the knowledge level and practices surrounding MDR-TB amongst HCWs at this health facility. It is hoped that the findings from the study could be used by decision makers and institutional managers so as to design and implement interventions to address the shortcomings that were identified.

Research methods and design

Study design

This cross-sectional study was conducted by means of a questionnaire designed for the study, taking into account other published questionnaires and the World Health Organization's MDR-TB management guidelines.[9] Besides sociodemographic and professional data, knowledge about MDR-TB was assessed by asking questions about the definition of MDR-TB, its aetiology, diagnosis, symptoms and treatment modalities. The knowledge level was categorised as good if a respondent scored at least 80%; and insufficient if the score was less than 80%. Participants' practices with regard to MDR-TB were assessed by asking them whether they possessed a copy of the MDR-TB treatment guidelines, whether they referred to these guidelines, whether they were involved in educating patients on MDR-TB and whether they reported using protective masks whilst attending to patients with MDR-TB.

Study population

This questionnaire was semi-structured, anonymous and self-administered. Given the small number of the targeted population, the questionnaire was sent to all 130 HCWs working at Botsabelo hospital, based on the information from the hospital human resources database. This referral hospital in Maseru district has 24 beds for MDR-TB patients and serves nine other districts.

Specially-designed collection boxes were placed in convenient places for participants to drop off the completed questionnaires. The boxes were in place from 23 September to 15 October 2010.

Data analysis

The field worker collected the returned questionnaires from the boxes, checked each one of them for completeness and numbered them. Data were captured into a Microsoft Excel® spreadsheet and imported into STATA 10 (www.stata.com 2007) for data analysis. Cross-tabulation was performed in order to assess the association between variables. The level of statistical significance was set at < 0.05.[10]

Ethical considerations

The Medunsa Research Ethics Committee of the University of Limpopo approved the study (Reference: MREC/H/99/2010: PG) and the permission to conduct the survey at the study site was obtained from the managers at the institution.

Results

Sociodemographic profile of participants

Of the 130 participants who received the questionnaire, 110 returned completed questionnaires – a response rate of 84.6%. The majority of participants were women (*n* = 66; 60%), married (*n* = 79; 71.8%) and nursing staff (*n* = 82; 74.5%). The mean age of participants was 30.76 ± 6.84 years old, with ages ranging from 20 to 56 years. Two age categories were

TABLE 1: Sociodemographic details of the participants.

Variables	*n*	%
Age category		
< 30 years old	64	58.2
> 30 years old	46	41.8
Gender		
Male	44	40.0
Female	66	60.0
Professional category		
Medical doctors	12	10.9
Nurses	82	74.5
Pharmacists	9	8.2
Counsellors	7	6.4
Work experience category		
Five years or less	60	54.5
Over 5 years	50	45.5
Marital status		
Single	28	25.5
Married	79	71.8
Divorced	2	1.8
Widowed	1	0.9
Knowledge level		
Good knowledge level	52	47.3
Insufficient knowledge level	58	52.7

created based on the median age of 30 years; the majority of participants (n = 64; 58.2%) were younger than 30 years of age, with 60 (54.5%) having five or less years of working experience, as is shown in Table 1.

Participants' knowledge about multidrug-resistant tuberculosis

The mean knowledge score of the participants was 74% ± 14.3%, ranging from 40% to 100% of correct answers. Overall, less than half (47.3%) of participants had good knowledge about MDR-TB. Participants gave incorrect answers about what constituted MDR-TB, how it is diagnosed, and the duration of treatment. As shown in Table 2, the level of knowledge differed based on the age and professional category of the participants.

There were no significant differences between male and female participants, or between those with different numbers of years of work experience (p > 0.05), as is shown in Table 3.

With regard to professional category, medical doctors showed a significantly better level of knowledge about MDR-TB than nurses and counsellors, but the difference was not significant when compared with pharmacists (p = 0.09).

Participants' practices with regard to multidrug-resistant tuberculosis

With regard to practice, about 83% (n = 91) of the participants stated that they used protective masks whilst attending to MDR-TB patients. About two-thirds (n = 73; 66.4%) of the participants reported being involved in educating patients about MDR-TB. Moreover, some 61.8% (n = 68) reported having their own copy of the MDR-TB treatment guidelines; and about 55% (n = 60) stated that they referred to these guidelines. These practices differed based on the professional category and other characteristics of the participants. For instance, 11 (91.7%) of the medical doctors and 74 (90.2%) of the nurses reported wearing protective masks; in contrast, only four (57.1%) of the counsellors and two (22.2%) of the pharmacists reported doing so. Moreover, pharmacists were the least involved in educating patients about MDR-TB –

TABLE 3: Odd ratios of features associated with good knowledge level.

Variables	Odds ratio (95% CI)	p-value
Age (Over 30 years vs. < 30 years old)	1.21 (0.56, 2.59)	0.63
Working experience (< 5 years vs. > 5 years)	1.09 (0.51, 2.35)	0.81
Male versus female	1.03 (0.48, 2.23)	0.94
Doctors versus nurses	6.28 (1.42, 44.40)	0.01
Doctors versus pharmacists	5.66 (0.77, 57.56)	0.09
Doctors versus counsellors	10.46 (1.22, 132.40)	0.03

more than half of them (n = 5; 55.6%) reported not being involved. On the contrary, 71.4% (n = 5) of the counsellors were involved in educating patients as well as 69.5% (n = 57) of the nurses and 58.8% (n = 7) of the medical doctors.

It is noteworthy that participants with a good level of knowledge about MDR-TB were more involved in educating patients about the disease as compared with those with insufficient knowledge (n = 48, 75% versus n = 19, 58.5%; p = 0.07). In contrast, 41.2% (n =14) of participants with an insufficient level of knowledge about MRD-TB did not participate in educating patients, whilst a quarter of those with insufficient level of knowledge did not wear protective masks when attending to MDR-TB patients (n = 7, 25.9% versus n = 4, 7.7%; p = 0.01).

Furthermore, based on the professional category, all of the counsellors reported that they do not refer to the MDR-TB treatment guidelines, whereas three-quarters of the medical doctors (n = 9; 75%) reported doing so, as did 56.1% (n = 46) of the nurses and 55.6% (n = 5) of the pharmacists. Interestingly, it was found that participants with a good level of knowledge referred to the MDR-TB management guidelines more significantly than those with an insufficient level of knowledge (n = 50, 66% versus n = 15, 44.1%; p = 0.03). Overall, participants older than 30 years, men and those with more than five years of work experience, referred more to the MDR-TB treatment guidelines than their counterparts, but the differences were not of statistical significance (p > 0.05).

Discussion

The findings from this study show that the majority of participants were women, young adults and nurses.

TABLE 2: Participants' level of knowledge.

Variables	Good level of knowledge		Insufficient level of knowledge		Total	
	n	%	n	%	n	%
Age category						
Less than 30 years	29	45.3	35	54.7	64	100
30 years and above	23	50	23	50	46	100
Gender						
Male	21	47.7	23	52.3	44	100
Female	31	47	35	53	66	100
Professional category						
Doctors	10	83.3	2	16.7	12	100
Nurses	36	43.9	46	56.1	82	100
Pharmacists	4	44.4	5	55.6	9	100
Counsellors	2	28.6	5	71.4	7	100
Work experience category						
5 years or less	29	48.3	31	51.7	60	100
Over 5 years	23	46	27	54	50	100

This distribution is consistent with the composition of the healthcare workforce in Lesotho, where 73.3% are nurses and mostly women.[11]

In line with the purpose of the study, it is disappointing to note that less than half of the participants had a good level of knowledge about MDR-TB. The deficits in knowledge identified were about what constituted MDR-TB, how it is diagnosed and the duration of its treatment. These knowledge gaps are similar to what had been reported by other investigators.[4,5,8,12,13]

Based on personal characteristics such as age, gender and number of years of working experience, there is no evidence from this study to suggest that there was any statistically-significant difference amongst participants with regard to their knowledge of MDR-TB. However, based on professional category, more nurses and pharmacists had an insufficient level of knowledge as compared with medical doctors. This deficit in knowledge was even more pronounced amongst counsellors, as 71.4% of them had insufficient level of knowledge about MDR-TB. These findings are similar to reports by other investigators such as Kiefer et al.[5] and Ahmed et al.,[12] raising some concerns in that counsellors who educate patients about MDR-TB are themselves not so knowledgeable about it. This observation suggests that there is an urgent need for counsellors to be educated on MDR-TB and other aspects regarding tuberculosis treatment and care.

With regard to other practices relating to MDR-TB, given the usefulness of treatment management guidelines, it is unacceptable that about 40% of participants reported not having their own copy of the treatment guidelines. This situation is unacceptable because the guidelines are documents that every HCW should possess in order to ensure consistency and quality in the delivery of healthcare and services.[14,15,16] It is important that institutional managers address this issue by making the guidelines available to all HCWs at the study site and at other healthcare facilities in the country.

With regard to the practice of using protective masks, although this study did not investigate whether these masks were purchased regularly and always available to staff members, about 17% of the participants reported that they did not used protective masks when they were in contact with MDR-TB patients. This is not acceptable, as all HCWs should use protective masks when dealing with MDR-TB patients. This is particularly important for pharmacists and counsellors who, routinely, are not provided with protective masks and are thus exposed to infection. This situation should be remedied because by protecting these HCWs, their family members and all other persons they interact with will be also protected.[17,18]

An important and encouraging finding from this study is that participants with good knowledge about MDR-TB were reported to use protective masks more significantly than those with an insufficient level of knowledge about MDR-TB

($p = 0.01$). This finding suggests that by increasing the level of knowledge it is possible to get a higher compliance with preventive interventions amongst HCWs. This is of utmost importance in order to avoid an increase in the burden of tuberculosis as an occupational disease amongst HCWs in Lesotho, as has been reported in other settings such as China.[19]

With regard to educating patients about MDR-TB, although two-thirds (66.4%) of the participants reported being involved in patient education, it is disconcerting that the majority of pharmacists were not involved in this important public heath activity. Whether this is due to increased workload or lack of initiative, it is critical that pharmacists participate in educating patients about MDR-TB, particularly regarding the pharmacotherapeutic aspects of the disease.[20] This is even more important given the finding from this study that counselors, as community health workers with a high school education, displayed an insufficient level of knowledge about MDR-TB but were reportedly educating patients about the disease.

With regard to the practice of referring to the treatment guidelines, about 55% of the participants reported that they referred to them. This is a worrying finding; even more so in that none of the counsellors reported *ever* referring to these guidelines. Although this finding is consistent with a report by several other investigators who stated that a good number of healthcare practitioners fail to comply with clinical practice guidelines, this needs to be corrected.[21,22,23] Although it is not established whether the guidelines manuals were purchased and made available to HCWs at the study site, institutional managers ought to ensure that clinical practice and management guidelines, including the MDR-TB treatment guidelines, should be made available to every HCW in the healthcare system. The above findings present the situation about MDR-TB at the time the study was conducted and may not be a permanent feature at the study site and throughout the country. Another limitation is that since this was a cross-sectional survey, causal relationships could not be established.

Conclusion

In conclusion, the level of knowledge about MDR-TB amongst HCWs, especially amongst nursing and allied health staff members as compared to medical doctors at the study site, was not at an acceptable level. The insufficient level of knowledge was associated with unsafe practices, such as not wearing protective masks, as well as not owning and not referring to the MDR-TB treatment guidelines. An educational intervention is recommended as well as an allocation of funds for the purchase of required protective equipment and clinical practice management guidelines and manuals.

Acknowledgements

All staff members at the study site are gratefully acknowledged for their contribution to this work.

Competing interests

The authors declare that they have no financial or personal relationship(s) that may have inappropriately influenced them in writing this article.

Authors' contributions

D.O. (University of Limpopo) completed the field work and N.M. (University of Limpopo) analysed the data and drafted the manuscript. Both authors conceptualised the research and provided intellectual input for the manuscript.

References

1. World Health Organization. WHO report 2009: global tuberculosis control. Epidemiology, strategy, financing [document on the Internet]. c2009 [cited 2009 Nov 24]. Available from: http://whqlibdoc.who.int/publications/2009/9789241563802_eng_doc.pdf

2. Satti H, McLaughlin MM, Hedt-Gauthier B, et al. Outcomes of multidrug-resistant tuberculosis treatment with early initiation of antiretroviral therapy for HIV co-infected patients in Lesotho. PLoS ONE. 2012;7(10):e46943. http://dx.doi.org/10.1371/journal.pone.0046943

3. Seung KJ, Omatayo DB, Keshavjee S, et al. Early outcomes of MDR-TB treatment in a high HIV-prevalence setting in Southern Africa. PLoS ONE. 2009;4(9):e7186. http://dx.doi.org/10.1371/journal.pone.0007186

4. Al-Maniri AA, Al-Rawas OA, Al-Ajmi F, et al. Tuberculosis suspicion and knowledge among private and public general practitioners: questionnaire based study in Oman. BMC Public Health. 2008;8:177. http://dx.doi.org/10.1186/1471-2458-8-177

5. Kiefer E, Shao T, Carasquillo O, et al. Knowledge and attitudes of tuberculosis management in San Juan de Lurigancho district of Lima, Peru. J Infect Dev Ctries. 2009;3(10):783–788.

6. Loveday M, Thomson L, Chopra M, et al. A health systems assessment of the KwaZulu-Natal tuberculosis programme in the context of increasing drug resistance. Int J Tuberc Lung Dis. 2008;12(9):1042–1047.

7. Naidoo S, Taylor M, Jinabhal CC. Critical risk factors driving the tuberculosis epidemic in Kwazulu-Natal, South Africa. South Afr J Infect Dis. 2007;22(2/3):45–49.

8. Vandan N, Ali M, Prasad R, et al. Assessment of doctors' knowledge regarding tuberculosis management in Lucknow, India: A public-private sector comparison. Public Health. 2009;123(7):484–489. http://dx.doi.org/10.1016/j.puhe.2009.05.004

9. World Health Organization. Management of MDR-TB: A field guide. A companion document to Guidelines for the programmatic management of drug-resistant tuberculosis [document on the Internet]. c2008 [cited 2009 Nov 24]. Available from: http://whqlibdoc.who.int/publications/2009/9789241547765_eng.pdf

10. Somekh B. Educational research. In: Somekh B, Lewin C, editors. Research methods in the social sciences. London: Sage Publications Ltd., 2005; pp. 7–8.

11. Mwase T, Kariisa E, Doherty J, et al. Lesotho health systems assessment 2010. Bethesda, MD: Health Systems 20/20, Abt Associates Inc.

12. Ahmed M, Fatmi Z, Ali S, et al. Knowledge, attitude and practice of private practitioners regarding TB-DOTS in a rural district of Sindh, Pakistan. J Ayub Med Coll Abbottabad. 2009;21(1):28–31.

13. Jurcev Savicević A. Gaps in tuberculosis knowledge among primary health care physicians in Croatia: Epidemiological study. Coll Antropol. 2009;33(2):481–486.

14. Richardson NL. Evaluating provider prescribing practices for the treatment of tuberculosis in Virginia, 1995 to 1998: An assessment of educational need. J Contin Educ Health Prof. 2000;20(3):146–155. http://dx.doi.org/10.1002/chp.1340200303

15. Gai R, Xu L, Wang X, et al. The role of village doctors on tuberculosis control and the DOTS strategy in Shandong Province, China. Biosci Trends. 2008;2(5):181–186.

16. World Health Organization. Guidelines for the programmatic management of drug-resistant tuberculosis: 2011 update [document on the Internet]. c2011 [cited 2013 Nov 26]. Available from: http://www.whqlibdoc.who.int/publications/2011/9789241501583_eng.pdf

17. Schaaf HS, Moll AP, Dheda K. Multidrug- and extensively drug-resistant tuberculosis in Africa and South America: Epidemiology, diagnosis and management in adults and children. Clin Chest Med. 2009;30(4):667–683. http://dx.doi.org/10.1016/j.ccm.2009.08.019

18. Zhao M, Li X, Xu P, et al. Transmission of MDR and XDR tuberculosis in Shanghai, China. PLoS ONE. 2009;4(2):e4370. http://dx.doi.org/10.1371/journal.pone.0004370

19. Chai JS, Mattingly DC, Varma JK. Protecting health care workers from tuberculosis in China: A review of policy and practice in China and the United States. Health Policy Plan. 2013;28(1):100–109. http://dx.doi.org/10.1093/heapol/czs029

20. World Health Organization/International Pharmaceutical Federation. Joint statement on the role of pharmacists in tuberculosis care and control [document on the Internet]. c2011 [cited 2012 Mar 20]. Available from: http://www.who.int/tb/features_archive/who_fip_joint_statement.pdf

21. Cabana MD, Rand CS, Powe NR, et al. Why don't physicians follow clinical practice guidelines? A framework for improvement. JAMA. 1999;282(15):1458–1465. http://dx.doi.org/10.1001/jama.282.15.1458

22. Holtz TH, Lancester J, Laserson KF, et al. Risk factors associated with default from multidrug-resistant tuberculosis treatment. Int J Tuberc Lung Dis. 2006;10(6):649–655.

23. Hoa NP, Diwan VK, Thorson AE. Diagnosis and treatment of pulmonary tuberculosis at basic health care facilities in rural Vietnam: A survey of knowledge and reported practices among health staff. Health Policy. 2005;72(1):1–8. http://dx.doi.org/10.1016/j.healthpol.2004.02.013

9

A survey to assess the extent of public-private mix DOTS in the management of tuberculosis in Zambia

Authors:
Gershom Chongwe[1]
Nathan Kapata[2]
Mwendaweli Maboshe[3]
Charles Michelo[1]
Olusegun Babaniyi[3]

Affiliations:
[1]University of Zambia, School of Medicine, Department of Public Health, Zambia

[2]Ministry of Health, National TB/Leprosy Control Program, Zambia

[3]World Health Organization Country Office, Zambia

Correspondence to:
Gershom Chongwe

Email:
gchongwe@gmail.com

Postal address:
PO Box 50110, Lusaka, Zambia

Background: Involving all relevant healthcare providers in tuberculosis (TB) management through public-private mix (PPM) approaches is a vital element in the World Health Organization's (WHO) Stop TB Strategy. The control of TB in Zambia is mainly done in the public health sector, despite the high overall incidence rates.

Aim: We conducted a survey to determine the extent of private-sector capacity, participation, practices and adherence to national guidelines in the control of TB.

Setting: This survey was done in the year 2012 in 157 facilities in three provinces of Zambia where approximately 85% of the country's private health facilities are found.

Methods: We used a structured questionnaire to interview the heads of private health facilities to assess the participation of the private health sector in TB diagnosis, management and prevention activities.

Results: Out of 157 facilities surveyed, 40.5% were from the Copperbelt, 4.4% from Central province and 55.1% from Lusaka province. Only 23.8% of the facilities were able to provide full diagnosis and management of TB patients. Although 47.4% of the facilities reported that they do notify their cases to the National TB control programme, the majority (62.7%) of these facilities did not show evidence of notifications.

Conclusion: Our results show that the majority of the facilities that diagnose and manage TB in the private sector do not report their TB activities to the National TB Control Programme (NTP). There is a need for the NTP to improve collaboration with the private sector with respect to TB control activities and PPM for Directly Observed Treatment, Short Course (DOTS).

Une étude pour évaluer l'étendue des DOTS combinés publics-privés dans la gestion de la tuberculose en Zambie.

Contexte: La participation de tous les professionnels de santé concernés dans la gestion de la tuberculose (TB) par une approche combinée publique-privée (PPM) est un élément capital de la Stratégie « Halte à la Tuberculose (TB) » de l'Organisation mondiale de la Santé (OMS). Le contrôle de la tuberculose en Zambie se fait principalement dans le secteur de la santé publique, malgré le taux d'incidence global élevé.

Objectif: Nous avons mené une enquête pour déterminer l'importance de la capacité, participation, pratiques et adhésion du secteur privé aux directives nationales pour le contrôle de la tuberculose.

Cadre: Cette enquête a été faite en 2012 dans 157 établissements de santé dans trois provinces de la Zambie où se trouvent environ 85% des services de santé privés du pays.

Méthodes: Nous avons utilisé un questionnaire structuré pour interviewer les directeurs des établissements sanitaires privés afin d'évaluer la participation du secteur de santé privé dans le diagnostic, la gestion et la prévention de la tuberculose.

Résultats: Sur les 157 établissements examinés, 40.5% provenaient de la Copperbelt, 4.4% de la Province Centrale et 55.1% de la province de Lusaka. Seuls 23.8% des établissements pouvaient faire un diagnostic complet et gérer les tuberculeux. Bien que 47.4% des établissements aient déclaré qu'ils avaient signalé leurs patients au programme national de contrôle de la tuberculose, la majorité (62.7%) de ces établissements n'a pas pu donner de preuve de notifications.

Conclusion: Nos résultats montrent que la majorité des établissements qui diagnostiquent et gèrent la tuberculose dans le secteur privé ne déclarent pas leurs activités concernant la tuberculose au programme de contrôle national de la tuberculose (NTP). Il faut que le NTP améliore sa collaboration avec le secteur privé par rapport aux activités de contrôle de la tuberculose et le PPM pour le Traitement de brève Durée sous Surveillance directe (DOTS).

Introduction

Involving all relevant healthcare providers in tuberculosis (TB) care and control through public–private mix (PPM) approaches is a vital element in the World Health Organization's (WHO) Stop TB Strategy. PPM refers to the activities that link all healthcare facilities within the private and public sectors to national TB programmes for the expansion of Directly Observed Treatment, Short Course (DOTS) activities.[1] The approach is one of the tools employed in the implementation of the International Standards for TB Care (ISTC) in order to achieve national as well as global TB targets. The use of private health providers has been shown to increase notification rates of smear-positive pulmonary TB by between 10% and 60%.[2]

The WHO estimates that there were 9 million new cases of TB in 2011, with 1.4 million TB deaths worldwide.[3] Zambia is amongst the WHO's African Region TB high-burden countries. It is estimated that in 2012, there were 40 726 new TB case notifications (including relapse cases in Zambia), or 289/100 000 population. In the southern African region, only South Africa, Swaziland, Lesotho and Botswana notified more cases per 100 000 population compared with Zambia in the year 2012.[4]

Increasing private-sector participation in TB control services has been shown to be a cost-effective way of improving care as well as notification rates of TB.[5,6,7] The improved notification rates are generally seen following greater collaboration between the National TB Control Programme (NTP) and the private sector;[8,9] however, other studies have suggested that consulting the private sector after the commencement of TB-related signs and symptoms may result in diagnostic and treatment delay.[10,11,12,13] The extent of the PPM for TB care and control in Zambia is not known.

Whilst the scale up of TB/HIV collaborative activities in Zambia has increased over the past decade, challenges still remain in getting service delivery points, including private healthcare providers, to adhere to recommended standards.[14] Private healthcare facilities are expected to take part in TB and HIV control activities such as diagnosis of cases, treatment and notification of cases. Information on the capacity to diagnose TB in the private health facilities, notification of cases to the authorities, the outcomes of treatment, as well as adherence to national treatment guidelines, is not available.

The scaling up of TB and/or HIV collaborative activities is one of the strategies of the Global Plan to Stop TB. According to the WHO world TB report for 2012, Zambia was amongst the countries that reported HIV testing rates of more than 85% in the year 2011.[3] With the prevalence of HIV amongst TB patients in Zambia estimated at 65% – 68%,[3,15] testing all TB patients for HIV is vital as it ensures that patients receive the appropriate care, which may include prophylactic Cotrimoxazole and/or antiretroviral therapy.

Aims and objectives

We carried out a survey to determine the extent of private-sector capacity and participation in the provision of tuberculosis control services in Zambia, as well as to assess the private provider practices and adherence to national guidelines.

Research methods and design

Study design and setting

A cross-sectional survey was done in Lusaka, Central and Copperbelt provinces, where about 85% of all private healthcare facilities in Zambia are found. There were two survey teams, one for Lusaka and another for the Central and Copperbelt provinces. Team members comprised public health-sector workers serving as TB focal point persons. The team members were trained on how to use a validated semi-structured questionnaire (see Annexure 1) which was used to collect information from the heads of the private health facilities. The questionnaire included questions on: staff availability; capacity to diagnose TB using chest X-ray, smear microscopy or culture methods; and ability to manage a case of TB by providing drugs and other services. The data were collected between September and October 2012 as part of operations research on behalf of the NTP.

Sampling strategy

A list of health facilities obtained from the Health Professions Council of Zambia, the body responsible for the licensing and regulation of all private health facilities in the country, was used as a sampling frame. Out of a total of 423 facilities on the list, 243 were in Lusaka and 180 from the Copperbelt province. We included facilities that offered general medical services regardless of their size.

Facilities such as dental clinics, optician clinics as well as clinics offering only reproductive health services were excluded. We also excluded mine underground clinics as well as first aid clinics within the mining plants and in workplaces. A number of facilities could not be located, mainly because they had closed or had moved to another area. After this process, the survey was conducted in the remaining 157 facilities, 87 of them in Lusaka, 63 from the Copperbelt province and 7 in the Central province.

Data analysis

The data was entered into a questionnaire in Epidata statistical software, then analysed using STATA 11.2 software (StataCorp 2011). Proportions were expressed as percentages with corresponding 95% confidence intervals.

Ethical considerations

A waiver was obtained from the University of Zambia Biomedical Research Ethics Committee to use these results arising from an operations research study by the National TB Control Programme.

Results

Out of 157 facilities, 63 (40.5%) facilities were from the Copperbelt province, 7 (4.4%) from Central province and 87 (55.1%) from Lusaka province. Eighty-nine per cent (n = 139) of the facilities were privately owned, 5.1% (n = 8) owned by faith-based institutions and 6.4% (n = 10) owned by quasi-government or parastatal (or semi-autonomous, government-supported) institutions. More than 90% (n = 142) of the facilities were manned by at least one doctor. However, the number of doctors working in the facilities ranged from zero in 9.5% (n = 15) of the facilities to 17 doctors found in one of the largest facilities. Furthermore, 38.6% (n = 140) of the facilities had at least one inpatient bed for admission of patients.

Management of tuberculosis cases

Only 23.8% (n = 151 [95% CI 17.0, 30.7]) of the facilities are able to fully diagnose and manage TB patients by conducting sputum smears or culture, chest X-ray examinations, as well as providing anti-TB drugs. Over half of the facilities (78 of 151; 51.7% [95% CI 43.6, 59.7]) reported that they routinely referred their suspected TB patients to the public sector whenever a case of TB is suspected, whereas 24.5% (n = 37 [95% CI 17.6, 31.4]) referred patients only after making the diagnosis. All the facilities that manage TB patients reported that they were able to provide TB drugs to their patients. Of these, 27.3% (n = 12) said they obtained their drugs from their own suppliers, whereas 72.7% (n = 32) of the providers obtained their drugs from the NTP through the respective district medical offices.

Notification of tuberculosis

Although 47.4% (n = 36 [95% CI 34.6, 57.5]) of the facilities reported that they do notify their cases to the NTP, 62.7% (n = 47 [95% CI 51.5, 73.9]) of these could not show evidence of this when asked to produce a treatment register.

Treatment guidelines

Only 36% (n = 48 [95% CI 27.8, 44.2]) of the respondents said they had been trained in the use of the national treatment guidelines, 79.2% (n = 38) of whom were trained through their respective district medical offices. Other training was provided by non-governmental organisations (NGOs). A total of 32 (66.7%) were trained using the latest guidelines introduced in 2007, whilst 16 (33.3%) were trained before the latest guidelines. Sixty-seven per cent (n = 63 [95% CI 57.3, 76.7]) of the respondents reported following the treatment guidelines when managing their patients.

Capacity to diagnose tuberculosis

We investigated the capacity for diagnosis of TB in the private health sector. Of all the facilities visited, only 42 (26.9%) had capacity to examine sputum smears (95% CI 20.1, 34.6). When disaggregated according to the type of facility, 5 of the 10 (50%) parastatal or government supported facilities had such capacity, compared with only 36 of the 139 (30%) private facilities and one (12.5%) of the faith-based institutions. Further, only 9 facilities (6.7% [95% CI 2.6, 10.7]) had the capacity to culture sputum for mycobacteria. X-ray facilities were available in 21.1% (n = 30 [95% CI 13.4, 26.3]) of the facilities, with parastatal and private facilities having similar capacity at 20.0% (n = 2) and 21.7% (n = 35) respectively. This is shown in Table 1. A few of the facilities[3] reported using rapid tests for TB diagnosis.

Tuberculosis and/or HIV collaborative services

Cotrimoxazole prophylaxis is provided to 58.8% (n = 77 [95% CI 49.8, 67.3]) of HIV patients. When asked whether they test their TB patients for HIV, 83 (66.4%) of the facilities replied in the affirmative (95% CI 57.4.0, 74.6). On the other hand, only 57.3% (n = 67 [95% CI 47.8, 66.4]) of the respondents reported screening their HIV patients for TB. Over 43% (n = 57 [95% CI 34.9, 52.4]) of the facilities reported the ability to provide antiretroviral (ARV) drugs to their patients. The proportion of facilities providing ARVs was higher in the parastatal health facilities than in those owned by faith-based institutions or private individuals, as is shown in Table 2.

Discussion
Key findings

Our results have shown that only a quarter of the private health facilities have a self-reported capacity to diagnose

TABLE 1: Availability of diagnostic services in private health facilities.

Type of facility	Perform sputum smear n (%)	Perform sputum culture n (%)	Chest X-ray n (%)	Provide tuberculosis drugs n (%)
Parastatal (N = 10)	5 (50.0)	1 (11.1)	2 (20.0)	6 (60.0)
Faith-based facility (N = 8)	1 (12.5)	0 (0.0)	1 (12.5)	3 (50.0)
Private (N = 139)	36 (30.0)	8 (6.7)	35 (21.7)	35 (29.7)
Total (N = 156)	**42 (26.9)**	**9 (6.7)**	**30 (21.1)**	**44 (32.8)**

TABLE 2: Availability of tuberculosis/HIV collaborative services in private health facilities.

Type of facility	Provide Cotrimoxazole prophylaxis n (%)	Screen HIV patients for tuberculosis n (%)	Test tuberculosis patients for HIV n (%)	Provide anti-HIV drugs n (%)
Parastatal (N = 10)	7 (70.0)	7 (70.0)	7 (70.0)	7 (70.0)
Faith-based facility (N = 8)	4 (57.1)	3 (60.0)	4 (80.0)	3 (42.9)
Private (N = 139)	66 (57.9)	57 (51.8)	72 (70.6)	47 (41.2)
Total (N = 156)	**77 (58.8)**	**67 (57.3)**	**83 (66.4)**	**57 (43.5)**

and manage TB cases in Zambia. Over three quarters of the facilities did not have capacity to either diagnose or manage tuberculosis cases and referred their patients to the public sector. Some studies have suggested that consulting the private sector after the commencement of TB-related signs and symptoms may result in diagnostic and treatment delay.[10,11,12] Ensuring that private providers have the necessary skills to diagnose and manage TB patients will improve notifications, possibly improving treatment outcomes and preventing the development of multi-drug resistant TB.

The need to notify TB cases is essential for TB control. The lack of notification by almost two-thirds of the private-sector providers, despite this being a legal requirement, is an opportunity for the NTP and other partners to engage private practitioners through the respective district medical offices on the need to notify TB cases. A well-established PPM strategy has the potential to improve case notifications by between 10% – 60%.[2] An analysis of different PPM models for TB control in Pakistan in order to estimate the contribution of the various private providers to TB case notification showed that the NGO model made the greatest contribution to case notification (58.3%), followed by the hospital-based model at 18.9%.[16]

Discussion of key findings

The scaling up of TB and/or HIV collaborative activities is one of the strategies of the Global Plan to Stop TB. According to the WHO world TB report for 2012, Zambia was amongst the countries that reported HIV testing rates of more than 85% in 2011.[3] These data are collected mainly from the public health sector. Our study has shown that only 70.5% of TB patients are tested for HIV in the private sector. With the prevalence of HIV amongst TB patients in Zambia estimated at 65% – 68%,[3,15] testing all TB patients for HIV is vital as it ensures that patients receive the appropriate care, which may include prophylactic Cotrimoxazole and/or anti-retroviral therapy.

Strengths and limitations

This is the first report on PPM DOTs in Zambia. Although many patients in Zambia seek medical attention from a myriad of practitioners, ranging from traditional healers to formal western-oriented medical practitioners, our study did not investigate the role played by traditional practitioners. It is not known what proportion of Zambians with TB seek medical attention from traditional practitioners, nor do we know what their practices are with regard to patients presenting with symptoms suggestive of TB. There is therefore a need to investigate the role of traditional health practitioners in TB care in Zambia, as it has been shown that up to 30% – 40% of TB patients would have been seen by a traditional healer prior to a TB diagnosis in other places.[17,18] The results could also have been affected by the differences in the size and capabilities of the facilities that were included in the survey as well as the presence of NTP staff amongst the data collectors.

Recommendations

There is need for the NTP to improve collaboration with the private sector with respect to TB control activities and PPM, especially seeing that the majority of the facilities do not report their cases to the national programme.

There is also a need to improve training of the private health practitioners in the latest TB treatment guidelines. All necessary efforts must be made by the NTP and stakeholders to ensure that knowledge transfer of the most effective, latest and evidence-based treatment guidelines are disseminated widely to the private sector if TB control is to be achieved. District medical offices must improve collaboration and oversight roles in order to improve notification of TB cases by the private sector. TB and/or HIV collaborative activities in the private sector need to be enhanced as part of the PPM activities and the NTP must make efforts to ensure that every practitioner adheres to the ISTC.[19]

Conclusion

Our results have shown that private sector participation in TB control and care is suboptimal. Whilst all the private facilities participate in the national TB programme either by diagnosing patients or referring them to other facilities for further management, the majority of the facilities did not show evidence of notification of cases to the NTP.

Acknowledgements

The authors would like to express their gratitude to the WHO and the University of Zambia Medical Education Partnership Initiative (MEPI) for funding this work. We further acknowledge the invaluable support rendered by the following individuals during the conduction of the survey and report writing: Ms Queen Chisanga, Ms Priscilla Mlauzi, Ms Mercy Musanide Mwale, Ms Josephine Ndoweka, Ms Sharon Musakanya, Ms Grace Banda, Mr Anderson Mumba, Ms Kunda Chisalaba, Mr Weston Mwanza, Mr Tenard Luhanga, Mr Silvester Chanda and Mr Minyoi Maimbolwa.

Special thanks go to the national, provincial and district levels of the Ministry of Health for facilitating the smooth running of this exercise and to all the private facilities that gave their valuable time to participate in this survey.

Competing interests

This work was funded by the WHO Country Office for Zambia. The authors declare that they have no financial or personal relationship(s) that may have inappropriately influenced them in writing this article.

Authors' contributions

G.C. (University of Zambia), N.K. (Ministry of Health, Zambia) and M.M. (WHO Country Office, Zambia) took part in the planning of the study, data collection, analysis and writing of the manuscript. C.M. (University of Zambia) and

O.B. (WHO Country Office, Zambia) took part in the data analysis and report writing and reviewed the manuscript.

References

1. Uplekar M. Involving private health care providers in delivery of TB care: Global strategy. Tuberculosis. 2003;83(1–3):156–164. http://dx.doi.org/10.1016/S1472-9792(02)00073-2

2. World Health Organization. Public-private mix for DOTS: Towards scaling up.WHO/HTM/TB/2005.356 [document on the Internet]. c2005 [cited 2014 Jul 19]. Available from: http://whqlibdoc.who.int/hq/2005/WHO_HTM_TB_2005.356.pdf?ua=1

3. World Health Organization. 2012 Global tuberculosis control. WHO/HTM/TB/2012.6 report[document on the Internet]. c2012 [cited 2013 Oct 10]. Available from: http://www.who.int/tb/publications/global_report/gtbr12_main.pdf [URL no longer available]

4. World Health Organization. Global tuberculosis report 2013 [document on the Internet]. c2013 [cited 2015 Feb 01]. Available from: http://apps.who.int/iris/bitstream/10665/91355/1/9789241564656_eng.pdf

5. Floyd K, Arora VK, Murthy KJR, et al. Cost and cost-effectiveness of PPM-DOTS for tuberculosis control: Evidence from India. Bull World Health Organ. 2006;84(6):437–445. http://dx.doi.org/10.2471/BLT.05.024109

6. Sinanovic E, Kumaranayake L. Sharing the burden of TB/HIV? Costs and financing of public–private partnerships for tuberculosis treatment in South Africa. Trop Med Int Health. 2006;11(9):1466–1474. http://dx.doi.org/10.1111/j.1365-3156.2006.01686.x

7. Ambe G, Lönnroth K, Dholakia Y, et al. Every provider counts: Effect of a comprehensive public–private mix approach for TB control in a large metropolitan area in India. Int J Tuberc Lung Dis. 2005;9(5):562–568.

8. Lal SS, Sahu S, Wares F, et al. Intensified scale-up of public–private mix: A systems approach to tuberculosis care and control in India. Int J Tuberc Lung Dis. 2011;15(1):97–104.

9. Lienhardt C, Glaziou P, Uplekar M, et al. Global tuberculosis control: Lessons learnt and future prospects. Nat Rev Microbiol. 2012;10(6):407–416.

10. Tobgay KJ, Sarma PS, Thankappan KR. Predictors of treatment delays for tuberculosis in Sikkim. Natl Med J India. 2006;19(2):60–63.

11. Van Wyk SS, Enarson DA, Beyers N, et al. Consulting private health care providers aggravates treatment delay in urban South African tuberculosis patients. Int J Tuberc Lung Dis. 2011;15(8):1069–1076. http://dx.doi.org/10.5588/ijtld.10.0615

12. Storla DG, Yimer S, Bjune GA. A systematic review of delay in the diagnosis and treatment of tuberculosis. BMC Public Health. 2008;8:15. http://dx.doi.org/10.1186/1471-2458-8-15

13. Godfrey-Faussett P, Kaunda H, Kamanga J, et al. Why do patients with a cough delay seeking care at Lusaka urban health centres? A health systems research approach. Int J Tuberc Lung Dis. 2002;6(9):796–805.

14. Kapata N, Chanda-Kapata P, Grobusch MP, et al. Scale-up of TB and HIV programme collaborative activities in Zambia – a 10-year review. Trop Med Int Health. 2012;17(6):760–766. http://dx.doi.org/10.1111/j.1365-3156.2012.02981.x

15. UNAIDS. Global report: UNAIDS report on the global AIDS epidemic 2010 [homepage on the Internet]. c2010 [cited 2015 Jan 29]. Available from: http://www.unaids.org/globalreport/Global_report.htm

16. Chughtai AA, Qadeer E, Khan W, et al. Estimation of the contribution of private providers in tuberculosis case notification and treatment outcome in Pakistan. East Mediterr Health J. 2013;19(3):213–218.

17. Salaniponi FML, Harries AD, Banda HT, et al. Care seeking behaviour and diagnostic processes in patients with smear-positive pulmonary tuberculosis in Malawi. Int J Tuberc Lung Dis. 2000;4(4):327–332.

18. Wilkinson D, Gcabashe L, Lurie M. Traditional healers as tuberculosis treatment supervisors: precedent and potential [Planning and Practice]. Int J Tuberc Lung Dis. 1999;3(9):838–842.

19. Hopewell PC, Pai M, Maher D, et al. International standards for tuberculosis care. Lancet Infect Dis. 2006;6(11):710–725. http://dx.doi.org/10.1016/S1473-3099(06)70628-4

Appendix 1: TB services public-private mix questionnaire.
Ministry of Health

1. District _____

2. Facility name _____

3. Type of facility

       a. Parastatal   ☐
       b. Faith based   ☐
       c. Company owned   ☐
       d. Privately owned   ☐

4. Date of interview _____/_____/_____ [dd/mm/yy]

5. Name of officer interviewed Prof/Dr/Mr/Ms_____

6. Interviewer's name _____

7. How long has the facility been operating? _____ Years

8. How many clinical staff work here?

       a. Doctors   ☐
       b. Clinical officers   ☐
       c. Nurses   ☐

9. How many inpatient beds does this facility have, if any _____

TB Services

10. What do you do when you have a suspected TB patient?

        a. Diagnose then refer   ☐
        b. Diagnose and manage
        c. Refer

11. If you manage TB patients, do you follow the national TB regimen?

        a. Yes   ☐
        b. No

12. Please describe the drugs provided and the period of treatment:

Drug	Duration of administration
a	
b	
c	
d	
e	

13. Have you been trained in using the national TB treatment guidelines?

        a. Yes   ☐
        b. No

    13.1 If yes, who trained you? _____
    13.2 If yes, which year was the training? _____

14. Do you follow the national treatment guidelines?

        a. Yes   ☐
        b. No

15. If you are involved in managing TB cases, do you notify the cases to the Ministry of Health authorities?

        a. Yes   ☐
        b. No

16. If yes where do you report?

        a. District Medical Office   ☐
        b. Provincial Medical Office
        c. Ministry of Health headquarters

17. Ask to see a notification form

    a. Present
    b. Absent

18. If no notifications are done, state why:

    a. Not aware
    b. Too much work
    c. Too busy
    d. Not applicable
    e. Other (specify) _____

19. Would you be willing to start notifying your cases to the MOH?

    a. Yes
    b. No

20. Do you provide TB drugs to your patients?

    a. Yes
    b. No

21. If yes, where do you obtain the drugs?

    a. Buy from our suppliers
    b. Obtain supplies from District Medical office
    c. Other (specify) _____

22. Are your TB patients tested for HIV?

    a. Yes
    b. No

23. Are your HIV patients screened for TB?

    a. Yes
    b. No.

24. Do you provide Cotrimoxazole prophylaxis to your HIV patients?

    a. Yes
    b. No.

25. Are you providing ARVs to your patients?

    a. Yes
    b. No.

Laboratory Services

26. Do you have capacity to examine sputum smears for TB?

    a. Yes
    b. No

27. Do you have capacity to culture sputum for TB?

    a. Yes
    b. No

28. Do you have chest X-ray facilities?

    a. Yes
    b. No

29. Do you have any other tests for TB? Please explain what they are:

    a. _____
    b. _____
    c. _____

10

A discourse analysis of male sexuality in the magazine *Intimacy*

Author:
Rory du Plessis[1]

Affiliation:
[1]Department of Visual Arts, University of Pretoria, South Africa

Correspondence to:
Rory du Plessis

Email:
rory.duplessis@up.ac.za

Postal address:
Private Bag X20, Hatfield 0028, South Africa

Background: The World Health Organization's publication, *Developing sexual health programmes*, states that the media is an important source of information about sexuality. Although the media can promote awareness of sexual health issues, it also acts as a vehicle for defining and regulating sex norms. In other words, the standards of 'normal' sex are in part defined by the media. Accordingly, it has become imperative to analyse the media's construction of sexual norms in order to reveal how they are related to specific ideological views. For the purposes of this study, the focus will be limited to analysing the South African publication *Intimacy*.

Aim: The study aims to reveal how the sex advice articles written in *Intimacy* for women in regard to their male partner's sexuality reflect patriarchal and phallocentric ideologies.

Method: A discourse analysis of the sex advice articles in the magazine *Intimacy* was conducted. It was informed by feminist theories of sexuality that seek to examine the ways in which texts are associated with male-centred versions of sexual pleasure.

Results: The discourse analysis identified a number of key themes regarding male sexuality. These include: (1) biological accounts of male sexuality; (2) phallocentric scripting of the sex act; and (3) the melodramatic penis.

Conclusion: Constructions of male sexuality require the inclusion of alternative modes of male erotic pleasure. This requires texts that encourage men to explore and also to experiment with pleasurable feelings associated with non-genital erogenous zones of the body.

Contexte: La publication de l'Organisation mondiale de la Santé, *Développement de programmes de santé sexuelle*, déclare que les médias sont une source importante d'informations sur la sexualité. Bien que les médias sensibilisent les gens aux problèmes de santé sexuelle, ils servent aussi de véhicule pour définir et réglementer les normes sexuelles. Autrement dit, les normes sexuelles 'normales' sont en partie définies par les médias. Ainsi, il est donc impératif d'analyser la construction des normes sexuelles des médias pour montrer leur corrélation par rapport à des points de vue idéologiques. Pour les besoins de cette étude, nous nous limiterons à l'analyse de la revue sud-africaine *Intimacy*.

Objet: L'étude a pour but de montrer comment les articles du magazine *Intimacy* qui donnent des conseils sur la sexualité aux femmes à l'égard de la sexualité de leur partenaire masculin reflètent des idéologies patriarcales et phallocentriques.

Méthode: Une analyse a été faite du discours des articles qui donnent des conseils sur la sexualité dans le magazine *Intimacy*. Il est influencé par les théories féministes sur la sexualité qui cherchent à examiner de quelle manière les textes sont centrés sur le plaisir sexuel des hommes.

Résultats: L'analyse du discours a identifié un certain nombre de thèmes clés concernant la sexualité masculine. Ce sont: (1) les récits naturalistes biologiques de la sexualité masculine; (2) les scénarios phallocentriques de l'acte sexuel; et (3) le pénis mélodramatique.

Conclusion: Les construits de la sexualité masculine requièrent l'inclusion de modes alternatifs de plaisir érotique masculin. Cela demande des textes qui encouragent les hommes à explorer et aussi à expérimenter des sentiments agréables associés aux zones érogènes non génitales du corps.

Introduction

The World Health Organization's publication, *Developing sexual health programmes*, states that the media is an important source of information about sexuality.[1] Although the media can promote awareness of sexual health issues, it also acts as a vehicle for producing normative notions of sex and, consequently, it plays a role in regulating current trends in sexual practices.[2] It is precisely in this role of being a major vehicle for the display and explanation of sexuality that the media has come to replace religious and moral leaders as sexual authorities in the public's pursuit of sexual 'normalcy'.[3] In other words, the standards of 'normal' sex are, in part, defined by the media.[2,3] Accordingly, it has become imperative to analyse the media's construction of sexual norms in order to reveal how they are related to specific ideological views.[3] Recent South African scholarship has focused specifically on investigating the role of magazines and print media in the construction and dissemination of normative notions of sex.[4,5,6] This study endeavours to continue in a similar vein as such scholarship by analysing the South African magazine publication, *Intimacy*.

The publication in question endeavours to provide its readers with information for a healthy, sensual and passionate lifestyle (Fernandez J 2008, personal communication, August 27). In particular, it intends to empower women to take control of their sex life.[7] This is underscored in the publication discussing 'all intimate and health issues woman face daily – How to put the passion back in your relationship, contraceptives, pregnancy, infertility, Breast cancer, Menopause, low libido, cervical cancer, etc.' (Fernandez J 2008, personal communication, August 27). As will be shown in the analysis that follows, such discussions which embody the hallmarks of female sexual empowerment[8] are obstructed by descriptions of male sexuality, found within the same publication, that both accept and reinforce dominant gender and sex norms. To elucidate further, although the magazine celebrates the right of women to desire sex and experience sexual pleasure, the sex advice written in *Intimacy* for women relating to their male partner's sexuality is limited to male-centred sex acts and sexual practices that are based on traditional gender roles, ideals and expectations.[8]

To put it succinctly, the study aims to reveal how the sex advice articles written for women regarding male sexuality reflect patriarchal and phallocentric ideologies. These ideologies ensure that sexuality is male-centred, which results in the precedence of male sexual needs. The key themes that contribute to the aforementioned ideologies include:

- Patriarchal: female submission to the sexual needs of men whilst at the same time providing emotional support to them. In other words, women are tasked with not only pleasing a man sexually but also caring for his self-esteem.[8,9,10]
- Phallocentric: penile erections are viewed as being the essence of male sexuality and satisfaction. Furthermore, 'real' sex is limited and valorised to a coital scenario – the penetration of the vagina by the penis.[2,3,8,11]

Such ideological underpinnings perpetuate narrow ideas of sex, sexuality and gender relations whilst delimiting the sexual act, female sexuality and male sexuality to predefined potentials and gender relations.[2] In view of this, the study takes a 'sex critical'[12] approach that seeks to analyse all forms of sexuality and sexual practices in order to reveal the presence of any normative values that perpetuate and uphold patriarchal ideologies.[12]

The research methodology of this study is a discursive analysis of the text in question. Discourse analysis does not seek to validate the 'truth' about male and female sexuality in this particular case but rather reveals the ways in which these 'truths' and our knowledge of sexuality are structured by ideology.[2,13] Accordingly, discourse analysis problematises purely biological accounts of human sexuality and instead argues that our understanding and interpretation of sexuality are shaped by ideological, socio-cultural and historical influences. As such, a discourse analysis of the given text aims to reveal the ways in which ideologies are embodied, manifested and reflected in the discussion of sexual acts (how the various sex acts are defined, classified and promoted), as well as the ways in which the sexual acts are connected to governing the conduct and relations between men and women.

In this discourse analysis, a number of key themes regarding male sexuality which reflect a patriarchal and phallocentric agenda are identified. These are: (1) biological accounts of male sexuality: that the 'needs' of the male sex drive dictate the sexual encounter; (2) phallocentric scripting of the sex act: male sexuality described exclusively in terms of the penis and the need for penetration; and (3) the melodramatic penis: descriptions that enshrine the penis as a revered icon of sexual pleasure for both men and women. A critical reading of an *Intimacy* article is offered under each theme in order to outline how it privileges both patriarchy and phallocentrism.

The study concludes by advocating for media texts to include alternative modes of male erotic pleasure as well as underscoring the role of primary care professionals with regard to promoting alternative forms of sex:

> [A]cts that acknowledge the legitimacy and potential of non-genital erogenous zones for orgasm and/or pleasure. In doing so, patients are encouraged to explore sexual sensations and experiment with pleasurable feelings associated with the whole body.[14]

Background

Sexuality has been a central concern of both the feminist movement and feminist scholarship.[2,3] In particular, this concern has taken the form of a number of studies that have revealed that the scientific investigations and theories of sexological research have a gender bias and basis in which male-centred versions of sex are valorised.[2] This is not just a peripheral idiosyncrasy but is argued to be the mainstay of the scientific basis of sexology which, from the early and late twentieth century, constructed a model of sexuality that purported to be both objective and scientific but, in fact, reflected and promoted the interests of patriarchy.[3,15] In other words, the model of sexuality provided by scientific texts reflects patriarchal values by defining sex in male terms and, consequently, it controls and restricts women to specific expressions of sexuality.[15]

Yet, as suggested previously, science is not the only underlying contributing factor accountable for this viewpoint as the media is equally influential in producing normative notions of sex. These notions regulate current trends in sexual practices and result in the denial or denigration of sexual practices that depart from patriarchal norms.[2] To this end, a number of feminist studies have also revealed that popular texts are reflective of patriarchal ideology.[2,16] In exposing the patriarchal ideology, a number of shared themes are present and recur in popular texts, namely: male sexuality prioritised over female sexuality; and the favouring of penetrative sex over other sexual activities.[2] In reviewing these themes, the reverberating finding is that popular texts articulate a set of sex and gender norms that serve patriarchy.[2]

This theorisation illustrates that there is a need for strengthening and expanding existing literature on sex – both scientific and popular – to offer an alternative version of female sexuality that does not imitate and/or epitomise patriarchal values. One attempt to do so is outlined by Rebecca Chalker, who advocates providing women with accurate and comprehensive information about their bodies and their sexuality.[17] In terms of popular sex advice literature, this includes offering a broader definition of what constitutes sex and promoting a wider range of sexually pleasurable activities that are less reflective of a male-centred model of sexuality, instead exploring the specificities of female sexual pleasures.[8,17] Explicit in this framework is that the possibility of an alternative and empowered female sexuality in heterosexual relationships requires male sexuality to depart from both patriarchal and phallocentric ideologies.[2] Therefore, only by engaging with the promotion of alternative modes of male sexuality can an empowered female sexuality occur.[2,8]

Although *Intimacy* provides wide-ranging information on female health, well-being and sexual health issues, whilst also encouraging women to recognise themselves as sexual beings and to accept, assert and explore their sexual desires, the publication does not necessarily advocate sexual agency and individual autonomy for women.[8] Instead, any identification of an 'active' or 'empowered' female sexuality is frequently oriented toward satisfying the pleasures and desires of a male-centred model of sex.[8] Thus, whilst the magazine aims to empower women to take control of their sex life,[7] this very attempt is hampered by the privileging and prioritisation of male sexual needs and desires.

Research methods and design
Sample

Intimacy is the English duplicate of the Afrikaans publication, *Intiem*. *Intimacy* was launched as a print publication but later adopted a solely web-based platform titled *INTIMACY4US*. The Afrikaans version, *Intiem*, continues in a print format. The sample consisted of the English bi-monthly issues of *Intimacy* from the July–September 2008 issue to the December 2009 – January 2010 issue, as well as the online

articles accessed up until July 2011. *Intimacy*, as with most other magazines, contains a number of article types. These include, amongst others, feature articles, advertorials, advice columns, editorials, human interest, opinion articles, interviews, profiles and expert-authored texts. In order to narrow this down and produce a more focused analysis, the study consisted only of articles pertaining to the genre of an 'informative content type' (articles in which the focus on sexuality adopts the format of: what-to, how-to, when-to, why-to, etc.).

Data analysis

Discourse analysis was utilised to identify the key themes that constitute *Intimacy*'s construction of male and female sexuality. The discourse analysis of the articles drew upon the method and guidelines suggested by Parker[18] and the sample was coded into themes through a process of repeated reading. Through this strategy, interpretations and connections were developed, themes were refined and reworked and sub-themes were identified. To this end, each time a particular concept was identified in an article, all the other articles in the sample were re-read and re-examined in order to expand the concept into a specific theme or assign it to a sub-theme.

The analysis was informed by feminist theories of sexuality that examine the ways in which texts are associated with male-centred versions of sexual pleasure.[2,3,8,15] However, this study makes no claim that this is the only possible reading of the articles in *Intimacy*. A fundamental feature of discourse analysis is that it acknowledges that there will always be the prospect of generating more appropriate or convincing interpretations.[19] Moreover, alternative interpretations are to be expected by deploying a different theoretical framework or by sampling a different genre of articles from *Intimacy*. As indicated previously, *Intimacy* has many types of articles featured in each issue, from advertorials, to agony aunt columns, letters to the editor and even articles authored by experts in the field. Each respective article type holds the potential for a reading that departs from this study's findings.

Results

As already indicated, three key themes regarding male sexuality have been identified in *Intimacy*. In the following section, the exploration of each theme will include a critical reading of one specific article in order to show how it reflects both patriarchal and phallocentric ideologies.

Discussion
Biological accounts of male sexuality

In the article, '20 ways a woman can superglue her marriage',[20] women are encouraged to be 'actively involved in the bedroom' and to improve their 'sexual repertoire'.[20] Such advice suggests that *Intimacy* advocates a degree of sexual agency for women. To elucidate further, the article encourages women to '[b]ecome comfortable with your sexuality and accept your body unconditionally. Know what stimulates you sexually, what you like and don't like, and communicate this to your mate'.[20] Such statements are salutary as they highlight the importance of sexual communication in constituting an empowered female sexuality. However, the potential to produce a fully-fledged sexual empowerment for women is limited by facets of male sexuality that are deemed to be non-negotiable and, consequently, waive the need for sexual communication. As will be argued below, these features of male sexuality are defined by *Intimacy* as being natural and biological facts and pivot primarily around the notion that men have an incessant need and desire for sex. For feminist theories of sexuality, such accounts are not objective or based on biological fact, but are instead patriarchal myths that are reinforced and perpetuated in popular, medical and sexological texts. Such myths maintain sexual privilege for men – that the 'needs' of the biological male sex drive dictate the sexual encounter.[3] In turn, by upholding such myths, any consideration afforded the female partner or communication from her is silenced by stern warnings and rebuke.

To explore these points, a critical reading of the article 'Do you refuse to have sex?'[21] is offered. In the following quote, women are obliged to accept and satisfy their husband's biologically-entrenched drive and innate need for sex:

> Withholding sex from your husband deprives him of a deep-rooted need as basic as your own need to receive love from him regularly. He feels loved by you when you care enough about him to meet his physical needs and desire him enough to want physical relations.[21]

Here, women are urged to accept these features of male sexuality without discussion or reflection – to unconditionally accept his *biological* needs and wants. Equally problematic is the fact that the article cautions women against denying their husband this need and desire for sex as it will result in detrimental consequences for the marriage:

> Your husband is mad about sex and thinks about it more than you do. Since the average man is more interested in sex than the average woman ... he is more likely to: have strong sexual urges, take sexual risks – despite the consequences – be unfaithful or try commercial sex services. If you realise that merely the sight of your low neckline, your rounded bottom or the scent of your perfume can unleash this primitive instinct, you can't help but realise that you should celebrate this ultimate attraction, as ignoring it could hold grave consequences for your marriage.[21]

In the above passage, male sexual satisfaction is acknowledged as an important means through which women can guarantee that men will remain unfailingly faithful to them. This places women in the role and responsibility of ensuring the 'sexual upkeep'[8] of men: women are urged to be willing and accepting of male sexual urges and constantly seek to satisfy them. In sum, female sexual communication is precluded when addressing the male sex drive. This holds significant repercussions for the extent to which women can be regarded

as active and empowered in their sexuality. They may be able to communicate what they find sexually pleasing but are bound in having to submit to the dictates and prioritisation of the male sex drive.

Phallocentric scripting of the sex act

Sex advice literature has been critiqued for denying the multiplicity of female sexuality – in particular, in reducing the female erogenous zones to only the vagina so as to comply with the coital imperative.[15] However, in *Intimacy* a plethora of articles explore the multiple erogenous zones of a women's body – all of which have orgasmic potential. A number of these articles are especially written for men with a view to enabling them to sexually please their wives. These include: '22 things you need to know about your wife's body'[22] that explores a number of non-genital erogenous zones that women find stimulating (including the neck, ears and navel); 'Your wife's beautiful body ...',[23] which lists a staggering 20 erogenous zones that hold the potential for female arousal and stimulation; and 'Men only: How to be a man'[24] that reiterates that 'the vagina isn't a woman's only erogenous zone. Don't forget about (amongst others) the ears, feet, neck, lips, thighs, eyelids, buttocks, nipples and breasts ... and her brain'.[24] Furthermore, a number of articles are related to coaching men in ways to ensure that their wives reach orgasm. Two examples are 'When the "Big O" plays hide and seek ...'[25] that outlines a list of steps for husbands to follow to ensure that their wives reach orgasm; and 'Men only: help her ride the waves!',[26] which stipulates the steps for men to follow in order to ensure that their wives experience multiple orgasms.

In contrast to the above, it will be argued that the sex advice written in *Intimacy* for women regarding their male partner's sexuality is limited to the penis and penetrative sex. Anything departing from this is deemed foreplay. To elucidate further, in articles such as 'What he really wants in bed ...',[27] which encourages women to explore their husband's erotic zones, the accomplishment of this task is limited to exploring the genital erogenous zones.[27] What is missing is the very discovery of a man's non-genital erogenous zones. Furthermore, the article in question also impedes the enactment of potential non-phallic sex acts by displaying an inordinate focus and attention on the penis. What becomes comprehensible is that the penis becomes enshrined in copious consideration as an organ *par excellence*. A further compelling example of this ongoing relentless focus on the penis is evident in the article 'Don't forget your mouth!'[28] that encourages women to kiss, caress and love the penis.[28]

When women are encouraged to explore a man's non-genital erogenous zones, it is exclusively in terms of foreplay. In 'Foreplay for those who've forgotten how...',[29] it is stated that:

> [w]e are so inclined to pay most of our attention to the "typical" erogenous zones that we forget there are other just as sensual parts of the body. Decide to lavish attention on alternative zones, such as your mate's legs.[29]

Yet, this whole exercise in foreplay is only enacted to supposedly increase the 'explosive force'[29] of the subsequent penetrative sex act and the culminating orgasm. This aspect, in which foreplay is limited to increasing the 'venting force' of an orgasm during the sex act, is underscored later in the very same article:

> Ask your mate to choose one non-erogenous zone on his body (for example his neck, ankles or tummy). Focus on this body part only, for the next 24 hours. Kiss that body part, tickle it, blow on it and cuddle it … be creative! Your goal should be to see how worked up you can get him in order to make your next session as explosive as possible![29]

For male sexuality, foreplay is relegated solely to amplifying the pleasure linked to the final penetrative sex act. Foreplay is accorded no significance as a legitimate, genuine and noteworthy sexual act in its own right. To this end, foreplay is merely added to the standard phallocentric script: intercourse is still the main event and anything else is considered foreplay. Additionally, this standard scripting also sees that sex is construed as a linear process in which foreplay is followed by penetration.[30] Consequently, both female and male sex acts are channelled into a limited form of expression in which sex takes on a particular linear pattern or sequence. Coitus remains the focus and endpoint in this sequence.[11,31]

Considering this section's findings, a number of critiques of *Intimacy*'s construction of male sexuality are perceptible. Although female sexuality is understood and heralded in its plurality and pervasive distribution of erogenous zones – all of which hold the possibilities for multiple orgasms – the converse is true for men. Male sexuality is described exclusively in terms of the penis and the need for penetration. For feminist theories of sexuality, this construct of male sexuality is reflective of phallocentric ideals. In this persistence of phallocentrism, vaginal intercourse is still deemed to be the sex act; everything else is relegated to foreplay. Thus, sex in such a framework lacks flexibility and non-penetrative, non-phallic possibilities.

The melodramatic penis

In the previous sections, male sexuality was outlined as phallocentric (in relation to prizing coital sex) and patriarchal (female submission to the needs of the male sex drive). However, the phallocentrism presented in *Intimacy* also displays a significant departure from standard accounts addressed to men that enshrine penis size as of a high value for female pleasure and masculine ideals. For instance, in the article, 'Men only: how to be a man',[24] the size of the penis is proclaimed as being insignificant for mutual sexual pleasure:

> Quality matters more than quantity: only the first 7,62 cm of the vagina benefits from stimulation, so you don't need much more than that. When it comes to mutual sexual pleasure, penis length and girth mean nothing compared to the quality of foreplay, the sensitivity of touch, and the depth of intimacy in the relationship.[24]

In addition, the article continues to state that in regard to penis size that 'Nobody cares: it's best to accept and appreciate what you have'.[24] These quotes are helpful in offering a departure from standard phallocentric scripts that accord a larger penis size with the ability to provide a higher degree of female satisfaction. However, the advice written for women regarding the issue of penis size perpetuates a number of other phallocentric associations. These links are not explicitly apparent but are revealed in the contextualisation of sex, male sexuality and marital relations that following conventional/patriarchal gender norms and associations. To delineate further, in 'A small problem',[32] the article commences with the following statement:

> On honeymoon, you wake up on the morning following a SECOND night without sex. When you peek under the sheets at your sleeping mate, you discover that he is … um … under-endowed. What next?[32]

Such a sensational proclamation is premised on a number of hegemonic accounts of male sexuality – for example, that normal men are sexually potent and incessantly require sex. Yet, even more perturbing, is that the statement is reductive: the lack of sex is based on the man's small penis; not on the man in question – his values, desires, psychology and interpersonal factors that are reflected in his sexual needs, frequency and responsiveness. Although the quote may be argued to be qualified in a more grounded and sensible account in later paragraphs, it is still based on an unwavering persistence of patriarchal ideals of male sexuality evident in the use of the term 'virility':

> If you suspect that your husband is a little self-conscious about the 'tools' under his belt, share the following facts with him … the length and width of a man's penis has nothing to do with his virility.[32]

In this account, the use of the term 'virility' is a propagation of patriarchal definition and values. Furthermore, the quote also reveals marital relations that are ascribed according to gendered divisions and roles. Women are provided with guidance in order to support their husbands. As such, the patriarchal description of women as a 'helper' for her man includes offering support to shore up and reassure him against any feelings of inadequacy or inferiority that he may have regarding his penis size. This is unmistakably noticeable in the following quote:

> If hubby feels intimidated by what he has seen in blue movies, comfort him with the information that only men with unusually large penises are used as actors and even then, their 'equipment' is made to look bigger using make-up and special photographic effects.[32]

The advice written for women regarding penis size can be discerned to reflect patriarchal views: the continuation of essentialist accounts of male sexuality (that men have an unrelentingly high sex drive and sexual responsiveness that is without a bearing on individual/interpersonal aspects and external factors); patriarchal terminology (male virility); and marital relations (the wife as the support and comfort for her husband). Yet, these very accounts do not construct the penis in terms of either a phallic spectacle (big, powerful and impressive) or as pitiful and shameful stemming from its disjuncture from the phallus (small and weak). As such, it departs from the polarity which structures the dominant discourse of the penis in the West: the dichotomy of phallic versus non-phallic.[33] Rather, the penis reflects a third category, termed the 'melodramatic penis'.[33] Peter Lehman coins the term 'melodramatic penis' to account for the discourses of the penis that do not polarise the penis as phallic/non-phallic but continue to affirm the spectacular importance of the penis.[33]

The discourse of the melodramatic penis includes a number of characteristics which will be explored further. Firstly, the melodramatic penis can be read in a positive manner as avoiding the simple structuring dichotomies of the large, awesome phallic spectacle versus its abject antithesis. In this sense, the penis is removed from either the ideal phallic spectacle or the ridicule of the ineptitudes of real penises. Secondly, although not presented within a dichotomy, the discourse of the melodramatic penis persists in defining the penis in terms of monumental importance – the penis is seen to be manifest in connotations associated with male sexuality, health and well-being that continue to block a penis from merely being a penis.[33] In this regard, the penis is no longer fixed in a dichotomy of phallic and non-phallic but it is still marked as connoting extraordinary meaning.[33] Thus, the discourse of the melodramatic penis challenges conventional representations, yet it remains a troubled site of representation as it continues to frame the penis in awe and mystique.[33] In other words, the melodramatic penis defies traditional dichotomies (phallic versus non-phallic) whilst maintaining and securing its importance in the sex script which continues to preclude the penis from being just a penis.[33]

To return to the article in question, the discourse of the melodramatic penis is apparent in the advice written for women, in which there is an appeal to the emotions of women to provide comfort and support for men in order to quell any lack of penis-confidence that they may have. Additionally, rather than merely being a body part, the penis is framed in terms of virility. It is also treated as a default conjecture in assessing the lack of male desire for sex and sexual responsiveness. Yet, what most epitomises the melodrama of the penis is the lack of the very identification of it as penis, an organ and not an extension of masculinity and gender stereotypes: an organ rather than a symbol that is embedded and assigned meaning in terms of virility; an organ rather than a motif of anxiety and feelings of insecurity; and an organ that is inconsequential to mutual sexual pleasure. Even in the closing remarks of the article in question, the melodrama of the penis is present:

> So, if your wedding night is coming up and you are wondering what's in your lucky dip, don't be anxious. You probably won't get a good look at your husband's penis on the first night – but, hopefully, you will find out what this wonderful apparatus can do for you! If he is skilful, there is little chance that you will ever guess its true size.[32]

The use of the term 'lucky dip' continues to mask the penis from being exactly what it is. In perpetuating such descriptions, the penis becomes a metaphor for pleasure and satisfaction; as tools, equipment and apparatuses for both female and male sexuality. Such metaphors persist in framing pleasure as a quality or capability of the penis. This is at the expense of outlining accounts of male and female sexuality in terms of mutual pleasure derived not from the penis or penetration but from contact, connection and the closeness of a sexual/relationship bond.

In sum, the discourse of the melodramatic penis is a departure from the dichotomist construction of the ideal, potent phallus set against the fallibility inherent in attempting to live up to this ideal. However, it still enshrines the penis with astounding importance in terms of offering pleasure for both men and women. Thus, even though the phallic qualities of large penis size are not present in the article, the discourses of the melodramatic penis continue to reinforce phallocentric descriptions of sex (the penis as an organ of pleasure for both sexes) and patriarchal relations (woman as a man's aid, offering him both support and reassurance in regard to penis size).[9]

Conclusion

The study has revealed that *Intimacy*'s aim to 'empower you as its reader and give you permission to take control of your sex life',[34] is, at best, only a pseudo-empowerment for women in heterosexual relations.[8] It can only ever promote an illusory sense of female control and pleasure as it persists in defining male sexuality according to patriarchal standards. The patriarchal underpinning of male sexuality in *Intimacy* has been revealed to delimit the sexual act, female sexuality and men to predefined potentials and gender relations: restriction of male sexual expression to the erect penis; notions of 'real' sex as penile-vaginal penetration (at the expense of diverse erotic experiences derived from non-genital erogenous zones); biological accounts of the male sex drive (that negate acts of communication and negotiation); the relegation of any sexual act that departs from coitus to foreplay (and thus of secondary importance); and the continual description of the penis as a revered icon of sexual pleasure for both men and women.

To offer a departure from the above findings, constructions of male sexuality require the inclusion of alternative modes of male erotic pleasure. This requires media texts and primary care professionals to encourage men to explore and also to experiment with pleasurable feelings associated with non-genital erogenous zones of the body.[2] Accordingly, in the case of primary care professionals, their role is to 'reintroduce sex [*within*] ... as wide a definition possible'[35] in order to propose an expansive view of male sexuality that affirms pleasure over the whole body. Such transformation is not to expose the inadequacies and limitations of male sexuality, but to disestablish the dominance of patriarchal and phallocentric versions of sex.[2] In doing so, it holds the potential of changing the sexual act via the exploration of non-phallicised versions of sex and sexuality, as well as empowering female and male sexuality to unlimited potential within a relationship based on mutual respect and sexual communication.

Acknowledgements

A slightly different version of this article was originally presented at the conference on: 'Work/Force: South African masculinities in the media' held at Stellenbosch University from 13–14 September 2012.

Competing interests

The author declares that no financial or personal relationship(s) have inappropriately influenced the writing of this article.

References

1. World Health Organization. Developing sexual health programmes: A framework for action [homepage on the Internet]. c2010 [cited 2014 Mar 25]. Available from: http://www.who.int/reproductivehealth/publications/sexual_health/rhr_hrp_10_22/en/

2. Potts A. The science/fiction of sex. Feminist deconstruction and the vocabularies of heterosex. New York: Routledge; 2002.

3. Tiefer L. Sex is not a natural act and other essays. 2nd ed. Boulder: Westview Press; 2004.

4. Schneider V, Cockcroft K, Hook D. The fallible phallus: A discourse analysis of male sexuality in a South African men's interest magazine. S Afr J Psychol. 2008;38(1):136–151. http://dx.doi.org/10.1177/008124630803800108

5. Wilbraham L. Dear Doctor Delve-in: A feminist analysis of a sex advice column for women. Agenda. 1996;12(30):51–65. http://dx.doi.org/10.2307/4065783

6. Wilbraham L. The psychologization of monogamy in advice columns: Surveillance, subjectivity and resistance. In: Burman E, Kottler A, Levett A, Parker I, editors. Culture, power and difference: Discourse analysis in South Africa. London: Zed Books, 1997; pp. 65–82.

7. Intimacy4Us. Welcome to INTIMACY4US: the website that celebrates sex, love, life and everything in-between! [homepage on the Internet]. No date [cited 2015 Jan 25]. Available from: http://www.intimacy4us.com/about-us.html

8. Farvid P, Braun V. 'Most of us guys are raring to go anytime, anyplace, anywhere': Male and female sexuality in Cleo and Cosmo. Sex Roles. 2006;55:295–310. http://dx.doi.org/10.1007/s11199-006-9084-1

9. Gill R. Postfeminist media culture: Elements of a sensibility. Euro J Cult Stud. 2007;10(2):147–166. http://dx.doi.org/10.1177/1367549407075898

10. Gill R. Mediated intimacy and postfeminism: A discourse analytic examination of sex and relationships advice in a women's magazine. Discourse Commun. 2009;3(4):345–369. http://dx.doi.org/10.1177/1750481309343870

11. Hite S. Oedipus revisited. Sexual behaviour in the human male today. London: Arcadia Books; 2005.

12. Downing L. Safewording! Kinkphobia and gender normativity in Fifty Shades of Grey. Psychol Sex. 2013;4(1):92–102. http://dx.doi.org/10.1080/19419899.2012.740067

13. Mills S. Discourse (the new critical idiom). London and New York: Routledge; 2004.

14. Du Plessis R. Exposing and countering sexual myths perpetuated in films. Medical Chronicle. 2012; July:72.

15. Du Plessis R. The sites/citing of female sexuality: An Irigarayan reading of Sex positive. Communicatio. 2010; 36(3):309–326. http://dx.doi.org/10.1080/02500167.2010.518786

16. Maass VS. Facing the complexities of women's sexual desire. New York: Springer; 2007. http://dx.doi.org/10.1007/978-0-387-33169-0

17. Chalker R. The clitoral truth: The secret world at your fingertips. New York: Seven Stories Press; 2000.

18. Parker I. Discourse dynamics: Critical analysis for social and individual psychology. London: Routledge; 1992.

19. Keller R. Doing discourse research: An introduction for social scientists. Translated by B. Jenner. London: Sage; 2013.

20. 20 ways a woman can superglue her marriage. Intimacy December 2008–January 2009; pp. 42–46.

21. Do you refuse to have sex? Intimacy. July–September 2008; pp. 30–35.

22. 22 things you need to know about your wife's body. Intimacy. July–September 2008; pp. 105–109.

23. Your wife's beautiful body... Intimacy. August–September 2009; pp. 96–101.

24. Men only. How to be a man. Intimacy. April–May 2009; pp. 91–94.

25. When the 'Big O' plays hide and seek ... Intimacy. February–March 2009; pp. 86–92.

26. Men only: Help her ride the waves! Intimacy. Oct–Nov 2008; p. 52–54.

27. Steyn A. What he really wants in bed ... [homepage on the Internet]. c2009 [cited 2011 Jul 5]. Available from: http://www.intimacy4us.com/bed/ [URL no longer available]

28. Joubert H. Don't forget your mouth! [homepage on the Internet]. c2009 [cited 2011 Jul 5]. Available from: http://www.intimacy4us.com/forget-mouth/ [URL no longer available]

29. Steyn A. Foreplay for those who've forgotten how... [homepage on the Internet]. c2010 [cited 2011 Jul 5]. Available from: http://www.intimacy4us.com/foreplay-whove-forgotten/ [URL no longer available]

30. Jackson S, Scott, S. Embodying orgasm: Gendered power relations and sexual pleasure. Women & Therapy. 2001;24(1–2):99–110.

31. Braun V, Gavey N, McPhillips K. The 'Fair Deal'? Unpacking accounts of reciprocity in heterosex. Sexualities. 2003;6(2):237–261. http://dx.doi.org/10.1177/1363460703006002005

32. A small problem. Intimacy. October–November 2008; pp. 52–54.

33. Lehman P. Running scared: Masculinity and the representation of the male body. Detroit: Wayne State University Press; 2007.

34. Welcome to intimacy. Intimacy. July–September 2008; p. 4.

35. Boynton P. Better dicks through drugs? The penis as a pharmaceutical target. Scan [online journal]. c2004 [cited 2015 Feb 01. Available from: http://scan.net.au/scan/journal/display.php?journal_id=37

11

Review of the Umthombo Youth Development Foundation scholarship scheme, 1999–2013

Authors:
Andrew Ross[1]
Gavin MacGregor[2]
Laura Campbell[1]

Affiliations:
[1]Department of Family Medicine, University of KwaZulu-Natal, South Africa

[2]Umthombo Youth Development Foundation, South Africa

Correspondence to:
Andrew Ross

Email:
rossa@ukzn.ac.za

Postal address:
Department of Family Medicine, University of KwaZulu-Natal, 24 Jupiter Road, Westville 3629, South Africa

Introduction: Staffing of rural and remote facilities is a challenge throughout the world. Umthombo Youth Development Foundation (UYDF) has been running a rurally based scholarship scheme since 1999. The aim of this review is to present data on the number of students selected, their progress, graduation and work placement from inception of the scheme until 2013.

Methods: Data were extracted from the UYDF data base using a data collection template to ensure all important information was captured.

Results: Since 1999, 430 rural students across 15 health disciplines have been supported by UYDF. The annual pass rate has been greater than 89%, and less than 10% of students have been excluded from university. All graduates have spent time working in rural areas (excluding the 32 currently doing internships) and 72% (52/73) of those with no work-back obligation continue to work in rural areas.

Discussion and conclusion: The UYDF model is built around local selection, compulsory academic and peer mentoring and social support, comprehensive financial support and experiential holiday work. The results are encouraging and highlight the fact that rural students can succeed at university and will come back and work in rural areas. With 46% of the South African population situated rurally, greater thought and effort must be put into the recruitment and training of rural scholars as a possible solution to the staffing of rural healthcare facilities. The UYDF provides a model which could be replicated in other parts of South Africa.

Examen du Programme de Bourses de la Fondation Umthombo pour le Développement de la Jeunesse, 1999–2013.

Introduction: La dotation en personnel des institutions en zones rurales et lointaines est un défi dans le monde entier. La Fondation Umthombo pour le Développement de la Jeunesse (UYDF) a organisé un programme de bourses en milieu rural depuis 1999. Le but de cet examen est de fournir des données sur le nombre d'étudiants sélectionnés, leurs progrès, l'obtention de leur diplôme et leur placement professionnel depuis le début du programme jusqu'à 2013.

Méthodes: Les données proviennent de la base de données de l'UYDF en se servant d'un modèle de collecte de données afin que toutes les informations importantes soient saisies.

Résultats: Depuis 1999, 430 étudiants ruraux dans 15 disciplines de la santé ont été aidés par l'UYDF. Le taux de réussite annuel était de plus de 89%, et moins de 10% des étudiants ont été exclus de l'université. Tous les diplômés ont travaillé en zone rurale (à l'exception des 32 qui sont en train de faire leur stage) et 72% (52/73) de ceux qui n'ont pas à rembourser leur bourse par le travail continuent à travailler dans les zones rurales.

Discussion et conclusion: Le modèle de l'UYDF s'articule autour de la sélection locale, du mentorat académique et par les pairs, et du soutien social, un soutient financier complet et du travail expérientiel de vacances. Les résultats sont encourageants et montrent que les étudiants ruraux peuvent réussir à l'université et reviendront travailler dans les zones rurales. Avec 46% de la population sud-africaine vivant à la campagne, il faut s'efforcer de recruter et de former d'avantage d'étudiants ruraux comme solution possible pour pourvoir en personnel les services de santé ruraux. L'UYDF fournit un modèle qui pourrait être reproduit dans d'autres parties de l'Afrique du Sud.

Background

Staffing of rural and remote health facilities is a challenge throughout the world. The World Health Organization (WHO) estimates that there is a global shortage of 4.3 million doctors and nurses, with up to 1 billion people without access to healthcare workers.[1] The Department of

Health in its *Human Resources for Health for South Africa 2030* estimated that there is a shortage of 14 932 professional nurses, 4145 doctors, 778 pharmacists, 1777 social workers and 345 physiotherapist in South Africa (SA), with rural areas impacted by staff shortages more than urban areas.[2]

In Australia, Canada and the United States of America, recruiting rural origin scholars who return to work in rural areas after training has been shown to be an effective strategy for increasing staffing levels at rural and remote facilities.[3,4] Using the pipeline metaphor, various strategies have been employed to increase the number of rural origin students in these countries. These include the promotion of careers in medicine at high schools, reservation of a certain percentage of places for rural origin students at medical schools, increasing the rural content and exposure to rural medicine at university, and recently the development of rurally located medical schools.[5]

Although there is substantial evidence from First World countries, there is relatively little evidence from developing countries that rural recruitment impacts on staffing levels at rural facilities. In 2003 a South African study reviewed where 138 rural origin and 140 urban origin students where working as health care professionals (HCPs). This study concluded that rural students were more likely to work in rural areas than urban origin students (38% vs. 12% respectively).[6] In 2003 Ross and Reid reviewed a number of HCPs who remained at a rural district hospital (DH) post-community service and found that the numbers who remained were small (22/278; 8%). The authors concluded that rural origin HCPs and those with provincial work-back obligations were more like to stay at a rural DH than those who grew up in an urban area or those without any contractual obligations.[7]

Currently there appear to be no systematic efforts to promote health science careers in rural areas of SA, and dysfunctional schools make entry into and success at medical school a challenge.[8] Most South African healthcare training institutions currently have a race-based admission policy to address the imbalances of the apartheid past. The University of KwaZulu-Natal has recently introduced a policy of admitting 28% quintile 1 and 2 students to the medical school to increase representation from these schools. Although many rural schools may be represented by quintile 1 and 2 schools this is an incidental consideration and not a policy to ensure adequate selection of rural origin students. Tumbo's 2009 study, which looked at rural representation at the nine health education facilities in SA, showed that rural origin students accounted for 27.4%, 22.4%, 26.7%, and 24.8% in medicine, physiotherapy, occupational therapy and dentistry respectively – significantly lower than the national rural population ratio.[9] As such, the recruitment of rural origin students could be considered to be an issue of social justice, important for the provision of health services in rural areas.

With 46% of the South African population situated rurally,[10] it would appear that geographical origin must become an important selection consideration at health training institutions. Greater effort should be put into the recruitment of rural scholars, the prioritisation of places for them to study at medical school and other health training institutions, provision of adequate support to enable them to succeed, as well as creation of posts, and other postgraduate career opportunities in rural areas.

Umthombo Youth Development Foundation (UYDF) has been running a rurally based scholarship scheme since 1999. The scholarships scheme was initially established to address staff shortages at a rural DH. The conceptualisation of the scheme was based on evidence from studies in Australia and Canada which showed that rural origin students are more likely to work in rural areas than urban origin students.[11,12] UYDF students are selected by the local hospital selection committee and sign a year-for-year work-back contract with UYDF. UYDF provides comprehensive financial support at university and a compulsory structured peer, academic and social mentoring programme. The hospital provides opportunities for experiential holiday work experience and employment opportunities on completion of their degree. By any definition (geography, work opportunities, distance, population density, etc.) the students supported by UYDF would be considered to be rural.[13]

Aim and objective

The aim of this review is to present data on the number of students selected, their progress, graduation and work placement from inception of the UYDF scheme in 1999 until 2013. It is hoped that this review will stimulate debate on admission policies and indicate possible solutions to the staffing challenges at rural healthcare facilities.

Methods

Data were extracted from the UYDF data base using a data collection template to ensure that all important information was captured. All students supported by UYDF have been included (even those partially funded by UYDF and who received a provincial bursary or other funding during the course of their studies). Graduates were contacted by UYDF staff to verify the information available at the office and to obtain any outstanding information.

Ethical considerations

Ethical permission for this study was given by the Human and Social Science Ethics Committee of the University of KwaZulu-Natal (HSS/0228/014)

Results

Some health science courses are three years in duration (dental therapy, environmental health, radiography, biomedical technology), some four years (physiotherapy, pharmacy, nursing) and others six years (medicine). This means that intake rates do not necessarily correspond with graduation rates; see Table 1 for details. In 2007

TABLE 1: Student numbers supported by UYDF since 1999.

Year	New students	Cumulative total*	No. passed**	Number repeating	Number excluded	Number graduated	Pass rate (%)
1999	4	4	4	0	0	0	100
2000	5	9	8	1	0	0	89
2001	6	15	13	1	1	0	87
2002	22	36	29	1	6	2	81
2003	17	45	40	4	1	7	88
2004	12	49	47	2	0	5	96
2005	12	56	50	3	3	10	89
2006	11	54	47	4	3	12	87
2007	17	56	52	0	4	13	93
2008	26	65	53	10	2	7	82
2009	37	83	71	10	2	19	86
2010	36	108	97	9	2	15	90
2011	61	152	132	16	2	25	87
2012	56	181	166	15	8 + 2 (poor attitudes)	22	92
2013	42	191	179	8	4 + 1 (ill health)	48	94
2014	66	205	-	-		-	-
Total	-	**430**	-	-	**41 (9.5%)**	**185**	-

*, Cumulative total = new students + existing students − number graduated − number excluded.
**, Number passed = number of students who were able to progress (they may have been carrying some subjects).

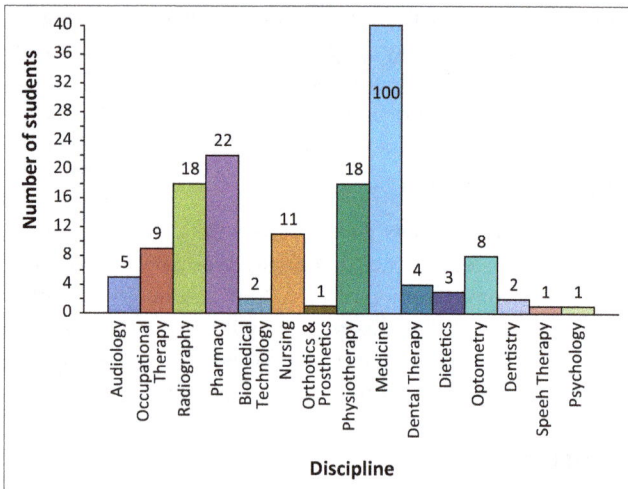

FIGURE 1: Current students by discipline (*n* = 205); there are 100 medical students (off the scale).

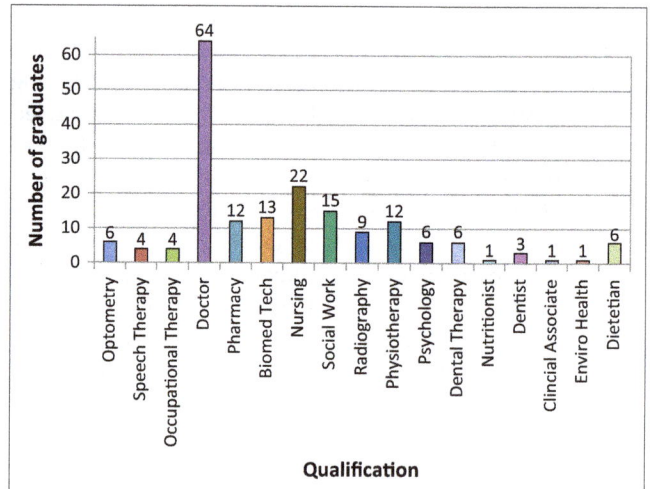

N = 183 (excludes the two who graduated in May 2014).
FIGURE 2: Breakdown of graduates by qualification.

UYDF moved from a voluntary run organisation to having full-time staff members (Director, full-time student mentor and administrative support), and the dramatic increase in the total number of students supported since 2008 can be attributed to this. Currently UYDF is supporting 205 students across 15 health disciplines, 65% of whom are women. A breakdown of students by discipline is presented in Figure 1.

As of May 2014 there are 185 UYDF graduates. A breakdown of graduates by discipline is presented in Figure 2.

Figure 3 shows the breakdown of graduates by current place of work

Some public sector hospitals are in urban areas, but most of the non-governmental organisations (NGOs) and some private practices where graduates work are in rural areas. Not all students are supported by UYDF for the duration of their training, as some students obtain a provincial

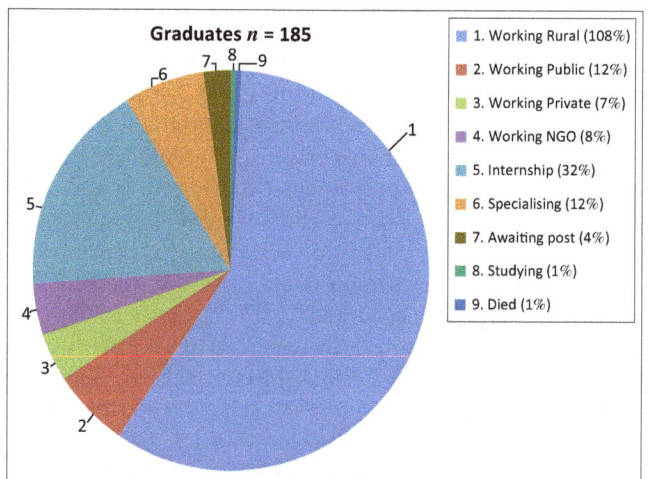

FIGURE 3: Current graduates by current place of work.

bursary during the course of their studies. The provincial bursary programme has different work-back obligations;

their graduates may work in any KwaZulu-Natal provincial hospital (including urban hospitals), and may engage in postgraduate training during their work-back obligation.

All graduates who received any support from UYDF have spent at least a year working at a rural DH (this excludes the 32 currently doing their internship, as it is not possible to do ones internship at a rural DH in SA). Nine graduates have bought themselves out of a portion of their UYDF contract, and only one has defaulted on their contractual obligations. Of the 73 graduates who have completed their contractual obligations to UYDF, 52 (71%) continue to practice in a rural area, 42 in rural DHs, and the balance are working for rural NGOs or in rural private practice. A breakdown of these graduates by location is presented in Figure 4.

Currently 57% (106/185) of the graduates are women, and qualification by gender is presented in Figure 5. Slightly more women than men have qualified as doctors and pharmacists, whilst numbers are equal for nursing and

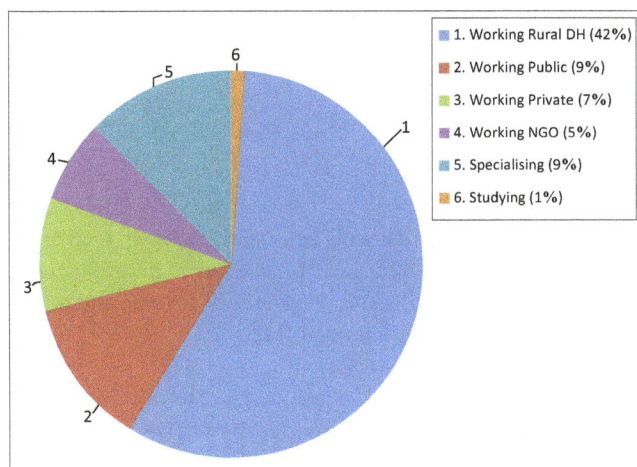

occupational therapy. More men than women have trained as biomedical technologists, nutritionists, dentists and clinical associates.

Discussion

The UYDF results are significant, particularly within the current SA context, and more so because of the rural origin of these students. With a pass rate of greater than 89% over a 15-year period and less than 10% of students being excluded from training institutions, these figures highlight the latent potential of rural scholars. These figures are also in sharp contrast to the national experience where, despite the number of black students at institutes of higher learning (IHL) rising from 30% in 1999 to 66% in 2010, this has not translated into an increased number of black graduates.

Cohort studies have shown that the completion rates of black African students at contact universities in the life sciences, mathematics and physical sciences is only about 33%, which is about half the completion rate of white students.[14] Other scholarship programmes have had varied student success, with the Rural Education Access Program (REAP) reporting 57% – 66% student completion rates of the 131 students supported in 2002.[15]

The success of the UYDF model may be related to several factors, including the following: (a) local hospital participation; (b) academic and peer mentoring; (c) social support; and (d) the reintegration and support of graduates into the hospitals once they have completed their training. These aspects are depicted in Figure 6.

The local DH is at the heart of the UYDF model, as the scholarship scheme started as a response to the need for staff at a rural DH. To ensure that the scheme is responsive to the needs of the hospital, the hospital selection committee is responsible for the promotion of a career in health through open days, and selection of health science students according to hospital priorities. UYDF students are also expected to do four weeks of experiential holiday work at the local hospital each year. This enables students to consolidate their theoretical knowledge in a practical way, and to apply their knowledge at a DH level, work alongside local HCPs and strengthen relationships with one another, with management at the hospital and with community members. This holiday work also prepares them for working at a DH as they understand the local conditions, challenges and resource constraints at such hospitals as well as what is expected of them as HCPs. Career-specific work experience is recognised as an important motivating influence for students at IHL and can contribute to students persisting and achieving academic success at IHL.[14] Experiential holiday work is an integral aspect of the UYDF model.

UYDF is responsible for facilitating the academic and peer mentoring and the social support at university. Rural students often feel alienated when they first attend IHL,

UYDF, Youth Development Foundation.
FIGURE 4: Work placement of graduates with no work-back obligation to UYDF (*n* = 73).

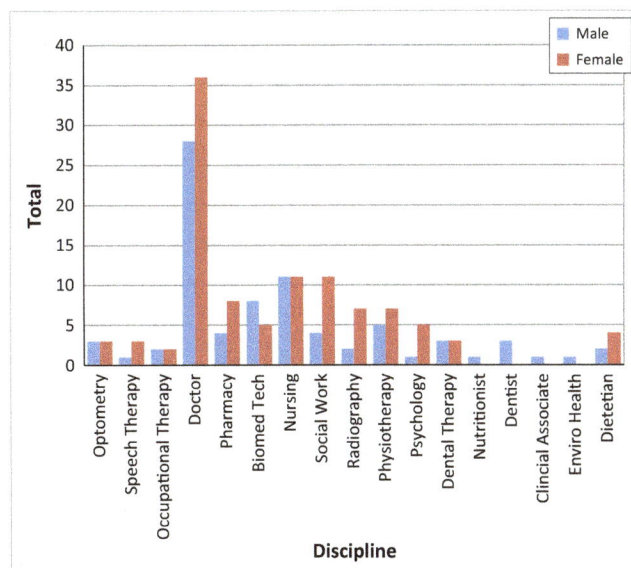

Legend:
1. Working Rural DH (42%)
2. Working Public (9%)
3. Working Private (7%)
4. Working NGO (5%)
5. Specialising (9%)
6. Studying (1%)

FIGURE 5: Breakdown of graduates by gender.

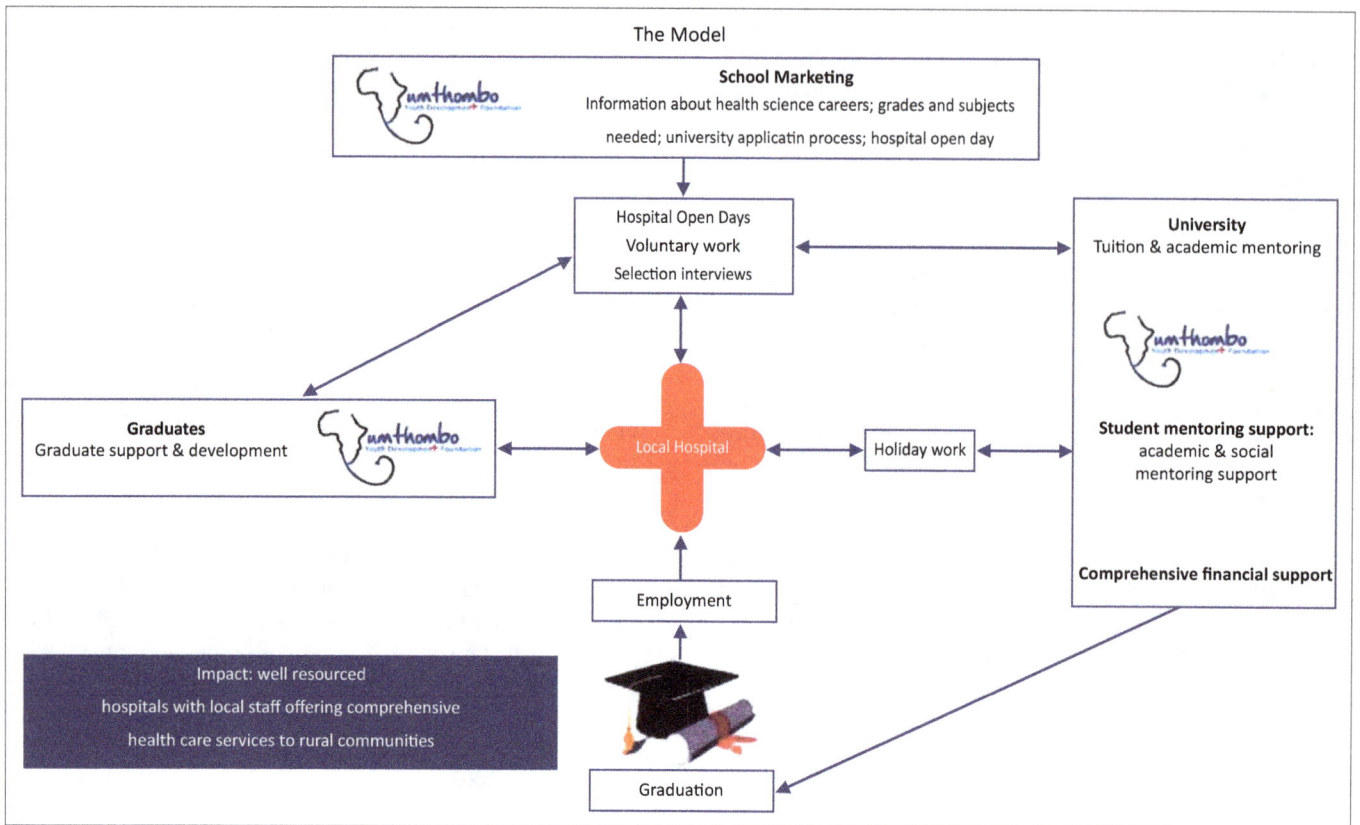

UYDF, Youth Development Foundation.
FIGURE 6: The UYDF model for student selection and support.

and this contributes to their social isolation and inability to access social and academic support.[16] The UYDF provides a 'family' of other rural origin students who help each other to adapt to the challenges of university and city life. TM, a UYDF graduate, put it this way: 'I would mentor new students. Not teaching them maths and physics, but I would mentor them in terms of social life, and how to handle the situation, knowing their background. So it was easier for the new guys to adapt in that environment, because I was there.'

Social and academic engagement has been identified by Tinto as critical to student success at IHL.[17] Academic mentoring and support is provided by UYDF mentors who meet regularly with UYDF students to review their progress and ensure that academic and social issues are being addressed. This accountability encourages and supports students to find solutions to any challenges they might face at university. The academic mentoring also communicates a belief that students have the potential to succeed and that they belong at an IHL.

Other studies have shown that when students believe that they have the ability to succeed and that they belong or deserve to be at an IHL this contributes to their success.[18] Laude at the University of Texas found that the introduction of small classes, mentorship and support which communicated to students that they had the ability to succeed and that they belong at university, influenced success of students who traditionally failed.[19] The academic

and peer mentoring as well as social support facilitated by UYDF is considered key to students' success, as it enables them to identify and overcome academic and social challenges in order to succeed at IHL.

Comprehensive financial support is also an important component of the support provided by UYDF, which may assist in the success of the scheme by allowing students to focus more on the academic challenges at university. Inadequate finances have been identified as an important reason why students in SA fail at IHL.[16,20] A criticism of the current NSFAS (National Student Financial Aid Scheme) funding model is that students only receive partial financial support, which covers fees and residence with only a small food and book allowance. This NSFAS model is based on the assumption that parents should make a family contribution towards these costs. However, for many rural students the family contribution is not forthcoming, and hunger and their limited access to the necessary resources distract from academic work and may contribute to their high failure rate. The Rural Education Access Programme, which supports many disadvantaged students, has recommended a review of the current funding model for NSFAS to ensure comprehensive funding for financially needy students at IHL.[16]

Recommendation

The UYDF provides a model which could be replicated in other parts of SA. However, further studies are needed to identify and understand the key aspects of the UYDF model and whether or not this model can be taken to scale.

Conclusion

Results from the last 15 years of the UYDF are significant and highlight that rural students can succeed at university with appropriate support. Whilst numbers are still small, all graduates have spent time working at rural hospitals, thus helping to ensure services are provided at these facilities. With 71% of those who have completed their work-back obligation having remained in rural sites, these numbers are encouraging and support data from other countries that rural origin students will return to work in rural areas.

As most of the current literature around the recruitment and training of rural origin students to provide services in rural areas is based on Australian and Canadian studies, this study adds to the body of literature by showing that even in developing countries, strategies to identify and support rural origin students to train as healthcare providers can contribute to the staffing of rural healthcare facilities.

Acknowledgements

With thanks to the staff of UYDF for the help in collecting the data and to Prof. and Dr S.M. Ross for the numerous reads and rereads of drafts.

Competing interests

The authors declare that they have no financial or personal relationship(s) that may have inappropriately influenced them in writing this article.

Authors' contributions

A.R. (University of KwaZulu-Natal) was responsible for conceptualising the research project, analysing the data and writing the article. G.M. (Umthombo Youth Development Foundation) was responsible for collecting and collating the data and contributed to the analysis and writing of the article. L.C. (University of KwaZulu-Natal) contributed to the writing and reviewing of the article.

References

1. Crisp N, Chen L. Global Supply of Health Professionals. N Engl J Med. 2014;370(10):950–957. http://dx.doi.org/10.1056/NEJMra1111610

2. Department of Health. Human Resources for Health for South Africa 2030. Pretoria: South African National Department of Health; 2011.

3. Sen Gupta T, Woolley T, Murray R, Hays RD, McCloskey T. Positive impacts on rural and regional workforce from the first seven cohorts of James Cook University medical graduates. Rural Remote Hlth. 2014;14(2657):1–14.

4. CS Winn CS, Chisolm BA, Hummelbrunner JA. Factors affecting recruitment and retention of rehabilitation professionals in Northern Ontario, Canada: A cross-sectional study. Rural Remote Hlth. 2014;14(2619):1–7.

5. World Organization of National Colleges, Academies and Academic Associations of General Practitioners/Family Physicians.Rural Medical Education Guidebook [WONCA online], WONCA; 2014. Available from: www.globalfamilydoctor.com

6. De Vries E, Reid SJ. Do South African medical students of rural origin return to rural practice? S AfrMed J. 2003;10(93):789–793.

7. Ross A, Reid SJ. The retention of community service officers for an additional year at district hospitals in KwaZulu Natal and the Eastern Cape and Limpopo Provinces. SA Fam Pract. 2009;51(3):249–253. http://dx.doi.org/10.1080/20786204.2009.10873856

8. Bloch G. The toxic mix: What's wrong with South Africa's schools and how to fix it. Cape Town Tafelberg; 2009.

9. Tumbo JM, Couper ID, Hugo JF. Rural-origin health science students at South African universities. S Afr Med J. 2009;99(1):54-56.

10. Statistics South Africa. Census South Africa 2001. Pretoria Statistics South Africa; 2001.

11. Wilson NW, Couper ID, De Vries E, Reid S, Fish T, Marais BJ. A critical review of interventions to redress the inequitable distribution of healthcare professionals to rural and remote areas. Rural Remote Hlth. 2009;9(2):1060.

12. Laven G, Wilkinson D. Rural doctors and rural background: How strong is the evidence? A systematic review. Austr J Rural Hlth. 2003;11(6):277–284. http://dx.doi.org/10.1111/j.1440-1584.2003.00534.x

13. Couper ID. Rural hospital focus: Defining rural. Rural Remote Hlth. 2003;3(2):205.

14. Lubben F, Davidowitz B, Buffler A, Allie S, Scott I. Factors influencing access students' persistence in an undergraduate science programme: A South African case study. Int J Educ Dev. 2010;30(4):351–358. http://dx.doi.org/10.1016/j.ijedudev.2009.11.009

15. Hartnack A. Humble beginnings, bright future: A tracking study of the first full intake of students on the rural education access programme. A decade on. Cape Town: Rural Education Access Programme; 2011.

16. Wickham S, Jones B, Coetzee G, Bailey T. Factors that facilitate success for disadvantaged higher education students. An investigation into approaches used by REAP, NSFAS and selected higher education institutions. Cape Town: Rural Education Access Program (REAP); 2008.

17. Tinto V, Pusser B. Moving From Theory to Action: Building a Model of Institutional Action for Student Success2006 28 June 2012. Available from: http://cpe.ky.gov/NR/rdonlyres/D7EE04D0-EE8C-4ACD-90F6-5BB3C8BC8E05/0/SS_related_info_6_22_3_Moving_from_Theory_to_Action.pdf

18. Yeager DS, Walton GM. Social-psychological interventions in education. They're not magic. Rev Educ Res. 2011;81(2):267–301. http://dx.doi.org/10.3102/0034654311405999

19. Tough P. Who Gets to Graduate? The New York Times 2014, May 15 [cited 2015 Mar 10]. Available from: http://www.nytimes.com/2014/05/18/magazine/who-gets-to-graduate.html?_r=0

20. Letseka M, Maile S. High university drop-out rates: A threat to South Africa's future. 2008 Mar [cited 2012 May 10]. Available from: http://www.hsrc.ac.za/Document-2717.phtml

12

Adherence of doctors to a clinical guideline for hypertension in Bojanala district, North-West Province, South Africa

Authors:
Asafa R. Adedeji[1]
John Tumbo[1]
Indiran Govender[1]

Affiliations:
[1]Department of Family Medicine and Primary Health Care, Sefako Makgatho Health Sciences University, South Africa

Correspondence to:
Indiran Govender

Email:
indiran.govender@gmail.com

Postal address:
PO Box 222, Medunsa 0204, South Africa

Background: Clinical guidelines are systematically developed statements that assist practitioners and patients to make healthcare decisions for specific clinical circumstances. Non-adherence of doctors to guidelines is thought to contribute significantly to poor delivery of clinical care, resulting in poor clinical outcomes.

Aim: To investigate adherence of doctors in rural district hospitals to clinical guidelines using the South African Hypertension Guideline 2006 as an example.

Setting: Four district hospitals in Bojanala district of North-West Province, South Africa.

Methods: A cross-sectional study determined adherence practices of doctors from records of patients with established hypertension seen at the four district hospitals.

Results: Of the 490 total records documented by 29 doctors, screening for co-morbidity or associated factors was carried out as follows: diabetes mellitus 99.2%, obesity 6.1%, smoking 53.5%, dyslipidaemia 36.9%, abdominal circumference 3.3%; organ damage: eye 0, kidney 82%, heart 43.5%, chronic kidney disease 38.2%, stroke/transient ischaemic attack 15.9%, heart failure 23.5%, advanced retinopathy 0.2%, coronary heart disease 23.7%, peripheral arterial disease 13.9%. Critical tests/measurements were documented in the following proportions: blood pressure 99.8%, weight 85.3%, height 65.7%, body mass index 3.1%, urinalysis 74.5%, lipogram 76.1%, urea/creatinine 80.4%, electrocardiogram 42.9%, blood glucose 100%; risk determination and grading: diagnosis by hypertension severity 19%, low added risk 57.1%, moderate added risk 64.7%, high added risk 89.6%, very high added risk 89.2%. Adherence to therapies was as follows: first-line guideline drugs 69.4%, second line 84.7%, third line 87.8% and fourth-line 89.6%.

Conclusion: Overall adherence of doctors to treatment guidelines for hypertension was found to be low (51.9%). Low adherence rates were related to age (older doctors) and less clinical experience, and differed with regard to various aspects of the guidelines.

Adhésion des Docteurs à des directives cliniques pour l'Hypertension dans le district de Bojanala, dans la Province du Nord Ouest d'Afrique du Sud.

Contexte: Les directives cliniques sont des énoncés systématiquement développés pour aider les médecins et les patients à prendre des décisions sanitaires dans des circonstances cliniques particulières. On les utilise pour normaliser les soins médicaux, promouvoir l'uniformité dans la pratique, améliorer la qualité des soins et réduire les risques liés aux soins cliniques. La non-adhérence des médecins aux directives contribue considérablement à la mauvaise prestation des soins cliniques ce qui entraine de mauvais résultats cliniques. L'étude avait pour but d'examiner l'adhésion dans la pratique des docteurs des hôpitaux de districts ruraux aux directives cliniques, en prenant comme exemple les directives sud-africaines de 2006 pour l'Hypertension.

Méthodes: On a fait une étude dans quatre hôpitaux du district de Bojanala dans la Province du Nord Ouest. On a déterminé l'adhésion aux pratiques des médecins à partir des dossiers des patients souffrant d'hypertension qui ont fréquenté les quatre hôpitaux de district. On a saisi les données sur une fiche de collecte de donnée. On a fait une analyse statistique descriptive sur SAS, Release 9.2.

Résultats: Sur les 490 dossiers documentés par 29 docteurs nous avons trouvé: dépistage de comorbidité ou des facteurs associés: DM 486 patients (99.2%), obésité 30 (6.1%), tabagisme 262 (53.5%), dyslipidémie 181 (36.9%), circonférence abdominale 16 (3.3 %), lésions aux organes: yeux 0, reins 402 (82%), cœur 213(43.5%), CKD 187 (38.2 %), attaque/TIA 78 (15.9%), insuffisance cardiaque 115 (23.5%), rétinopathie avancée 1 (0.2%), maladie cardiovasculaire 116 (23.7%), artériopathie périphérique 68 (13.9%). Les tests critiques et évaluations ont été documentés dans les proportions suivantes: Tension artérielle 489 (99.8%), Poids 418 (85.3%), Taille 322 (65.7%), BMI 15 (3.1%), Analyse d'urine 365 (74.5%), Lipogramme 373 (76.1%), Urée/créatinine 394 (80.4%), ECG 210 (42.9%), GS 490 (100%). La détermination et le degré de risque ont été documentés dans les proportions suivantes: diagnostic par gravité de l'hypertension 93 (19%), risque additionnel faible 280 (57.1%), risque additionnel modéré 317 (64.7%), risque additionnel élevé 439 (89.6%), risque additionnel très élevé 437 (89.2%). Adhésion aux directives thérapeutiques dans 340 (69.4%) médicaments de première ligne 415 (84.7%) de deuxième ligne 430 (87.8%) de troisième ligne, et dans 439 (89.6%) thérapies de quatrième intention.

Conclusion: L'adhésion totale des médecins aux directives de traitement pour l'hypertension est faible (51.9%). Le faible taux d'adhésion est lié à l'âge et à l'expérience clinique du médecin et diffère selon les différents aspects des directives.

Introduction

Clinical practice guidelines are systematically developed statements that assist practitioners and patients to make healthcare decisions for specific clinical circumstances.[1] Guidelines can be further defined as a document that streamlines particular processes according to a regular routine.[1] In the medical context it refers to a document which seeks to guide decisions and criteria regarding diagnosis, management/treatment in specific areas of healthcare.[2] They are derived from synthesised evidence that have been translated into specific practice-oriented recommendations.[3] Guidelines identify, summarise and evaluate evidence of the highest quality and the most up-to-date data about prevention, diagnosis, prognosis, therapy including dosages of medications, risk/benefit and cost-effectiveness.[4]

Objectives of clinical guidelines are to standardise medical care and promote uniformity in practice as it relates to care, in order to raise quality of care, reduce several kinds of risk (to the patient, healthcare provider, medical insurers and health plans) and achieve the best balance between cost and medical parameters such as effectiveness, specificity, sensitivity, availability and stakeholders' preferences. Overall the central role of guidelines is to help clinicians make better decisions.[1]

There has been increasing concern globally regarding poor adherence of clinicians to clinical guidelines. Various reasons have been advanced as barriers to adherence to clinical guidelines amongst medical practitioners.[5,6] These include the clinicians' lack of requisite skill and expertise to implement recommended action, lack of the mandatory equipment or staff to implement a guideline recommendation, not being aware of the existence of the guidelines, unfamiliarity or disagreement with the recommendations of the guidelines, lack of confidence in ability to implement the guideline, inability to overcome the inertia of previous practice, the presence of external barriers to following recommendations, a lack of expectancy that adherence to guidelines will lead to the desired process of health care, or simply forgetting to use it.[7] Poor adherence to clinical guidelines has been reported to contribute to poor health outcomes, compromised quality of care and increased risks, with resultant adverse events.

In the Bojanala district of North-West Province, South Africa, we observed diversity and inconsistency in clinical decisions made by medical practitioners in district hospitals, attributable to erratic adherence to guidelines. In our opinion lack of standardised clinical management of patients may lead to adverse outcomes. Analysis of surveillance data conducted by the Patients Safety Group in North-West Province shows an increasing trend in preventable adverse events resulting from poor adherence of clinicians to guidelines.[8]

A host of clinical management guidelines are readily available in all district hospitals in Bojanala district. Prominent amongst these are management guidelines for hypertension, diabetes mellitus, asthma and epilepsy. As the doctors are not only aware of the existence but also the location of guidelines, it was of interest to the researchers to describe their adherence to guidelines using the 2006 hypertension clinical management guidelines[9] (still the most recent hypertension guidelines at the time of this study) as a case study.

In the period prior to 2006 there were parallel guidelines produced by the Southern African Hypertension Society and the South African Department of Health, but the 2006 South African Hypertension Guideline is a joint effort by the two bodies.[9] The guideline outlined the different broad aspects that practitioners need to concentrate on in order to achieve effective blood pressure (BP) control, starting from the initial patient risk screening/profiling, measurements and investigations to be done, risk categorisation and holistic management of hypertensive patients with or without co-morbidities, to their follow up and ongoing care plan.

Our study sought to investigate adherence practices of doctors to the use of clinical/practice guidelines in four district hospitals in Bojanala district, North-West Province. We chose the 2006 Hypertension Guideline as an example as it is freely available at the facilities.

Research methods and design

A descriptive cross-sectional study using existing patient records was conducted. Records of patients registered as hypertensive in the chronic diseases registers at four rural district hospitals in Bojanala district of North-West Province, South Africa, were evaluated. The four hospitals had 48, 250, 32 and 40 beds, and also conducted outpatient clinics for chronic illnesses, including hypertension. Patient records completed by 29 doctors (general practitioners) at the four hospitals were evaluated.

The formula for calculation of the sample size used was $n = p(1-p)(1.96/a)^2$, where n is the sample size, $p = 0.75$ (assumed adherence rate which is 75% [see below] and $a = 0.04$ (accuracy of ± 4%). The 0.75 is halfway between 0.7 (70%) and 0.8 (80%);if the acceptable minimum level of adherence is in the range of 70% – 80%, the precision of the 95% confidence interval, that is the distance from the percentage calculated from the sample to the interval limits, will be ± 4% (which is also the a). This calculation yielded $n = 450$. We oversampled to 484 to allow for missing data, and this was proportionately distributed to the four hospitals as 110, 95, 95 and 184 cases respectively. At each hospital files were consecutively selected until the desired sample size was achieved. Files with missing, illegible or incomplete records were excluded.

The following variables were evaluated for adherence to the hypertension management guideline:

1. Screening for major risk factors: diabetes mellitus, smoking, obesity (body mass index – BMI), dyslipidaemia and abdominal obesity.
2. Grading of risk.
3. Performance of scheduled investigations including fundoscopy, urea and electrolytes, urine dipsticks and electrocardiogram (ECG).

4. Screening for complications, including peripheral arterial disease, heart failure, chronic renal failure, stroke, transient ischaemic attack, advanced retinopathy and coronary heart disease.
5. Routine measurements of the BP (taken at least twice in one consultation, in sitting position), weight, height, BMI, abdominal circumference, urine dipsticks or urinalysis, lipogram, urea and electrolyte levels, ECG and blood glucose level.
6. Documentation of lifestyle modification methods, such as exercise, dietary modification, quitting smoking, alcohol intake.
7. Adherence to prescriptions according to guidelines.
8. Review of treatment and care strategies.
9. Evidence of scheduled review dates.

These data were captured into a data collection sheet. Adherence to each variable was classified as complete (C), partial (P) or non-adherent (N) compared with the reference Hypertension Guideline. Complete adherence referred to an adherence level above 65% and partial adherence to 50 – 64.9%, whereas adherence levels of less than 49.9% were classified as non-adherent. Descriptive statistical analysis was performed using SAS software, version 9.2.

Ethical considerations

Ethical approval for the study was obtained from the Medunsa Research Ethics Committee (MREC/M/147/2011: PG).

Results

There were 29 full-time doctors. Doctors in the district hospitals who were considered to have additional qualifications were those with any type of postgraduate medical diploma/fellowship or MMed/college fellowship qualification in Family Medicine. In the four hospitals the mean age of the doctors was 43.9 years (range 29-67 years). There were more males (18) than females (11). The mean length of experience was 15 years (range 4-39 years). More doctors (16) obtained their basic degree locally, whilst 13 had foreign qualifications. Table 1 lists the characteristics of the participating doctors.

Adherence to screening for major cardiovascular risk factors was high for diabetes mellitus (n = 486, 99.2%), moderate

for smoking (n = 262, 53.5%), low for obesity (n = 30, 6.1%), dyslipidemias (n = 181, 36.9%) and abdominal obesity (n = 30, 6.2%) (Table 2).

Adherence to measurement aspects of the guidelines was high for BP (n = 489, 99.8%), whilst adherence to staging of the severity in accordance with the guideline was low (n = 93, 19.0%).

Adherence to lifestyle modification/non-drug treatment recommendations was low for physical activity (n = 152, 31.2%), dietary modification (n = 228, 46.5%), and advice on stopping/reduction of alcohol intake (n = 169, 34.5%) and stopping smoking (n = 231, 47.2%). Adherence to the ongoing care aspect was high for referral (n = 385, 78.6%), whilst adherence to discussion of review date was low (n = 26, 5.3%).

When all of the items which were evaluated were considered in totality, overall adherence was found to be 51.9% (Table 3).

Discussion

This study found a generally low adherence of doctors to clinical management guidelines, using the Hypertension Guideline 2006 as an example. Considering all of the different aspects of the guidelines together, the doctors demonstrated complete adherence to 46.7%, partial adherence to 5.2% and non-adherence to 48.1%.

The overall results of our study are comparable to those of another conducted in Pretoria, South Africa, which found that overall adherence to the hypertension practice guideline used by generalists in private practice was 55%, whilst in public service primary care doctors it was 56.4%.[10]

Several determinants of adherence practice, including demographic characteristics of practitioners, training background, experience and the different aspects of the guideline, were investigated in this study. There were more males (62%), foreign qualified doctors (52.2%), those having a basic medical degree (76%), and those with less than 10 years' experience (56.2%) with average experience of 11.4 years. In addition the doctors were predominantly young, most being in the age range 20–39 years (55.2%), with a mean age of 43.9 years.

TABLE 1: Characteristics of the participating doctors.

Variable	Categories					Total (n)
Age (years)	**21–30 (%)**	**31–40 (%)**	**41–50 (%)**	**51–60 (%)**	**> 60 (%)**	
	5 (17.2)	11 (37.9)	7 (24.1)	4 (13.8)	2 (6.9)	29
Sex	**Male (%)**		**Female (%)**			
	18 (62.1)		11 (37.9)			29
Qualifications	**Basic medical degree only (%)**		**Medical degree and postgraduate qualification (%)**			
	22 (75.9)		7 (24.1)			29
Where qualification obtained	**Locally (%)**		**Foreign (%)**			
	16 (55.2)		13 (44.8)			29
Years of Experience	**< 5 (%)**		**6–10 (%)**		**> 10 (%)**	
	11 (37.9)		5 (17.3)		13 (44.8)	29

TABLE 2: Evidence of adherence to the hypertension guidelines.

Variable	Categories assessed	Patient records assessed		
		Adherent (%)	Partially adherent (%)	Non-adherent (%)
Screening for major cardiovascular risk factors	Diabetes mellitus	411 (83.9)	75 (15.3)	4 (0.8)
	Smoking	177 (36.1)	85 (17.4)	228 (46.5)
	Obesity	30 (6.1)	0	460 (93.9)
	Dyslipidaemia	181 (36.9)	0	309 (63.1)
	Abdominal girth	15 (3.1)	15 (3.1)	460 (93.8)
Screening for target organ damage	Eyes	0	0	490 (100)
	Kidneys	402 (82)	0	88 (18)
	Heart	213 (43.5)	0	277 (56.5)
Documentation of measurements done	BP	2 (0.4)	487 (99.4)	1 (0.2)
	Weight	418 (85.3)	0	72 (14.7)
	Height	322 (65.7)	0	168 (34.3)
	BMI	15 (3.1)	0	475 (96.9)
	Abdominal circumference	16 (3.3)	0	474 (96.7)
Documentation of routine investigations	Urinalysis	365 (74.5)	0	125 (25.5)
	Lipogram	373 (76.1)	0	117 (23.9)
	Urea and electrolytes	394 (80.4)	0	96 (19.6)
	ECG	210 (42.9)		280 (57.1)
	Blood glucose	490 (100)	0	0
Documented severity grading	Severity staging of condition according to guideline	93 (19)	0	397 (81)
Documented care	Lifestyle modification advice was documented	435 (22.2)	345 (17.6)	1180 (60.2)
Documentation of ongoing care	Referral	385 (78.6)	0	105 (21.4)
	Discussed review date	26 (5.3)	0	464 (94.7)
	Given review date	454 (92.7)	0	36 (7.3)
	Support home visits	2 (0.4)	0	488 (99.6)
Medication	Appropriateness of medication prescribed according to staging	340 (69.4)	0	150 (30.6)
	Review and adjustment of medicine relative to response	256 (52.2)	0	234 (47.8)

TABLE 3: Overall adherence to items on the hypertension management guideline.

Hospital	C (%)	P (%)	N (%)	Total items evaluated
A	2323 (47)	249 (5.0)	2373 (48.0)	4945
B	1953 (47.3)	208 (5.0)	1967 (47.7)	4128
C	3624 (46.3)	388 (5.0)	3813 (48.7)	7825
D	1931 (46.4)	248 (6.0)	1984 (47.7)	4163
All hospitals	**9831 (46.7)**	**1093 (5.2)**	**10137 (48.1)**	**21061**

P-value for values from all four hospitals is 0.2623

The average duration of clinical experience found in this study was comparable to the 12 years' experience of doctors working in the rural public health sector reported in another study in South Africa.[10] Evidence from literature points to the fact that doctors' demographic characteristics affect their attitude to the uptake and adoption of guidelines.[11] Some of these characteristics are number of years since graduation, age of the doctor, participation in postgraduate education, where the medical degree was obtained, and additional qualifications.[10,12] Another study on adherence to hypertension clinical guidelines in Saudi Arabia found that 98.1% of rural district primary care physicians were foreign-trained, which was postulated to have influenced their hypertensive guideline adherence.[12]

With regard to adherence specific to various aspects of the hypertension guideline, our study demonstrated no significant interhospital variations. Excluding screening for diabetes mellitus as a major risk factor and screening for target organ damage in the kidney, which showed high (83.9% and 82% respectively) adherence at district level, all of the other variables revealed poor adherence to guideline recommendations. The study from Saudi Arabia reported high to very high (from 88.8% to 99.4%) adherence to all aspects of screening for major risk factors and target organ damage, which agrees only in small part with the present study. Another South African survey of hypertensive patients found much lower adherence than our study, in that doctors reported silent renal disease in 6% of female patients and left ventricular hypertrophy in 35% of the patients.[13]

Adherence to the guideline recommendations on generic parameter measurements and investigations also illustrated poor utilisation of recommendations on BP measurement. Only one BP reading was taken in sitting position in 99.4% of the patients, and BP was taken in both sitting and standing positions in only 0.4% of patients, consistent with partial adherence and complete non-adherence respectively in the present study. This is comparable with the results of the Saudi Arabia study, which established that doctors only measured BP in both sitting and standing positions in 5.6% of patients.[12] This similarity may be explained by comparable doctors' profiles in the Saudi and the current study. Another study in Europe also found low adherence (not quantified) to BP measurement guidelines.[14] Inconsistencies in adherence to BP measurement requirements raise questions about the reliability of hypertension diagnosis.[15] In one study all patients (100%) reviewed had defective BP measurements taken.[15] This finding agrees with low adherence figures of the current study on BP measurement, but differs in the type of error committed. Our study confirmed findings from other studies that found that doctors do not measure BP correctly.

The BP and other measurements, such as weight, height, urine dipsticks and blood glucose, are usually done by the nursing staff before the doctors' consultation with the patients, and they were all done at a high level of compliance. Adherence to performance of other tests/measurements like BMI/abdominal circumference (3.1/3.3% respectively) and ECG (42.9%) were low. The performance of ECGs in our study concurs with the finding of Ardery et al.[16] (41.5% adherent). The findings of the current study contrasts with the results of the study by Al-Gelban et al.,[12] which reported that doctors calculated BMI in up to 90.1% and performed ECG in 87.9% of patients that they managed, whereas adherence to lipogram (89.8%), urea and electrolytes (88.2%) and urine analysis (95.7%) measurement in the same study were high to very high, consistent with those in our study. The variation in results between Al-Gelban study and the current study might be due to differences in data collection methods. The Al-Gelban study employed a standardised questionnaire for data collection, which may have made it possible to gather more information about doctors' adherence; the record review employed by the current study was limited by the quality of documentation.[12] Conversely, a South African study reported that urinalysis was performed in 49.7% of patients, ECG was not done at all (100% non-adherence rate), whilst BMI and waist circumference were calculated in almost all the patients in the study.[15]

Adherence to the guideline recommendations on diagnosis according to hypertension staging or degree of severity/normality and grading of risk was very low in all the four hospitals (19% for the whole district). This is comparable to the Saudi Arabia study, which reported that 25% of doctors surveyed could not grade the risks of hypertension correctly in the general population.[12] This similarity may again be explained by comparable doctors' profiles in the Saudi study and the current study. Adherence to grading of risk aspect of the guidelines was either average or high in all four hospitals (district totals of 57.1%, 64.7%, 89.6% and 89.2% for low added risk, moderate added risk, high added risk and very high added risk respectively). This is comparable to the findings of an European study where 68.5% of participating physicians used a global risk assessment tool whilst another 69.4% reported that they used charts to grade risk.[17] The tool and the charts were designed using information contained in the 7th Joint National Committee hypertension guidelines from which the 2006 South African Hypertension Guideline was adapted. This may explain the similarity in these findings.

Assessment of documented practice on guideline recommendations regarding the management aspect also demonstrated poor adherence to all four components of lifestyle modification. There were low adherence levels for dynamic exercises (3.1%), dietary modification (21%), advice on stopping smoking (37.8%) and stopping or reducing alcohol intake (26.9%). These findings concur with results from other studies[14,18] which reported low adherence to recommendations on lifestyle modification and non-pharmacological management. In contrast the Saudi study reported adherence to recommendations on dietary modification at 98.8%, but this study did not address other components of lifestyle modification.[12]

This study revealed generally high adherence to drug treatment recommendations. Adherence to the prescription of first-line treatment (diuretics) when indicated was found to be 69.4%, which is higher than reported in another South African study which found 58.8% adherence to prescription of diuretics by public service doctors when indicated.[10] Other studies reported reduced use of diuretics,[12,18] particularly in countries with a trend of increased use of second-line drugs such as angiotensin-converting enzyme inhibitors (ACEIs) and calcium-channel blockers (CCBs).[19]

Adherence to prescription of second-line treatment (ACEI) when indicated was also high, at 84.7%. This is also in keeping with the findings of the Pretoria study, which reported 73.5% adherence amongst public service doctors in patients with compelling indications.[10] Contrasting adherence data were reported by the Saudi Arabia study (17.7%).[12] Adherence to prescription of third-line treatment (CCB) when indicated was also high, at 87.8%. This contrasted with both Ernst's[10] and the Saudi study,[12] which reported 26.1% and 13.0% adherence respectively to CCB prescription when indicated. Adherence to prescription of a fourth-line treatment (beta blocker) when indicated/necessary was also found to be high, at 89.6% for the district. This correlated with results of the study by Ernst,[10] which reported a high adherence (73.5%) by public service doctors to use of beta blockers when indicated. In contrast, the study by Al-Gelban et al. reported a low adherence of 47.2%.[12]

The present study demonstrated average adherence (52.2%) to drug/treatment review/adjustment which is comparable with results of the study by Ardery,[16] that reported medication dose adjustment in 55.9% of applicable cases. The present study differs from the study by Berlowitz et al.,[20] which reported only 25.6% adherence to treatment review when indicated.

Adherence in terms of appropriate referrals of patients was generally high, with values generally ≥ 75%. The adherence figures of medical records, where review dates were discussed and given, were incongruous with each other – review dates were almost always given (adherence figures > 85% in all four hospitals), whilst adherence to discussion of review date was low (less than 10% – extremely low for all four hospitals). This may be attributed to poor documentation on the part of the doctors, although Dickerson et al.[14] also reported low adherence to follow-up appointment dates. Almost no doctors followed guideline recommendations on ongoing care for follow-up of hypertensive patients (district non-adherence figures stood at 99.6%) in the hospitals.

Limitations of the study

The confined setting of the study in a single district limits the generalisability of the findings to other settings dissimilar to this one.

Conclusion

This study found that doctors in rural district hospitals of North-West Province generally have poor adherence to clinical guidelines. Adherence rates to guidelines are related to the age and clinical experience of the practitioner, and differ with regard to the various aspects of the recommendations. There is a need to enhance some of the practical skills necessary for appropriate screening in order to improve adherence to guidelines and improve clinical outcomes.

Acknowledgements

The authors would like to thank Mrs Louise Erasmus for her assistance in the literature searches. We would like to place on record our sincere appreciation to the Department of Family Medicine and Primary Health Care at Sefako Makgatho Health Sciences University for its assistance with the publication fee.

Competing interests

The authors declare that they have no financial or personal relationship(s) that may have inappropriately influenced them in writing this article.

Authors' contributions

A.R.A. (Sefako Makgatho Health Sciences University) conceived the original research idea, collected data and edited the final manuscript, J.T. (Sefako Makgatho Health Sciences University) drafted the research protocol, collected and analysed data and edited the final manuscript, and I.G. (Sefako Makgatho Health Sciences University) was involved in drawing up the protocol for the research, data analysis, and wrote up the research article.

References

1. Cabana MD, Rand CS, Powe NR, et al. Why don't physicians follow clinical practice guidelines? A framework for improvement. JAMA. 1999;282:1458–1465. http://dx.doi.org/10.1001/jama.282.15.1458

2. Harrison MB, Legare F, Graham LD, Fervers B. Adapting clinical practice guidelines to local context and assessing barriers to their use. CMAJ. 2010;182:E78-E84. http://dx.doi.org/10.1503/cmaj.081232

3. Straus SE, Richardson WS, Glasziou P, Haynes RB. Evidence-based medicine: How to practice and teach EBM. 3rd ed. Edinburgh: Elsevier, 2005; pp. 247–261.

4. Cluzeau FA, Burgers JS, Brouwers M. The AGREE Collaboration. Development and validation of an international appraisal instrument for assessing the quality of clinical practice guidelines: The AGREE project. Qual Saf Health Care. 2003;12:18–23. http://dx.doi.org/10.1136/qhc.12.1.18

5. Espeland A, Baerheim A.Factors affecting general practitioners' decisions about plain radiography for back pain: Implications for classification of guideline barriers – a qualitative study.BMC Health Serv Res. 2003;3:8. http://dx.doi.org/10.1186/1472-6963-3-8

6. Shiffman RN, Shekelle P, Overhage JM, Slutsky J, Grimshaw J, Deshpande AM. Standardized reporting of clinical practice guidelines: A proposal from the Conference on Guideline Standardization. Ann Intern Med. 2003;139:493–498. http://dx.doi.org/10.7326/0003-4819-139-6-200309160-00013

7. Rogers EM. Diffusion of innovations. 4th ed. New York,: The Free Press; 1995.

8. North West Department of Health Provincial Ethical and Patient Safety Group. 2009 patient safety report; 2009. Available from: http://www.rhap.org.za/wp-content/uploads/2014/05/National-Core-Standards-2011-1.pdf

9. Seedat YK, Croasdale MA, Milne FJ. South African hypertension guidelines. SAMJ. 2006;96(4):337–362.

10. Ernst S. Hypertension guideline adherence by private practitioners and primary health care physicians in Pretoria. SA Fam Pract. 2005;47(3):51-54. http://dx.doi.org/10.1080/20786204.2005.10873202

11. Anderson RM, Donelly MB, Dedrick RF, Conrad CP. The attitudes of nurses, dieticians and physicians toward diabetes. Diabetes Educ. 1991;17:261–264. http://dx.doi.org/10.1177/014572179101700407

12. Al-Gelban SK, Khan MY, Al-Khaldi YM, et al. Adherence of primary care physicians to hypertension management guidelines in the Aseer region of Saudi Arabia. Saudi J Kidney Dis Transpl. 2011;22(5):941–948.

13. Peer N, Dennison CR, Lombard C, Levitt N, Steyn K, Hill MN. Target organ damage in black South African patients with hypertension. J Clin Hypertens. 2006;8:A174.

14. Dickerson JE, Garratt CJ, Brown MJ. Management of hypertension in general practice: Agreements with and variations from the British Hypertension Society guidelines. J Hum Hypertens. 1995;9:835– 839.

15. Rayner B, Blockman M, Baines D, Trinder Y.2007.A survey of hypertensive practices at two community health centres in Cape Town. SAMJ. 2007;97(4):280–284.

16. Ardery G, Carter BL, Milchak JL, et al. Explicit and implicit evaluation of physician adherence to hypertension guidelines. J Clin Hypertension 2007; 9(2):113-119. http://dx.doi.org/10.1111/j.1524-6175.2007.06112.x

17. McAlister FA, Teo KK, Lewanczuk RZ, Wells G, Montague TJ. Contemporary practice patterns in the management of newly diagnosed hypertension. CMAJ. 1997;157:23–30.

18. Cuspidi C, Michev I, Lonati L, et al.Compliance to hypertension guidelines in clinical practice: a multicentre pilot study in Italy. J Hum Hypertens. 2002;16:699–703. http://dx.doi.org/10.1038/sj.jhh.1001468

19. Campbell NR, McAlister FA, Brant R, et al. Temporal trends in antihypertensive drug prescriptions in Canada before and after introduction of the Canadian Hypertension Education Program.SJ Hypertens. 2003;21:1591–15 http://dx.doi.org/10.1097/00004872-200308000-0002597

20. Berlowitz DR, Ash AS, Hickey EC, Friedman RH, Glickman M, Kader B, et al. Inadequate management of blood pressure in a hypertensive population. N Engl J Med. 1998; 339:1957–1963. http://dx.doi.org/10.1056/NEJM199812313392701

Rural Zulu women's knowledge of and attitudes towards medical male circumcision

Authors:
Joseph N. Ikwegbue[1]
Andrew Ross[1]
Harbor Ogbonnaya[1]

Affiliations:
[1]Department of Family Medicine, University of KwaZulu-Natal, South Africa

Correspondence to:
Joseph Ikwegbue

Email:
jossy73uk@yahoo.co.uk

Postal address:
PO Box 10814, Empangeni, South Africa

Background: Medical male circumcision (MMC) is a key strategy in the South African HIV infection prevention package. Women may have a potentially powerful role in supporting such a strategy. Circumcision is not a traditional part of Zulu society, and Zulu women may have limited knowledge and ambivalent or negative attitudes towards MMC.

Aim: This study employs quantitative data to expand insight into rural Zulu women's knowledge of and attitudes towards MMC, and is important as women could potentially yield a powerful positive or negative influence over the decisions of their partners and sons.

Setting: A hospital-based antenatal clinic in rural KwaZulu-Natal.

Methods: Participants were 590 pregnant, mostly isiZulu-speaking women. Data on their knowledge of and attitude towards MMC were collected using a questionnaire and were analysed descriptively.

Results: The majority of the women supported MMC; however, knowledge of the potential benefits was generally poor. Most would encourage their partners and sons to undergo MMC. The preferred place for the procedure was a hospital.

Conclusion: Zulu participants supported MMC and would support their partners and children being circumcised. Knowledge around potential benefits was worryingly poor, and further research into disseminating information is essential. The findings highlight the need for an expanded campaign of health education for women, and innovative means are suggested to enhance information accessibility. Reasons for preferring that MMC be carried out in hospital need to be explored further.

Connaissances et attitudes des femmes zouloues de la campagne à l'égard de la circoncision médicale masculine.

Contexte: La circoncision médicale masculine (MMC) est une stratégie clé du programme sud-africain de prévention du VIH. Les femmes ont un rôle potentiellement important de soutien dans cette stratégie. La circoncision n'est pas une tradition zouloue et les femmes zouloues ont une connaissance limitée et des attitudes ambivalentes ou négatives envers la MMC.

Méthode: Les 590 participantes étaient des femmes enceintes, en majorité d'expression isiZulu qui fréquentaient une clinique prénatale d'un hôpital de campagne au KwaZulu-Natal. Les données sur leurs connaissances et leur attitude envers la MMC ont été collectées au moyen d'un questionnaire et analysées de façon descriptive.

Résultats: La majorité était en faveur de la MMC, mais elles avaient peu de connaissances des avantages potentiels de la procédure. La plupart voulaient encourager leur partenaire et leurs fils à subir la MMC. L'hôpital était l'endroit préféré pour subir l'opération.

Discussion: Les résultats montrent fortement le besoin de faire une campagne élargie d'éducation sanitaire pour les femmes et des moyens innovants sont proposés pour améliorer l'accessibilité de l'information. Il faudra explorer d'avantage pour quelles raisons elles préfèrent que la MMC soit faite dans les hôpitaux.

Conclusion: Les participantes zouloues sont pour la MMC et encourageraient leur partenaire et leurs fils à être circoncis. Les avantages potentiels de la procédure étaient peu connus et il faudra absolument chercher à diffuser des informations.

Introduction

In 2007 the World Health Organization (WHO) estimated that 33 million people worldwide were HIV positive and that 35% lived in sub-Saharan Africa.[1] In South Africa a Department of Health report in 2014 estimated that 5.7 million South Africans were HIV positive, representing 12% of the South African population.[2] Numerous international studies indicate that medical male circumcision (MMC) can significantly reduce the incidence of HIV infection in males.[3] Local South African studies report a 60% reduction in risk of HIV infection in men who have been circumcised.[4]

In 2007 the WHO and UNAIDS recommended that MMC should be a priority HIV prevention intervention in countries with a high HIV infection prevalence and low prevalence of male circumcision.[5] As South Africa meets these criteria, the South African National Department of Health adopted MMC as a key preventative initiative. In 2010 a campaign was initiated to roll out MMC, aiming to circumcise 5.7 million or 80% of men aged 15–49 years over a 5-year period.[6] Historically male circumcision is already a cultural practice amongst sectors of the mainly rural population of South Africa, including in the Xhosa-, Venda- and Sotho-speaking ethnic groups.[7] However, literature reports that circumcision is not part of Zulu cultural traditional practices.[8,9] Although the practice of male circumcision was supported by the Zulu king in 2010, the practice is still considered somewhat alien amongst the isiZulu-speaking population.[9] As a consequence Zulu men may be potentially reluctant to undergo MMC as it is not part of their culture.

Willingness to undergo MMC may also be influenced by knowledge of the procedure and its potential benefits and challenges. A qualitative study in rural KwaZulu-Natal in 2012 reported that men generally did have adequate knowledge of the potential benefits of MMC and expressed willingness to undergo the procedure.[10] Interestingly, the study reported that 'men's positive attitude could be enhanced by women's endorsement and increased participation in MMC promotion'.[10]

It is encouraging that women could play a potentially positive role in supporting the MMC campaign. However, as circumcision is culturally unfamiliar, Zulu women may have an ambivalent or somewhat negative attitude towards supporting men in carrying out MMC. There may also be some ambiguity or negativity around MCC for other reasons, including that it may be associated with a negative effect on sexual pleasure.[11,12] Rural women's knowledge around potential benefits and challenges of MMC may be lacking, as they may have poor access to health information in general and about MMC in particular. A large multi-centre international study found that although women generally support MMC programmes, they often lack factual knowledge about the benefits and risks of MMC and its role in HIV infection prevention.[13] A study of information availability and utilisation by rural women in KwaZulu-Natal reported a need for suitable media where information on issues such as health, agriculture, education, business and legal matters could be made more readily available.[14]

The majority of studies on MMC have comprised male participants and there is correspondingly less literature available on the knowledge and opinions of women about MMC. A meta-analysis of 13 studies indicated that only four included women participants.[16] A small study in rural KwaZulu-Natal included 44 women and reported that 68% of the sample was in favour of male circumcision, and that 73% would circumcise their young sons.[10]

The main predictors of support of circumcision revolved around the women's knowledge about the relationship between male circumcision status and reduction of acquisition of sexually transmitted infections, including HIV; a higher knowledge was associated with an increased likelihood of MMC support. The greatest logistical barrier to MMC that was identified was that circumcision could only be carried out by trained hospital doctors.[15] This restraint may be particularly pertinent in rural areas, as hospitals may not be readily accessible.

It cannot be assumed that rural women have knowledge of circumcision; for example, a knowledge, attitude and practice study in South Africa revealed that one-third of the female participants could not identify a circumcised penis.[17] It is also of concern that 3% of participants in this study thought that circumcised men were fully protected against HIV; as a result of such misconceptions, women may not request their partners to use condoms during sexual intercourse.

It is pertinent to expand the literature around rural Zulu women's knowledge of MMC for several reasons, including the following: they may not know of the potential benefits; their cultural norms may mitigate against it; they may feel that MMC would have a negative effect on, for example. sexual pleasure. Rural women may be particularly naive about the potential benefits of MMC as they may have poor access to technology, the media and health information. They may be less willing than their urban counterparts to support MMC as hospitals may be far from their homes and access may be logistically and financially challenging.

A literature review indicates that there has been a qualitative review of the knowledge and attitudes of women around MMC in rural KwaZulu-Natal.[10] This current study employs quantitative data to expand the knowledge, and is important as women could potentially yield a powerful positive or negative influence over the decisions of their partners and sons.

Research methods and design
Study design

This was an exploratory study; such studies are carried in areas of research where there is little existing information.[18] The study was observational, descriptive and cross-sectional and ran from April to August 2012.

Setting

The study site was an antenatal clinic at the regional obstetric hospital in rural northern KwaZulu-Natal. The site was specifically selected as the study intended to assess the knowledge and attitudes of rural women.

Study population and sampling strategy

The study population was mostly isiZulu-speaking African women attending the antenatal clinic over the study period. This population was purposively selected as being potentially information-rich key informants.[18] It is particularly important to study these women as they may be having unprotected intercourse and are at risk of HIV infection. On average 1000 women attend the antenatal clinic at the study site every month. A sample size of 600 women, representing 60% of the study population, was considered to be sufficient for this exploratory study (exploratory studies typically sample 30% of the study population).[18] All women attending the antenatal clinic were invited by the clinic nurse to partake in the study. During routine antenatal health education sessions, the purpose of the study was explained by the nurse to the women. Potential pressure to join the study was thus minimised, as the nurse was not a member of the research team. Women were presented with a Study Information Sheet and Consent Form, both of which were available in English and isiZulu. Women were invited to participate until the required sample size was reached.

Data collection

Data were collected using a structured questionnaire which was based on the findings of a qualitative study carried out a nearby study site.[10] This qualitative review involved 44 women and data were collected using focus group discussion. The themes arising from this study were summarised as a questionnaire, and initial content analysis by members of the research team and nurses at the study site indicated that potential participants would be able to understand it and respond to the questions. The questionnaire included information on demographic features (age, marital status, education level). Questions generated from the earlier qualitative study considered the following:

- Do you feel that MMC protects men against HIV?
- Would you support your partner to go for MCC?
- Do you feel that MMC improves sexual satisfaction?
- Does MMC protect your partner from HIV?
- Would you support MMC for a cultural reason?
- Would you circumcise a male child?
- Where would you prefer MMC to be held?
- Do you think MMC should be part of HIV prevention?
- Do you feel that MMC increases male promiscuity?
- Do you feel that MMC will cause sexual problems?

The questionnaire was available in both English and isiZulu and was distributed to participants who consented to participate in the study. A research assistant and nurse were available to assist women if they reported difficulty in understanding the questions. A box was left in the antenatal clinic where completed questionnaires were dropped off and later collected by a research assistant. A total of 590 questionnaires were returned out of the 620 distributed.

Data analysis

Data were entered into Excel and analysed descriptively using SPSS version 21.

Ethical considerations

Ethical permission for the study was given by the Biomedical Research Ethics Committee of the University of KwaZulu-Natal (BE136/11), the study site (hospital) ethics committee and the Provincial Department of Health.

Results

The results are presented as follows: (a) demographic features; and (b) knowledge and attitudes.

Demographic features

The majority of the participants were in the age range 20–39 years (86%), 15.7% were married, a quarter (23.2%) had only primary school education, and half (53%) had completed matric. In terms of ethnic background, 98% considered themselves to be Zulus, with two Xhosas and two Sothos. This and other demographic information is presented in Table 1a and Table 1b.

Knowledge and attitudes

Table 2 summarises aspects of knowledge and attitudes of MMC amongst women who participated in the study. Two-thirds (64%) reported that they knew the meaning of MMC. Only half (47.9%) felt that MMC could protect men against HIV infection. Interestingly, despite this reported low level of knowledge about the potential benefits, most (82.4%) responded that they would encourage their partner to go for MCC. Most did not relate MMC to improvements in sexual satisfaction (91.5%). Two-thirds (66%) were supportive

TABLE 1a: Demographic profile of participants.

Age group (yrs)	Frequency (%)	Educational status	Frequency (%)
10–19	65 (11.3%)	University/higher institution	111 (19.3%)
20–29	337 (58.7%)	Matric	313 (53.1%)
30–39	157 (27.4 %)	Primary	137 (23.6%)
40–49	15 (2.6%)	None	15 (2.6%)
Missing data	16	-	15
Total	574	-	575

TABLE 1b: Demographic profile of participants.

Marital status	Frequency (%)	Employment status	Frequency (%)
Married	90 (15.7%)	Employed	90 (15.3%)
Not married	484 (84.3%)	Unemployed	500 (84.7%)
Missing data	16	-	-
Total	574	-	590

TABLE 2: Knowledge and attitudes.

MCC amongst woman	Answer	Frequency
Knows the meaning of MMC	Yes	380 (64.4)
	No	210 (35.5)
Total		**590**
Supports MMC to protect partner from HIV infection	Yes	391 (66.3)
	No	199 (33.7)
Total		**590**
Feels that MMC protects men against HIV infection	Yes	271 (47.9)
	No	64 (11.3)
	Not sure	231 (40.8)
	Missing data	24
Total		**566**
Supports MMC for cultural reasons	Yes	55 (9.3)
	No	535 (90.7)
Total		**590**
Supports partner going for MMC	Yes	459 (82.4)
	No	25 (4.5)
	Not sure	73 (13.1)
	Missing data	33
Total		**557**
Effect of MMC on sexual pleasure	Increase	158 (29)
	Decrease	45 (8.3)
	Not sure	341 (62.7)
	Missing data	46
Total		**544**
Believes MMC will improve sexual satisfaction	Yes	50 (8.5)
	No	540 (91.5)
Total		**590**
Would circumcise male child	Yes	471 (83.7)
	No	36 (6.4)
	Not sure	56 (9.9)
	Missing data	27
Total		**563**
Preferred place for circumcision	Hospital	480 (86.5)
	Surgery	45 (8.1)
	Traditional	20 (3.6)
	Others	10 (1.8)
	Missing data	35
Total		**555**
Supports MMC being integrated into HIV prevention package	Yes	418 (70.8)
	No	18 (3.1)
	Not sure	103 (19.1)
	Others	-
	Missing data	51
Total		**539**
Feels MMC will increase male promiscuity	Yes	56 (9.5)
	No	534 (90.5)
Total		**590**
Feels MMC will cause sexual problems	Yes	5 (0.8)
	No	585 (99.2)
Total		**590**

MMC, Medical male circumcision.

of the MMC programme to protect their partners from HIV infection. Most did not support MMC as a cultural practice (90%). Encouragingly, most (83.7%) would take their son for circumcision. The preferred place for circumcision was a hospital (86.5%). It was of concern that 90% felt that MMC may increase male promiscuity. The Pearson Chi-square test

showed a significant association between level of education and the meaning of male circumcision ($p = 0.009$) and an inverse association between level of education and understanding that MMC protects against HIV ($p = 0.004$).

Discussion

The demographic profile of the participants is similar to that of other studies on antenatal clinic attendance at district hospitals in South Africa, with the majority of women in the 20–29 years age group (58.7%) and 11% in the 10–19 years age group.[19] Most of the women in this study were unemployed and unmarried. It is of concern to note that 24% (137/575) of the women that responded had only primary education and that only 19% (111/575) had exposure to higher education. Although education is seen as a priority by many rural communities, a report by the Global Movement for Children[20] highlighted the barriers to female education in many rural communities, including the preference for male education in most families. This finding is significant, as a meta-analysis sponsored by the World Bank suggested that female education increases women's negotiating power, narrows the inequality between men and women and improves the overall health status of women, including their ability to negotiate condom use.[21]

It is reassuring that participants reported a high level of support for circumcision, and this finding is consistent with other local studies which have shown MMC to be an acceptable preventative intervention amongst female pharmacy and nursing students.[20] A high level of women's support for MMC is reflected in other international studies.[16]

Participants displayed a poor knowledge of the role of MMC in prevention of HIV infection transmission, with only half of the participants aware that MMC is important for prevention of HIV infection. This lack of knowledge is consistent with the findings of other studies.[23] Analysis showed a positive association between level of education and the reported knowledge of the meaning of male circumcision ($p = 0.009$). It was somewhat surprising that a higher level of education had an inverse relationship with the knowledge that male circumcision protects against HIV infection ($p = 0.004$). Further studies are needed to review issues around this unexpected finding.

These findings highlight the need for expanded dissemination of information about the benefits of MMC to women. There is an urgent need to employ strategies to enhance women's access to knowledge around MMC. Existing literature also stresses the importance of finding suitable media for dissemination of health information to rural women.[14,24] In rural KwaZulu-Natal there is a unique intervention around increasing information accessibility found in the Mpilonhle Project. This project makes use of mobile health and education units in rural schools and communities in KwaZulu-Natal to provide medical and social services, give HIV counselling and education, and assist people to improve their computer skills.[25] Such existing projects could be sourced and encouraged to introduce information-sharing for women around MMC in the range of interventions available.

It was encouraging that despite a lack of knowledge about the benefits of MMC most participants were supportive of the MMC programme and would encourage their partners and sons to be circumcised. The high level of support for childhood male circumcision is similar to the findings of studies carried out elsewhere.[26] This important finding must be further investigated, as studies suggest that infant circumcision is also an effective strategy for prevention of transmission of HIV infection and other sexually transmitted infections.[28]

A positive finding was that a minority thought that MMC would reduce sexual pleasure and that most did not expect MMC to cause any sexual problems nor lead to greater promiscuity amongst men. These are reassuring findings, because if circumcision was perceived to reduce sexual pleasure, cause sexual dysfunction or lead to greater promiscuity, women's support for the roll out of MMC may be lessened.

The preferred place for the MMC procedure was in a hospital, and this is significant since a rural population may have poor access to a hospital facility. That there was a preference for hospitals may reflect that circumcision is not routinely carried out as a traditional practice in this rural Zulu community. It would be interesting to compare this finding to that amongst potential Xhosa participants in the Eastern Cape where circumcisions are commonly carried out in the community. However, Xhosa women may also support circumcision in a hospital due to the high mortality and morbidity associated with community-based circumcision.[25,26,27]

The majority of respondents supported the integration of MMC into an HIV prevention package, and this finding is consistent with those of other studies, and may reflect the support for any programme aimed at preventing HIV and/or AIDS.[29,30]

Limitations

A limitation in the study lay in the data collection method. Questions only assessed whether women thought they knew about MMC, and an actual knowledge assessment did not occur. Further studies on actual knowledge and not reported knowledge are required. The views of those who did not agree to participate were not explored, and this may be significant as women who have particularly strong negative views of circumcision may have refused to participate.

Conclusion

It was reassuring that women supported MMC and would advocate it. The low level of knowledge of the potential benefits of MMC was concerning and points towards a need for expansion of information accessibility for these women. The preference for hospital-based MMC may limit access, and further study is required to assess whether this finding is particular to this Zulu sample.

Acknowledgements

A big thanks to the nursing staff of Lower Umfolozi Hospital high-risk clinic for their assistance and co-operation. Special thanks to research assistant Sinhle Sibande, the isiZulu translator, Mr Tlou, who assisted with the analysis, and Dr Kambaran, Dr Clara and Zanele Sithebe.

Competing interests

The authors declare that they have no financial or personal relationship(s) that may have inappropriately influenced them in writing this article.

Authors' contributions

I.J. (University of KwaZulu-Natal) conceived, designed, collected and collated data, then interpreted and wrote the article, including literature reviews. A.R. (University of KwaZulu-Natal) provided guidance and mentorship at every stage of the research, including corrections, suggestions and critiques of the article. H.O. (University of KwaZulu-Natal) provided mentorship, support and guidance throughout.

References

1. UNAIDS 2008. Report on the global AIDS epidemic [cited 2012 January 03]. Geneva: UNAIDS. Available from: http://data.unaids.org/pub/globalreport/2008/20080715-fs-regions-en.pdf

2. Central Intelligence Agency. The World Fact Book: HIV/AIDS in South Africa [cited 2014, January 28]. Available at: https://cia.gov/library/publications/the-world-factbook/geos/sf.html

3. Wawer MJ, Makumbi F, Kigozi G. Circumcision in HIV-infected men & its effects on HIV transmission to female partners. Lancet. 2009;374(9685):229–237. http://dx.doi.org/10.1016/S0140-6736(09)60998-3

4. Anova Health Institute. Orange Farm: Bophelo pele [cited 2011, June 28]. Available at: http://www.anovahealth.co.za/projects/entry/orange-farm Accessed on 28/06/2011

5. World Health Organization. Fact sheet: Voluntary medical male circumcision for HIV prevention [July 2012; cited 2014, November 26]. Available at: http://www.who.int/hiv/topics/malecircumcision/fact_sheet/en/

6. Treatment Action Campaign. TAC Briefing on Adult adolescent voluntary medical male circumcision (VMMC) [cited 2015, Mar 10]. Available at: http://www.tac.org.za/community/node/3190#_ft8

7. Kruger National Park. Venda [cited 2014, Mar 09]. Available at: http://krugerpark.co.za/africa_venda.html. accessed on 09/03/2014

8. Caldwell JC, Caldwell P. 1994. The neglect of an epidemiological explanation for distribution of HIV/AIDS in sub-Saharan Africa: Exploring the male circumcision hypothesis. Health Trans Rev. 1994;4:23–45.

9. Tshapa N. Zulu men and circumcision in South Africa [cited 2014, 09 Mar]. Available at: www.ulwazi.org/index.php5?title=zulu_men_and_circumcision_in_south_africa

10. Scott BE, Weiss HA, Viljoen JI. 2005. The acceptability of male circumcision as HIV intervention among a rural Zulu population, KwaZulu Natal, South Africa [cited 2011, Apr 15]. Available at: http://www.ncbi.nih.gov/pubmed/15832878

11. O'Hara K, O'Hara J. The effects of male circumcision on the sexual enjoyment of the female partner [1999; cited 2010, Sept 5]. Available at: http://www.circumcision.org/studies.htm

12. Bensley G. Effects of male circumcision on female arousal and orgasm [2003; cited 2010, Aug 10]. Available at: http://www.circumcision.org/studies.htm

13. Arnott J, Kehler J: Male medical circumcision for HIV prevention: Are women ready? http://www.malecircumcision.org/advocacy/documents/SA_MMC_women_ready.pdf. Accessed on 25/11/2014

14. Jiyane GV. An Exploratory Study of the Information Availability and Utilization by the Rural Women of Melmoth, Kwazulu Natal [2002; cited 2014 Nov 25]. Available at: http://uzspace.uzulu.ac.za/bitstream/handle/10530/169/An+exploratory+study+of+the+information+availability+and+utilization+by+the+rural+women+of+Melmot.pdf;jsessionid=2C1FF363BF33BB8E29F76868E9F8FC1B?sequence=1

15. Mattson C, Robert C. Bailey, R. Muga, et al. Acceptability of male circumcision and predictors of circumcision preference among men and women in Nyanza Province, Kenya. AIDS Care. 2005;17(3):182-194. http://dx.doi.org/10.1080/09540120512331325671

16. Weiss H.A, Halperin D, Bailey R.C, et al. Male circumcision for HIV prevention: From evidence to action? AIDS. 2008;22(5):567-574. http://dx.doi.org/10.1097/QAD.0b013e3282f3f406

17. Lissouba P, Taljaard D, Rech D, et al. Knowledge, attitude and practices of women toward male circumcision after three years of roll-out in Orange farm, South Africa [cited 2014, Feb 2]. Available at: http:// Pag.ias2011.org/Abstracts.aspx?AID=935

18. Terre Blanche M, Durrheim K, Painter D, editors. Research in practice. Applied methods for the social sciences. Cape Town: University of Cape Town; 2006.

19. Statistics on children in South Africa. HIV and health – teenage pregnancy [2010 July; cited 2014, Mr 10]. Available at: www.childrencount.ci.org.za/indicator.php?id=5&indicator=27

20. Global Movement for Children. PERU: Rural girls face barriers to education [cited 2015, Mar 10]. Available at: http://www.ipsnews.net/2011/02/peru-rural-girls-face-barriers-to-education/

21. World Bank. Impact of investments in female education [cited 2014, Mar 23]. Available at: http://siteresources.worldbank.org/INTGENDER/Resources/ImpactInvestmentsFemaleEdu.pdf

22. Naidoo PV, Dawood F, Driver C, Narainsamy M, Ndlovu S, Ndlovu V. Knowledge, attitudes and perceptions of pharmacy and nursing students towards male circumcision and HIV in a KwaZulu-Natal University, South Africa. Afr J Prm Health Care Fam Med. 2012;4(1), Art. #327, 7 pages. http://dx.doi.org/10.4102/phcfm.v4i1.327

23. Lukobo MD, Bailey RC. Acceptability of male circumcision for prevention of HIV infection in Zambia. AIDS Care. 2007;19(4):471-477. http://dx.doi.org/10.1080/09540120601163250

24. Ariyo OC, Ariyo MO, Okelola OE, et al. 2013. Assessment of the role of mass media in dissemination of agricultural technologies among farmers in Kaduna North Local Government Area of Kaduna State, Nigeria. J Biol Agric Health Care. 2013;3(6):19-28.

25. Erasmus J. Mobile HIV testing in KZN: The Mpilonhle Project [cited 2014, Sept 22]. Available at: http://www.mediaclubsouthafrica.com/land-and-people/886-mpilonhle-171208#ixzz3DezTmWBE

26. Madhivanan P, Krupp K, Chandrasekaran V, Karat SC, Reingold AL, Klausner JD. Acceptability of male circumcision among mothers with male children in Mysore, India [cited 2014, Mar 10]. Available at: www.ncbi.nlm.nih.gov/pubmed/18453858

27. Circumcision Deaths – Mail & Guardian. http://mg.co.za/tag/circumcision-deaths. Accessed on 10/03/2014

28. Morris BJ, Wodak AD, Mindel A, et al. Infant male circumcision: An evidence-based policy statement [cited 2014, Mar 10]. Available at: www.scirp.org/journals/paperinformation.aspx?paperid=17415

29. Westercamp N, Bailey RC. Acceptability of male circumcision for prevention of HIV/AIDS in sub-Saharan Africa – a review [cited 2014, Mar 11]. Available at: http://www.medscape.com/viewarticle/556572

30. Scott BE, Weiss HA, Viljoen JI. The Acceptability of male circumcision as an HIV intervention among a rural Zulu population, Kwazulu-Natal, South Africa [cited 2014, Mar 10]. Available at: http://www.global-campaign.org/clientfiles/scott%20male%20circumcision.pdf

14

Does counselling improve uptake of long-term and permanent contraceptive methods in a high HIV-prevalence setting?

Authors:
Amon Siveregi[1]
Lilian Dudley[2]
Courage Makumucha[3]
Phatisizwe Dlamini[1]
Sihle Moyo[4]
Sibongiseni Bhembe[5]

Affiliations:
[1]Mankayane Government Hospital, Swaziland

[2]Division of Community Health, Department of Interdisciplinary Health Sciences, Stellenbosch University, South Africa

[3]Institute of Development Management, Mbabane, Swaziland

[4]Hlatikhulu Government Hospital, Swaziland

[5]Piggs Peak Government Hospital, Swaziland

Correspondence to:
Amon Siveregi

Email:
amonsiveregi@yahoo.co.uk

Postal address:
PO Box 06, Mankayane, Swaziland

Background: Studies have shown a reduced uptake of contraceptive methods in HIV-positive women of childbearing age, mainly because of unmet needs that may be a result of poor promotion of available methods of contraception, especially long-term and permanent methods (LTPM).

Aim: To compare the uptake of contraceptive methods, and particularly LTPM, by HIV-positive and HIV-negative post-partum mothers, and to assess the effects of counselling on contraceptive choices.

Setting: Three government district hospitals in Swaziland.

Methods: Interviews were conducted using a structured questionnaire, before and after counselling HIV-negative and HIV-positive post-partum women in LTPM use, unintended pregnancy rates, future fertility and reasons for contraceptive choices.

Results: A total of 711 women, of whom half were HIV-positive, participated in the study. Most (72.3% HIV-negative and 84% HIV-positive) were on modern methods of contraception, with the majority using 2-monthly and 3-monthly injectables. Intended use of any contraceptive increased to 99% after counselling. LTPM use was 7.0% in HIV-negative mothers and 15.3% in HIV-positive mothers before counselling, compared with 41.3% and 42.4% in HIV-negative and HIV-positive mothers, respectively, after counselling. Pregnancy intentions and counselling on future fertility were significantly associated with current use of contraception, whilst current LTPM use and level of education were significantly associated with LTPM post-counselling.

Conclusion: Counselling on all methods including LTPM reduced unmet needs in contraception in HIV-positive and HIV-negative mothers and could improve contraceptive uptake and reduce unintended pregnancies. Health workers do not always remember to include LTPM when they counsel clients, which could result in a low uptake of these methods. Further experimental studies should be conducted to validate these results.

Les services de conseils contribuent-ils à améliorer l'utilisation permanente et à long terme des méthodes de contraception dans les zones à forte prévalence de VIH?

Contexte: Les études ont montré une diminution de l'utilisation des méthodes contraceptives chez les femmes séropositives en âge d'avoir des enfants, surtout en raison des besoins non satisfaits résultant de la mauvaise promotion des méthodes de contraception disponibles, notamment les méthodes permanentes et à long terme (MPLT).

Objectif: Comparer l'utilisation des méthodes contraceptives, notamment les MPLT, par les mères séropositives et séronégatives venant d'accoucher, et évaluer les effets des conseils donnés sur le choix de contraceptif.

Lieu: Trois hôpitaux de district gouvernementaux au Swaziland.

Méthodes: On a mené des entrevues à l'aide d'un questionnaire structuré, avant et après avoir conseillé les femmes séropositives et séronégatives venant d'accoucher dans l'utilisation des MPLT, sur les taux de grossesses non voulues, la fécondité ultérieure et les raisons du choix de contraception.

Résultats: 711 femmes, dont la moitié était séropositives, ont participé à l'étude. La plupart d'entre elles (72.3% séronégatives et 84% séropositives) utilisaient des méthodes modernes de contraception, avec la majorité utilisant des médicaments injectables to les 2 ou 3 mois. Après consultations, l'usage prévu des contraceptifs a augmenté à 99%. L'utilisation des MPLT était de 7.0% chez les mères séronégatives et de 15.3% chez les mères séropositives avant la séance de conseil, comparé à 41.3% de mères séronégatives et 42.4% de mères séropositives, respectivement après la séance de conseils. Les intentions de grossesse et les conseils sur la fécondité ultérieure étaient liés considérablement à l'utilisation actuelle de contraception, alors que l'utilisation actuelle des MPLT et le niveau d'éducation étaient liés considérablement aux MPLT après la consultation.

Conclusion: Les conseils donnés sur toutes les méthodes, y compris les MPLT ont réduit les besoins de contraception non satisfaits chez les mères séropositives et séronégatives t pourrait améliorer la prise de contraceptifs et réduire les grossesses non volontaires. Le personnel de santé ne se souvient pas toujours de parler des MPLT quand ils conseillent leurs clients, ce qui pourrait causer la faible utilisation de ces méthodes. Il faudra faire d'autres études expérimentales pour valider ces résultats.

Background

Strategies for controlling the HIV and AIDS pandemic include reduction of the spread occurring through sexual intercourse, prevention of mother-to-child transmission (PMTCT), treatment of sexually transmitted infections, reduction in gender-based violence and prevention of unwanted pregnancies.[1,2] An unintended pregnancy is a pregnancy that is mistimed, unplanned or unwanted at the time of conception.[2] Globally, up to 50% of pregnancies are unintended, and as many as one-third of the 357 000 maternal deaths have been attributed to unintended pregnancies; despite its impact on maternal and child health, the contraceptive aspect of HIV prevention has been neglected.[3] Preventing unintended pregnancies by contraception reduces perinatal transmission of HIV and is a cost-effective component of PMTCT.[2] A study in eight African countries showed that a moderate decrease in the number of pregnancies in HIV-positive women resulted in the same number of HIV-infected births averted, as a result of the current PMTCT efforts by using nevirapine.[4]

Before the advent of antiretrovirals (ARVs), HIV-positive women had a short and poor quality of life, and most would not consider having children because of poor health or would not be fertile because of the disease.[5] With ARVs, their quality and duration of life have improved.[5] Fertility has also been shown to improve as immunological function improves.[6] Many HIV-positive women choose, or are pressurised by family members, to have children.[7] HIV-positive women of childbearing age are, however, not adequately counselled on sexuality and fertility intentions,[2,8] resulting in unintended pregnancies and leading to unsafe abortions or deterioration of health, especially when the mother's viral load is high. It is therefore important that healthcare workers counsel HIV-positive women on future fertility plans and suitable contraception methods to avoid unintended pregnancies.

Underuse and inconsistent use of contraceptives contribute to unintended pregnancies.[9] Evidence is lacking on the best method of contraception for HIV-positive women, but most authorities advocate long-term and permanent methods (LTPM) of contraception such as the intrauterine device (IUD), implants and sterilisation.[5] A study in England showed a decrease in unintended pregnancies between 1998 and 2011, and a statistically significant association between the decrease and the use of LTPM was found.[10] In 2012, the American College of Obstetricians and Gynaecologists recommended the use of LTPM for all women.[11] These methods are safe, non-user-dependent and have the highest continuation rates compared with other methods.[12] With LTPM, fertility can be delayed to a time when the couple feels ready, or when the woman's immune system has improved, without the risk of forgetting to take a pill or without having to come for 2-monthly injections.[8] LTPM also has the advantage of reducing the pill burden as some of the HIV-positive women will be taking additional medication for comorbidities.

LTPMs are underutilised because of poor promotion of these methods by healthcare workers, with most women, especially those living with HIV and AIDS, using injectables and pills.[13] Studies have, however, shown that proper counselling by healthcare providers improves acceptability of these methods.[9,14,15] A study in Rwanda and Zambia showed an increased uptake of LTPM of up to 36% after contraceptive and fertility counselling in post-partum mothers.[16] A randomised control study (RCT) was conducted in North Carolina, where post-partum mothers were randomised to receiving a script with LTPM information whilst the other group was not given anything. At follow-up, no significant difference was noted in the uptake of LTPM between the two groups.[17] A similar RCT was conducted in Chicago, where participants were randomised to watching a video with LTPM information or a placebo video. The uptake of LTPM was also not significantly different between the two groups.[18] We therefore chose to do face-to-face interviews with participants, giving them information on LTPMs and all the other contraceptive methods.

Swaziland has an HIV-prevalence of 26% in adults, with 31% in women of reproductive age and 42% in pregnant women.[19] Women account for approximately 60% of cases, and there is a high rate of discordant couples.[20] Approximately 50% of Swazi women of childbearing age are on contraceptives, with only 1.3% of these on IUDs, and 5.7% have been sterilised.[20] Studies have shown a higher percentage of contraceptive uptake in women who have disclosed their statuses to spouses than those who have not.[21] Disclosure is difficult for many women in Swaziland who are not in stable relationships.[19,22]

Female sterilisation is actively promoted in HIV-positive women in Swaziland government hospitals to an extent that some women feel coerced and regret having been sterilised.[7] Promotion of IUDs and implants is neglected in both HIV-positive and -negative women.[15]

The present study therefore sought to describe the current use of contraceptive methods, particularly LTPMs, amongst post-partum HIV-positive and HIV-negative women in Swaziland, and to assess whether counselling improved the preference for future use of LTPMs.

Methods
Study design and setting

This was a before-and-after observational-analytic study of contraception uptake and factors associated with contraceptive uptake (mainly LTPMs) amongst HIV-positive and HIV-negative post-partum mothers going for treatment to three district hospitals in Swaziland. The three hospitals, in Mankayane, Hlatikhulu and Piggs Peak, have a burden of HIV of up to 42% in pregnant mothers.[11] These are the only government district hospitals in the country that attend to similar patients in terms of numbers and characteristics. Pills, injectables, condoms, implants, IUDs and sterilisation are available at the three hospitals, with all contraceptives being given by nurses, except for sterilisation, which is performed in theatre by medical officers.

Contraceptive and LTPM preferences were measured before and after a 20-minute face-to-face counselling session on all available contraceptives by trained counsellors. The counsellors, who were also nurses from different departments of the same hospital, were trained for a week at Mankayane Government Hospital on all available contraceptives, advantages and disadvantages of each method, and indications and contraindications. They were also trained on standardised counselling techniques. A post-test was given after the course, which they all passed.

Sample and study population

The study population included all women going to the public health units of the three hospitals for post-partum and child immunisation services up to 3 months post-partum. The trained data collectors screened the mothers coming to the facilities and included all who met the inclusion criteria and consented to participate. Mothers who had undergone hysterectomy were excluded.

Inclusion criteria

Women coming to the hospitals' public health units for a postnatal review and immunisation of babies up to 3 months were included in the study.

Exclusion criteria

Women who did not test their HIV status in the previous pregnancy and those who underwent hysterectomy were excluded from the study.

Sampling technique

A convenience sample of all consecutive women going to the hospitals for their 7 days' and 6 weeks' postnatal review and immunisation of their children up to 3 months were recruited and counselled until the required sample size was attained.

The attending women included those who had used PMTCT facilities in the previous pregnancy (the pregnancy for which they were attending postnatal services) and were presumed to be HIV-positive. PMTCT facilities have a testing rate above 99% for pregnant women and provide ARVs during pregnancy and labour and nevirapine to the babies. Inclusion criteria were the same for HIV-positive and HIV-negative mothers.

A sample size of 690 participants was calculated to detect a 2.5% difference in the use of LTPM between HIV-positive and HIV-negative mothers and a 10% difference in the uptake of LTPM before and after counselling. Previous studies have estimated the prevalence of LTPM to be around 7% in HIV-positive women and 5% in HIV-negative women.[6]

Data collection

A staff nurse from each hospital was trained to conduct interviews with participants, in the patient's home language using a structured questionnaire. Study participants were interviewed by a separate trained data collector in each site before and after the counselling session. Data collected included demographics, time since last pregnancy, unintended pregnancy, previous exposure to contraceptive and LTPM counselling, and regret about using LTPM. Data were entered into Microsoft Excel by a data entry technician and checked by the principal investigator. Data were collected between February and May 2014.

Data analysis

Data analysis was carried out using STATA 12 software. Medians, interquartile ranges and frequencies were used to describe the data. Fisher's exact test was used to compare the baseline characteristics between HIV-positive and HIV-negative women. Differences in contraceptive use between HIV-positive and HIV-negative women were compared by using Fisher's exact test. LTPM use before, and LTPM preference after, counselling were compared between HIV-positive and HIV-negative participants using chi-squared tests. Univariate and logistic regression analyses were performed to analyse factors associated with LTPM use before, and LTPM preference after, counselling. Univariate analysis was carried out using factors associated with the use of LTPM in the literature. Factors found to be associated with the outcome were included in the regression model. Missing values were excluded from the analysis.

Ethics

The research was approved by the Stellenbosch University Ethics Committee (Reference number: S13/07/131) and Ministry of Health Swaziland Ethics Committee (Reference number: MH/599c/FWA00015267/IRB00009688).

Results

A total of 711 women, of whom 359 were HIV-negative and 352 HIV-positive, participated in the study. The study participants were between 13 and 55 years old, with HIV-positive mothers being significantly older than the HIV-negative mothers (Table 1). More HIV-positive women were either formally employed or self-employed, knew their partners' status and had more children than the HIV-negative women. Time since last pregnancy was the same between the two groups (Table 1).

Current use of contraception

Current contraception use was higher in HIV-positive mothers (84.1%) than in HIV-negative mothers (72.4%) (Table 2). Most of the women (90.5% HIV-negative and 86.2% HIV-positive mothers) were using short-term contraception. The 2-monthly and 3-monthly injectables were the most commonly used methods, with relatively low condom use

TABLE 1: Summary characteristics of HIV-positive and HIV-negative mothers seeking post-partum services.

Characteristic	Response	HIV-positive n (%)	HIV-negative n (%)	Total n	p-value
Participants	-	352	359	711	-
Age in years	< 25	113 (35.0)	210 (65.0)	323	< 0.0001
Median 26 (interquartile range 21–31)	25–40	222 (61.)	142 (39.0)	364	
	> 40	17 (70.8)	7 (29.2)	24	
Employment status	Employed/sed/u	128 (54.2)	108 (45.8)	236	0.003
	Self-employed	60 (60.0)	40 (40.0)	100	
	Unemployed	164 (43.7)	211 (56.3)	375	
Level of education	Primary/s/t	93 (54.1)	79 (45.9)	172	0.035
	Secondary	158 (44.6)	196 (55.4)	354	
	Tertiary	101 (54.6)	84 (45.4)	185	
Relationship status	Single/m	44 (37.6)	73 (62.)	117	< 0.0001
	Married	211 (62.8)	125 (37.2)	336	
	Divorced	8 (80.0)	2 (20.0)	10	
	Widowed	8 (61.5)	5 (38.5)	13	
	In a relationship	81 (34.5)	154 (65.5)	235	
Number of children alive	None	13 (17.8)	60 (82.2)	73	< 0.0001
	1 or 2	172 (42.2)	236 (57.8)	408	
	More than 2	167 (72.7)	63 (27.3)	230	
Time since last delivery	< 4 weeks	88 (44.3)	111 (55.7)	199	0.058
	4–6 weeks	75 (44.9)	92 (55.1)	167	
	6–10 weeks	94 (54.6)	78 (45.4)	172	
	10–12 weeks	95 (54.9)	78 (45.1)	173	
Knowledge of partner's HIV status	No	89 (35.2)	164 (64.8)	253	< 0.0001
	Yes	263 (57.4)	195 (42.5)	458	
Pregnancy intentions	Within 2 years	5 (27.8)	1372.2 ()	18	< 0.0001
	2–5 years	47 (29.0)	113 (71.0)	160	
	Never again	176 (64.7)	96 (35.3)	272	
	Not sure	124 (47.5)	137 (52.5)	261	
Planned pregnancy	No	185 (49.0)	192 (51.0)	377	0.274
	Yes	162 (53.3)	142 (46.7)	304	
Satisfaction with sterilisation	Dissatisfied/v	1 (33.3)	2 (66.7)	3	0.799
	Satisfied	1 (50.0)	1 (50.0)	2	
	Very satisfied	9 (81.8)	2 (18.2)	11	

TABLE 2: Current contraceptive use in HIV-positive and HIV-negative post-partum women.

Characteristic	Value	HIV-positive n (%)	HIV-negative n (%)	n	p-value
Total participants	-	352	358	710	-
Current contraceptive use	No	56 (15.9)	99 (27.6)	155	< 0.0001
	Yes	296 (84.0)	259 (72.3)	515	
Current contraception method	Barrier	50 (16.8)	57 (21.5)	107	< 0.0001
	Combined pill	26 (8.7)	24 (9.1)	50	
	Combined injectable	59 (19.9)	59 (22.4)	118	
	Progesterone-only pill	29 (9.8)	38 (14.4)	67	
	Progesterone injectable	78 (26.3)	61 (23.1)	139	
	IUD	15 (5.1)	4 (1.5)	19	
	Implant	26 (8.8)	18 (6.8)	44	
	Sterilisation	13 (4.4)	3 (1.1)	16	
Reasons for using method	Easy to use	142 (47.8)	122 (46.2)	264	< 0.0001
	Efficacy	44 (14.8)	49 (18.6)	93	
	Low risk of side-effects	30 (10.1)	45 (17.1)	75	
	Recommended by health worker	81 (27.2)	48 (18.1)	129	

in both groups. Very few women (7.0% HIV-negative and 15.3% HIV-positive mothers) were on long-term methods, which included IUD, implant and sterilisation (Figure 1), with significantly more HIV-positive mothers on LTPM than HIV-negative mothers before the counselling intervention (Table 3).

Ease of use was an important factor in the choice of contraception for many women (46.2% of HIV-negative and 47.8% of HIV-positive women). More HIV-negative women (17.1%) than HIV-positive women (10.1%) chose contraception methods because of the low risk of side-effects. More HIV-positive women (27.2%) than HIV-negative

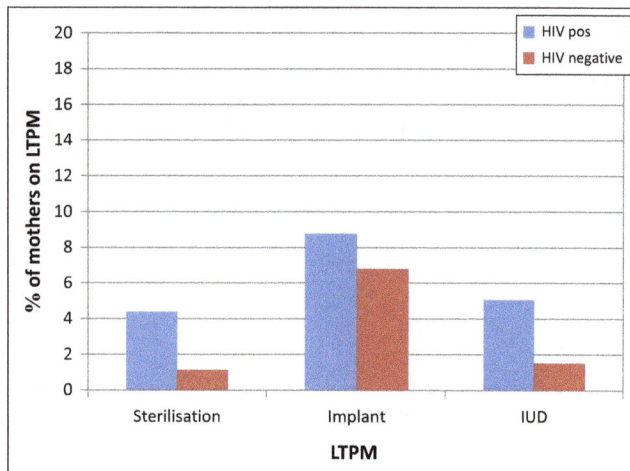

LTPM, Long-term and permanent methods; IUD, intrauterine device.

FIGURE 1: Long-term and permanent methods method use in HIV-positive and HIV-negative post-partum mothers before counselling.

women (18.2%) chose their method following advice from health workers (Table 2).

Education increased the likelihood that participants would prefer LTPM after counselling (Table 4). Thirty-nine per cent of those with primary schooling, 41% of those with secondary schooling, and 61% of those with tertiary education preferred LTPM after counselling.

Counselling on long-term and permanent methods

Most of the mothers had received contraceptive counselling during their recent pregnancy, with more counselling received by HIV-positive women (93.7%) than HIV-negative women (81.4%) (Figure 2). HIV-positive women also received more counselling than HIV-negative mothers on IUDs (71.1% and 55.0%) and implants (84.5% and 72.5%, respectively). Although very few women had undergone sterilisation, more HIV-positive (65.6%) than HIV-negative (42.0%) mothers reported prior counselling on sterilisation. Unintended pregnancies were high in both the groups (53.3% in HIV-positive and 57.5% in HIV-negative mothers), with

no significant difference between them. Only 13.3% of HIV-positive mothers who had undergone sterilisation regretted it, compared with 25% in HIV-negative mothers. There was no significant difference in the levels of satisfaction between the two groups (Table 1).

Only 1.4% of HIV-positive and 3.6% of HIV-negative mothers wanted to conceive within 2 years, and 50% of HIV-positive mothers and 26.7% of HIV-negative mothers did not want to become pregnant again (Table 1).

Long-term and permanent methods before counselling

Before counselling, 15.3% of HIV-positive mothers used LTPM compared with 7.0% in HIV-negative mothers, with a statistically significant difference (Table 5).

Long-term and permanent methods preference after counselling

After counselling, 42.4% of HIV-positive mothers and 41.3% of HIV-negative mothers preferred to be on LTPM (Figure 3, Tables 3 and 5).

Factors associated with current use of long-term and permanent methods

In the univariate analysis, marital status, HIV status, counselling on future fertility, age, the number of children alive, time since last pregnancy and pregnancy intentions were all associated with being on LTPM. In the logistic regression, only previous counselling on future fertility and pregnancy intentions were significantly associated with being on LTPM. Previous counselling on fertility had a logistic regression coefficient of 0.91 and a p-value of 0.002, indicating that participants who had prior fertility counselling were 2.5 times more likely to be on LTPM than those who did not have prior counselling. Mothers who wanted to wait for more than 2 years or did not want to become pregnant were 1.25 times more likely to be on LTPM than those who wanted to become pregnant within 2 years, with a coefficient of 0.23 and a p- value of 0.045 (Tables 6 and 7).

TABLE 3: Prior long-term and permanent methods counselling and preferred method of contraception after counselling intervention.

Variable	Response	HIV-positive (N = 352) n (%)	HIV-negative (N = 359) n (%)	p-value
Prior counselling on sterilisation	No	120 (34.3)	196 (57.9)	< 0.0001
	Yes	229 (65.6)	142 (42.0)	
Prior counselling on implant	No	54 (15.5)	93 (27.5)	< 0.0001
	Yes	294 (84.4)	245 (72.6)	
Prior counselling on IUD	No	101 (28.8)	152 (45.01)	< 0.0001
	Yes	249 (71.1)	86 (53.0)	
Preferred method after counselling	Barrier	40 (11.5)	50 (14.0)	< 0.0001
	Combined pill	8 (2.3)	20 (5.6)	
	Combined injectable	58 (16.7)	60 (16.9)	
	Progesterone-only pill	13 (3.8)	15 (4.2)	
	Progesterone injectable	81 (23.3)	64 (18.0)	
	IUD	21 (6.1)	14 (3.9)	
	Implant	67 (19.3)	115 (32.3)	
	Sterilisation	59 (17.0)	18 (5.1)	

TABLE 4: Long-term and permanent methods preference after counselling, and level of education of mothers.

Preference	Primary n (%)	Secondary n (%)	Tertiary n (%)
LTPM preference after counselling	65 (39)	145 (41)	112 (64)
Total	168	351	184

LTPM, Long-term and permanent methods.

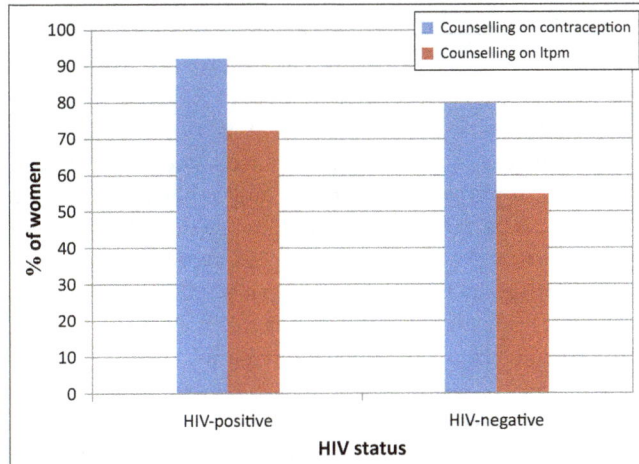

LTPM, Long-term and permanent methods.

FIGURE 2: Prior contraceptive and long-term and permanent methods counselling in HIV-positive and HIV-negative post-partum women.

TABLE 5: Long-term and permanent methods use before and preference after counselling.

Methods	HIV-positive n (%)	HIV-negative n (%)	Total	p-value
LTPM use before counselling	54 (15.3)	25 (7.0)	79	0.003
LTPM preference after counselling	147 (41.8)	147 (40.9)	294	0.872

LTPM, Long-term and permanent methods.

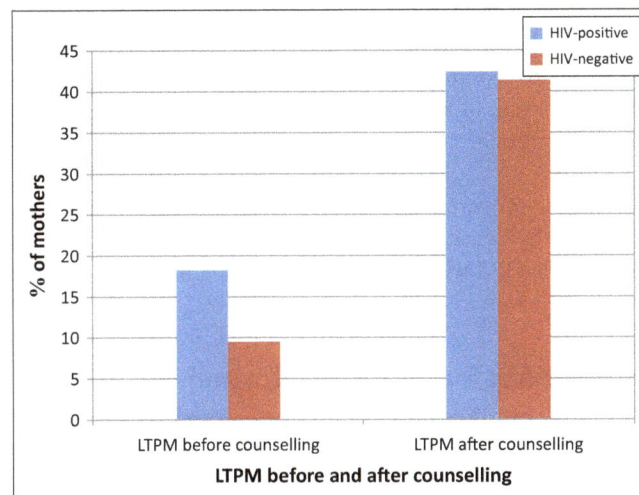

LTPM, Long-term and permanent methods.

FIGURE 3: Long-term and permanent methods use before counselling and long-term and permanent methods preference after counselling in HIV-positive and HIV-negative mothers.

Factors associated with long-term and permanent methods preference after counselling

In the univariate analysis, participants' age, future pregnancy intentions, prior LTPM use, level of education and the number of children alive were all associated with LTPM

TABLE 6: Univariate analysis of factors associated with being on long-term and permanent methods before counselling intervention.

Variable	Odds ratio	p-value	Confidence interval
Pregnancy intention	0.61	0.001	0.51–0.75
Time since last pregnancy in weeks	1.29	0.029	1.02–1.62
Number of children alive	2.44	0.001	1.55–3.80
Counselling on future fertility	3.90	0.001	2.29–6.30
Previous use of PMTCT services	2.13	0.003	1.29–3.54
Marital status	0.79	0.007	0.66–0.93
Age	1.08	0.0001	1.05–1.10
Previous contraceptive counselling	1.89	0.23	0.66–5.40
Level of education	1.25	0.179	0.90–1.80

LTPM, Long-term and permanent methods.

preference after counselling. In the logistic regression, only the level of education and prior LTPM use were associated with LTPM preference after counselling. Those who were on LTPM were 12 times more likely to prefer it after counselling than those who were not (Tables 8 and 9).

Discussion

LTPM use was very low in both HIV-positive and HIV-negative mothers, which is consistent with prior studies in Zambia and South Africa.[1,15] As in the other studies, our results show that a high percentage of women were on injectable contraceptives, citing ease of use and convenience as important reasons for choosing their methods. We found, however, that LTPM use before counselling was significantly higher in HIV-positive mothers, which was not reported in the earlier studies. This finding is not unexpected in our setting, where most health workers still believe that HIV-positive women should not become pregnant because of their sero-status and recommend long-term or permanent methods. Counselling on all LTPMs was significantly higher in HIV-positive than HIV-negative mothers. More than 65% of women had counselling on an LTPM method prior to the study, but only 14.1% used LTPM. After the trained interviewer's counselling on all available contraceptives, there was a significant increase in the number of women preferring to be on LTPM. In the South African study, 78% of mothers preferred to be on LTPM after the counselling intervention, which demonstrates that mothers are willing to be on LTPM if it supports their fertility desires.

LTPM use before counselling was associated with prior counselling on future fertility and pregnancy intentions, which was in agreement with the South African study.[15] Post-counselling LTPM preference was associated with the level of education and the current use of LTPM. The more educated the women, the more they preferred to be on LTPM, which was also in agreement with the above-cited South African study.

However, even after counselling, only 6.1% of HIV-positive women and 3.9% of HIV-negative women preferred to use an IUD. Previous studies[2] have cited fear of infection and procedures involved[15] as the main reasons why women, especially those who were HIV-positive, shunned IUDs.

TABLE 7: Logistic regression of factors associated with use of long-term and permanent methods prior to counselling.

Variable	Regression coefficient	Odds ratio	p-value	Confidence interval
Pregnancy intention	−0.2335	0.79	0.045	0.63–0.99
Time since last pregnancy in weeks	0.1832	1.20	0.146	0.93–1.53
Number of children alive	−0.036	1.00	0.991	0.54–1.80
Counselling on future fertility	0.9105	2.49	0.002	1.39–4.46
Previous use of PMTCT	0.2329	1.26	0.412	0.72–1.06
Marital status	0.1338	0.8748	0.181	0.72–1.06
Age in years	0.0446	1.046	0.056	0.99–1.09

LTPM, Long-term and permanent methods.

TABLE 8: Univariate analysis of factors associated with long-term and permanent methods preference after counselling.

Variable	Odds ratio	p-value	Confidence interval
Age in years	1.04	0.001	1.03–1.06
Level of education	1.59	0.0001	1.30–1.98
Employment status	0.99	0.862	0.83–1.16
Marital status	1.00	0.864	0.91–1.10
Partner's status	0.87	0.38	0.63–1.19
LTPM use before counselling	13.27	0.001	5.9–29.5
Pregnancy intention	0.80	0.001	0.71–0.81
Number of children alive	1.34	0.017	1.05–1.71

LTPM, Long-term and permanent methods.

TABLE 9: Logistic regression of factors associated with use of long-term and permanent methods after counselling.

Variable	Odds ratio	p-value	Confidence interval
Age in years	1.00	0.716	0.97–1.04
Level of education	1.48	0.04	1.13–1.97
Number of children alive	0.77	0.227	0.51–1.21
LTPM use before counselling	12.3	0.0001	5.45–27.3
Pregnancy intention	0.870	0.085	0.75–1.90

LTPM, Long-term and permanent methods.

These fears were addressed in the counselling sessions. The IUD has been found to be safe in HIV-positive mothers who are healthy,[23] is very convenient, with a quick return to fertility after removal[24] and does not require repeated contact with health services. It is potentially more reliable than injectables, which women may forget to return for, or suspend the use of.[25]

The high unintended pregnancy rates in HIV-positive and HIV-negative mothers suggest that there is still an unmet need. Despite the high levels of counselling on contraception, LTPM counselling levels were lower, particularly in HIV-negative women. LTPM appears to be a lower priority in counselling sessions by health workers, which could contribute to the poor uptake of this method.

Those who wanted to delay pregnancy by more than 2 years or did not want another child were more likely to be on LTPM. Prior counselling on future fertility was also associated with being on LTPM. This finding was in agreement with the South African study,[10] which showed higher chances of being on LTPM for mothers who had prior counselling on future fertility. Consequently, there is a need for broader counselling in post-partum mothers to include their future fertility intentions and all contraceptives available to reduce unintended pregnancy rates.

Limitations

Because of fear of reprimand by nurses who acted as data collectors, some of the mothers might have given false responses, especially on future pregnancy intentions and on the current use of contraceptives. The expressed preferred contraceptive method of participants after counselling was one of our main outcomes, but this may, however, not translate into actual use by the participants.

Because we used a convenience sample, there could be other confounding factors leading to spurious results. Contraceptive use could be different in clients who present during a different time period than the one used for data collection. In addition, our interviewers were not blinded and hence could have biased the study results. Staff nurses who acted as data collectors could also have introduced bias because they were working at the same hospital. They could easily interact with nurses working in these departments, causing them to change the way they offer contraceptive counselling and contraceptives.

As a before-and-after study without a control, there might have been other factors that influenced the mothers outside of our counselling intervention, which we did not measure. If we had had a control group, we might have detected that the routine consultations could in fact also have had an impact on LTPM uptake.

Our follow-up period was short, and hence we were unable to confirm whether the changes in contraceptive preference and uptake of LTPM were sustained and whether this translated into a reduction in unplanned pregnancies.

Implications for future practice and research

Future efforts should focus on increasing women's knowledge on safe, long-term contraceptive methods so that they can make informed choices. Future research should use control groups to assess whether these interventions really increase LTPM and reduce unintended pregnancy rates.

Conclusion

Although the reported use of contraceptives was very high, LTPM uptake was still very low, which was reflected in unintended pregnancies that were very high in both HIV-positive and HIV-negative mothers, suggesting that strategies to prevent unwanted pregnancies and vertical transmission of HIV in HIV-positive mothers need strengthening. Women who were counselled on, and offered a wider range of, contraception services expressed a high preference for future use of LTPM. Prior to the intervention, women who had been previously counselled on future fertility intentions were more likely to use LTPM than those who had not been counselled. This finding shows the importance of counselling mothers on the uptake of LTPM. Post-counselling, current use of LTPM and level of education were associated with a preference for LTPM, indicating that promoting women's education can also go a long way to reduce unmet needs in contraception, and hence unintended pregnancies. Most of the women who were on LTPM still preferred LTPM post-counselling, showing that this method is convenient and suited most mothers' fertility intentions, who wanted to wait for more than 2 years before becoming pregnant.

Of concern were the low IUD preference levels even after counselling. If promoted actively, this method would be very important in this setting where most mothers are willing to wait for more than 2 years without becoming pregnant. Further research on the acceptability of interventions to increase IUD uptake is needed in high HIV-prevalence settings.

We recommend that a study with a longer follow-up be conducted to assess whether the effects of the intervention were sustained and whether increased use of LTPM would reduce unintended pregnancies.

Acknowledgements

Funding from the US President's Emergency Plan for AIDS Relief (PEPFAR) through Health Resources and Services Administration (HRSA) under the terms of grant T84HA21652 via the Stellenbosch University Rural Medical Education Partnership Initiative (SURMEPI) is gratefully acknowledged.

The authors also acknowledge Professor Lilian Dudley, their research supervisor, who gave technical support from protocol development to the completion of the write up; Stellenbosch University's Biostatistics Department which helped the authors with sample size calculations and provided support for data analysis; Phatisizwe Dlamini, Sihle Moyo and Sibongiseni Bhembe, the data collectors, and Courage Makumucha, the data entry technician; the Swaziland Ministry of Health; and the hospital management and staff at the hospitals where they collected data.

Competing interests

The authors declare that they have no financial or personal relationship(s) that may have inappropriately influenced them in the writing of this article.

Authors' contributions

A.S. (Mankayane Hospital) was the principal investigator. L.D. (Stellenbosch University) was the research supervisor.

P.D. (Mankayane Hospital), S.M. (Hlatikhulu Hospital) and S.B. (Piggs Peak Hospital) were data collectors. C.M. was the data entry technician.

References

1. Chibwesha CJ, Li MS, Matoba CK, et al. Modern contraceptive and dual method use among HIV-infected women in Lusaka, Zambia. Infect Dis Obstet Gynecol. 2011, article ID 261453, 8 pages. PMID: 22007138. http://dx.doi.org/10.1155/2011/261453

2. Johnson KB, Akwara P, Rutstein SO, Bernstein S. Fertility preferences and the need for contraception among women living with HIV: The basis for a joint action agenda. AIDS. 2009;23 Suppl 1:S7–S17. PMID: 20081391. http://dx.doi.org/10.1097/01.aids.0000363773.83753.27

3. de Vos M. Integrating sexual and reproductive health and rights and HIV/AIDS in South Africa. HIV/AIDS Policy Law Rev. 2010;15:52–53. PMID: 21413629.

4. Sweeney S, Obure CD, Maier CB, Greener R, Dehne K, Vassall A. Costs and efficiency of integrating HIV/AIDS services with other health services: A systematic review of evidence and experience. Sex Transm Infect. 2012;88:85–99. PMID: 22158934. http://dx.doi.org/10.1136/sextrans-2011-050199

5. Brou H, Viho I, Djohan G, et al. Pratiques contraceptives et incidence des grossesses chez des femmes apres un depistage VIH a Abidjan, Cote d'Ivoire [Contraceptive use and incidence of pregnancy among women after HIV testing in Abidjan, Ivory Coast]. Rev Epidemiol Med Soc Sante Publique. 2009;57:77–86. PMID: 19304422. http://dx.doi.org/10.1016/j.respe.2008.12.011

6. Schwartz SR, Rees H, Mehta S, Venter WD, Taha TE, Black V. High incidence of unplanned pregnancy after antiretroviral therapy initiation: Findings from a prospective cohort study in South Africa. PloS One. 2012;7:e36039. PMID: 22558319. http://dx.doi.org/10.1371/journal.pone.0036039

7. Badell ML, Lathrop E, Haddad LB, Goedken P, Nguyen ML, Cwiak CA. Reproductive healthcare needs and desires in a cohort of HIV-positive women. Infect Dis Obstet Gynecol. 2012;107878. PMID: 22761541. http://dx.doi.org/10.1155/2012/107878

8. Gamazina K, Mogilevkina I, Parkhomenko Z, Bishop A, Coffey PS, Brazg T. Improving quality of prevention of mother-to-child HIV transmission services in Ukraine: A focus on provider communication skills and linkages to community-based non-governmental organizations. Central Eur J Public Health. 2009;17:20–24. PMID: 19418715.

9. Dehlendorf C, Kimport K, Levy K, Steinauer J. A qualitative analysis of approaches to contraceptive counseling. Perspect Sex Reprod Health. 2014;46:233–240. PMID: 25040686. http://dx.doi.org/10.1363/46e2114

10. Connolly A, Pietri G, Yu J, Humphreys S. Association between long-acting reversible contraceptive use, teenage pregnancy, and abortion rates in England. Int J Womens Health. 2014;6:961–974. eCollection 2014. PMID: 25473316. http://dx.doi.org/10.2147/IJWH.S64431

11. Sundstrom B, Baker-Whitcomb, DeMaria AL. A qualitative analysis of long-acting reversible contraception. Matern Child Health J. 2014;26 November [Epub ahead of print]. PMID: 25424456. http://dx.doi.org/10.1007/s10995-014-1655-0

12. Hathaway M, Torres L, Vollett-Krech J, Wohltjen H. Increasing LARC utilization: Any woman, any place, any time. Clin Obstet Gynecol. 2014;57:718–730. PMID: 25314089. http://dx.doi.org/10.1097/GRF.0000000000000071

13. Okpo E, Allerton L, Brechin S. 'But you can't reverse a hysterectomy!' Perceptions of long acting reversible contraception (LARC) among young women aged 16–24 years: A qualitative study. Public Health. 2014;128:934–939. PMID: 25369357. http://dx.doi.org/10.1016/j.puhe.2014.08.012

14. Andia I, Kaida A, Maier M, et al. Highly active antiretroviral therapy and increased use of contraceptiv es among HIV-positive women during expanding access to antiretroviral therapy in Mbarara, Uganda. Am J Public Health. 2009;99:340–347. PMID: 19059862. http://dx.doi.org/10.2105/AJPH.2007.129528

15. Crede S, Hoke T, Constant D, Green MS, Moodley J, Harries J. Factors impacting knowledge and use of long acting and permanent contraceptive methods by postpartum HIV positive and negative women in Cape Town, South Africa: A cross-sectional study. BMC Public Health. 2012;12:197. PMID: 22424141. http://dx.doi.org/10.1186/1471-2458-12-197

16. Tang JH, Dominik RC, Zerden ML, Verbiest SB, Brody SC, Stuart GS. Effect of an educational script on postpartum contraceptive use: A randomized controlled trial. Contraception. 2014;90:162–167. PMID: 24833047. http://dx.doi.org/10.1016/j.contraception.2014.03.017

17. Davidson AS, Whitaker AK, Martins SL, et al. Impact of a theory-based video on initiation of long-acting reversible contraception after abortion. Am J Obstet Gynecol. 2015;212:310.e1–7. PMID: 25265403. http://dx.doi.org/10.1016/j.ajog.2014.09.027

18. Khu NH, Vwalika B, Karita E, et al. Fertility goal-based counseling increases contraceptive implant and IUD use in HIV-discordant couples in Rwanda and Zambia. Contraception. 2013;88:74–82. PMID: 23153896. http://dx.doi.org/10.1016/j.contraception.2012.10.004

19. Central Statistical Office (Swaziland) and Macro International, Inc. Swaziland demographic and health survey 2006–07. Mbabane: Central Statistical Office and Macro International, Inc; 2008.

20. Macro International, Inc. HIV prevalence estimates from the demographic and health surveys. Available from: http://www.measuredhs.com/pubs/pdf/OD51/OD51.pdf. Calverton, MD: Macro International, Inc.; 2008.

21. Antelman, G, Fawzi S, Mary C, et al. Associated factors of HIV-1 status disclosure: A prospective study among HIV-infected pregnant women in Dar es Salaam, Tanzania. AIDS. 2001;15:1865–1874.

22. Fanquhar C, Ngacha D, Bosire R, Nduati RW, Kreiss J, John G. Prevalence and correlates of partner notification regarding HIV-1 in an antenatal setting in Nairobi, Kenya. Paper presented at: XIII International AIDS Conference; 2000 July 9–14; Durban, South Africa.

23. Thonneau PF, Almont T, Almond TE. Contraceptive efficacy of intrauterine devices. Am J Obstet Gynecol. 2008;198:248. PMID: 18221924. http://dx.doi.org/10.1016/j.ajog.2007.10.787

24. World Health Organization. Improving access to quality care in family planning: Medical eligibility criteria for contraceptive use. 3rd ed. Geneva: World Health Organization; 2004.

25. Baumgartner JN, Morroni C, Mlobeli RD, et al. Timeliness of contraceptive reinjections in South Africa and its relation to unintentional discontinuation. Int Fam Plan Perspect. 2007;33:66–74. PMID: 17588850.

15

Medical education and the quality improvement spiral: A case study from Mpumalanga, South Africa

Authors:
Martin Bac[1]
Anne-Marie Bergh[2]
Mama E. Etsane[2]
Jannie Hugo[1]

Affiliations:
[1]Faculty of Health Sciences, Department of Family Medicine, University of Pretoria, South Africa

[2]MRC Unit for Maternal and Infant Health Care Strategies, Faculty of Health Sciences, University of Pretoria, South Africa

Correspondence to:
Martin Bac

Email:
martin.bac@up.ac.za

Postal address:
Private Bag X323, Arcadia 0007, South Africa

Background: The short timeframe of medical students' rotations is not always conducive to successful, in-depth quality-improvement projects requiring a more longitudinal approach.

Aim: To describe the process of inducting students into a longitudinal quality-improvement project, using the topic of the Mother- and Baby-Friendly Initiative as a case study; and to explore the possible contribution of a quality-improvement project to the development of student competencies.

Setting: Mpumalanga clinical learning centres, where University of Pretoria medical students did their district health rotations.

Method: Consecutive student groups had to engage with a hospital's compliance with specific steps of the Ten Steps to Successful Breastfeeding that form the standards for the Mother- and Baby-Friendly Initiative. Primary data sources included an on-site PowerPoint group presentation ($n = 42$), a written group report ($n = 42$) and notes of individual interviews in an end-of-rotation objectively structured clinical examination station ($n = 139$).

Results: Activities in each rotation varied according to the needs identified through the application of the quality-improvement cycle in consultation with the local health team. The development of student competencies is described according to the roles of a medical expert in the CanMEDS framework: collaborator, health advocate, scholar, communicator, manager and professional. The exposure to the real-life situation in South African public hospitals had a great influence on many students, who also acted as catalysts for transforming practice.

Conclusion: Service learning and quality-improvement projects can be successfully integrated in one rotation and can contribute to the development of the different roles of a medical expert. More studies could provide insight into the potential of this approach in transforming institutions and student learning.

Education médicale et amélioration de sa qualité: une étude de cas au Mpumalanga, Afrique du Sud.

Contexte: La courte durée des roulements des étudiants médicaux ne favorise pas la réussite des projets approfondis d'amélioration de la qualité qui nécessitent une approche plus longitudinale.

Objectif: Décrire le processus d'intronisation des étudiants dans un projet longitudinal d'amélioration de la qualité, au moyen du thème de l'Initiative des Hôpitaux amis de la Mère et des Bébés comme étude de cas; et examiner la contribution possible d'un projet d'amélioration de la qualité au développement des compétences des étudiants.

Lieu: Les centres de formation clinique du Mpumalanga où les étudiants médicaux de l'Université de Pretoria ont fait leurs roulements dans les districts sanitaires.

Méthode: Des groupes consécutifs d'étudiants ont dû, avec l'autorisation de l'hôpital, s'engager à suivre les mesures spécifiques des Dix Conditions pour le Succès de l'Allaitement maternel qui est la norme de l'Initiative des Hôpitaux amis de la Mère et des Bébés. Les sources de données primaires comprenaient une présentation PowerPoint du groupe sur le terrain ($n = 42$), un rapport écrit du groupe ($n = 42$) et les notes des entrevues individuelles dans une station d'examen Clinique structuré objectivement à la fin du roulement ($n = 139$).

Résultats: Les activités de chaque roulement changeaient selon les besoins identifiés par l'application du cycle d'amélioration de la qualité en consultation avec l'équipe de santé locale. Le développement des compétences des étudiants est décrit selon les rôles d'un expert médical dans le cadre du CanMEDS: collaborateur, promoteur de la santé, érudit, communicateur, gérant et professionnel. L'exposition à la situation réelle dans les hôpitaux publics sud-africains a eu une grande influence sur beaucoup d'étudiants, qui ont aussi été les catalyseurs du changement de pratique.

Conclusion: L'apprentissage par le service et les projets d'amélioration de la qualité peuvent être intégrés avec succès dans un roulement et peuvent contribuer au développement des différents rôles d'un expert médical. Un plus grand nombre d'études pourra donner un aperçu des possibilités de cette approche et transformer les institutions et l'apprentissage des étudiants.

Introduction

The report of the Global Independent Commission on the Education of Health Professionals for the 21st Century recommends health education reforms that make provision for transformative learning in academic systems of hospitals and primary care networks rather than in academic centres.[1] Universities are urged to incorporate innovative forms of learning beyond the classroom. The report states that:

> [t]he education of health professionals in the 21st century must focus less on memorising and transmitting facts and more on promotion of the reasoning and communication skills that will enable the professional to be an effective partner, facilitator, adviser, and advocate. (p. 1945)[1]

Students should also be prepared for effective teamwork in the health system and be able to use global resources to address local priorities.[1]

Various models exist for describing the competencies of medical practitioners and how to develop them. Different sets of competencies that are applied in different countries, in undergraduate and postgraduate medical education and in different disciplines show many overlaps, with the core competencies being essentially similar. The Royal College of Physicians and Surgeons of Canada proposes the CanMEDS framework to develop leadership attributes and competencies.[2] This model describes the different roles performed by a competent medical expert: collaborator, health advocate, scholar, communicator, manager and professional.[2] The Accreditation Council for Graduate Medical Education (ACGME) divides the core competencies for residents into six areas: patient care and procedural skills; medical knowledge; interpersonal and communication skills; professionalism; practice-based learning and improvement (PBLI); and systems-based practice (SBP).[3]

Skills in quality improvement (QI) are regarded a necessary competency for family physicians[3,4] and South African medical schools also recognise the importance of including QI skills in the medical curriculum for general practitioners.[5] Medical schools in six European countries developed a framework for effective quality improvement for general practitioners and family medicine physicians based on the assumption that core QI tasks are applicable across multiple contexts, including the United States and Canada.[6] The following domains (comprising 35 competencies) emerged from their qualitative study: patient care and safety; effectiveness and efficiency; equity and ethical practice; methods and tools; development (continuing professional education); and leadership and management.[6]

Wong et al.[7] organised QI curricula with medical students and postgraduate trainees as targets in three main categories: formal curriculum activities for teaching concepts and methods; educational activities related to specific QI skills; and initiatives requiring participation from students. According to Van Deventer and Sondzaba, QI helps to extend students' awareness of health systems issues beyond the traditional clinical medicine.[5] The focus is therefore not only on clinical care, but also on issues related to organisation, ethics and patient safety.[6]

Quality improvement in medical education at the University of Pretoria

The Department of Family Medicine at the University of Pretoria (UP) is responsible for exposing undergraduate medical students to theoretical QI concepts and methods. Students get theoretical exposure to QI at various points in the medical programme and have specific skills-development assignments to facilitate their preparation for QI initiatives. In the final 18 months of internship they are further immersed in real-life clinical practice in public hospitals and are challenged to look for opportunities to improve patient safety and patient care. During this period, students do a seven-week district health and community obstetrics rotation in a number of clinical learning centres (CLCs) attached to six district hospitals and three provincial referral hospitals in Mpumalanga Province. The purpose of this rotation is to engage them in the district health system. Students are allocated in pairs to the centres and there are usually between two and six students per CLC, with one student fulfilling the role of group leader. They also live together in the same accommodation and get to know each other socially.

One of the learning opportunities in this rotation is a compulsory QI group assignment in which students are required to be active participants in a project with a specific topic or in a specific field of study. Until 2010, students selected their own topics per rotation. The short time frame of one rotation was not conducive to the completion of all the steps in the QI cycle. Since then a more focused approach has been followed by concentrating on the same area of improvement for a longer period of time, with each group of students contributing to an on-site longitudinal QI project. A previous study of the impact of brief QI projects by medical students found that the overall outcome of a QI project was strengthened by revisiting the same topic.[5]

The objective of this article is: (a) to describe the process of inducting students into a longitudinal QI project, using the topic of the Mother- and Baby-Friendly Initiative (MBFI) as case study; and (b) to explore the possible contribution of a QI project to the development of student competencies.

Research methods and design
Ethical considerations

Ethical approval for studying this approach to QI was obtained from the Research Ethics Committee of the UP's Faculty of Health Sciences (S160/2009) and the Provincial Health and Research Ethics Committee of the Mpumalanga Department of Health. The purpose of the study was explained to students during their orientation for the rotation.

Choice of focus and study period

For 2012, the topic selected for the students' QI projects was infant feeding, with special attention on hospital activities to become designated as mother- and baby-friendly, according to the World Health Organization (WHO)/UNICEF guidelines.[8] The choice of this topic followed on previous student activities related to the integration of maternal and child health services[9,10,11,12] and as a response to South Africa's poor performance on the achievement of the Millennium Development Goals (MDGs) 4 and 5.[13] A further impetus was the August 2011 Tshwane Declaration of Support for Breastfeeding in South Africa, which called for the accreditation – by 2015 – of all public hospitals and health facilities according to the standards of the MBFI.[14] A number of the hospitals where students do rotations had lost their mother- and baby-friendly status in the recent past, mostly as a result of not fully complying with steps 1 (written breastfeeding policy), 2 (training of all staff) and 10 (mother support groups). Furthermore, in April 2012, a national policy directive regarding the implementation of the 2010 WHO prevention of mother-to-child transmission (PMTCT) guidelines came into effect and the provision of free formula on demand for HIV-exposed infants was stopped.[15]

The MBFI QI programme was conducted in Mpumalanga Province over a period of one year (2012), with a follow-up study in the last rotation of 2013. The study included 139 students in six rotations and nine clinical learning centres in 2012 and 32 students in eight CLCs in the last rotation of 2013.

The educational learning experience

Students received face-to-face orientation and a written guideline on their project. They were also taken through the QI cycle (Figure 1) to illustrate how their assignment featured as part of a spiral. They were instructed to form a team with relevant role players. The team ideally included their on-site mentor and key personnel in the hospital, clinic and/or sub-district (dieticians, nurses, midwives, doctors and managers). For the MBFI, the standards had already been set in the form of the 10 steps to successful breastfeeding and the three additional criteria derived for South Africa from the revised international guidelines for the Baby-Friendly Hospital Initiative (BFHI) (see Figure 2).[8] Students' main function was to assess present practice and improvement in the adherence to the national and international standards. By reflecting on present practice they were then expected to make recommendations to address the detected discrepancies between the standard practice and current practice. The next group would then be required to follow up on the implementation of recommendations and work on further improvement:

> 'Our project was part of the "Plan and Change" step of the QI cycle. The groups before us had already identified the standards and measured the current practices in place and so it was our role to implement change using their insight as our driver.' (HospH Rot3)

In the first rotation, students started out by exploring the reasons for the hospitals' loss of mother- and baby-friendly status, where applicable, and other problems related to infant

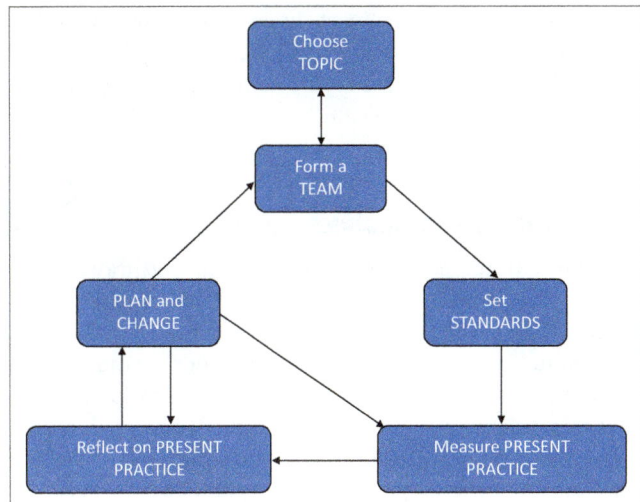

FIGURE 1: The quality improvement cycle used for the student projects.[16]

Ten steps to successful breastfeeding

Every facility providing maternity services and care for newborn infants should:

- Have a written breastfeeding policy that is routinely communicated to all healthcare staff.
- Train all healthcare staff in skills necessary to implement this policy.
- Inform all pregnant women about the benefits and management of breastfeeding.
- Help mothers initiate breastfeeding within half an hour of birth.
- Show mothers how to breastfeed, and how to maintain lactation even if they should be separated from their infants.
- Give newborn infants no food or drink other than breastmilk, unless medically indicated.
- Practise rooming-in – that is, allow mothers and infants to remain together – 24 hours a day.
- Encourage breastfeeding on demand.
- Give no artificial teats or pacifiers (also called dummies or soothers) to breastfeeding infants.
- Foster the establishment of breastfeeding support groups and refer mothers to them on discharge from the hospital or clinic.

Three additional criteria

Compliance with the Code of Marketing of Breastmilk Substitutes

Mother-friendly care (labour practices and birth companions)

HIV and infant feeding

FIGURE 2: Standards for mother- and baby-friendly hospitals.[8]

feeding. Students focused on the first step that pertains to the facility's breastfeeding policy. In the second rotation, the focus was on training (step 2). In all rotations, students had to observe skin-to-skin practices in the labour ward and report on progress. In some rotations, students did infant-feeding surveys by means of standard questionnaires and interview guides provided by the university. In the last rotation of 2012 and of 2013, students had to interview health workers on their views regarding breastfeeding policies, how policy changes affected their work, what they considered major infant-feeding challenges and recommendations with regard to the latest infant-feeding policy.

For the first two rotations, the guidelines were fairly uniform but started to diversify per centre as each QI project developed a 'life of its own', determined by the context and staff needs. From the second rotation onwards, students also received copies of the reports from previous groups for the purpose of continuity and to build on work already done. One example of project diversification was Hospital A, where students could not make headway with the work required for steps 1 and 2 and, as a result, went on to step 10 by assisting the establishment of breastfeeding support groups in the community.

Data sources and analysis

Specific requirements for student groups and individuals at the end of each rotation included an on-site group presentation in PowerPoint, a written group report and a six-minute individual interview at a station of the end-of-rotation objectively structured clinical examination (OSCE) (with an interviewer and a note taker). These documents were the primary data sources for our analysis. In 2012, a total of 139 students participated in the OSCE interviews. There were 34 reports and presentations in 2012 and eight in the single rotation in 2013. Three hospitals had students for all six rotations in 2012; two had students for four rotations; two for three rotations; and two for one rotation only.

Three researchers studied the reports and presentations before each OSCE. Thereafter, two researchers immersed themselves in the reading and re-reading of the reports to identify the different roles performed by students according to the CanMEDS framework. OSCE notes were then checked for any insights that could complement the results from the analysis of the reports and presentations.

Trustworthiness[17] was pursued by means of triangulation of data sources (different sites; different rotations) and utilising two data analysts. Credibility was further enhanced by the group report and the verification of individual students' involvement in the QI project in the OSCE interviews. Rich descriptions in the form of direct quotations from students' reports and references to interviews indicate the authentic voices of individual participants and groups and allow for transferability and confirmability. The detailed description of the educational learning experience should enable other researchers to conduct a similar study and contributes to dependability.

Results
Student roles and competencies

We used the CanMEDS framework to describe the ideal of the different roles students had to perform in developing their competency to conduct QI inquiries and to reflect on the extent to which students were able to practise these competencies. The QI project contributed to the development of students as *medical experts*. The MBFI is a patient-centred initiative, which enabled students to become health advocates and integrate their knowledge, clinical skills, procedural skills and professional attitudes linked with a public health perspective and non-clinical roles.[5] The focus was therefore on bridging the gap between evidence, policy and practice.[4] With the limited resources available, students had to come up with feasible proposals to manage and improve patient care within the specific context where they worked. Students also had to learn how to collaborate and use their personal communication skills in a scholarly manner within the constraints of the public health system.

Collaborator

The role of the collaborator is to work effectively 'within a healthcare team to achieve optimal patient care' (p. 5).[2] Teamwork was the essence of the QI projects:

'We took the role of members of the quality improvement team … We couldn't have achieved our goal without the help and support of our various team members and are thankful for the role they play in our, but also in the patient's lives. We aim to work together as a great team to achieve ultimate Baby Friendly Status.' (HospA Rot5)

The challenge students faced was working across groups of professionals in different sections of the hospital, such as the labour and postnatal wards and the neonatal unit. They also had to collaborate with dieticians, quality assurance officers and managers. In some rotations, student QI activities extended to adjacent clinics, schools and communities:

'We didn't encounter much [sic] obstacles, everyone worked together very well. The only thing that was a bit of a problem was the clinics' involvement in the breastfeeding policy … The clinics are functioning very well individually, but they must realise what more they could achieve by working as the bigger A [*town name*] team …' (HospA Rot2)

Although students were required to act as collaborators, they experienced professional boundaries and hierarchies as important obstacles in the smooth functioning of interprofessional activities – 'We have arranged a meeting in the hope of having as many multidisciplinary attending as possible; unfortunately only the dieticians attended' (HospA Rot3). For some centres, students described their reception as welcoming and inclusive – 'Upon arrival at Clinic Z [*a community health centre*] we were greeted as old friends and we felt warm in our hearts' (HospH Rot4). At Hospital H, students also became ex-officio members of the breastfeeding committee working towards regaining the hospital's mother- and baby-friendly status. At other centres, students felt they had a hostile reception and struggled to form a team with the health professionals; *inter alia* as a result of strained interprofessional relationships:

'We followed the steps of the cycle and found some of the shortcomings to be: lack of staff motivation, no multidisciplinary involvement, inadequate communication, overall apathy towards breastfeeding importance and lack of commitment.' (HospG Rot1)

Similarly, students sometimes found the good attendance of their end-of-rotation presentation by staff members 'overwhelming' (OSCE HospH Rot2), whereas in other instances 'attendance of the presentation was poorer than expected. … We had hoped that the Maternity Staff would attend, and we were rather shocked that not one was present' (HospA Rot2).

Health advocate

The health-advocacy role entailed the students' immersing themselves in the national and international literature and taking this vision to the hospital where they were placed. Despite staff ignorance and resistance, they had to play the role of advocates on behalf of mothers and babies to make the health services more mother and baby friendly. One of their first activities was to determine the current status of the hospital's breastfeeding policy (step 1). In the majority of the hospitals that had lost their mother- and baby-friendly status, the existing policy had been found inadequate. Students' advocacy role included assistance with up-dating the policy or continuous enquiry into the state of policy development where there had been no or slow progress over time:

> 'We first consulted with the labour ward matron concerning their policy of a baby friendly hospital and the implementation of this policy. There is, in fact, a policy in the hospital, but we found it has not been strictly adhered to and poorly implemented. The policy is in fact outdated and the BFHI committee is in the process of reviewing and writing up a new policy meeting the standards set for the BFHI. We reviewed the 10 steps to successful breastfeeding and noted the points of concern for hospital H and where they need to work on and improve.' (HospH Rot1)

Students also had the role of enquiring about the activities of the breastfeeding committee, which was defunct in a number of the hospitals:

> 'We were lucky to have the chance to attend the first two meetings of a new committee that included the dieticians for the first time, the postnatal staff and paediatric staff.' (HospA Rot1)

> 'It was found that the last proper training session and documentation of breastfeed training at Provincial Hospital B took place in 2006. This was obviously not sufficient and an investigation to get to the root of the problem was launched.' (HospB Rot5)

At individual sites, a number of other advocacy roles were observed. As part of their project students had to enquire about and observe skin-to-skin practices immediately after birth during all rotations. At some sites they had to lead by example when doing their own deliveries to illustrate that skin-to-skin contact was feasible, even if they had not always been able to change midwifery practices in general:

> 'With each patient we managed, we were successful in counselling and initiating both breastfeeding and skin-to-skin care. After practising it ourselves we informed the nursing staff that it was possible. In spite of this, the beliefs of the staff have remained unchanged.' (HospG Rot3)

In one instance, students discovered that free formula was still being issued by the hospital after the introduction of the new infant feeding policy on 01 April 2012. After the matter had been reported, the practice was stopped.

Scholar

The scholarly activities of students included reading up about the MBFI and breastfeeding, as well as doing small surveys on infant-feeding intentions and/or practices in pregnancy, the immediate post-partum period and at postnatal follow up between six weeks and six months after birth:

> 'To accomplish these goals [*setting up a support group, developing a breastfeeding counselling checklist*] we had to consult literature concerning skin-to-skin care, breastfeeding and quality improvement methods from sources such as the WHO, Medline and Cochrane. This data was utilised to design the breastfeeding pamphlet, develop our literature review and support some [*of*] our recommendations.' (HospA Rot4)

Students had to disseminate their findings and recommendations at the end of each rotation in a presentation and report to local management, the breastfeeding team and other stakeholders. In this way they had to transform the literature reviewed and the data collected into new knowledge that could be applied to the local situation. Scholarly activities had an influence on both students and healthcare workers:

> 'We also found that the babies aren't placed on the mother's chest at all until they reach Post Natal Ward, thus revealing that skin[-*to-skin*] care is not really practised … This raised awareness in us as the advantages of skin to skin care are numerous … and therefore emphasis should be placed on promoting skin-to-skin care.' (HospA Rot5)

> 'Sr. Sithole* did not have a written guideline for the exact method of performing adequate skin to skin contact and we therefore undertook a literature review to seek answers. Our plan was mainly aimed at educating healthcare workers in the district.' (HospD Rot5) (Pseudonym*)

Communicator

In the guidelines that the students received at the beginning of the rotation, the importance of good communication with the local facilitator and other key role players was emphasised in order to establish rapport and trust. In their project reports, students were also required to give feedback on their consultation process with the health team. Intra-group communication amongst students had to be facilitated by the group leader in order to have good collaborative learning:

> 'Our group leader was exceptionally proficient and guided the group with no difficulty. Whilst being steady and fair, he was also accommodating and considerate. He skilfully directed the project and assigned tasks with seemingly no effort, masterfully considering the strengths and capabilities of each team member. This ensured that the best possible result was produced in the shortest amount of time.' (HospH 2013)

Delivering information and reaching a mutual understanding are important components of good communication. In this regard students acted as informants, educators and trainers. At some sites they did their compulsory skills-training session on MBFI-related topics. They were also involved in staff training sessions that were part of some hospitals' MBFI training (step 2). Good communication skills were required in cases where students met with resistance and conflict within the health team. Students also learned about poor intra- and inter-institutional communication in the health system that led to inertia with regard to training and the inability to involve clinics in the MBFI:

'One very noted point that was received with a lot of anger and agreement [*during the presentation*] was the one pertaining to shifting of [*training*] responsibility [*between labour ward and postnatal ward staff*]. It was the one point of total agreement and has been promised to be rectified.' (HospB 2013)

'We have noted in discussions with both members of the breastfeeding committee and in a Subdistrict PHC [*primary healthcare*] unit managers meeting, that there is a degree of blameshifting between the two parties [*hospital and clinics*].' (HospA 2013)

Manager

The QI project demanded from students the use of different skills as managers. Decision making was a golden thread throughout. Students had to schedule and harmonise their individual and group activities with the other requirements and compulsory activities within the rotation. This required good time management and leadership in public health settings where these qualities are often lacking. Some students commented on the unexpected workload accompanying the QI project, which posed a challenge to individuals to complete their tasks and to the group to prioritise appropriately:

'Our Quality Improvement Report took longer than expected to write up but we are proud of the end result. We did not anticipate how much time it required, perhaps we would have started sooner if we had some foresight.' (HospD Rot5)

Visiting different clinics to collect data for the surveys required logistical coordination. Data capturing and analysis had to be organised and responsibilities allocated. In the case of poster and pamphlet development, printing and distribution of material had to be costed and managed:

'As we identified that individual "Feeding the Future" cards are not economically feasible, we opted for larger posters to be prominently displayed in the relevant wards and clinics. Time will be set aside to educate sisters of the above mentioned clinics on the importance of the "Feeding the Future" poster and how they can use it to educate mothers on breastfeeding at every antenatal care visit.' (HospH Rot4)

The ability to bring all the threads together at the end of the rotation into a coherent presentation and report demonstrated a group's ability to execute tasks collaboratively. The group report had to list individual student contributions and in the OSCE students were probed in such a way that the issue(s) discussed would demonstrate identification with and intimate involvement in the project as a whole. Only one student demonstrated involvement of less than 5/10.

Professional

In the MBFI QI project, students expanded their role as professionals by discovering that the art of medicine is much more than the care for individual patients:

'While assessing what the focus of our QI project would be, we reviewed the quality improvement cycle and the principles of quality improvement in district hospitals. In doing this we

decided to take three main mantras to heart, being: Focus on the patient; Start small; and Seek solutions.' (HospA Rot3)

During their project, students not only became more knowledgeable about breastfeeding and the importance of sound infant-feeding practices, but also developed realism and professional insight in matters related to public health and provider and client behavior:

'We are of the view that if the focus is shifted from regaining status to making an impact on the lives of the mothers and children passing through the hospital and clinic system, it would foster the environment that MBFI aims to achieve.' (HospA 2013)

'One of the mothers unfortunately didn't receive the breastfeeding message with similar enthusiasm due to her HIV status. She had read in the package insert … contraindicated to breastfeed … she was unyielding to change her decision. This was an important lesson for all the group members as we realised the impact of HIV related stigma. This type of stigma may be more deeply entrenched in the community than we at first thought.' (HospH Rot3)

Achievements, challenges and limitations

It was not possible to measure the effect of students' involvement in QI quantitatively in terms of organisational changes or patient outcomes, as the projects were embedded in the specific context of a complex healthcare setting, sometimes with many underlying problems where students landed in the proverbial cross-fire of different hospital factions:

'The presentation initiated a heated discussion between the staff from the labour ward, postnatal ward, family medicine practitioners, dieticians and the matron. This discussion culminated in the formation of a new approach to the QIP for the next group.' (HospG Rot4)

Students at two sites concluded at the end of 2012 that little progress had been made with the MBFI:

'It seems that from the start of this extended quality improvement little progress has been made with the BFHI.' (HospB Rot5)

On the other hand, many students commented on the meaningfulness of their experience, even in hospitals where MBFI progress was perceived to be slow or absent – 'You can make a difference in a place like this' (OSCE HospG Rot3).

'Despite the challenges we faced we are proud of the work we produced and the contributions we made to Hospital D. We are grateful for the learning experience!' (Hosp D Rot5)

'"That's one small step for man, one giant leap for mankind." It was a great privilege to play even a minor role in such a massive worldwide venture. We realised that even a small group of people can make a massive difference.' (HospA Rot5)

Students were exposed to the planning and implementation of change and, although they were mostly not champions leading change, they demonstrated the possibility of being temporary change agents[3] or catalysts working together with local change agents in one team – 'During our … rotation we met a lot of passionate people, which is the most important ingredient to success' (HospA Rot5).

> 'In attendance [*at our presentation*] was the head matron, whom it seemed we reached with our presentation … The matron was the only person out of all that attended that felt like she could make a difference from here on and that, after we've left, she can continue with all the previous groups' and our efforts … Overall we were happy with the reaction to our presentation, though most of it was negative, a discussion did ensued [*sic*] and critical thinking processes were started.' (HospA Rot6)

Although not generalisable, students contributed to the MBFI by working on the shortcomings identified in previous internal and external hospital assessments – 'Ultimately our progress as a group lay in the realisation that the previous groups have instilled a good backbone for skin-to-skin support and [*MBFI*] implementation' (HospA 2013).

> 'The breastfeeding committee expressed a great amount of gratitude as it relates to the contributions of the previous group[*s*] in 2012. They explained that the majority of the input was made in the relevant wards, where practices were changed significantly. They also explained that the hospital's breastfeeding committee received extremely helpful recommendations from this group of students.' (HospH 2013)

Students' influence and contribution were visible in a variety of activities and events – 'We made headway in policy approval, reforming a committee, organising staff training, educating staff at the rural clinics and initiating patient education' (HospG Rot3).

Probably the most rewarding for students was the independent reaccreditation of two institutions in 2012 and the continued role they could play in the MBFI in 2013:

> 'There is no better way to summarise what we have been trying to do at Hospital H than to acknowledge the reinstatement of their 'Baby-Friendly' status as of November 2012. The endorsement of the External Provincial Assessment report clearly shows that the interventions focussed upon by this year's students in breastfeeding and skin-to-skin care have made a positive and lasting impact for Hospital H and its patients and employees.' (HospH Rot3)

> 'We became part of the team as the men (and women) on the ground. We assisted with the monitoring and observation of the implementation of the policies put in place in labour ward and post natal ward. We were good for the role as the staff carried on with their duties without altering them for our sake as compared to if any of the MBFI members were to walk in. The other role we played was to evaluate the real circumstances and how possible it is to implement all the policies in the real situations in the wards. This made us realise that students form an invaluable part of the MBFI committee even though each group is present in the hospital for only six weeks, especially in short-staffed hospitals like Hospital F.' (HospF 2013)

Other achievements included the following:

- Revival of and participation in breastfeeding committees (albeit with variations in lasting results).
- Attendance of other decision-making meetings.
- Participating in internal assessments at the request of a breastfeeding committee or a nursing manager.
- Update of policies.
- Inputs in the initiation and/or overhaul of training programmes.
- Development of educational materials (3 breastfeeding pamphlets, 3 posters, 1 'Feeding the Future' motivational card for mothers, 2 breastfeeding counselling checklists).
- Active participation in breastfeeding week/month activities (3 sites).

> 'The most positive change that we noticed was the fact that more counselling on breastfeeding was taking place now.' (HospB 2013)

Three important lessons
Top-down themes and topics

The organisation of the QI projects for the MBFI was an attempt by the university to align with recent government developments to promote the achievement of MDG 4. For the programme coordinators, the ability to guide students in a more uniform manner was attractive. However, this approach led to diverse responses at hospital level, with some hospitals embracing student participation and others showing little or no interest. In the welcoming hospitals there was a direct need to prepare for reaccreditation in 2012 and 2013.

> 'For us to be given the opportunity to present our case and findings for people as respected and high up as the head matron … and the CEO [*chief executive officer*] of the hospital show how serious Hospital H is about regaining this BFHI recognition. We contributed on various levels of the quality improvement cycle and process.' (HospH Rot1)

> 'The only problem with the implementation of the 10 steps with regards to the committee is that the committee only reassures the implementation of the 10 steps when there is an evaluation and it is not constantly checked upon.' (HospD 2013)

Ownership of quality improvement

Through the student reports we observed different degrees of hospital ownership of the MBFI – 'No ownership of projects' (OSCE HospA Rot 2). The fact that the topic of MBFI was chosen by the university in consultation with the provincial health department might have influenced ownership of QI positively or negatively. Students as 'outsiders' bringing a topic not selected by the local hospital appeared to be less welcome in certain hospitals – 'Matron forgets meeting appointment' (OSCE HospG Rot 2). This illustrates a challenge of bridging the policy-practice gap in hospitals lagging behind in their MBFI efforts. The selection of local topics related to specific public health policies, in consultation with the on-site university facilitator and other key personnel, may improve local ownership and involvement of students in an on-going QI programme of the hospital.

> 'The other major problem is the lack of an active chairperson to lead the breastfeeding committee. No-one is involved to ensure continuous progress monitoring or the implementation of trainings, meetings, etc. We raised this topic with the

dieticians who agreed with our observation and decided that as it was an internal matter is [*sic*] should be dealt with internally.' (HospA Rot3)

Short versus longitudinal projects

Six rotations on the same theme were too long for some of the hospitals and we observed fluctuating enthusiasm amongst the student groups and 'topic fatigue' from the on-site health team toward the end.

> 'We got the impression that they [*clinic staff*] are either tired of students interfering and would lie to get rid of us or that they are scared that we would report them to some authority for not being up to the required standard.' (HospA Rot6)

For 2013, hospitals also identified shorter QI projects on a broad range of topics. Having a mix of short- and long-term QI projects (single or multiple QI cycles and/or spirals) can improve the ownership and responsibility of the local health team to implement the recommendations originating from the student projects. This mix has already shown potential for more intensive collaboration between students and the health team in projects for the improvement of pain control during labour and modifiable factors contributing to maternal mortality.

Discussion

The study of final year medical students' longitudinal QI projects demonstrated that these projects could be part of their normal curriculum for developing their non-clinical competencies. Students acted as triggers to facilitate the implementation of new policies in the form of the MBFI guidelines and to narrow the gap between policy and practice. For many students this was a first-time experience in hospitals outside metropolitan areas and they gained new perspective on the role doctors should be able to play. Vildbrad and Lyhne[18] suggest that non-medical expert roles are often neglected in the medical curriculum and that medical schools should create opportunities for students to develop these competencies. QI projects, especially those related to system-based practice, should be integrated in the normal curriculum in medical schools[19] and should not only be on a voluntary basis for those with an interest.

When applied to the ACGME core competencies, most of our students' activities were related to PBLI and SBP.[3] These competencies contribute to empowering 'learners with the skills to plan, lead, and execute health care systems improvement efforts' (p. 93).[20] There is evidence that the study participants developed and practised these skills successfully and with enthusiasm, thereby fulfilling their professional role. The phrase 'making a difference' was frequently used to describe QI project experiences. This is similar to the outcomes of a Joint Royal College of Physician Training Board project that demonstrated the ability of trainees to lead small-scale change that can contribute to improving multidisciplinary teamwork, clinical practice and patient care.[21] The positive student experiences reflected a

sense of student group ownership,[22] even if there were QI ownership issues at some of the learning sites.

Choudhery et al.[23] identified five practical areas to make QI projects valuable learning experiences: more awareness of QI and ideas for projects; promoting faculty mentorship and publication; education on project design and implementation; resources (e.g. books and funds); and dedicated time allowed. Vaux[21] refers to an enabling infrastructure to be able to make a difference. Our QI programme in an under-resourced provincial public health system was made possible by the infrastructure provided through the CLCs and the on-site mentors who received sufficient information to further guide and support students during their rotation. Guidance students received on the areas of MBFI to address in their activities included aspects of design and implementation. Students received resources in the form of academic and website references and had access to the university library, although the focus was more on teamwork and sharing their learning with the health workers on site.[24] As part of their compulsory activities, students had to spend time on their QI activities, and this provided a unique opportunity to familiarise students and hospital staff with new policy developments and translate them to local protocols. The longitudinal nature of the QI programme provided for a longer time frame to complete the individual site projects and allowed for continuity in learning experiences. The interdisciplinary nature of this programme and the intensive group work challenged students to excel in utilising and further developing their non-clinical skills.

Varkey and Karlapudi[20] refer to programme experiences on the challenges to implement PBLI and SBP curricula because of lack of time and resources and a perception that PBLI and SBP are not relevant to future careers. Our students found challenges in the following forms: resistance to change practice (especially skin-to-skin care); interpersonal tensions; slow progress on the uptake of student recommendations in some of the learning centres with the implementation of certain of the 10 steps to successful breastfeeding; high workload as a result of staff shortages; insufficient continuity of staff in management positions and in membership of breastfeeding committees; poor interdisciplinary collaboration; and lack of integration between extra- and intra-mural health services. Some of these challenges are similar to the findings of a study by Watts et al.[25] that identified the following major challenges: staff turnover; competing priorities; no clear sense of focus; no link to performance assessment; no clear sense of added value; inability to translate provided tools into viable projects; and incomplete teams. The authors stated that sustainable, continuous QI initiatives needed more than dedicated leadership support, formal education sessions and dedicated non-clinical time.

Research limitations were the relatively small number of hospitals participating, the single focus on MBFI and the time period that did not allow for drawing conclusions on the long-term impact. Students do not have the authority and power to implement their recommendations and even with a longitudinal QI approach this remains a major limitation in achieving significant change in some hospitals. Studies are needed on how this type of experiential service learning contributes to transformational learning in order to be able to make recommendations to other medical schools with regard to longitudinal approaches to QI in medical education. Further studies on the ideal mix between single and longitudinal QI projects may provide more insights into improving the service-learning experience of students and how to improve the local ownership. Whereas the current study focused on the student experiences of their QI projects, views of health care providers on the longitudinal QI approach should also be elicited more systematically. Notice should also be taken of other maternal and child health interventions promoted by current initiatives such as the Priority Cost Effective Lessons for System Strengthening South Africa (PRICELESS SA).[26]

Conclusion

This study illustrates how QI projects carried out in a platform of hospitals contributed to the development of the non-medical competencies of a medical expert, especially where there is a clear focus, explicit instruction and adequate mentorship. The experience with the MBFI QI projects illustrated how the third QI curriculum category requiring active student participation[7] can be implemented in a meaningful manner. Students were required to initiate projects in consultation with the health team and to be the 'conscience' in cases where progress with the implementation of the MBFI steps was slow. The exposure to the real-life situation in South African public hospitals had a great influence on many students as expressed in their personal reflections on the rotation. In addition to contributing to the development of their competencies, it could be argued that the QI projects transformed the students as well as the institutions. Turning individual QI projects into a longitudinal QI programme may have contributed to sustain some of the changes achieved.

Acknowledgements

The enthusiastic support from and facilitation by Ms Maria van der Merwe, Provincial Nutrition Programme Manager, and Ms Duduzile Mdluli, Director: Maternal, Child and Women's Health and Nutrition of the Mpumalanga Department of Health is acknowledged with thanks. Without the contributions of all the students, the facilitators and staff members at the hospitals and learning centres this work would not have been possible. A special thank you goes to the family physicians for their contributions: Drs L. Nkombua, J.J. Ongole, S. Ukpe, V. Antia, R. Chundu, F. Tiamiyu, C. Bondo, A. Angelova and C. Eche. Barbara English of the Research Office of the Faculty of Health Sciences, UP is thanked for editorial and language support. We would also like to thank the anonymous reviewers for their constructive suggestions.

Competing interests

The authors declare that they have no financial or personal relationship(s) that may have inappropriately influenced them in writing this article.

Authors' contributions

M.B. (Department of Family Medicine, University of Pretoria), AM.B., M.E.E. (both MRC Unit for Maternal and Infant Health Care Strategies, University of Pretoria) and J.H. (Department of Family Medicine, University of Pretoria) all contributed to the design of the QI programme. M.B., in collaboration with J.H., was in charge of the programme. A.M.B. and M.E.E. collated most of the data sources. M.B. and A.M.B. drafted the first version of the manuscript on which M.E.E. and J.H. gave inputs and approved the final version.

References

1. Frenk J, Chen L, Bhutta ZA, et al. Health professionals for a new century: Transforming education to strengthen health systems in an interdependent world. Lancet. 2010;376(9756):1923–1958. http://dx.doi.org/10.1016/S0140-6736(10)61854-5

2. The Royal College of Physicians and Surgeons of Canada. CanMEDS framework 2005 [document on the Internet]. c2005 [cited 2014 Apr 17]. Available from: http://www.royalcollege.ca/portal/page/portal/rc/common/documents/canmeds/framework/the_7_canmeds_roles_e.pdf

3. Accreditation Council for Graduate Medical Education. ACGME Common Program Requirements [document on the Internet]. c2013 [cited 2014 Dec 23]. Available from: www.acgme.org/acgmeweb/Portals/0/PFAssets/ProgramRequirements/CPRs2013.pdf

4. Van Deventer C, Mash B. African primary care research: Quality improvement cycles. Afr J Prm Health Care Fam Med. 2014;6(1):Art. #598. 7 pages.

5. Van Deventer C, Sondzaba N. The impact of brief quality improvement (QI) projects by medical students in primary care. Afr J Prm Health Care Fam Med. 2012;4(1):Art. #383, 6 pages.

6. Czabanowska K, Klemenc-Ketis Z, Potter A, et al. Development of a competency framework for quality improvement in family medicine: A qualitative study. J Contin Educ Health Prof. 2012;32(3):174–180. http://dx.doi.org/10.1002/chp.21142

7. Wong BM, Levinson W, Shojania GH. Quality improvement in medical education: Current state and future directions. Med Educ. 2012;46(1):107–119. http://dx.doi.org/10.1111/j.1365-2923.2011.04154.x

8. World Health Organization, UNICEF. Baby-friendly hospital initiative: Revised, updated and expanded for integrated care. Section 1, Background and implementation. Geneva: World Health Organization; 2009.

9. Bergh A-M, Cilliers C, Pattinson R, et al. A gap survey on PMTCT. Proceedings of the 28th Conference on Priorities in Perinatal Care in Southern Africa (held at Champagne Sports Castle, KwaZulu-Natal, 2009 Mar 10–13) [document on the Internet]. c2009 [cited 2014 Apr 18]. Available from: http://www.perinatalpriorities.co.za/proceedings-database/

10. Cilliers C, Bergh A-M, Pattinson R, et al. On the impossibility of infant feeding counselling. Proceedings of the 28th Conference on Priorities in Perinatal Care in Southern Africa (held at Champagne Sports Castle, KwaZulu-Natal, 2009 Mar 10–13) [document on the Internet]. c2009 [cited 2014 Apr 18]. Available from: http://www.perinatalpriorities.co.za/proceedings-database/

11. Etsane E, Bergh A-M, Pattinson R, et al. A survey on the implementation of BANC in Mpumalanga. Proceedings of the 30th Conference on Priorities in Perinatal Care in Southern Africa (held in Polokwane, 2011 Mar 8–11) [document on the Internet]. c2011 [cited 2014 Apr 18]. Available from: http://www.perinatalpriorities.co.za/proceedings-database/

12. Etsane E, Bergh A-M, Pattinson R, et al. Evaluation of the use of the postnatal card in MACH I sub-districts in Mpumalanga. Proceedings of the 31st Conference on Priorities in Perinatal Care in Southern Africa (held at Kruger Gate, 2012 Mar 6–9) [document on the Internet]. c2012 [cited 2014 Apr 18]. Available from: http://www.perinatalpriorities.co.za/proceedings-database/

13. Republic of South Africa. Millennium Development Goals Country Report 2010 [document on the Internet]. c2010 [cited 2014 Apr 18]. Available from: http://beta2.statssa.gov.za/MDG/MDGR_2010.pdf

14. The Tshwane declaration of support for breastfeeding in South Africa. S Afr J Clin Nutr. 2011;24(4):214.

15. Middelton L. Breastfeeding, not formula, for South Africa's HIV-positive mothers. Inter Press Service News Agency, 2012 April 1 [page on the Internet]. c2012 [cited 2014 Apr 17]. Available from: http://www.ipsnews.net/2012/04/breastfeeding-not-formula-for-south-africas-hiv-positive-mothers/

16. De Villiers M, Couper I, Conradie H, et al. The guidebook for district hospital managers. Durban: Health Systems Trust; 2005.

17. Shenton AK. Strategies for ensuring trustworthiness in qualitative research projects. Edu Inf. 2004;22:63–75.

18. Vildbrad MD, Lyhne JH. Improvements in the CanMEDS competencies for medical students in an interdisciplinary and voluntary setting. Adv Med Educ Pract. 2014;5:499-505. http://dx.doi.org/10.2147/AMEP.S74876

19. Chen CA, Park RJ, Hegde JV, et al. How we used a patient visit tracker tool to advance experiential learning in systems-based practice and quality improvement in a medical student clinic. Med Teach. 2014;Nov 17:1–5. http://dx.doi.org/10.31 09/0142159X.2014.975193

20. Varkey P, Karlapudi SP. Lessons learned from a 5-year experience with a 4-week experiential quality improvement curriculum in a preventive medicine fellowship. J Grad Med Educ. 2009;1(1):93–99. http://dx.doi. org/10.4300/01.01.0015

21. Vaux E, Went S, Norris M, et al. Learning to make a difference: Introducing quality improvement methods to core medical trainees. Clin Med. 2012;12(6):520–525. http://dx.doi.org/10.7861/clinmedicine.12-6-520

22. Weeks WB, Robinson JL, Brooks WB, et al. Using early clinical experiences to integrate quality-improvement learning into medical education. Acad Med. 2000;75(1):81–84. http://dx.doi.org/10.1097/00001888-200001000-00020

23. Choudhery S, Richter M, Anene A, et al. Practice quality improvement during residency: Where do we stand and where can we improve? Acad Radiol. 2014;21(7):851–858. http://dx.doi.org/10.1016/j.acra.2013.11.021

24. Shaw EK, Chase SM, Howard J, et al. More black box to explore: How quality improvement collaboratives shape practice change. J Am Board Fam Med. 2012;25(2):149–157. http://dx.doi.org/10.3122/jabfm.2012.02.110090

25. Watts B, Lawrence RH, Singh S, et al. Implementation of quality improvement skills by primary care teams: Case study of a large academic practice. J Prim Care Community Health. 2014;5(2):101–106. http://dx.doi. org/10.1177/2150131913520601

26. Priceless SA. Priority Cost Effective Lessons for System Strengthening South Africa [page on the Internet]. c2014 [cited 2015 Jan 20]. Available from: http://www. pricelesssa.ac.za/

16

Clinical Associate students' perception of the educational environment at the University of the Witwatersrand, Johannesburg

Authors:
Abigail Dreyer[1]
Audrey Gibbs[1]
Scott Smalley[1]
Motlatso Mlambo[1]
Himani Pandya[1,2]

Affiliations:
[1]Centre for Rural Health,
Department of Family
Medicine, Faculty of Health
Sciences, University of the
Witwatersrand, South Africa

[2]Faculty of Health Sciences,
Department of Paediatrics
and Child Health, Division
of Community Paediatrics,
University of the
Witwatersrand, South Africa

Correspondence to:
Abigail Dreyer

Email:
abigail.dreyer@wits.ac.za

Postal address:
Private Bag 03,
Witwatersrand 2050,
South Africa

Background: An important determinant of a student's behaviour and performance is the school's teaching and learning environment. Evaluation of such an environment can explore methods to improve educational curricula and academic atmosphere.

Aim: To evaluate the educational environment of the Bachelor of Clinical Medicine Practice programme as perceived by students at the University of the Witwatersrand, South Africa.

Setting: This cross-sectional study was conducted with all final-year students ($n = 25$) enrolled in 2011, with a response rate of 88% ($n = 22$). Students were in two groups based in the Gauteng and North-West provinces.

Methods: Data were collected using the Dundee Ready Educational Environmental Measure questionnaire, which was administered to all students. Total and mean scores for all questions were calculated for both groups.

Results: The learning environment was given an average score of 130/196 by the students. Individual subscales show that 'Academic self-perception' was rated the highest (25/32), whilst 'Social self-perception' had the lowest score (13/24). Positive aspects of the academic climate included: student competence and confidence development; student participation in class; constructive criticism provided; empathy in medical profession; and friendships created. Areas for improvement included: feedback provision to students; course time-tables; ensure non-stressful course; provision of good support systems for students; and social life improvement.

Conclusion: Students' perceptions of their learning environment were 'more positive' than negative. Results from this study will be used to draw lessons for improving the curriculum and learning environment, improve administrative processes and develop student support mechanisms in order to improve their academic experience.

Perception des étudiants assistants de clinique de l'environnement éducatif à l'Université du Witwatersrand.

Contexte: Un déterminant important du comportement et de la performance d'un étudiant est l'environnement scolaire d'enseignement et d'apprentissage. L'évaluation de cet environnement peut permettre de développer des moyens pour améliorer les programmes d'enseignement et l'atmosphère académique.

Objectif: Evaluer l'environnement éducatif du programme de Licence en Pratique de Médecine clinique, tel que le perçoivent les étudiants de l'Université du Witwatersrand, en Afrique du Sud.

Cadre: Cette étude transversale a été faite avec tous les étudiants de dernière année ($n = 25$) inscrits en 2011 avec un taux de réponse de 88% ($n = 22$). Les étudiants étaient dans deux groupes dans les provinces du Gauteng et du Nord Ouest, respectivement.

Méthodes: Les données ont été collectées au moyen du questionnaire de Mesure environnementale éducative de Dundee Ready qui a été distribué à tous les étudiants. On a calculé les notes totales et moyennes de toutes les questions des deux groupes.

Résultats: Les étudiants ont donné une note moyenne de 130/196 à l'environnement d'apprentissage. Les sous-domaines individuels montrent que 'la perception académique de soi-même' était la plus élevée (25/32) alors que 'la perception sociale de soi-même' avait la note la plus basse (13/24). Les aspects positifs du climat académique comprenaient: le développement de l'assurance et des compétences des étudiants; la participation des étudiants en classe; les critiques constructives formulées; la compassion dans la profession médicale; les amitiés créées. Les domaines à améliorer étaient notamment: les feed-back aux étudiants; l'horaire des cours; assurer des cours non-stressants; donner de bons systèmes de soutien aux étudiants; l'amélioration de la vie sociale.

Conclusion: La perception des étudiants de leur environnement d'apprentissage était 'plus positive'. Les résultats de cette étude seront utilisés pour tirer des leçons afin d'améliorer le programme scolaire et l'environnement d'apprentissage, de parfaire les processus administratifs et de développer les mécanismes de soutien aux étudiants pour améliorer leur expérience universitaire.

Introduction

An important determinant of a student's behaviour and performance is the school's teaching and learning environment.[1] Evidence suggests that a positive learning environment as perceived by students impacts their academic performance and can lead to increased success in both the academic and professional domains.[2] Innovations in medical curricula (which include a blend of classroom, workplace, clinical and community-based learning) and increasing diversity of the student population in medical courses have led to increased recognition of a need to evaluate the educational environment of medical schools. Evaluation helps to assess if these curricula are beneficial to students and adding to their skills as compared to the traditional counterparts, and to draw lessons for continuous improvement.[3]

The combination of workforce shortages, increasing burden of chronic disease, more treatable conditions, advances in medical technology and an ageing population have led to increasing demands on the healthcare system.[4] The inequitable distribution of healthcare workers with shortages in rural communities presents a major area of concern for addressing the global burden of diseases and quality healthcare delivery with universal coverage.[5] Mostly, urban areas show a heavy concentration of healthcare workers whilst the population in rural areas experiences a greater burden of diseases.

As evident from the literature, there have been recommendations in the past that new models of healthcare delivery should be examined to address these issues.[4] Staffing health facilities with sufficient numbers of appropriately trained health professionals is a major challenge and a prerequisite to implement the National Health Insurance successfully in South Africa.[6] To fulfil the National Department of Health's vision of 'Health care for all' it is necessary to develop and employ new health professional cadres to meet the health needs of the population, ensure retention and improve workforce productivity.[7]

Whilst mid-level health workers have been successfully addressing medical workforce shortage in high-income countries such as the United States of America, Europe and Australia,[4,8,9] they hold great potential for addressing human resources shortages in low- and middle-income countries, as suggested by evidence from mid-level practitioner employment in countries like Uganda, Tanzania, Kenya, Malawi and Mozambique.[10]

With this in mind, South Africa has developed a new cadre of mid-level health professionals called Clinical Associates, with the aim of improving quality of health care at hospitals, revitalising primary health care at district level and universalising health coverage in the country.[10] Formation of this cadre in South Africa led to development of a 3-year Bachelor of Clinical Medicine Practice (BCMP) degree programme resulting in qualification as a Clinical Associate. The BCMP was started by three universities in South Africa,

with the University of the Witwatersrand (Wits) launching its programme in 2009.[11]

The BCMP course structure is based on the principle of developing a sound knowledge of medical and clinical sciences to enable students to understand medical conditions of patients and their management strategies with a patient-centred approach. The curriculum follows an integrated approach with a combination of teaching modalities delivered in the classroom, skills laboratory and district hospitals led by family medicine practitioners and clinical associate tutors.

During this evaluation the third-year BCMP students were placed at various district and provincial hospitals in Gauteng and North-West provinces for clinical rotations. In 2011 the hospitals used in Gauteng included the Kopanong and South Rand District Hospitals and Natalspruit Hospital, whilst those in North-West included Taung District Hospital and Rustenburg and Mafikeng Provincial Hospitals. As per the curriculum, students needed to complete 5-week clinical rotations in the following departments during their third year in 2011: (1) Surgery, (2) Emergency Medicine, (3) Paediatrics, (4) In-patient Medicine, (5) Out-patient Medicine and HIV, and (6) Elective (can choose any department from the above five again or a different department). Students are allowed to remain in one hospital for more than one rotation, generally spending 5–15 weeks at one hospital.

As evident from the literature, many evaluations (qualitative and quantitative) have been conducted globally to measure the academic environment of health sciences programmes (undergraduate and postgraduate) by utilising different methodologies. These evaluations include assessment of medicine, nursing, physiotherapy, dental science, chiropractic and other related programmes.[12] In order to gather information on whether the programme was meeting the expectations of students in terms of a better learning environment, and if its design was student-centred, an initial evaluation was required to guide course organisers for better development of the programme. It was therefore decided to evaluate the educational environment of the BCMP in 2011 with the rationale of quality improvement, to incorporate students' feedback in course development and provide a better academic experience for future Clinical Associate students.

This study is a preliminary evaluation which was conducted with the first cohort of third-year students (placed in Gauteng and North-West provinces) who graduated in 2011 as Clinical Associates. Our objectives were firstly to understand and evaluate students' (Clinical Associates) perceptions and/or experiences of the educational environment in the BCMP programme by using the Dundee Ready Education Environment Measure (DREEM); secondly, to generate a profile of students' perceptions in terms of the strengths and weaknesses of the educational environment by exploring individual item scores; and lastly, to utilise results to draw lessons for improving the curriculum and learning environment and develop student support mechanisms in order to improve the academic experience.

Research methods and design

Study design and setting

This cross-sectional quantitative survey was conducted in 2011 amongst third-year (final-year) Wits BCMP students (based in North-West and Gauteng provinces) who graduated in 2011 as Clinical Associates.

Whilst the overall response rate was 88% ($n = 22/25$), there was an item-specific response rate where items 1, 13, 16 and 28 were responded to by 10 out of 11 students from Gauteng. Although the demographic characteristics of respondents (such as gender and age) were not captured through the questionnaire, we assumed that any differences in these did not have a significant influence on their views about the learning environment of the BCMP. In addition, we assumed that due to small sample size the exclusion of respondents' demographic information would ensure that their identity was concealed and that no information would be easily identifiable to us.[13]

Data collection

Data were collected using the self-administered DREEM questionnaire consisting of 50 items to be answered on a 5-point Likert scale ranging from 'strongly agree' to 'strongly disagree'. The questionnaire was administered within a classroom setting after the lecture. Before conducting the study and selecting the instrument we assumed that the learning environment as perceived by students was not restricted to the third year (final-year) of their clinical rotations when they answered the questions, but pertained to the overall environment throughout the three years of the course. We assumed that whilst answering the questions students perceived the terms in the questionnaire as follows:

- 'Teaching' – overall teaching including classroom and hospital based;
- 'Teachers' – all staff members involved with BCMP including course organisers, lecturers, tutors, clinical supervisors, hospital-based doctors and nurse mentors;
- 'Atmosphere' – both classrooms based at Wits as well as clinical based at hospitals in Gauteng and North-West; and
- 'School'/'teaching sessions'/'tutorials'/'classes' – pertains to both Wits University and hospitals outside Wits (for clinical rotations).

The universal DREEM tool consists of 50 items with a global score of 200.[14] Our modified DREEM tool consists of 49 items which measure aspects of the academic climate. The DREEM scoring tool is divided into five subscales (categorised below) which consist of a set of questions/items and get a separate score. Scores for all five subscales contribute towards the total DREEM score of 196 as follows:

- Students' perception of learning/teaching (12 questions with a maximum score of 48);
- Students' perception of teachers/course organisers (11 questions with a maximum score of 44);
- Academic self-perception (8 questions with a maximum score of 32);
- Perception of atmosphere (12 questions with a maximum score of 48); and
- Social self-perception (6 questions with a maximum score of 24).

Modification of the DREEM tool was done by removing question 46, that is 'my accommodation is pleasant' (under the subscale social self-perception) since the accommodation of all students from Gauteng and North-West varied enormously during the third year. Hence 49 out of 50 questions were selected (resulting in a maximum DREEM score of 196 instead of 200) and scoring for this subscale (left with 6 instead of 7 questions) was modified in the following way: 0–6 = miserable; 7–12 = not a nice place; 13–18 = not too bad and 19–24 = very good socially. The overall DREEM score was interpreted using the following guidelines: 0–49 = very poor; 50–98 = plenty of problems; 99–147 = more positive than negative; and 148–196 = excellent.[14]

Data analysis

Data were analysed using Microsoft Excel 2010 and interpreted to draw conclusions about the educational environment in the BCMP programme in the following ways:

- Average DREEM score and average scores for five subscales (North-West + Gauteng).
- DREEM score and subscale scores for both Gauteng and North-West student groups separately.
- Mean scores for all 49 questions – average scores out of 49 and separately for two groups (individual indicators with high and low scores highlighted).
- Total percentage scores: agreement (calculated by adding responses of students who 'strongly agree' and 'agree' categories); uncertain (calculated by giving a percentage to all student responses which indicated uncertain/unsure); and disagreement (calculated by adding responses of students who 'strongly disagree' and 'disagree').

Data were scored as per the scoring guide by Roff et al.[14] All 49 items are in the form of statements pertaining to the student's learning environment. Out of 49, the positive items (such as 'teaching helps to develop my confidence') are rated on a 5-point Likert scale scored as 4 for 'Strongly agree', 3 for 'Agree', 2 for 'Uncertain', 1 for 'Disagree' and 0 for 'Strongly disagree'. In addition to that, 9 out of 49 are negative items/worded negatively (such as 'I find the experience disappointing') and are reverse scored as 0 for 'Strongly agree', 1 for 'Agree', 2 for 'Uncertain', 3 for 'Disagree' and 4 for 'Strongly disagree'.[14]

Apart from five subscale scores, all 49 items are given an individual mean score out of a maximum of 4 to 'pinpoint specific strengths and weaknesses';[15] 'Items that have a mean score of 3.5 and over are real positive points'; 'Items with a mean between 2 and 3 are aspects of the climate which could be enhanced', and 'Any items with a mean score of 2 or less need to be examined more closely as they indicate "problem areas"'.[15] For example, a mean score of 3.5 for a positive statement ('teaching helps to develop my confidence') would imply that students positively perceive that teaching develops their confidence, whilst the same score on a negative item (e.g. 'teachers ridicule the students') implies that students disagree that teachers ridicule them. Similarly, a mean score of 2 or less for a positive item (e.g. 'teaching is well focused') implies that students do not perceive teaching as well focused, whilst the same score on a negative item (I find the experience disappointing) implies that students are not happy with the experience and find it disappointing.

Ethical considerations

This study received ethics clearance from the Human Research Ethics Committee, Faculty of Health Sciences, University of Witwatersrand, South Africa (Protocol M10802).

Results

Table 1 shows a summary of scores for both groups along with subscale scores, average DREEM scores and their inference. The average DREEM score for both groups was 130 out of 196, with individual scores of 129 and 131 for Gauteng and North-West students respectively. The subscale which was scored highest by both groups is 'academic self-perception' (76.6%), which inferred a feeling more on the positive side, followed by 'perception of atmosphere' (66.6%) inferring a more positive attitude. Table 1 further shows that the subscale with a lowest score is 'social self-perception' (54.4%), inferring that this aspect of the programme is not too bad.

Table 2 reflects that the item with the highest mean score in the 'students' perception of learning' subscale is number 21 ('Teaching helps to develop my confidence') for the Gauteng group (mean = 3.2) and 16 ('Teaching helps to develop my competence') for the North-West group (mean = 3.4). The lowest score (reverse score, mean = 1.3) was given to item 25 ('Teaching over-emphasises factual learning') by North-West students. The highest scores in the 'students' perception of teachers' subscale were given to items 32 ('Teachers provide constructive criticism') and 37 ('Teachers give clear examples') by Gauteng students (mean score 2.9 for both) and item 39 ('Teachers get angry in class') by North-West students (reverse score, mean = 3.5). Item 29 ('Teachers are

good at providing feedback to students') was scored lowest by both groups (mean = 1.4 and 1).

Items that were scored highest in the 'academic self-perception' subscale include number 10 ('I am confident of passing this year') for the Gauteng group (mean score = 3.9) and 31 ('I have learnt a lot about empathy in my profession') and 45 ('much of what I have to learn seems relevant to a career in health care') for the North-West group (mean score = 3.5). Individual items with the highest mean scores in the 'perception of atmosphere' subscale include number 49 ('I feel able to ask the questions I want') for both Gauteng and North-West, with means of 3.5 and 3.4 respectively, whilst those with the lowest scores include item 12 ('this school is well time-tabled') for Gauteng (mean = 1.7) and 42 ('the enjoyment outweighs the stress of this course') for North-West students (mean = 1.6). Social self-perception has the maximum items with mean scores of less than 2, namely items 3 ('there is a good support system for students who get stressed'), 14 ('I am rarely bored on this course'), 19 ('my social life is good') and 28 ('I seldom feel lonely').

After the reverse scoring of the 9 negative items (numbers 4, 8, 9, 17, 25, 35, 39, 48 and 49), mean scores of all 49 items for both groups separately and combined were calculated along with per cent agreement, percent uncertain and percent disagreement scores (presented in Table 2). In terms of per cent scores from both groups (indicated as bold in Table 2), 86% of students agree that they are encouraged to participate in teaching sessions, teaching helps to develop their competence (81%) and confidence (86%), the teachers practise a patient-centric approach (86%) and give clear examples during teaching (82%). Almost 90% or more students are confident of passing this year and agree that they have learnt a lot about empathy in their profession (96%), their problem-solving skills are being well developed (91%), they are able to ask the questions they want (96%), the atmosphere is relaxed during lectures (91%), and that much of what they have learnt seems relevant to a career in health care (96%).

Insight into scores

With regard to mean scores for individual items in the DREEM inventory, 5/49 items for the Gauteng group and 8/49 items for the North-West group were marked at 2

TABLE 1: Average DREEM scores, subscale scores and their inference.

DREEM subscales and maximum scores	Students' perception of learning		Subscale inference	Students' perception of teachers		Subscale inference	Academic self-perception		Subscale inference	Perception of atmosphere		Subscale inference	Social self-perception		Subscale inference	DREEM scores
	48	%		44	%		32	%		48	%		24	%		Max. 196
Gauteng third year (N = 11)	31	64	A more positive perception	28	63	Moving in the right direction	24	77	Feeling more on the positive side	32	67	A more positive attitude	14	58	Not too bad	129
North-West third year (N = 11)	33	69	A more positive perception	31	69	Moving in the right direction	24	76	Feeling more on the positive side	32	66	A more positive attitude	12	51	Not a nice place	131
Average subscale scores for both cohorts and inference	32	66	A more positive perception	29	66	Moving in the right direction	24	77	Feeling more on the positive side	32	66	A more positive attitude	13	54	Not too bad	130

Overall interpretation = More positive than negative.
DREEM, Dundee Ready Education Environment Measure.

TABLE 2: Individual items in the DREEM inventory.

Subscale	Number	Question	Gauteng third year		North-West third year		Average of mean scores a+b/2	Total % of students in Gauteng and North-West third year		
			N1	Mean scores (a)	N2	Mean scores (b)		Agreement %	Uncertain %	Disagreement %
Students' perception of learning	1	I am encouraged to participate in class	10	3.1	11	3.3	3.2	85.9	14.1	0
	7	Teaching is often stimulating	11	2.1	11	2.6	2.4	54.5	27.3	18.2
	13	Teaching is student-centred	10	2.4	11	2.6	2.5	61.8	19.1	19.1
	16	The teaching helps to develop my competence	10	3.1	11	3.4	3.2	80.9	14.1	5
	20	The teaching is well focused	11	2.6	11	2.6	2.6	63.6	27.3	9.1
	21	The teaching helps to develop my confidence	11	3.2	11	3.0	3.1	86.4	4.5	9.1
	24	The teaching time is put to good use	11	2.5	11	2.8	2.6	72.7	9.1	18.2
	25	The teaching over emphasises factual learning	11	2.0	11	1.3	1.6	45.5	36.4	18.2
	38	I am clear about the learning objectives of the course	11	2.7	11	2.9	2.8	68.2	22.7	9.1
	44	The teaching encourages me to be an active learner	11	2.6	11	2.8	2.7	72.7	22.7	4.5
	47	Long-term learning is emphasised over short-term learning	11	2.5	11	2.9	2.7	68.2	27.3	4.5
	48	The teaching is too teacher-centred	11	2.6	11	2.6	2.6	4.5	36.4	59.1
Students' perception of teachers	2	The teachers are knowledgeable	11	2.6	11	3.0	2.8	72.7	27.3	0
	6	The teachers are patient with patients	11	2.8	11	3.4	3.1	86.4	4.5	9.1
	8	The teachers make fun of their students	11	2.9	11	3.1	3.0	9.1	9.1	81.8
	9	The teachers are strict and controlling	11	2.8	11	2.7	2.8	9.1	22.7	68.2
	18	The teachers appear to have effective communication skills with patients	11	2.2	11	2.5	2.3	54.5	27.3	18.2
	29	The teachers are good at providing feedback to students	11	1.4	11	1.0	1.2	18.2	13.6	68.2
	32	The teachers provide constructive criticism	11	2.9	11	2.7	2.8	68.2	27.3	4.5
	37	The teachers give clear examples	11	2.9	11	2.9	2.9	81.8	9.1	9.1
	39	The teachers get angry in teaching sessions	11	2.6	11	3.5	3.0	4.5	13.6	81.8
	40	The teachers are well prepared for their classes	11	2.3	11	3.1	2.7	72.7	13.6	13.6
	49	The students irritate and annoy the teachers	11	2.2	11	2.4	2.3	18.2	40.9	40.9
Academic self-perception	5	Learning strategies which worked for me before continue to work for me now	11	2.5	11	2.2	2.4	59.1	9.1	31.8
	10	I am confident about passing this year	11	3.9	11	3.3	3.6	90.9	9.1	0
	22	I feel I am being well prepared for my profession	11	2.5	11	3.0	2.8	63.6	27.3	9.1
	26	Last year's work has been a good preparation for this year's work	11	2.8	11	3.0	2.9	77.3	4.5	18.2
	27	I am able to memorise all I need	11	2.6	11	2.5	2.6	59.1	31.8	9.1
	31	I have learned a lot about empathy in my profession	11	3.4	11	3.5	3.5	95.5	0	4.5
	41	My problem-solving skills are being well developed	11	3.2	11	3.4	3.3	90.9	9.1	0
	45	Much of what I have to learn seems relevant to a career in healthcare	11	3.5	11	3.5	3.5	95.5	4.5	0
Perception of atmosphere	11	The atmosphere is relaxed during ward teaching	11	2.5	11	2.7	2.6	72.7	9.1	18.2
	12	This school is well time-tabled	11	1.7	11	1.7	1.7	40.9	4.5	54.5
	17	Cheating is a problem in this school	11	2.8	11	2.8	2.8	18.2	9.1	72.7
	23	The atmosphere is relaxed during teaching	11	2.9	11	3.2	3.0	90.9	4.5	4.5
	30	There are opportunities for me to develop interpersonal skills	11	3.3	11	2.8	3.0	77.3	18.2	4.5
	33	I feel comfortable in teaching sessions socially	11	3.1	11	2.6	2.9	68.2	22.7	9.1
	34	The atmosphere is relaxed during tutorials	11	2.5	11	3.1	2.8	72.7	22.7	4.5
	35	I find the experience disappointing	11	2.5	11	2.6	2.5	18.2	18.2	63.6
	36	I am able to concentrate well	11	2.6	11	2.5	2.6	63.6	22.7	13.6
	42	The enjoyment outweighs the stress of the course	11	2.5	11	1.6	2.0	36.4	27.3	36.4
	43	The atmosphere motivates me as a learner	11	2.5	11	2.4	2.5	63.6	18.2	18.2
	50	I feel able to ask the questions I want	11	3.5	11	3.4	3.4	95.5	4.5	0
Social self-perception	3	There is a good support system for students who get stressed	11	1.4	11	1.6	1.5	9.1	50	40.9
	4	I am too tired to enjoy this course	11	2.5	11	2.2	2.4	31.8	4.5	63.6
	14	I am rarely bored on this course	11	2.1	11	2.0	2.0	45.5	13.6	40.9
	15	I have good friends in this school	11	3.3	11	2.8	3.0	77.3	13.6	9.1
	19	My social life is good	11	3.0	11	1.8	2.4	59.1	13.6	27.3
	28	I seldom feel lonely	10	1.8	11	1.7	1.8	28.6	14.1	57.3

or less than 2 out of the maximum score of 4 (highlighted in Table 2 as bold). Most of these low scores are in 'social self-perception' for both groups. In addition to this, 33/49 individual items for both groups in the DREEM inventory have been marked with an average mean score of between 2 and 3, suggesting that some aspects of the BCMP programme could be enhanced. Majority of these middle scores (falling between 2 and 3) are in 'students' perception of teachers' and 'perception of atmosphere' for both groups. Lastly, Table 2 reveals that 3/49 individual items for both groups in the DREEM inventory have been marked with an average mean score of 3.5 and above out of the maximum score of 4. These are regarded as 'real positive points' for the BCMP programme. All of these high scores are in 'academic self-perception'.

Discussion

The educational climate of an institution or course reflects the academic offering and contributes to development of students as practitioners.[16] Evaluation of the BCMP was done as an exercise to provide initial feedback on the programme. The results provide a profile of students' perceptions of the BCMP programme, which highlights its strengths and weaknesses. Whilst the BCMP programme is new and thus still undergoing modification, this evaluation indicates that it is positively perceived by students.

The DREEM evaluation of the Wits BCMP programme shows an average score of 130/196 (with minor differences between North-West and Gauteng students), indicating a 'more positive than negative' educational environment. The global DREEM score reported by medical schools in countries such as the United Kingdom (124/200),[15] India (123/200),[17] Sri Lanka (108/200),[18] Nigeria (118/200)[1] and Iran (100/200)[19] were lower than in our study. The differences could be attributed to the fact that our total DREEM score was based on a single cohort of Clinical Associate students, whilst other studies either administered the DREEM questionnaire to a large number of undergraduate students at different years of enrolment,[17] administered the DREEM questionnaire to all students in medical schools,[15] or conducted comparative cross-sectional studies in a number of medical schools.[20]

There are other studies with a single cohort of students like our study which also had a lower DREEM score of 106/200[21] (Kuwait) and 118/200 (Malaysia).[22] The differences could also be attributed to the fact that the BCMP is a new programme which makes a learning environment exciting for Clinical Associates. Our DREEM score was similar to that found in a study conducted amongst medical schools in Nepal (130/200).[23]

The results demonstrate a positive perception of learning by the students, which reflects that the BCMP offers a favourable learning environment (32/48). The highest individual scores in this section indicate that teaching helps to develop the students' confidence (3.2) and competence (3.1), which are important traits needed in their future

professional settings. Students also believed that they were encouraged to participate in class (3.2), which is an indication of an open and interactive learning atmosphere. Contrary to our findings, a study conducted in Malaysia with second-year medical sciences students ($n = 67$) found a mean score of 1.88, which indicates that teaching does not provide enough experiences to help them to have confidence.[22]

One of the areas of concern perceived by students in the current study is that 'teaching over-emphasises factual learning' (45.5%). This finding is consistent with that of Arzumanet al.[22] We were unsure whether, whilst answering this question, students referred to class-based teaching (which includes factual learning) or hospital-based teaching (which is more of a hands-on experience). Hence due to lack of clarity the findings cannot be interpreted to draw a conclusion as to whether the BCMP programme stressed factual learning. Further exploration in this regard through qualitative research can provide a clear picture.

Two more results from this section need to be addressed. Only 54.5% of students agreed that 'teaching is often stimulating', and only 61.8% agreed that 'teaching is student-centred', with mean scores of 2.4 and 2.5 respectively. The latter is important as the BCMP curriculum focuses on student-centred learning and problem-solving. More emphasis in the curriculum on promoting student-centred learning is suggested.

The next area of the study demonstrates that educators in the BCMP programme are being perceived as moving in the right direction in terms of quality of their teaching. Students in the North-West group were more satisfied with their teachers than the Gauteng group. Best traits of teachers as perceived by students include providing constructive criticism, giving clear examples in class and not getting angry at students. This is encouraging for the BCMP programme, as the findings of a study conducted by Aghamolaei and Fazel[19] were that student perceptions of teachers were that they do not provide constructive criticism.

Our study highlights two areas that need to be addressed for this section. Results indicate a need for teachers to improve their communication with patients. This finding is in contrast with Arzuman et al.'s[22] study, which found that students indicated that their teachers had good communication skills. The greater area of concern is that only 18.2% agreed with the statement 'teachers are good at providing feedback to the students' (1.2), with 68.2% disagreeing with the statement. This question had the lowest mean score of the study. The understanding of the term 'feedback' may not be clear in this context. We are not sure if students referred to timely feedback in class, feedback on return of test marks, periodic feedback on their assignments and performance in exams and in clinics, including lack of clarity on the person who provided feedback (teachers in class, clinical mentors/tutors/course organisers). This area must be explored further through qualitative research for a better understanding, with steps being implemented to improve the process of teachers providing feedback.

Different to studies conducted in traditional and innovative medical schools, which found that academic self-perceptions and social self-perceptions were rated lower,[24] in our study 'Academic self-perception' was marked highest by both groups (24/32). Students strongly believed and were confident that they would pass (3.6, highest mean score of the study), they have learnt a lot about empathy in their profession, and much of what they have learnt seems relevant to a career in healthcare. They also perceive that their problem-solving skills are being well developed, which is an important objective of the BCMP programme and indicates that the learning environment is contributing to fulfilling the course objectives. The students' perceptions were proved accurate, because they all passed the course and are now working as Clinical Associates. The findings of our study differ from those of Hamid et al.,[25] who found that the subscale with the highest mean score was 'students' perception of learning' (27/48), and 'academic self-perception' had a lower score of 20/32. Our study reveals a more positive feeling amongst the students.

All students perceived their 'learning atmosphere' in the category of 'a more positive attitude', with a slightly higher score for Gauteng students compared to North-West students. The best perceived aspect of the learning atmosphere is that students from both groups were able to ask questions they wanted, which potentially enhanced their communication skills with and learning from teachers. The atmosphere was relaxed during teaching, thereby promoting teacher-student interaction and sharing of scientific and conceptual knowledge. Other studies also found that the overall learning atmosphere for the students was comfortable.[22]

Areas of concern included perceptions by both student groups that the course was not well time-tabled (1.7), which may be explained by the fact that the BCMP was newly introduced and undergoing modifications. Clearly the results indicate an area for coordinators to address. Similarly, other studies found that students' perceptions of atmosphere were that the school/course was not well time-tabled.[19,21] North-West students perceived that the course was too stressful for them to enjoy, which could be attributed to their placements in distant areas far from family and friends.

Although all of the students had different social environments at their places of clinical placements, their overall 'social self-perception' does not stand as an indicator with good scores. Students from Gauteng perceived their social environment as 'not too bad', whilst those from North-West perceived it as 'not a nice place' – which could be attributed to distant location and being away from home for a long time. A positive perception was that students had good friends within the groups, indicating that fellow students acted as supporters. This is similar to the findings by Arzuman et al.,[22] who found that students had a good social life, which was reflected by them having good friends on campus. Similar to other studies,[19] areas of concern include lack of good support systems for students who get stressed (mean score of 1.5, second lowest score), feeling lonely and lack of

a good social life. It was unclear as to what type of support system they referred to (academic/social/personal). In order to improve the social aspect and ensure that apart from academics students also enjoy their social life, we need to further explore this aspect through qualitative research and take measures accordingly.

Considering the nature of the BCMP, which is an innovative curriculum and combines both classroom-based learning as well as external hospital/clinic-based teaching, DREEM does have some limitations in this context. Terms such as 'course organisers/teachers', 'atmosphere' and 'learning/teaching' present ambiguity in terms of whether the students perceived these for classroom- or hospital-based learning environments. In this regard we are considering designing instruments that are suited to evaluate the learning environment at different stages of the BCMP degree, so that they can capture students' perceptions without ambiguity. The venue used to administer the questionnaire might have influenced the students' responses about the programme.

Conclusion

The DREEM evaluation study offers a preliminary introspection into the learning environment of the BCMP programme. Despite the sample size, this study tried to evaluate the overall educational climate of the innovative BCMP curriculum at Wits. Results from this study demonstrated that the BCMP programme was perceived as a positive learning environment, contributing to the course objectives. This study highlighted strengths and weaknesses in the programme that can guide course organisers to design/modify the course.

As this was the first cohort, future evaluations will need to be conducted periodically on a larger scale with an increased sample size and incorporating more variables, and a modified questionnaire better suited to the context of the BCMP learning environment, with an additional qualitative component for better exploration of students' perceptions.

Acknowledgements

A special thanks to all the BCMP third-year (final-year) students who completed the DREEM survey. We also want to acknowledge Ms Lilo du Toit for participating in the data collection, Prof. Ian Couper for editing the manuscripts before publication, and the BCMP tutors and preceptors at the clinical sites. Funding for this project was provided by a project grant from Atlantic Philanthropies.

Competing interests

The authors declare that they have no financial or personal relationship(s) that may have inappropriately influenced them in writing this article.

Authors' contributions

A.D. (University of the Witwatersrand) was the project manager at the Lehurutshe site, and participated in drafting the article, conceptual contributions and carried out data analysis, main writing of this article and editing in preparation for submission; A.G. (University of the Witwatersrand) made conceptual contributions and contributed to data analysis; S.S. (University of the Witwatersrand) made conceptual contributions and contributed to interpretation of the results. M.M. (University of the Witwatersrand) participated in writing this article and interpretation of the results; and H.P. (University of the Witwatersrand) made initial conceptual contributions and participated in the data analysis.

References

1. Genn J. AMEE Medical Education Guide No. 23 (Part 2): Curriculum, environment, climate, quality and change in medical education-a unifying perspective. Med Teach. 2001;23(5):445–454. http://dx.doi.org/10.1080/01421590120075661

2. Brown T, Williams B, Lynch M. The Australian DREEM: Evaluating student perceptions of academic learning environments within eight health science courses. Int J Med Educ. 2011;2:94–101. http://dx.doi.org/10.5116/ijme.4e66.1b37

3. Miles S. Changes in medical education: Examining the students' views. In: Cavenagh P, Leinster SJ, Miles S, editors. The changing face of medical education. Abingdon, UK: Miles Radcliffe Publishing Ltd, 2011; pp. 103–115.

4. Ho P, Pesicka D, Schafer A, Maddern G. Physician assistants: Trialling a new surgical health professional in Australia. ANZ J Surg. 2010;80(6):430–437. http://dx.doi.org/10.1111/j.1445-2197.2010.05311.x

5. Wilson N, Couper I, De Vries E, Reid S, Fish T, Marais B. A critical review of interventions to redress the inequitable distribution of healthcare professionals to rural and remote areas. Rural and Remote Health. 2009;9(2):1060.

6. Doherty J, Couper I, Fonn S. Issues in medicine: Will clinical associates be effective for South Africa? SAMJ. 2012;102(11):833–835. http://dx.doi.org/10.7196/samj.5960

7. National Department of Health. Human Resources for Health, South Africa. HRH strategy for the Health Sector: 2012/13-2016/17.Pretoria: National Department of Health; 2011, p. 7.

8. Cawley JF, Hooker RS. Physician assistants: Does the US experience have anything to offer other countries? J Health Serv Res Policy. 2003;8(2):65–67. http://dx.doi.org/10.1258/135581903321466012

9. Merkle F, Ritsema T, Bauer S, Kuilman L. The physician assistant: Shifting the paradigm of European medical practice? HSR Proc Intens Care Cardiovasc Anesth. 2011;3(4):255.

10. Doherty J, Conco D, Couper I, Fonn S. Developing a new mid-level health worker: Lessons from South Africa's experience with clinical associates. Global Health Action. 2013;6.

11. Couper I, Hugo H. Addressing the shortage of Health Professionals in South Africa through the development of a new cadre of health worker: The creation of Clinical Associates (unpublished).

12. Soemantri D, Herrera C, Riquelme A. Measuring the educational environment in health professions studies: A systematic review. Med Teach. 2010; 32(12): 947–952. http://dx.doi.org/10.3109/01421591003686229

13. Babbie E. The practice of social research. 11th ed. Belmont: Thomson Wadsworth; 2007.

14. Roff S, McAleer S, Harden RM, Al-Qahtani M, Ahmed AU, Deza H, et al. Development and validation of the Dundee ready education environment measure (DREEM). Med Teach. 1997;19(4):295–299. http://dx.doi.org/10.3109/01421599709034208

15. Dunne F, McAleer S, Roff S. Assessment of the undergraduate medical education environment in a large UK medical school. Health Educ J.2006;65:149. http://dx.doi.org/10.1177/001789690606500205

16. O'Brien AP, Chan TMF, Cho MAA. Investigating nursing students' perceptions of the changes in a nursing curriculum by means of the Dundee Ready Education Environment Measure (DREEM) inventory: Results of a cluster analysis. Int J Nurs Educ Scholarsh. 2008;5(1):1–18. http://dx.doi.org/10.2202/1548-923X.1503

17. Pai PG, Menezes V, Srikanta, Subramanian AM, Shenoy JP. Medical students' perception of their educational environment. J Clin Diagn Res. 2014;8(1):103–107. http://dx.doi.org/10.7860/JCDR/2014/5559.3944

18. Jiffry MTM, McAleer S, Fernandoo S, Marasinghe RB. Using DREEM questionnaire to gather baseline information on an evolving medical school in SriLanka. Med Teach. 2005;27:348–352. http://dx.doi.org/10.1080/01421590500151005

19. Aghamolaei T, Fazell. Medical students' perception of the educational environment at an Iranian Medical Sciences University. BMC Med Educ. 2010;10:87. http://dx.doi.org/10.1186/1472-6920-10-87

20. Jawaid M, Raheel S, Ahmed F, Aijaz H. Students' perceptions of educational environment at Public Sector Medical University of Pakistan. J Res in Med Sci. 2013;18(5):417–421.

21. Bouhaimed M, Thalib L, Doi S. Perception of the educational environment by medical students undergoing a curricular transition in Kuwait. Med Princ Pract. 2009;18:204–208. http://dx.doi.org/10.1159/000204351

22. Arzumzn H, Yussoff MSB, Chit SP. Big Sib students' perceptions of the educational environment at the school of medical sciences, University Sains Malaysia, using Dundee Ready Educational Environment Measure (DREEM) Inventory. Malays J Med Sci. 2010;17(3):40–47.

23. Roff S, McAleer S, Ifere OS, Bhattacharya S. A global diagnostic tool for measuring educational environment: Comparing Nigeria and Nepal. Med Teach. 2001;23(4):378–382. http://dx.doi.org/10.1080/01421590120043080

24. Al-Hazimi A, Zaini R, Al-hyiani A, Hassan N, Gunaid A, Ponnamperuma G, Karunathilake I, Roff S, McAleer S, Davis M. Educational environment in traditional and innovative medical schools: A study in four undergraduate medical schools. Edu Health. 17(2):192–203.

25. Hamid B, Faroulah A, Mohammadhosein B. Nursing students' perceptions of their educational environment based on DREEM model in an Iranian University. Malays J Med Sci.2013;20(4):56–63.

17

Erectile function in circumcised and uncircumcised men in Lusaka, Zambia: A cross-sectional study

Authors:
Evans Chinkoyo[1,2]
Michael Pather[1]

Affiliations:
[1]Faculty of Medicine and Health Sciences, Department of Interdisciplinary Health Sciences, Division of Family Medicine and Primary Care, University of Stellenbosch, South Africa

[2]Chipata Level 1 Hospital, Lusaka, Zambia

Correspondence to:
Michael Pather

Email:
mpather@sun.ac.za

Postal address:
PO Box 19063, Tygerberg 7505, South Africa

Background: Evidence from three randomised control trials in South Africa, Uganda and Kenya showing that male circumcision can reduce heterosexual transmission of human immunodeficiency virus (HIV) infection from infected females to their male partners by up to 60% has led to an increase in circumcisions in most African countries. This has created anxieties around possible deleterious effects of circumcision on erectile function (EF).

Aim: To compare EF in circumcised and uncircumcised men aged 18 years and older.

Setting: Four primary healthcare facilities in Lusaka, Zambia.

Methods: Using a cross-sectional survey 478 participants (242 circumcised and 236 uncircumcised) from four primary healthcare facilities in Lusaka, Zambia were asked to complete the IIEF-5 questionnaire. EF scores were calculated for the two groups, where normal EF constituted an IIEF-5 score ≥ 22 (out of 25).

Results: Circumcised men had higher average EF scores compared to their uncircumcised counterparts, ($p < 0.001$). The prevalence of erectile dysfunction was lower in circumcised men (56%) compared to uncircumcised men (68%) ($p < 0.05$). EF scores were similar in those circumcised in childhood and those who had the procedure in adulthood, ($p = 0.59$). The groups did not differ significantly in terms of age, relationship status, smoking, alcohol and medication use. A statistically significant difference was observed in education levels, with the circumcision group having higher levels of education ($p < 0.005$).

Conclusion: The higher EF scores in circumcised men show that circumcision does not confer adverse EF effects in men. These results suggest that circumcision can be considered safe in terms of EF. A definitive prospective study is needed to confirm these findings.

Fonction érectile chez les hommes circoncis et non circoncis à Lusaka, Zambie: Une étude transversale.

Contexte: Les preuves des trois essais contrôlés randomisés en Afrique du Sud, en Uganda et au Kenya montrent que la circoncision masculine peut réduire de 60% la transmission hétérosexuelle de l'infection VIH des femmes infectées à leur partenaire masculin ; cela a eu pour résultat une augmentation des circoncisions dans la plupart des pays africains. Mais cela a aussi causé des craintes sur les effets nuisibles possibles de la circoncision sur la fonction érectile (FE).

Objectif: Comparer la FE chez les hommes circoncis et non circoncis de 18 ans et plus.

Lieu: Quatre établissements de santé primaire à Lusaka, Zambie.

Méthodes: Au cours d'une étude transversale on a demandé à 478 participants (242 circoncis et 236 non circoncis) de quatre établissements de soins primaires à Lusaka, Zambie de remplir le questionnaire IIEF-5. Les résultats des deux groups ont été calculés, et on a constaté que la FE normale avait un résultat IIEF-5 ≥ 22 (sur 25).

Résultats: les résultats moyens de FE des hommes circoncis étaient plus élevés que ceux des non circoncis, ($p < 0.001$). La fréquence de dysfonctionnement érectile était moindre chez les hommes circoncis (56%) que chez les non circoncis (68%) ($p < 0.05$). Les résultats de la FE étaient semblables chez ceux qui avaient été circoncis dans leur enfance et ceux qui l'avaient été à l'âge adulte, ($p = 0.59$). Les groupes ne différaient pas énormément selon leur âge, leur situation sexuelle, le fait qu'ils fument ou qu'ils boivent de l'alcool et la prise de médicaments. On a observé une différence importante statistiquement dans le niveau d'éducation, où le groupe de circoncis avait un plus haut niveau d'éducation ($p < 0.005$).

Conclusion: Le résultat plus élevé de la FE chez les homes circoncis montre que la circoncision ne produit pas d'effets néfastes de la FE chez les hommes. Ces résultats suggèrent que la circoncision peut être considérée comme sans danger pour la FE. Il faudra faire une étude prospective définitive pour confirmer ces résultats.

Introduction

Male circumcision, defined as the surgical removal of the foreskin, has been practised for various reasons since time immemorial. In some cultures it is practised as a rite of passage and is accompanied by a period of initiation where newly circumcised boys are given life skills and lessons on how to live as responsible men later on in life. In parts of the world where circumcision is practised for religious purposes, this usually signifies a covenant with God and is performed in the neonatal period, or at some other time during childhood. Circumcision also has a role in medicine as treatment for some penile conditions and as a means of reducing the chance of acquiring some sexually transmitted infections and other non-communicable diseases of the penis.[1,2]

Whilst benefits of male circumcision are well documented, questions about its effects on erectile function (EF) continue to be asked. Most studies that have been conducted to explore the relationship between male circumcision and EF have yielded conflicting results.[3,4,5,6] This study aimed to compare EF in circumcised and uncircumcised men in Lusaka, Zambia.

Study rationale and motivation

The fear of developing sexual problems following circumcision has resulted in a lot of myths around the procedure. Studies conducted so far have failed to provide consensus on this issue. The evidence generated from this study will help people to understand what happens to them after circumcision, and will help them make informed choices regarding this procedure. The evidence will also help to inform international efforts during implementation of country circumcision programmes for prevention of HIV infection.

Aim and objectives

The aim of this study was to compare EF in circumcised and uncircumcised adult men aged 18 years and above in Lusaka, Zambia.

The research question in this study was 'Is there a difference in (erectile function) EF between circumcised and uncircumcised men in Lusaka, Zambia?'

The objectives of the study were as follows:

* To determine the prevalence of erectile dysfunction (ED) amongst circumcised and uncircumcised men aged 18 years and above.
* To compare the prevalence of ED in circumcised and uncircumcised men aged 18 years and above.
* To determine whether the age at which circumcision was performed in study participants had any effect on EF in adulthood.
* To make recommendations on how to respond to concerns regarding EF following circumcision.

The aims and objectives of the study were derived from the hypothesis that there was no significant difference in EF between circumcised and uncircumcised males.

Literature review

Male circumcision is increasingly being accepted as an additional viable strategy for the prevention of HIV transmission from infected females to their uninfected male partners. Three randomised clinical trials in South Africa, Kenya and Uganda have demonstrated that male circumcision can provide partial protection for heterosexual men against HIV infection from infected female sexual partners.[7] This has prompted Ministries of Health in most countries hard-hit by the HIV pandemic to consider male circumcision as an additional strategy for prevention of HIV infection. In Zambia a strategy to circumcise up to 2.5 million males between the ages of 13 and 39 years by 2020 has been launched and measures put in place to ensure its success.[8] Most countries in sub-Saharan Africa have also introduced plans to circumcise up to 80% of eligible males in their populations.[9] The expected outcome of these interventions is a reduction in new HIV infections.

Whilst emphasis is currently on prevention of HIV infection, there are several ongoing debates around the safety, relevance and human rights aspects of male circumcision.[10,11] Some of these discussions are centred around children, in view of their inability to consent to the procedure on their own and having to rely on adults to make decisions on their behalf.

Questions are also being asked about the effect of circumcision on sexual function and the ability of a circumcised man to initiate and maintain a satisfactory erection for normal sexual intercourse. Normal sexual function requires intact genitalia, good blood flow to pelvic organs, an intact neuro-endocrine system and a healthy psychological state.[12] Male circumcision interferes with the integrity of the genitalia by removing the foreskin together with its nerves and blood vessels. This partial denervation of the penis and the subsequent keratinisation of the exposed glans can potentially cause sensory changes resulting in altered ability to experience tactile stimulation, which is necessary for initiation and maintenance of a penile erection.

There have been several attempts to explore the relationship between male circumcision and sexual function, but they have yielded disparate results. In a study of the effect of circumcision on EF, penile sensitivity, sexual activity and satisfaction, Fink et al.[4] observed, amongst other findings, that adult circumcision appeared to result in worsened erectile function and decreased penile sensitivity. Several studies of this nature have been published and yielded similar results.[13,14] Other studies also reported reduced glans sensitivity following circumcision, but without any difference in EF.[15,16] A review of international evidence for benefits and risks of infant circumcision[17] concluded that male circumcision had no adverse effect on sexual function, penile sensation or satisfaction. In a randomised controlled study conducted in Uganda[6] circumcision did not appear to have any adverse effects on sexual function and satisfaction in men. However, this study had limitations in that blinding was not possible and therefore there was a possibility of both interviewer and reporting bias by participants.

Another study looking at the effect of circumcision on male sexual function in Kenya[7] also observed that circumcision did not have clinically important adverse effects on male sexual function in sexually active adults who underwent the procedure. This same result was echoed by systematic reviews and a meta-analysis of scientific literature on this subject which concluded that male circumcision has no adverse effect on sexual function, sensitivity, sexual sensation, or satisfaction.[18,19]

This lack of consensus at international level called for local exploration of the subject in order to establish whether similar results could be reproduced in Zambia, a country with a different cultural context. Since there had not been any formal studies to establish the prevalence of ED amongst Zambian men, the survey aimed to simultaneously measure the prevalence of ED amongst circumcised and uncircumcised men in order to compare the results. The study also sought to determine whether there was any difference in EF in those circumcised in childhood compared to those circumcised in adulthood.

Research methods and design

Study design

This was a descriptive cross-sectional survey. This study design was adequate for the main aim and objectives of the survey.

Setting

The study was conducted in outpatient departments of four primary healthcare facilities in Lusaka, Zambia between 01 June 2013 and 30 September 2013. The four healthcare facilities were the Matero, George, Kanyama and Chilenje Health Centres.

Study population

The population of interest for this study comprised circumcised and uncircumcised sexually active males older than 18 years living in Lusaka, Zambia.

The survey included all sexually active men older than 18 years who were visiting the study sites for various reasons, and those who had responded to requests to participate in the study (e.g. patients with minor ailments, men accompanying patients, employees and their partners, men previously circumcised at the centres).

Exclusion criteria were males younger than 18 years, men with mental and physical conditions that would have made it difficult for them to participate in the study (e.g. clinical depression, psychosis, serious physical illness, alcohol or other drug intoxication), lack of sexual experience, and refusal to participate in the study.

Sample size and sampling method

A convenience sample of an equal number of circumcised and uncircumcised men totalling a minimum of 460 individuals was chosen for the study. The sample size was calculated based on the assumption of 25% disease in the uncircumcised group and 37.5% in the circumcised one; two-sided confidence level 95%, power 80%. A total of 242 circumcised and 236 uncircumcised men took part in the study. The population that was accessible to the study consisted of all eligible adult males visiting Chilenje, Matero, Kanyama and George Health Centres during the study period. Since all the study sites also serve as circumcision centres, circumcision records with contact details dating back the last few years were also used as sampling frames to recruit willing participants into the study. Such candidates were non-randomly contacted by telephone with requests to participate. Participants were also requested to encourage their peers and family members to participate.

The four participating sites are scattered across Lusaka and generally receive people from different sections of society, and can therefore be reasonably considered representative of the population of interest. Chilenje Health Centre is located in a peri-urban township that has relatively higher education levels and income per household than the Kanyama and George compounds. Matero community falls somewhere in between Chilenje and the Kanyama and George compounds in terms of socio-economic development. The sampling frame was also representative of males who had undergone circumcision under the programme that stimulated interest for this study.

Data collection and measurement methods

Adult men visiting Matero, Kanyama, George and Chilenje Health Centres during the study period were approached with the request to participate in the survey. These included circumcised and uncircumcised male patients, employees, partners of female employees, men previously circumcised at the centres and others referred by participants themselves. Eligibility for the survey was ascertained first and the purpose of the study explained before requesting them to participate in the study. Those who agreed to participate were given participant information sheets containing details of the study. They were assured of confidentiality and each one of them gave written informed consent before enrolling into the study. All participants were given the freedom to decline to participate and to withdraw from the study at any point without fear of any reprisals. They were then handed the IIEF-5 questionnaire with seven demographic questions to complete.

The measure used in this study (IIEF-5 questionnaire)[20] is a well-known, abridged version of the International Index of EF questionnaire (IIEF).[21] The IIEF-5 questionnaire was administered to study participants as part of a structured interview during which other demographic data were also captured, for example age, level of education, relationship status, smoking habits, alcohol use, and use of medications, including sexual enhancers. This questionnaire comprises four questions from the EF domain and one question from the intercourse satisfaction domain of the IIEF. Each of the five items of the questionnaire can be scored from a minimum of 1 to a maximum of 5. The IIEF-5 score20 is the sum of the ordinal responses to the five items in the questionnaire. The following are the possible scores with their interpretations: 22–25 – no ED, 17–21 – mild ED, 12–16 – mild-to-moderate ED, 8–11 – moderate ED, and 5–7 – severe ED.

The IIEF-5 has been validated in several cultures and languages, and has been shown to have good reliability and discriminant validity.[22,23,24] Participants were divided into two groups, that is circumcised and uncircumcised. All participants received the same IIEF-5 questionnaire, and those who could not read and/or write were assisted to answer it in private. They were assured of confidentiality, and each one of them was only surveyed once.

Data and statistical analysis

Data were captured on paper-based questionnaires which were kept in locked cabinets. These data were subsequently entered into an Excel data set on a password-protected computer.

IIEF-5 scores were analysed to assess EF, whilst demographic data were evaluated to screen for confounding factors. Chi-square tests were used to examine differences in some categorical variables (alcohol use, cigarette smoking, relationship status and education level), whilst Mann-Whitney U-tests were used for comparison of the two groups by age, medication use and EF scores. Calculated probabilities of < 0.05 were considered to be significant and are quoted to three decimal places. All other statistical results are quoted to two decimal places.

Ethical considerations

This study was conducted with strict adherence to the ethics standards of the University of Stellenbosch Human Research Ethics Committee and the University of Zambia Biomedical Research Ethics Committee, and in accordance with the Helsinki Declaration of 1975, as revised in 2008.

Results

There were 478 participants in this study, 242 in the circumcised group and 236 in the uncircumcised one. There were very few differences between the two groups of participants in terms of age, relationship status, alcohol use, smoking and medication use. However, significant differences were observed in participants' levels of education and EF scores.

Erectile function evaluation

Figure 1 depicts IIEF-5 scores by group. Most of the scores for both groups (92%) were between 16 and 25, that is in the mild to no ED range.

Comparison of erectile function scores

Figure 2 shows IIEF-5 scores plotted against groups. The median in circumcised men was higher than in uncircumcised men. The two groups showed statistically significant differences to each other, with higher average scores observed in the circumcised group ($U = 23062.50$, $Z = 3.64$, $p < 0.001$).

Prevalence of erectile dysfunction

The prevalence of ED in all participants surveyed was around 62%. Amongst circumcised participants 44% registered normal EF compared to 32% in the uncircumcised

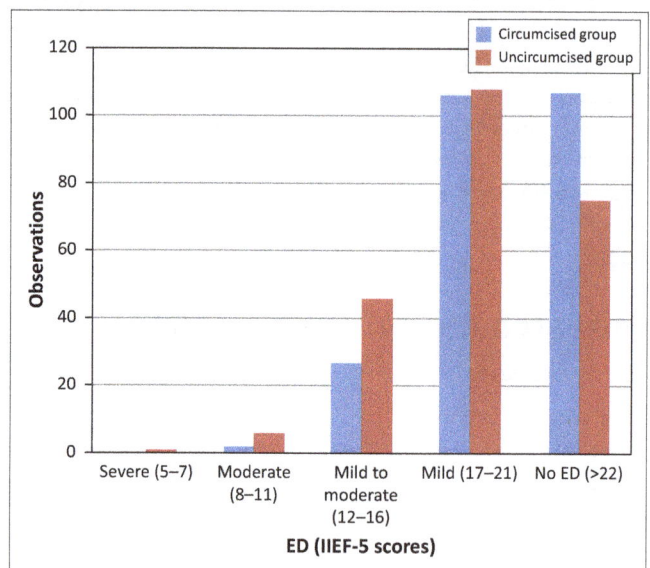

ED, erectile dysfunction.

FIGURE 1: ED scores in the circumcised and the non-circumcised groups, variable IIEF-5 scores.

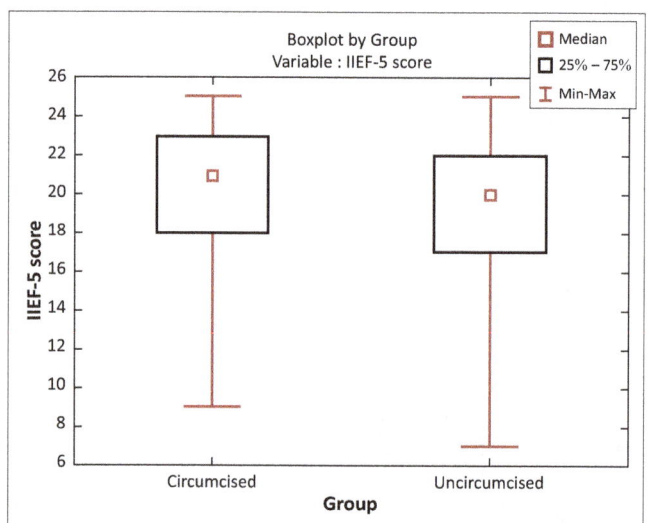

FIGURE 2: Boxplot by circumcised and uncircumcised group plotted against IIEF-5 scores.

group. These results imply that 56% of circumcised and 68% of uncircumcised participants had varying degrees of ED (Table 1).

Comparison of erectile dysfunction in the two groups

The observed difference in the prevalence of ED in the two groups was statistically significant (χ^2 [$N182$] = 7.83, df = 1, $p < 0.05$). More participants in the circumcised group had normal EF than participants in the uncircumcised group.

Education level

The circumcised group had significantly more participants with higher education levels than the uncircumcised group (χ^2 [$N478$] = 19.05, df = 6, $p < 0.005$) (Table 2).

Relationship between age at circumcision and erectile function

Table 3 shows the distribution of participants who were circumcised in childhood and those circumcised in adulthood. The prevalence of ED was around 58% and 56% in those circumcised in childhood and adulthood respectively. These results did not show any statistically significant difference between the two subgroups (χ^2 [$N242$] = 0.29, df = 1, $p = 0.59$).

Demographic characteristics

Age of participants

A review of participants' age ranges was conducted for all 478 patients in the study (Figure 3). The mean ages of the two groups did not differ significantly ($U = 26944.50$, $Z = 1\text{-}066976$, $p = 0.286$).

Relationship status

The majority of participants were either married (58%) or single (37%). About 3% were divorced, whilst those who were separated from their partners and widowers accounted for 1% each. No statistically significant difference was observed between the two groups in this respect (χ^2 [$N478$] = 6.69, df = 4, $p = 0.153$).

Alcohol use

About 53% of participants in the circumcision group admitted to using alcohol, whilst in the uncircumcised group 51% reported alcohol use. No statistically significant difference was found between the two groups in the use of alcohol (χ^2 [$N247$] = 0.10, df = 1, $p = 0.758$).

Smoking

Smokers represented 18% and 23% in the circumcised and uncircumcised groups respectively. There was no statistically significant difference in this category between the two groups (χ^2 [$N97$] = 1.41, df = 1, $p = 0.235$).

Medication use

In the circumcised group 7% reported use of antihypertensive drugs, whilst less than 1% indicated use of anti-diabetic medications. Almost 2% and less than 1% of participants from the uncircumcised group reported use of antihypertensives and anti-diabetic medications respectively. None of the participants reported use of medications for ED. These results did not present any significant difference between the two groups ($U = 26932.00$, $Z = 0.99$, $p = 0.318$).

Discussion

The results of this study showed higher average EF scores in circumcised men compared to uncircumcised men. The

TABLE 1: Two-way summary table of observed frequencies of IIEF-5 scores ≥ or < 22.

IIEF-5 score	Circumcision group n (%)	Uncircumcised group n (%)
≥ 22	107 (44.2%)	75 (31.8%)
< 22	135 (55.8%)	161 (68.2%)
Total	242 (100%)	236 (100%)

TABLE 2: Two-way summary table of observed frequencies of level of education.

Education level	Group-circumcised	Group uncircumcised	Row-totals
None	3	3	6
%	50	50	-
Primary (Grades 1–7)	20	29	49
%	40.82	59.18	-
Junior Secondary (Grades 8–9)	26	52	78
%	33.33	66.67	-
Senior Secondary (Grades 10–12)	76	70	146
%	52.05	47.95	-
College certificate or diploma	96	70	166
%	57.83	42.17	-
Undergraduate degree	20	9	29
%	68.97	31.03	-
Postgraduate degree	1	2	3
%	33.33	66.67	-
Missing data	0	1	1
%	0	100	-
Totals	242	236	478

TABLE 3: Age at circumcision.

Category	Number	%
Circumcised in childhood (< 18 years old)	107	44.2
Circumcised in adulthood (> 18 years old)	135	55.8
Total	242	100

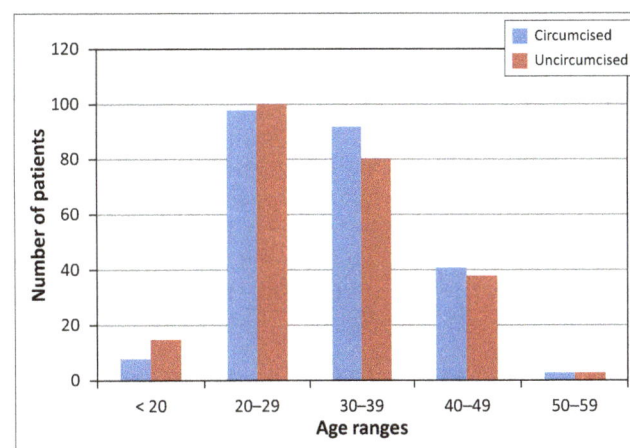

FIGURE 3: Age ranges in the circumcised and uncircumcised group.

prevalence of ED was correspondingly lower in circumcised participants than in uncircumcised ones. No difference was observed in the prevalence of ED between those circumcised in childhood and those circumcised in adulthood. There were no statistically significant differences between the groups in age, relationship status, smoking, alcohol use and medication use. However, a significant difference was observed in the education level category, which demonstrated more participants with higher levels of education in the circumcision group.

The higher IIEF-5 scores that were observed in the circumcised group implied that circumcision did not have significant adverse effects that could have worsened participants' EF. Again demographic characteristics of the two groups that were being compared were similar and only differed in the education level category, where circumcised men indicated higher education levels than their counterparts in the uncircumcised group. The observed differences in education levels between the two groups could not have had much impact on study results, as research assistants were at hand to help participants with difficulties in completing the questionnaire.

The finding in this research that circumcision does not worsen EF replicates the findings of Collins et al.,[13] who stated that the procedure did not appear to present any clinically important effects on EF in adults who underwent the procedure. Observed higher average IIEF-5 scores in the circumcised group present a different picture from what was observed in the study by Fink et al.[9] in which it was suggested that circumcision appeared to worsen EF. Similarities in EF in those circumcised in childhood and in adulthood agree with the findings of Aydur.[25]

There are several possible explanations for what was observed in this study. First, even if all efforts were made to assist participants with challenges in completing the questionnaire, it seems possible that the higher education levels observed in the circumcised group might have made it easier for them to understand instructions in the questionnaire and to answer them more objectively. Participants with lower education levels might have misread the questions and provided incorrect responses. It is also plausible that the opposite might have happened, with more literate participants providing misleading responses. This is especially so because the IIEF-5 tool is subjective in nature and can be reported differently by different individuals. Even if the questionnaire had been validated in other languages and cultures, this had not been done in Zambia, and this could have affected participants' interpretation of the tool. The other explanation for these results could be recall bias, with participants self-selecting the importance of their groups or only reporting those behaviours that they considered socially acceptable.

The clinical relevance of these findings is that they demonstrate that circumcised men have normal EF, with high average IIEF-5 scores. These findings may help clinicians to better counsel those wishing to undergo circumcision.

Limitations

In order to strengthen internal validity of this cross-sectional survey some predictor and confounding variables such as age, sexual partner relationship status, alcohol use and smoking habits were also included in the questionnaire. The measure used (IIEF-5) is a well-known international instrument with proven reliability and discriminant validity.

The study design did not allow for making conclusions about cause and effect, and it is prone to selection and measurement bias. The convenience sampling method used to recruit participants did not allow randomisation and therefore might not be representative of the male population in Lusaka. The IIEF-5 assessment tool for this survey has never been validated in Zambia. Its primary weakness is its subjective nature and reliance on self-reporting by participants. The quota sampling that was used to select some participants in the circumcised group was prone to recall bias in favour of reporting only socially acceptable outcomes. Circumcision status was not verified through physical examination. Literacy levels also differed, and this can lead to poor understanding of instructions in the IIEF-5 questionnaire, resulting in misleading responses.

One area that remains to be explored is the response of female partners of circumcised and uncircumcised men to gauge their assessment of their partners' EF. Considering that the IIEF-5 questionnaire was applied for the first time in Zambia, there is a need to validate it locally before using it for future studies.

Conclusion

The findings of this study show that circumcision does not confer adverse effects that could cause ED in men. These results suggest that circumcision can be considered safe in terms of EF. However, a definitive prospective study in a similar cultural context is needed to confirm these findings.

Acknowledgements

I had no financial conflicts of interest during the study. I had, however, previously served as a male circumcision technical advisor and had participated in drafting the WHO circumcision course notebook for trainers.[26]

Approval to conduct the study was obtained from the University of Stellenbosch Human Research Ethics Committee (HREC) (Ethics reference number N10/11/387) and the University of Zambia Biomedical Research Ethics Committee (Reference Nnmber: 005-11-12).

Dr Justin Harvey from the Stellenbosch University Centre for Statistical Consultation helped with data analysis and provided valuable statistical advice.

Competing interests

The authors declare that they have no financial or personal relationship(s) that may have inappropriately influenced them in writing this article.

Authors' contributions

E.C. (University of Stellenbosch and Chipata Level 1 Hospital) conceived the research idea, designed the study, performed a literature search, collected and analysed the data, and prepared the manuscript for submission. M.P. (University of Stellenbosch) supervised the whole process from conception to final submission.

References

1. Tobian AA, Gray RH, Quinn TC. Male circumcision for the prevention of acquisition and transmission of sexually transmitted infections: the case for neonatal circumcision. Arch Pediatr Adolesc Med. 2010;164(1):78–84. http://dx.doi.org/10.1001/archpediatrics.2009.232

2. Daling JR, Madeleine MM, Johnson LG, et al. Penile cancer: Importance of circumcision, human papillomavirus and smoking in in situ and invasive disease. Int J Cancer. 2005;116(4):606–616. http://dx.doi.org/10.1002/ijc.21009

3. Fink KS, Carson CC, DeVellis RF. Adult circumcision outcomes study: Effect on erectile function, penile sensitivity, sexual activity and satisfaction. J Urol. 2002;167(5):2113–2116. http://dx.doi.org/10.1016/S0022-5347(05)65098-7

4. Cortés-González JR, Arratia-Maqueo JA, Martínez-Montelongo R, Gómez-Guerra LS. Does circumcision affect male's perception of sexual satisfaction? Arch Esp Urol. 2009;62(9):733–736.

5. Kigozi G, Watya S, Polis CB, et al. The effect of male circumcision on sexual satisfaction and function, results from a randomized trial of male circumcision for human immunodeficiency virus prevention, Rakai, Uganda. BJU Int. 2008;101(1):65–70. http://dx.doi.org/10.1111/j.1464-410X.2007.07369.x

6. Krieger JN, Mehta SD, Bailey RC, et al. Adult male circumcision: Effects on sexual function and sexual satisfaction in Kisumu, Kenya. J Sex Med. 2008;5(11):2610–2622. http://dx.doi.org/10.1111/j.1743-6109.2008.00979.x

7. Mills E, Cooper C, Anema A, Guyatt G. Male circumcision for the prevention of heterosexually acquired HIV infection: A meta-analysis of randomized trials involving 11,050 men. HIV Med. 2008;9(6):332–335. http://dx.doi.org/10.1111/j.1468-1293.2008.00596.x

8. World Health Organisation, Regional Office for Africa. (30 July 2010). National Male Circumcision Strategy & Implementation Plan 2010–2020 [Press release]. c2009 [cited 30 June 2010]. Available from: http://www.afro.who.int/en/zambia/zambia-publications.html.

9. Nagelkerke NJ, Moses S, de Vlas SJ, Bailey RC. Modelling the public health impact of male circumcision for HIV prevention in high prevalence areas in Africa. BMC Infect Dis. 2007;7:16. http://dx.doi.org/10.1186/1471-2334-7-16

10. Bristol N. Male circumcision debate flares in the USA. Lancet. 2011;378(9806):1837. http://dx.doi.org/10.1016/S0140-6736(11)61796-0

11. Benatar M, Benatar D. Between Prophylaxis and child abuse: the ethics of neonatal male circumcision. Am J Bioethics. 2003;3(2):35–48. http://dx.doi.org/10.1162/152651603766436216

12. Fouad RK, Koussa VKT, Swerdloff RS. Male sexual function and its disorders: Physiology, pathophysiology, clinical investigation, and treatment. Endocrine Rev. 2001;22(3):342–388. http://dx.doi.org/10.1210/edrv.22.3.0430

13. Bronselaer GA, Schober JM, Meyer-Bahlburg HF, T'sjoen G, Vlietinck R, Hoebeke PB. Male circumcision decreases penile sensitivity as measured in a large cohort. BJU Int. 2013;111(5):820–827. http://dx.doi.org/10.1111/j.1464-410X.2012.11761.x

14. Sorrells ML, Snyder JL, Reiss MD, et al. Fine-touch pressure thresholds in the adult penis. BJU Int. 2007;99(4):864–869. http://dx.doi.org/10.1111/j.1464-410X.2006.06685.x

15. Collins S, Upshaw J, Rutchik S, Ohannessian C, Ortenberg J, Albertsen P. Effects of circumcision on male sexual function: debunking a myth? J Urol. 2002;167(5):2111–2112. http://dx.doi.org/10.1016/S0022-5347(05)65097-5

16. Senkul T, Iserl C, Sen B, Karademir K, Saracoglu F, Erden D. Circumcision in adults: effect on sexual function. Urology. 2004;63(1):155–158. http://dx.doi.org/10.1016/j.urology.2003.08.035

17. Morris BJ, Wodak AD, Mindel A, et al. Infant male circumcision: An evidence-based policy statement. Open J Prev Med. 2012;2(1):79–92. http://dx.doi.org/10.4236/ojpm.2012.21012

18. Morris BJ, Krieger JN. Does male circumcision affect sexual function, sensitivity, or satisfaction? A systematic review. J Sex Med. 2013. http://dx.doi.org/10.1111/jsm.12293

19. Tian Y, Liu W, Wang JZ, Wazir R, Yue X, Wang KJ. Effects of circumcision on male sexual function: a systematic review and meta-analysis. Asian J Androl. 2012;15(5):662–666. http://dx.doi.org/10.1038/aja.2013.47

20. Rosen RC, Cappelleri JC, Smith MD, Lipsky J, Pena BM. Development and evaluation of an abridged five-item version of the International Index of Erectile Function (IIEF-5) as a diagnostic tool for erectile dysfunction. Intl J Impot Res. 1999;11:319–326. http://dx.doi.org/10.1038/sj.ijir.3900472

21. Rosen RC, Riley A, Wagner G, Osterloh IH, Kirkpatrick J, Mishra A. The international index of erectile function (IIEF): A multidimensional scale for assessment of erectile dysfunction. Urology. 1997;49(6):822–830. http://dx.doi.org/10.1016/S0090-4295(97)00238-0

22. Lim TO, Das A, Rampal S, et al. Cross-cultural adaptation and validation of the English version of the International Index of Erectile Function (IIEF) for use in Malaysia. Int J Impot Res. 2003;15(5):329–336. http://dx.doi.org/10.1038/sj.ijir.3901009

23. Ahn TY, Lee DS, Kang WC, Hong JH, Kim YS. Validation of an Abridged Korean Version of the International Index of Erectile Function (IIEF-5) as a Diagnostic Tool for Erectile Dysfunction. Korean J Urol. 2001;42(5):535–540.

24. Mahmood MA, Rehman KU, Khan MA, Sultan T. Translation, cross-cultural adaptation, and psychometric validation of the 5-item International Index of Erectile Function (IIEF-5) into Urdu. J Sex Med. 2012;9:1900–1903. http://dx.doi.org/10.1111/j.1743-6109.2012.02714.x

25. 25.Aydur E, Gungor S, Ceyhan ST, Taiimaz L, Baser I. Effects of childhood circumcision age on adult male sexual functions. Int J Impot Res. 2007;19:424–431. http://dx.doi.org/10.1038/sj.ijir.3901545

26. 26.World Health Organisation, UNAIDS, Jhpiego. Male Circumcision under Local Anaesthesia: Course Notebook for Trainers [homepage on the Internet]. c2008 [cited 8 December 2013]. Available from: http://reprolineplus.org/resources/male-circumcision-under-local-anaesthesia-learning-package-course-notebook-trainers.

18

Alcohol use amongst learners in rural high school in South Africa

Authors:
Thembisile M. Chauke[1]
Hendry van der Heever[1]
Muhammad E. Hoque[2]

Affiliations:
[1]Department of Public Health, University of Limpopo, Medunsa Campus, South Africa

[2]Graduate School of Business and Leadership, University of KwaZulu-Natal, Westville Campus, South Africa

Correspondence to:
Muhammad Hoque

Email:
hoque@ukzn.ac.za

Postal address:
Private Bag X54001, Durban 4000, South Africa

Background: Drinking behaviour by adolescents is a significant public health challenge nationally and internationally. Alcohol use has serious challenges that continue to deprive adolescents of their normal child growth and development. Drinking is associated with dangers that include fighting, crime, unintentional accidents, unprotected sex, violence and others.

Aim: The aim of the study is to investigate drinking patterns, and factors contributing to drinking, amongst secondary school learners in South Africa.

Method: The sample included 177 male (46.6%) and 206 female (53.4%) respondents in the age range from 15–23 years, selected by stratified random sampling.

Results: The results indicated that 35.5% of male and 29.7% of female respondents used alcohol. Both male and female respondents consumed six or more alcohol units (binge drinking) within 30 days; on one occasion the consumption was 17.5% and 15.9% respectively. It was found that alcohol consumption increases with age, 32.2% of 15–17 year-olds and 53.2% of 18–20 year-olds consumed different types of alcohol. It was deduced that 28.9% respondents reported that one of the adults at home drank alcohol regularly, and 9.3% reported that both their parents drank alcohol daily. It was found that 27.6% of the respondents agreed that friends made them conform to drinking. The tenth and eleventh grade reported 15.2% of male and 13.9% of female respondents were aware that alcohol can be addictive.

Conclusion: This study found that age, gender, parental alcohol use and peer pressure were found to be the major contributing factors to alcohol use amongst learners Prevention campaigns such as introducing the harmful effects of alcohol use amongst learners are of utmost importance in reducing alcohol use amongst learners in South Africa.

La consommation d'alcool chez les élèves des collèges ruraux en Afrique du Sud.

Contexte: La consommation d'alcool chez les adolescents est un enjeu important de la santé publique sur le plan national et international. La consommation d'alcool pose des défis majeurs qui continuent à priver les adolescents d'une croissance et d'un développement normaux. L'abus d'alcool est associés à des dangers comme les bagarres, les crimes, les accidents involontaires, les rapports sexuels non protégés, la violence et autres.

Objectif: Le but de cette étude est d'examiner la consommation d'alcool, et les facteurs qui contribuent à l'abus d'alcool chez les élèves des écoles secondaires en Afrique du Sud.

Méthode: L'échantillon comprenait 177 hommes (46.6%) et 206 femmes (53.4%) dans la tranche d'âge de 15 à 23 ans, sélectionnés par échantillon aléatoire stratifié.

Résultats: les résultats ont indiqué que 35.5% des hommes et 29.7% des femmes consommaient de l'alcool. Les hommes aussi bien que les femmes interrogés buvaient six consommations ou plus (beuveries) en 30 jours; une fois la consommation était de 17.5% et 15.9% respectivement. On a remarqué que la consommation d'alcool augmentait avec l'âge, 32.2% des 15à 17 ans et 53.2% des 18 à 20 ans consommaient différents types d'alcool. On en a déduit que 28.9% des personnes interrogées ont répondu qu'un adulte chez eux buvait régulièrement de l'alcool, et 9.3% ont dit que leurs deux parents buvaient tous les jours de l'alcool. On a trouvé que 27.6% des personnes interrogées convenaient que les amis les entrainaient à boire. Les élèves de dixième et onzième année ont répondu que 15.2% des hommes et 13.9% des femmes savaient que l'alcool pouvait créer une dépendance.

Conclusion: Cette étude a trouvé que l'âge, le sexe, l'utilisation d'alcool par les parents et la pression des camarades étaient la cause majeure de consommation d'alcool chez les élèves. Il faudra organiser des campagnes de prévention parmi les élèves, soulignant les effets nocifs de l'alcool, si l'on veut diminuer la consommation d'alcool des élèves en Afrique du Sud.

Introduction

Substance use, particularly alcohol, is a common source of social and health problems in almost all countries in the world, South Africa included.[1] The World Health Organisation (WHO) (2004) states that the availability of alcohol to underage persons under different circumstances, such as alcoholic families or communities, parental permissiveness, poverty and peer pressure fuels adolescent alcohol use.[2] Learners also seem to have drinking problems, which pose global social and public health concern.[3] South Africa is also experiencing substantial change with the onset age of alcohol intake. According to studies conducted in South Africa it was reported that there is growing evidence that South African society experiences fairly widespread alcohol consumption amongst youth and adults.[4,5,6,7,8]

Alcohol has the potential to influence adolescents to engage in risky sexual behaviour such as multiple sex partners, and to become vulnerable to sexually transmitted infections, unintended pregnancy, and sexual violence.[9] When a young person is under the influence of alcohol, undoubtedly the body and mind are not functioning well as expected by norms and the decision-making power is weakened. Researchers have singled out outstanding risk factors such as scholastic problems, risky sexual behaviour, crime and violence, accidents and injury. The findings indicated that early adolescent alcohol use and the use of other substances had significant negative effects on cognitive and effective self-management strategies.[10]

In South Africa, as in other countries, the alcohol initiation age has reduced significantly. The review about prevalence data from five national surveys, which were collected over 12 years in South Africa, supports the mode that binge drinking amongst youth aged 15-24 years increased between 1998–2005 from 29% to 31%.[11] Recent studies reported high level of alcohol use amongst adolescents and high school learners in South Africa.[5,6,7,8,12] Many studies have reported on alcohol use amongst high school learners in South Africa. However, no study has been conducted in the northern township area of Gauteng province of South Africa. Therefore, this study aimed to investigate alcohol use amongst secondary school learners in the northern township of Gauteng province, with reference to their socio-demographics characteristics, drinking patterns and contributing factors regarding substance use.

Methodology

This was a quantitative cross-sectional descriptive study conducted at Makhosini Secondary School (MSS) in Soshanguve Township, outside the limits of the City of Tshwane Municipality in Gauteng Province, South Africa. MSS provides formal education to mainly Black African learners from neighbouring households. The school caters for learners of both sexes; Grades 10–12. The residents in the township in which the study was conducted reside in both formal and informal settlements and are of low socio-economic status.

A total of 792 students, who were in grades 10 and 11, was the population size of the study. Sample size for the study was calculated using the following information: from a population of 792 (learners) using an expected frequency of 50% and the worst expected frequency of 45% at 95 confidence level, the final sample size was 383. To prevent incomplete information the number was increased to 400 learners, the sample representative in grades 10 and 11 learners was increased to 225 and 175 respectively.

Stratified random sampling technique was used to select the sample. A table of random numbers was generated in this manner with no order of sequence, assigning a number to each of the population of 792 learners. Three hundred and ninety numbers were selected, using three digit numbers selected from the table of random numbers of three figures in columns of ten, commencing at any point in the table, accepting 30 numbers with three digits in each column horizontally, until the sample size was reached. If a number was encountered more than once, the number was skipped.

The self-administered questionnaire was developed based on previous research.[13] The questionnaire consisted of socio-demographic factors such as age, gender, grade, and religion; the drinking patterns amongst learners; factors contributing to the use of alcohol. All the questions were closed ended. The questionnaire was written in English because it is the language of teaching and learning in the school.

Data collection day was arranged with the school head master after obtaining permission to conduct the study from the Education Department, the school governing body and the principal. Data collection was executed on the same day in a school hall, which can accommodate more than 390 learners, with a sitting arrangement that simulated a classroom situation. Confidentiality was preserved; no staff member was present or involved during the administration of the questionnaire. The researcher monitored data collection and learners were asked to complete the questionnaire and drop it inside a box next to the door. This box had a small opening on top that could prevent anyone from tampering with the contents. It was anticipated that each learner would complete the question in 20 to 30 minutes.

The data collection tool was pre-tested in a different secondary school from the school in the main study. Ten learners composed of five boys and five girls in the same grade of study were asked to volunteer in the pre-test survey after obtaining permission from the school principal. Data collection occurred between November and December 2011.

Ethical approval for the study was obtained from the ethics committee of the University of Limpopo (Medunsa Campus). Also, permission to conduct research was approved by the Gauteng Education Department, the principal and the school governing body. Learners were asked to participate in the study after the purpose of the study was explained to them and were informed that participating in the study was voluntary and that they were free to withdraw from participating at any time. All the students who were younger than 18 years were given the consent form to give to their parents for approval. Informed consent was obtained from the participants who were over 18 years of age. The parents of the respondents who were under 18 years of age provided their signatures or (thumb prints as per their wish), thereby assuring them that confidentiality would be adhered to at all times.

Data were cleaned, coded and captured and then analysed through SPSS18 (Statistical Package for Social Science). Descriptive statistics were used to analyse socio-demographic information, including age, gender and grade level. The chi-square test was carried out to find the association between categorical variables. P-values < 0.05 were considered statistically significant.

Result

In the study 390 grade 10 and 11 learners took part in the study, but 383 respondents completed the questionnaire correctly. Table 1 summarises the learner's socio-demographic information. Results showed that the average age of the participants was 17.93 years with a standard deviation of 2.75 years. More than half (53.4%) were female, and 77.3% were in grade 10. Regarding religion, the majority (77.3%) were Christian followed by African Traditional (9.9%). When asked who they were currently living with, fewer than half (42.8%) of the learners responded that they were living with both parents during the study.

It was found that 35.5% male and 29.7% female students drank alcohol in their lifetime. Results indicated that all the

TABLE 1: Socio-demographics characteristics of the respondents.

Variables	Frequency	Percentage
Age group		
15–17 years	147	38.4
18–20 years	225	58.7
21–23 years	11	2.9
Mean age (SD)	17.93 (2.75) years	
Gender		
Male	177	46.6
Female	206	53.4
Grade		
Grade 10	217	56.7
Grade 11	166	43.3
Religion		
Christianity	296	77.3
Islam	14	3.7
African Traditional	38	9.9
Hindu	1	0.3
Other	34	8.9
Currently living with		
Both Parents	164	42.8
Single Parent	122	31.9
Guardian	30	8.9
Mother and step-father	34	7.8
Child-headed family	3	0.8
Grandparents	30	7.8

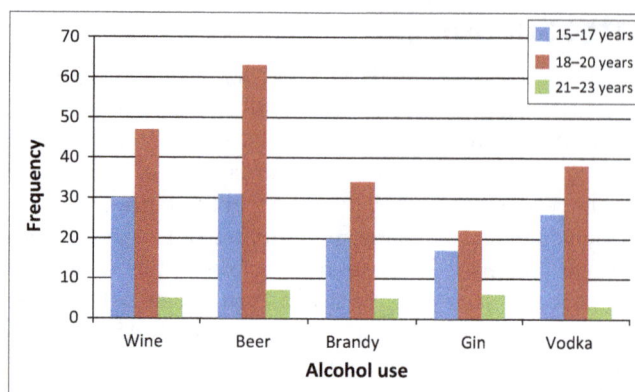

FIGURE 1: Types of alcohol used with regards to learners' age ($n = 354$).

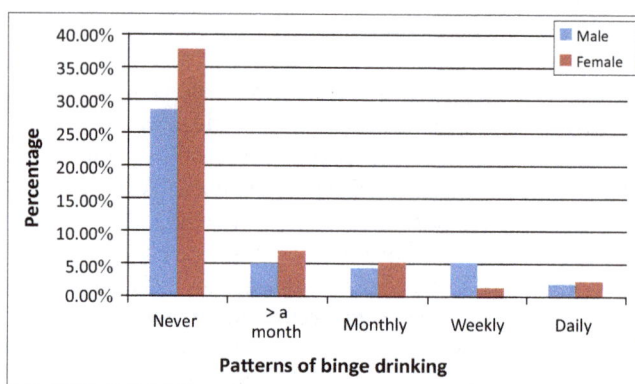

FIGURE 2: Patterns of binge drinking (six or more in one occasion) amongst the learners by gender.

TABLE 2: Effects of alcohol use amongst the learners.

Response	Male	Female	Total	p-value
Absenting self from school because of alcohol use				
Yes	26 (6.7%)	13 (3.3%)	39 (10.0%)	0.010
No	151 (39.4%)	193 (50.3%)	344 (89.8%)	
Embarrassment caused by drinking				
Yes	47 (12.3%)	78 (20.3%)	125 (32.6%)	0.02
No	130 (33.9%)	128 (33.4%)	258 (67.4%)	
Failure to do homework after alcohol consumption				
Yes	42 (11%)	29 (7.6%)	71 (18.5%)	0.015
No	135 (35.2%)	177 (46.2%)	312 (81.5%)	
Unable to study for a test after alcohol use				
Yes	37 (9.7%)	24 (6.3%)	61 (15.9%)	0.014
No	140 (36.6%)	182 (48.6%)	322 (84.1%)	

different age groups of learners used many different kinds of alcohol (Figure 1). With regards to binge drinking, 21.2% [95% CI: 12.7%–25.0%] reported binge drinking. Daily binge drinking was reported by nine male and eight female learners (Figure 2).

Table 2 summarises information about the effect of alcohol amongst the respondents according to gender. Thirty-nine (10.0%) of both gender reported that they did not attend school because of alcohol use. More male students (6.7%) were absent, failed to do homework (11.0%), and were unable to study for a test after alcohol consumption compared to female students (3.3%, 7.6%, and 6.3% respectively) ($p < 0.05$). It was also found that more females were embarrassed

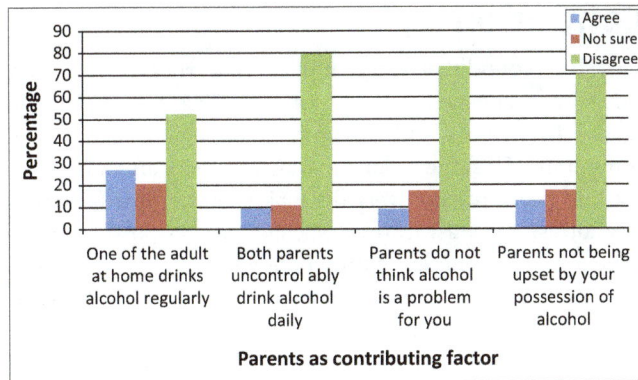

FIGURE 3: Parents as contributing factor to learners' alcohol use (*n* = 383).

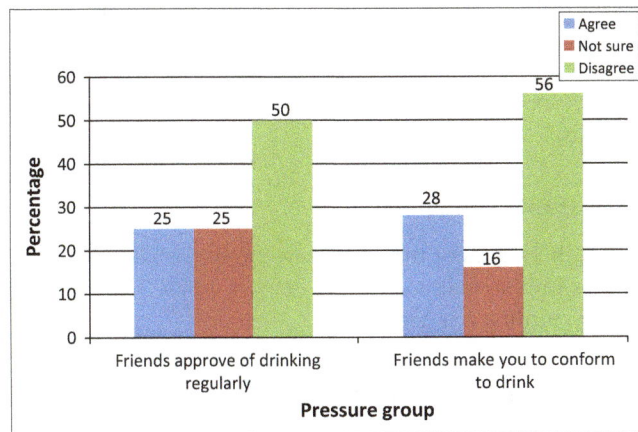

FIGURE 4: Alcohol consumption due to peer pressure group (*n* = 383).

(20.3%) than male students (12.3%) because of drinking alcohol ($p < 0.05$).

Figure 3 shows parental behaviours as a factor contributing to alcohol use by learners. Results highlighted that more than a quarter (26.9%) of the learners reported that there was an adult that drank alcohol regularly at home and 9.3% indicated that both parents were uncontrollably drinking alcohol daily. Most respondents (73.8%) indicated that parents were unhappy about them using alcohol. With regards to peer pressure, 27.6% respondents reported that friends required them to conform to drinking, whilst 56.1% disagreed with this statement (Figure 4).

Discussion

The present study investigated school learners' behaviour regarding alcohol use. Alcohol use involved drinking beer, wine or spirits. In this study alcohol use is defined as the amount (quantity) consumed, patterns of drinking and how often they drank various types of alcohol. The study found risky behaviour and that it impacted on their education. Sadly, the findings of the study suggest that education and other life factors are seriously jeopardised by the pressure of alcohol use amongst learners at MSS. Young and de Klerk indicated that learners (adolescents) are faced with alcohol-related harms associated with social, health and educational problems.[14] The study results found

that learners use alcohol following various patterns, from experimenting to binge drinking.

The study found that different types of alcohol (beer, wine, brandy, gin whisky and vodka) were consumed by learners across the spectrum. The study found that beer was the most consumed liquor, followed by wine and spirit. WHO indicated that wine, beer and spirit are mostly consumed in sub-Saharan Africa, whilst the type of alcohol consumed depends on geographical differences and the type of people practicing the behaviour.[15] A study conducted amongst adolescents in 35 European countries reported 90% of school learners used alcohol in their lifetime and 19% had engaged in illicit drug use.[16] Studies from the USA also reported different types of substance use by the adolescents.[17,18] The South African national Youth Risk Behaviour Survey (YRBS) reported lifetime prevalence rates for alcohol use as 50%, 13% for cannabis use and 12% for inhalants or prescription drug use.[5] These meant that the socio-economic factors do determine the type of alcohol consumed in the region.

Binge drinking is known to be hazardous drinking where the patterns of drinking increase the chances of alcohol-related risks. It involves rapid and excessive drinking over a short period of time.[14] The study found that both male and female respondents consumed six or more alcohol units within 30 days; on one occasion this was 17.5% and 15.9% respectively. Binge drinking has become problematic for teenagers and young people; previous studies have showed its growth in the country. There was an increase from 29% of current drinkers in 1998 to 31% in 2005 in the age group 15–24 years.[11] The study indicated that there was less gender difference in binge drinking. This could be because of availability, accessibility, socio-economic and environmental factors. The same study added that binge drinking is a national challenge; this was proven prevalent in 24% of men in the Western Cape, followed by the North-West with 20.0%, Gauteng 16.0% and the Free State with 15.0%.[11] This could be demonstrating how adults transfer the binge drinking behaviour to their children and society. Research conducted by the NSDUH on alcohol use and delinquent behaviour amongst adolescents aged 12–17 years found that 41.3% were involved in serious fighting at school, 22.4% had attacked someone with the intention of inflicting serious harm, and 12.4% were found carrying a handgun in the previous year. These have a negative impact on the public health.[19]

The present study illustrated that 28.9% respondents reported that one adult at home drank alcohol regularly, and 9.3% reported that both their parents drank alcohol daily. The findings indicated that parents, as role models for their children, influence their teenagers. It highlighted that parents who use alcohol have great influence on their adolescents drinking behaviour.[10] Adolescents who are exposed to such environments at home are likely to model it and consider it to be acceptable. Such parents spend less or no quantity or quality time with their children to give support and guidance. Researchers argued that parents, who spend most of their time drinking, are linked to those adolescents who use alcohol or drugs.[10]

It was also found that 8.8% parents thought that alcohol use was not a problem for their children, whereas 12.5% respondents reported that their parents were not upset by their being in possession of alcohol. In a study it was reported that parents, who are users of alcohol, may predetermine the future alcohol involvement of their child.[3] Parenting is a critical process during the developmental stages of a child. Most parents set boundaries clearly, for example telling their toddlers not to put things in their mouths. These set limits are necessary for a child's safety. All this changes when the child starts to talk; parents try to reason or use rewards to help their child to set and reach goals. Researchers have highlighted that adolescents that spend more time with friends than parents have greater opportunity for alcohol consumption. Parents with lower monitoring skills have a history of alcohol use.[10,20]

Some of the adolescents are involved in consumption because parents are not aware of their activities due to their lack of communication with their parents. Effective parenting is formed by the child-parent relationship. Parents' motivation, norms, beliefs, values and goals are imperative to modify behaviour of their adolescents. More importantly, parents must be monitors and managers of adolescents' behaviour.[20] Parents need to discuss the critical values they want to impart, such as hard work, goal setting, showing respect, spending time with elders, and being a responsible citizen.

It was evident from the study that 25.0% of the respondents enjoyed their friends' approval by drinking regularly; 27.6% agreed that friends made them conform to drinking. Teenagers want to be like their friends and they want to know that their friends accept them as part of the group. Adolescents pressurize each other to be homogeneous peer groups and their behaviour is sometimes outrageous. South African society is also said to be very tolerant towards alcohol and other substances. Adolescents are encouraged by some people and their peers to accept drinking, tell jokes about drinking, and wear T-shirts with slogans that promote drinking and smoking.[21]

Researchers also explain the social factors that lead adolescents to alcohol use. Curiosity and experimentation forms part of this as some see their peers becoming intoxicated with alcohol and other drugs. They also associate alcohol intake with graduating to adulthood. They also consider alcohol consumption to be normal within their peer or cultural groups.[19,21]

The population in this study comprised high school students from one school. This has implications for the generalisability of the findings. Since this is a cross-sectional study, causal inferences cannot be made from the results reported. The self-reported data are subject to bias but anonymity might have reduced this bias.

Conclusion

This study found that a large number of learners at MSS used alcohol and engaged in binge drinking. This may contribute to risk behaviours and disruptions amongst others or the community. This study found that age, gender, parental alcohol use and peer pressure were the major contributing factors to alcohol use amongst learners Alcohol use was also found to have a negative influence on school work (e.g., absenteeism, low performance, truancy and delinquency). Prevention campaigns, such as introducing the harmful effects of alcohol use amongst learners, are of utmost importance in reducing alcohol use amongst learners in South Africa. In future, explorative research needs to be conducted to investigate why high school learners engage in risky behaviours.

Acknowledgements

The authors wish to thank all the learners who voluntarily participated in the study.

Competing interests

The authors declare that they have no financial or personal relationship(s) that may have inappropriately influenced them in writing this article.

Authors' contributions

T.M.C. (University of Limpopo) and H.v.d.H. (University of Limpopo) conceptualised the topic. T.M.C., H.v.d.H., and M.E.H. (University of KwaZulu-Natal) developed the methodology. T.M.C. and M.E.H. analysed the data. H.v.d.H. and M.E.H. wrote the manuscript. M.E.H. wrote the manuscript but all the authors approved the final version of the manuscript.

References

1. Visser M, Routledges L. Substance abuse and psychological well-being of South African adolescents. South African J Psychol. 2007;37(3):595–615. http://dx.doi.org/10.1177/008124630703700313

2. World Health Organization. WHO Global status report on alcohol Geneva: World Health Organization [homepage on the Internet]. 2004 [cited 2010 Sep 28]. Available from: http://www.who.int/substance_abuse/publications/global_status_report_2004_overview.pdf.

3. Liddle HA, Rowe CL. Adolescent substance abuse: Research and clinical advances. New York: Cambridge University Press; 2006. http://dx.doi.org/10.1017/CBO9780511543968

4. Parry DH, Myers D, Morojele NK, et al. Trends in adolescent alcohol and other drug use: Findings from three sentinel sites in South Africa (1997-2001). J Adolesc. 2004;27:429–440. http://dx.doi.org/10.1016/j.adolescence.2003.11.013

5. Reddy SP, James S, Sewpaul R, et al. Umthente uhlaba usamila? The South African Youth Risk Behaviour Survey 2008. Cape Town: South African Medical Research Council, 2010; p. 1–172.

6. Carney T, Myers BJ, Louw J, Lombard C, Flisher AJ. The relationship between substance use and delinquency among high-school students in Cape Town, South Africa. J Adolesc. 2013;36:447–455. http://dx.doi.org/10.1016/j.adolescence.2013.01.004

7. Kaufman ZA, Braunschweig EN, Feeney J, et al. Sexual Risk behavior, alcohol use, and social media use among secondary school students in informal settlements in Cape Town and Port Elizabeth, South Africa. AIDS Behav. 2014;18:1661–1664. http://dx.doi.org/10.1007/s10461-014-0816-x

8. Myers B, Kline TL, Doherty IA, Carney T, Wechsberg WM. Perceived need for substance use treatment among young women from disadvantaged communities in Cape Town, South Africa. BMC Psychiatry. 2014;14:100. http://dx.doi.org/10.1186/1471-244X-14-100

9. Brown SA, McGue M, Maggs J, et al. A developmental perspective on alcohol and youth 16 to 20 year of age. Paediatrics 2008;121(4):290–310. http://dx.doi.org/10.1542/peds.2007-2243D

10. Morojele NK, Parry CDH, Brook JS. Substance abuse and the young: Taking action [homepage on the Internet]. 2009 [cited 2010 Sep 23]. Available from: http://www.sahealthinfo.org/admodule/substance2009.pdf.

11. Peltzer K, Ramlagan S. Alcohol use trends in South Africa. J Soc Sci. 2009; 18(1):1–12.

12. Hoque M, Ghuman S. Do parents still matter regarding adolescents' alcohol drinking? Experience from South Africa. Int J Environ Res Public Health. 2012;9:110–122. http://dx.doi.org/10.3390/ijerph9010110

13. Engs RC. The student alcohol questionnaire (SAQ) [homepage on the Internet]. 2007 [cited 2010 Jan 27]. Available from: www.indiana.edu/-engs/quest/saq.html.

14. Young C, de Klerk V. Pattern of alcohol use on a South African University Campus: The findings of two annual drinking surveys. Afr J Drug Alcohol Stud. 2008;7(2):10–112.

15. World Health Organization. Global strategy to reduce the harmful use of alcohol [homepage on the Internet]. 2010 [cited 2011 May 30]. Available from: http://www.who.int/substance_abuse/msbalcstragegy.pdf.

16. Hibell B, Guttormsson U. The 2011 ESPAD Report: Substance use among students in 36 European Countries. ESPAD Report. 2012.

17. Eaton DK, Kann L, Kinchen S, et al. Youth risk behavior surveillance United States, 2011. Centers for Disease Control and Prevention 2009. MMWR. 2012;61(4):1–162.

18. Johnston LD, O'Malley PM, Bachman JG, Schulenberg JE. Monitoring the future national results on drug use: 2012 overview, key findings on adolescent drug use. Ann Arbor, MI: Institute for Social Research, University of Michigan; 2013.

19. NSDUH Report (National Survey on Drug Use and Health, Substance Abuse and Mental Health Service Administration (SAMHSA)), Office of Studies. Alcohol use and delinquent behaviours among youths [homepage on the Internet]. 2005 [cited 2010 Jan 27]. Available from: http://oas.samhsa.gov/.

20. Hayes L, Smart D, Toumbourou JW, Sanson A. Parental influences of adolescent alcohol. Research Report [homepage on the Internet]. 2004; 10 [cited 2011 May 28]. Available from: http://www.myoutofcontrolteen.com/files/Parenting_Influences_on_Teen_Alcohol_Use.pdf.

21. Hartman A. Millennium life orientation grade 9 learner's book. Paarl, South Africa: Action Publisher; 2006.

19

Non-allopathic adjuvant management of osteoarthritis by alkalinisation of the diet

Authors:
David P. van Velden[1]
Helmuth Reuter[2]
Martin Kidd[3]
F. Otto Müller[4]

Affiliations:
[1]Department of Pathology, Faculty of Medicine and Health Sciences, Department of Pathology, Stellenbosch University, South Africa

[2]Winelands Medical Research Centre, South Africa

[3]Centre for Statistical Consultation, Department of Statistics and Actuarial Sciences, Stellenbosch University, South Africa

[4]Clinical Trials and Drug Development Consultant, George, South Africa

Correspondence to:
David van Velden

Email:
dpvv@sun.ac.za

Postal address:
Erf 5B, De Zalze Winelands Golf Estate, Stellenbosch 7600, South Africa

Background: Osteoarthritis (OA) is a chronic condition. Nonsteroidal anti-inflammatory drugs recommended for treatment have serious adverse effects. A compelling body of anecdotal evidence alerted the authors to the therapeutic potential of dietary supplementation with Multiforce® (MF) Alkaline Powder for relief of OA symptoms.

Aim: The aim of the study was to test the hypothesis that dietary supplementation with MF relieves clinical signs and symptoms of OA of the hands.

Setting: The study was done at the MEDSAC hospital in Somerset West, Western Cape, South Africa.

Methods: The research was conducted in two stages. An open interventional study ($n = 40$) confirmed the notion that MF 7.5 g twice daily is likely to be an effective alternative or adjunct for relief of symptoms of OA of the hands. The main study was conducted with 100 eligible, consenting volunteers (aged 47–89 years) according to a randomised, placebo-controlled, crossover design. Study duration was 56 days, 28 days per regimen; crossover to alternate regimens took place on day 28.

Results: Compared to placebo, MF intake over 28 days was associated with significant reductions ($p < 0.005$) in pain, tenderness and stiffness of interphalangeal and metacarpophalangeal joints of the hand. Confirmation of systemic alkalinisation by MF, which is rich in organic anions in the form of citrate salts, was reflected by a significant and sustained increase in urine pH.

Conclusion: A dietary supplement, Multiforce® Alkaline Powder, containing citrate salts which are converted into bicarbonate *in vivo*, was efficacious and safe as sole therapeutic intervention, significantly attenuating OA-associated signs and symptoms of the hands.

Gestion adjuvante non-allopathique de l'ostéoarthrite par alcalinisation de l'alimentation.

Introduction: L'ostéoarthrite (OA) est une condition chronique. Les médicaments anti-inflammatoires non-stéroïdes – piliers du soulagement symptomatique – peuvent causer des effets nocifs graves, surtout chez les personnes âgées. Un ensemble de preuves anecdotiques probantes ont attiré l'attention des auteurs sur le potentiel thérapeutique du supplément alimentaire du Multiforce® Alkaline Powder (MF) pour le soulagement des symptômes d'ostéoarthrite.

Objectifs: Le but de l'étude était de tester, au moyen d'essais contrôlés randomisés, l'hypothèse que le supplément alimentaire avec MF soulage les signes et les symptômes cliniques de l'OA des mains.

Méthodes: La recherché a été faite en deux phases. Une étude ouverte interventionnelle ($n = 40$) a confirmé la notion que 7.5 g de MF deux fois par jour est une alternative ou un supplément efficace pour le soulagement des symptômes d'ostéoarthrite des mains. Là-dessus l'étude principale a été faite sur 100 volontaires admissibles et consentants (47–89 ans), selon un plan croisé, randomisé et contrôlé par placebo; $n = 50$ par groupe de traitement A et B (verum $n = 50$- groupe A, et placebo $n = 50$- groupe B, spécifiant quel traitement a été fait en premier). La durée de l'étude était de 56 jours, 28 jours par régime. La transition aux régimes alternés s'est faite le 28ème jour. Les visites cliniques ont eu lieu tous les quinze jours.

Résultats: Comparativement au placebo, la prise de MF pendant 28 jours a montré des réductions significatives des douleurs ($p < 0.005$), de la sensibilité et de la raideur des articulations inter-phalangiennes et métacarpo-phalangiennes de la main. La confirmation d'une alcalinisation par MF, riche en anions organiques sous forme de sels de citrate, a été vérifiée par une augmentation importante et prolongée du pH de l'urine. La prise de MF a été bien tolérée.

Conclusion: Le supplément alimentaire, Multiforce® Alkaline Powder, contenant des sels de citrate qui sont convertis en bicarbonate in vivo, est efficace et sans danger quand il sert de seule thérapie, et il atténue considérablement les signes et les symptômes associés à l'ostéoarthrite des mains.

Introduction

Osteo-arthritis (OA) is a major cause of morbidity, affecting 60% of men and 70% of women over the age of 65 years.[1] Current therapeutic approaches, including allopathic (Western) medicine, fail to prevent initiation and progression of OA, and some have life-threatening side-effects. The rapidly rising rates of complex, chronic disease are creating an unsustainable burden on the national economy in both direct (e.g. treatment) and indirect (e.g. lost productivity) costs.

These chronic and degenerative diseases cannot be effectively treated with drugs alone. As a matter of fact, chronic drug use for these conditions is not only costly but often has serious side-effects. Popular analgesics and nonsteroidal anti-inflammatory drugs (NSAIDs) such as celecoxib, diclofenac, ibobrufen, naproxen and aspirin have confirmed risk for heart disease and internal bleeding.[2,3] Paracetamol can damage the liver. Allopathic medicines often do not cure these diseases, but rather mask the symptoms.

The incidence of OA increases with age, and ageing patients present with comorbidities that add to the complexity of treatment. Degeneration of joint cartilage is still the most important pathophysiological feature of OA. Tissues surrounding the joints, such as muscles, bones, tendons and ligaments, are also involved in the disease process. Recommendations for management of OA comprise non-pharmacological and pharmacological approaches. Non-pharmacological interventions include education and self-management, referral to a physical therapist, aerobic muscle-strengthening and water-based exercises, weight reduction, diet interventions, walking aids, knee braces, therapeutic footwear and insoles, thermal modalities, transcutaneous electrical nerve stimulation and acupuncture. Pharmacological treatments consist of paracetamol, systemic and topical cyclo-oxygenase-2 (COX-2) non-selective and selective inhibitors, classified as NSAIDs, topical capsaicin, intra-articular corticosteroids and hyaluronates, glucosamine and/or chondroitin sulphate and diacerin for possible structure-modifying effects, and use of opioid analgesics and tramadol for the treatment of refractory pain.[4,5] Methotrexate, which has immunosuppressive and anti-inflammatory effects, is promising, but this drug may have serious side-effects, including liver disease, lung inflammation, increased susceptibility to infection, and suppression of blood cell production in the bone marrow. Studies with disease-modifying drugs in management of OA, such as bisphosphonates with the aim of inhibiting increased bone turnover, did not produce positive results.[1]

Long-term use of systemic NSAIDs to relieve OA symptoms could cause serious adverse events, such as gastro-intestinal bleeding, renal damage, and induction or aggravation of bronchial asthma and cardiovascular complications.[2] The effect of COX-2 inhibitors on renal function is still tenuous. Of great concern has been the voluntary withdrawal of rofecoxib (Vioxx®) from the market in 2004 because of an increased risk of serious cardiovascular events, including heart attacks and stroke amongst patients taking Vioxx® compared to patients receiving placebo.[6]

Dietary considerations

The typical 'Western diet' is considered acidogenic due to the greater acid load contained in animal products, and is low in fruit and vegetables, resulting in a state of overlooked low-grade chronic, compensated metabolic acidosis.[7] The ensuing acidotic stress and hypoxia may play a role in the pathophysiology of OA.[8] In response to states of diet-derived metabolic acidosis, the kidney implements compensating mechanisms to restore the acid-base balance.

In South Africa there is compelling anecdotal evidence that an alkaline diet supplement, Multiforce® (MF) Alkaline Powder, has beneficial effects in patients with primary OA prompted this research to objectively explore the influence of dietary supplementation with MF on symptoms and signs of OA.

Aim

The aim of the study was to test, by means of a randomised controlled trial, the hypothesis that dietary supplementation with MF relieves clinical signs and symptoms of OA of the hands.

Research methods and design

The research comprised two stages, a pilot study and the main study.

In the pilot, a single-centre, open study of the efficacy and safety of MF in participants ($n = 40$) with OA revealed significant improvements ($p < 0.005$) in all parameters assessed. Side-effects were negligible (unpublished data).

The pilot study was followed by a single-centre, double-blind, placebo-controlled crossover study of the efficacy and safety of MF in participants with OA of the hands ($n = 100$), which is the subject of this article.

Both protocols were approved by the Ethics Committee for Human Research of Stellenbosch University (SU Ethics ref no: 10/02/009).

Study population

One hundred (100) consenting and responsible adult male and female volunteers (47–89 years of age; mean 65 years) with symptoms and signs of OA of the hands (left or right), with or without current allopathic treatment, fulfilling the inclusion criteria were recruited in Somerset West and surrounding areas.

For inclusion participants had to be able to understand and follow the instructions of the protocol; be mobile enough to attend visits to the clinic; give informed consent; be willing, committed, and able to return for all clinic visits and complete all study-related procedures; be able to engage in telephone communication; be compliant with the American Rheumatism Association classification of OA;[9] and be able to complete a daily pain visual analogue scale (VAS) and the validated Stanford Health Assessment Questionnaire (HAQ) 20-item disability scale at each of the six visits. The two-page HAQ-DI (disability index)[10] was used.

Exclusion criteria were, inter alia, gout or serum uric acid equal to or greater than 0.45 mmoL/L, rheumatoid arthritis or high-sensitivity C-reactive protein (hs-CRP) > 20 mg/dl, known or suspected current infection or recurrent infectious disease of a joint, immunosuppressive therapy, history of demyelinating disease or symptoms suggestive of multiple sclerosis, psoriasis, intra-articular, intramuscular or intravenous glucocorticoid therapy eight weeks prior to the screening visit, glomerular filtration rate of < 30 mL/min (as per the Modification of Diet in Renal Disease index), history of acute or recurrent urinary tract infections, 'abnormal' clinical chemistry and haematology values, such as serum transaminases and alkaline phosphatase > 2 x upper limit of normal, full blood count outside normal limits, and abnormal serum electrolyte levels.

In addition, patients with any other arthritic or medical condition that in the opinion of the investigator could compromise participation or interfere with evaluations were excluded, as were those with a history of drug abuse within the five years prior to the screening visit, a history of alcohol abuse or current intake of 21 or more alcohol-containing drinks per week, and any investigational drug taken within three months or five drug half-lives, whichever was the longer period, prior to screening.

Washout period

Prior to randomisation eligible participants were instructed to discontinue any medication (over-the-counter or prescription) used for relief of pain or stiffness of joints for 14 consecutive days, and preferably with the consent of a prescribing physician. At completion of the study patients could be switched back to their pre-study medication regimen.

Screening visit (visit 1)

At the screening visit participants provided informed consent and underwent clinical and laboratory evaluation for trial inclusion. In addition a urine dipstick analysis was performed and urine pH measured by means of a semi-automated colorimetric method (Siemens kit) within two hours of voiding. Patients were instructed not to change their diet in any way during the study period. Random urinary pH was an indication of the dietary acid load; 85% of study participants had a low urinary pH, indicating an acidogenic diet.[11]

Trial medication

Study-related medication (MF verum and matching placebo) was supplied by Bioforce SA Pty (Ltd). Each 7.5 g of MF Alkaline Powder (verum) contains magnesium hydrogenium phosphate 244 mg, calcium citrate 145 mg, potassium bicarbonate 783 mg, magnesium citrate 315 mg, potassium citrate 870 mg, dicalciumphosphate 2-hydrate 973 mg, organic plant calcium, acerola extract and mannitol, and delivers about 250 mg of elemental calcium. The placebo contained mannitol, polydextrose, pirosil, xanthan gum, maize starch and beetroot leaf mix, and was designed and manufactured by Powdermix Technologies (Pty) Ltd (www.powdermix.co.za).

Trial medication was provided in sachets containing 7.5 g of product. The contents of one sachet, suspended in 200 mL of non-carbonated water at room temperature, were ingested twice daily; that is 30 minutes before breakfast (am) and 30 minutes before supper (pm). Patients were instructed to take the medication (verum or placebo) for a period of 28 days, after which they immediately switched to the alternative treatment for another 28 days. The participants and evaluating physician were blinded regarding the identity of treatments.

Dietary intervention

Patients were encouraged to continue with their individual standard diets for the duration of the study, the only intervention being supplementation with MF.

Biochemical assessment of inflammation

At each visit hs-CRP measurement was performed to evaluate whether subjects with long-established OA had active inflammation, and to assess whether MF intervention had any anti-inflammatory effects.[12]

Assessment of joints

At the end of the washout period assessment of generalised pain was done according to a VAS. Pain assessment was done on a 10-point scale, which is a double-anchored horizontal line standardised to 15 centimetres in length, where each end represents opposite ends of a continuum. This line is labelled 0 = no pain at the left anchor point and 10 = severe pain at the right anchor point. Patients were instructed to place a vertical mark on the line to indicate the severity of their pain.

The interphalangeal or metacarpophalangeal joints of the hand were evaluated separately. One joint only served as outcome target; that is left or right hand (interphalangeal or metacarpophalangeal joints), whichever was the worst affected. The affected joints were assessed for tenderness on pressure, and for pain and stiffness upon active or passive movement. Tenderness, pain and stiffness were recorded on a 4-point scale as follows:

- 0 = Patient felt no tenderness/pain/stiffness.
- 1 = Patient complained of pain/stiffness.

- 2 = Patient complained of pain and winced.
- 3 = Patient complained of pain, winced and withdrew the hand.

Clinical assessments were performed by the same investigator throughout the study.

Rescue medication

Participants were allowed to use oral paracetamol up to a maximum of 2 g daily for pain during the washout and trial periods. In the event that the intake of maximum daily quantities was exceeded on five consecutive days, patients were to be withdrawn from the study as 'treatment failures'. No other analgesics or NSAIDs were allowed during the washout and trial periods. Reconciliation of rescue medication issued and used took place at visits 4, 5 and 6, and at any time of termination of participation.

Concomitant medication

Participants were allowed to continue with existing chronic medication if there was no suspected interaction between MF and such regimens.

Study flow sequence

Day 1 (visit 2)

Baseline clinical and biochemical data, including urine pH, were collected. Instruction was given regarding quality of life and VAS scale scoring. Randomisation was done to either MF verum or MF placebo ($n = 50$ per treatment group).

Day 14 (visit 3)

QOL and pain-scale data were collected. Joint parameters were clinically assessed. Urine pH was determined. Side-effects were recorded. Rescue medication was reconciled and reissued.

Day 28 (visit 4)

Clinical and biochemical evaluation was done as on day 1 (visit 2). Day 14 (visit 3) procedures were repeated with a crossover to the alternate regimen (verum ⇄ placebo).

Day 42 (visit 5)

Evaluations were done as on day 14 (visit 3).

Day 56 (visit 6)

This visit signalled the end of the study. Evaluations were done as per day 28 (visit 4). Patients who chose to do so switched back to pre-study pharmacotherapy.

Statistical analysis

For statistical analysis of the data a mixed-model repeated measures analysis of variance was conducted, with group and time as fixed effects and the patients as random effects. For post-hoc pairwise comparisons, Fisher's least significant difference (LSD) was used. Analyses were conducted using the VEPAC module of Statistica 12 data analysis software system (StatSoft, Inc., 2014; www.statsoft.com). A significance level of 5% ($p < 0.05$) was used as the guideline for determining significant changes.

Results

One hundred and fifty-nine patients were screened for OA of the hands, and 100 who fulfilled the inclusion criteria were enrolled in the study. They were randomly assigned into two groups, A and B (verum $n = 50$ group A, and placebo $n = 50$ group B, specifying which treatment came first). Drop-outs were not replaced. Two patients, one from each treatment group, dropped out because they relocated, and 98 patients completed the trial. Eighty-eight per cent of participants were female.

All participants had primary OA of the IP or MP joints of the hands.

Acceptability and tolerance of supplement

No serious adverse events occurred. Three patients reported mild diarrhoea whilst on the verum intervention. Overall acceptability was good.

Value of the Stanford HAQ

During the two-month intervention trial no significant changes were found in functional ability in dressing and grooming, arising, eating, walking, hygiene and reach. Most participants had only difficulty in grip strength (opening jars and taps) and in performing certain household activities and gardening. Although they did experience some improvement in the function of the hands on the verum, this was not statistically significant. It is clear that this questionnaire is more appropriate for patients with rheumatoid arthritis with severe functional disability, and it did not help in assessing the influence of the intervention on OA in those with longstanding OA and no other serious functional disabilities. Patients with OA of the hands have low functional disability not amenable to change.

Efficacy

The influence of the verum (MF) intervention compared to placebo on efficacy parameters is depicted in Figure 1 (a–d).

The MF verum regimen, prior to or following the placebo regimen, resulted in significant ($p < 0.005$) improvement in the four efficacy variables evaluated. Significance was reached within two weeks of treatment. Placebo did not exhibit any positive outcome ($p > 0.005$) at any time. Of note is the observation that switching from verum to placebo was not accompanied by worsening of the signs and symptoms of OA, and that verum treatment had apparently not reached optimum therapeutic efficacy after four weeks.

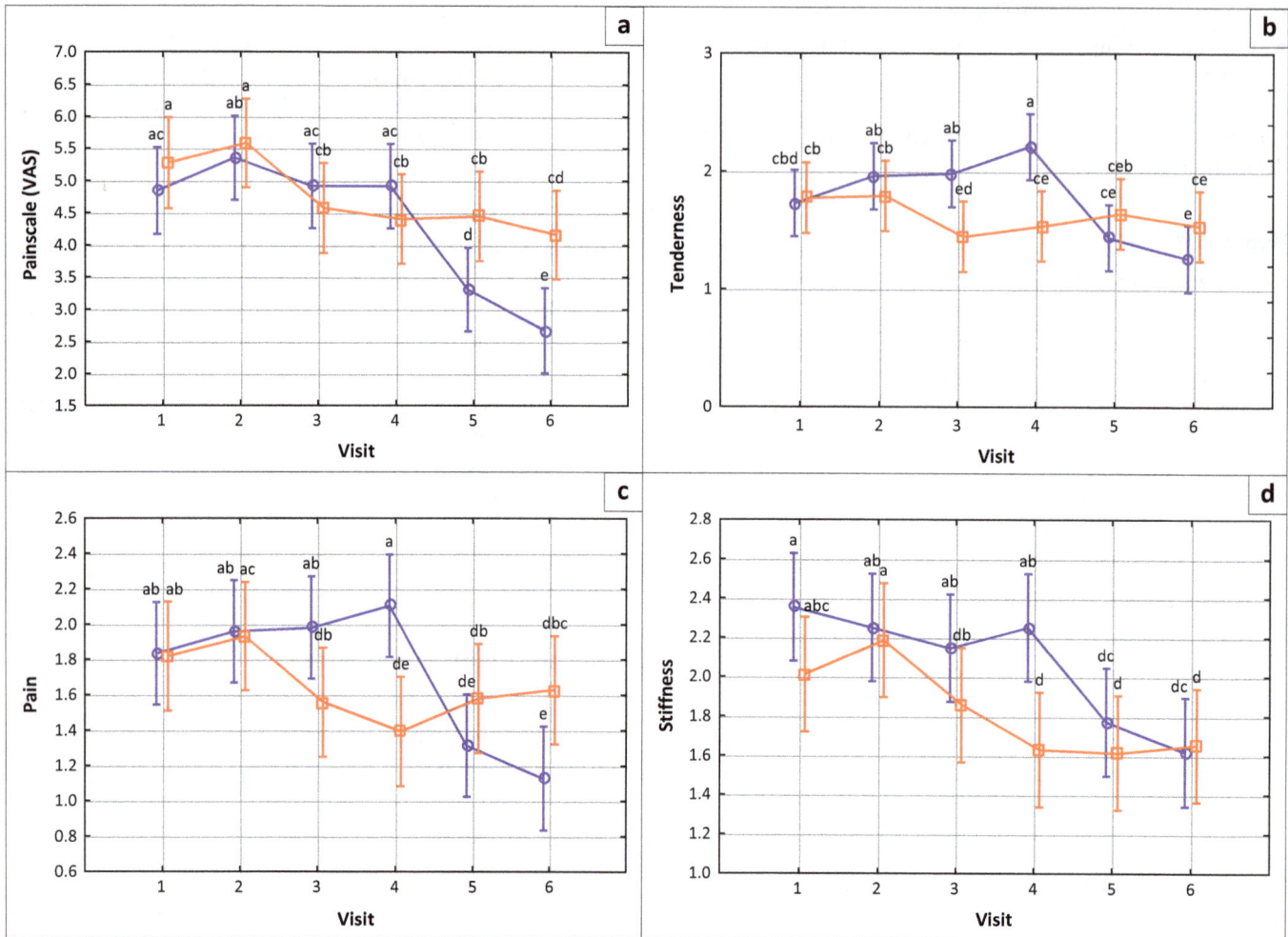

FIGURE 1: VAS pain score on 10-point scale, and clinical assessment of interphalangeal or metacarpophalangeal joint tenderness, pain, and stiffness on a 4-point scale (0–3). Vertical bars denote 0.95 confidence intervals. Blue: placebo followed by verum; red: verum followed by placebo. The letters on Figures 1 and 2 represent the results from the post hoc tests where all means were compared pairwise to determine possible significant differences. In this way any mean on the graph can be compared to any other mean. If the annotations share just one letter (e.g. a vs. a, b vs. b or a vs. ab), then the corresponding p-value comparing the two means will be > 0.05. If the annotations share no letters (e.g. a vs b or a vs bc) then the corresponding p-value comparing the two means will be < 0.05.

Urine pH

The group that received placebo first followed by a switch to verum after four weeks showed no significant change in urine pH, but the switch made after four weeks (visit 4) was followed by a significant and sustained increase in pH.

Conversely, in the group that received verum first, followed by placebo after four weeks, urine pH increased significantly, but when the switch to placebo was made (visit 4) urine pH returned to pre-verum values. These data clearly distinguished verum from placebo and served as a surrogate endpoint for gauging study compliance with regard to adherence to treatment regimens (see Figure 2).

Inflammatory marker

There was no change in hs-CRP during the study period of two months. The median value for hs-CRP at baseline was 2.9 mg/dL (25th – 75th percentile 0.3–23). Traditionally CRP has been used to distinguish systemic inflammatory disorders such as rheumatoid arthritis from OA. However, multiple studies have demonstrated that hs-CRP is

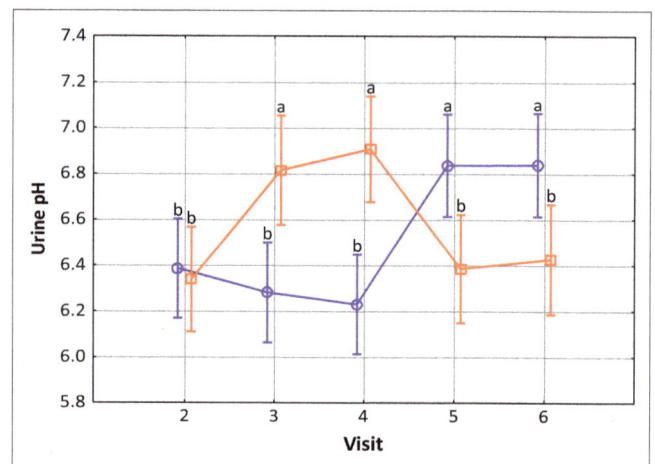

FIGURE 2: Mean urine pH values determined at baseline and subsequent fortnightly clinic visits. Blue: placebo followed by verum; red: verum followed by placebo.

modestly elevated in the plasma of patients with OA compared to age-matched controls. Whilst hs-CRP levels in rheumatoid arthritis are typically > 15 mg/L, levels in OA typically range from 3 to 8 mg/L.[12] This may indicate that the preparation does not influence inflammation, or it may be that the volume of the synovium in longstanding OA is too small to influence it.

Rescue medication

We investigated the use of the rescue medication and it was found not to be different in the placebo and verum groups.

Discussion

The results of this randomised placebo-controlled study involving 98 participants corroborate the findings of the pilot study, namely that the dietary supplement MF, at a dose of 7.5 g twice daily, reduces signs and symptoms of OA in hands significantly, and that ingestion of MF in this manner is associated with alkalinisation of urine. It is thus a tenable deduction that the pilot study was devoid of a placebo effect.

Efficacy of MF reached significance within two weeks and was sustained over the four weeks of treatment, regardless of the order of randomisation. It is also apparent that efficacy levels had not reached steady state after four weeks, which suggests that MF could provide even more pronounced relief if used continuously. This theory is supported by the observation that MF treatment appeared to result in a 'carry-over' effect, deduced from the finding that improvement in signs and symptoms of OA was sustained even after crossover from verum to placebo.

A limitation of the study is the short intervention time, and that we did not do a diet recall during the study. Dietary restrictions and modifications were not enforced in this study. Therefore it is reasonable to deduce that alterations in the OA signs and symptoms and urine pH were induced by dietary supplementation with MF, which is rich in organic anions, notably citrate salts, which are converted into bicarbonate systemically. Although the mechanism(s) whereby MF supplementation provided clinical relief of OA of the hands is not clear, the acidic extracellular environment may lead to increased intracellular acid loads experienced by chondrocytes. Extracellular factors such as acidosis may affect articular chondrocytes and this may have implications for disease progression and potential therapeutic intervention. Articular cartilage is a highly specialised tissue designed to allow pain-free, friction-less movement across joints. Mature cartilage is avascular, relatively hypoxic and acidic and thus provides an unusual and challenging environment to the resident cell, the chondrocyte.

In joint diseases such as OA and rheumatoid arthritis oxygen levels are reduced further from increased consumption by inflammatory cells, and reduced delivery of oxygen to synovial fluid due to joint capsule fibrosis and subchondral bone sclerosis. Alteration in the physical environment and release of inflammatory mediators by articular cells (under disease conditions) leads to acidosis. Cartilage matrix synthesis has a bimodal response to alterations in extracellular pH with optimal synthesis occurring between pH 7.0–7.2, and synovial fluid acidosis occurs in OA and rheumatoid arthritis, suggesting that pH and hypoxia may have an important role in maintaining cartilage integrity.[7] It is possible that 'correction' of underlying systemic metabolic acidosis resulting from 'Western-style' eating habits may play a role.[6,13,14]

Conclusion

Dietary supplementation with MF, which contains organic anions in the form of citrate salts, significantly relieved the symptoms and signs of OA of the hands. Based on the study outcome, MF may be considered a safe and effective, non-allopathic therapeutic modality, alone or as an adjunct to other interventions, in the management of this common degenerative disease. Further research based on comorbidity factors might be warranted. These are short-term findings, and long-term studies are required to evaluate the influence of MF on bone and joint physiology and pathology.

Acknowledgements

This was a contract research project conducted on behalf of South Africa Natural Products and supported by Bioforce (Pty) Ltd. The company only provided financial support in conducting the study, but the study design, data capturing and interpretation was carried out by the authors under the ethical supervision of the University of Stellenbosch. Statistical analysis was done by Prof. Martin Kidd of the Centre for Statistical Consultation, Department of Statistics and Actuarial Sciences, University of Stellenbosch. The authors did not receive any other sponsorship or other activities of the company. The authors declare no conflict of interest, and have no financial interest in the product.

Competing interests

The authors declare that they have no financial or personal relationship(s) that may have inappropriately influenced them in writing this article.

Authors' contributions

D.P.v.V. (University of Stellenbosch) was the principal investigator, and did all the clinical evaluations during the trial period in this single-centre investigation. After the untimely death of F.O.M. in 2014, the results were mainly compiled by D.P.v.V. and H.R. (Winelands Medical Research Centre) as a rheumatologist assisted in formulation of the protocol and interpretation of the data, whilst M.K. (Centre for Statistical Consultation, University of Stellenbosch) carried out statistical analysis of the results. F.O.M. (Clinical Trials and Drug Development, George), as a clinical pharmacologist, was instrumental in finalising the protocol and interpreting the findings.

References

1. Golding MB. Update on the biology of the chondrocyte and new approaches to treating cartilage diseases. Best Pract Res Clin Rheumatol. 2006;20(5):1003–1025. http://dx.doi.org/10.1016/j.berh.2006.06.003

2. Schellak N. Cardiovascular effects and the use of nonsteroidal anti-inflammatory drugs. S Afr Fam Pract. 2014;56(1):16–20. http://dx.doi.org/10.1080/20786204.2014.10844578

3. Van Schoor Jacky: An update on nonsteroidal anti-inflammatory drugs and gastrointestinal risk. S Afr Fam Pract. 2014;56(4):9–2.

4. Zhang W, Moskowitz RW, Nuki G, et al. OARSI recommendations for the management of hip and knee osteoarthritis, Part II: OARSI evidence-based, expert consensus guidelines. Osteoarthritis and Cartilage. 2008;16:137–162. http://dx.doi.org/10.1016/j.joca.2007.12.013

5. Hochberg MC, Altman RD, April KT, et al. American College of Rheumatology. 2012 Recommendations for the use of nonpharmacologic and pharmalogic therapies in osteoarthritis of the hand, hip, and knee. Arthritis Care Res. 2012;64(4):465–474. http://dx.doi.org/10.1002/acr.21596

6. US Food and Drug Administration. FDA issues Public Health Advisory on Vioxx® (rofecoxib) as its manufacturer voluntarily withdraws the product [archived content; first published 2014 Sept 30]. Available from: http://www.fda.gov/NewsEvents/Newsroom/PressAnnouncements/2004/ucm108361.htm

7. Adeva Maria M, Souto Gema. Diet-induced metabolic acidosis. Clin Nutr. 2011;30:416–421. http://dx.doi.org/10.1016/j.clnu.2011.03.008

8. Collins JA, Moots RJ, Winstanley R, et al. Oxygen and pH-sensitivity of human osteoarthritic chondrocytes in 3-D alginate bead culture system. Osteoarthritis and Cartilage. 2013;21:1790–1798. http://dx.doi.org/10.1016/j.joca.2013.06.028

9. Altman R, Alargon G, Appelrouth D, et al. The American College of Rheumatology criteria for the classification and reporting of osteoarthritis of the hand. Arthritis Rheum. 1990;33:1601–1610. http://dx.doi.org/10.1002/art.1780331101

10. Bruce B, Fries JF. The Stanford health assessment questionnaire (HAQ): A review of its history, issues, progress, and documentation. J Rheumatol. 2003;30(1):167–178.

11. Ausmann LM, Oliver, LM, Goldin BR, et al. Estimated net ash excretion inversely correlates with urine pH in vegans, lacto-ovo vegetarians, and omnivores. J Ren Nutr. 2008;18(5):456–465. http://dx.doi.org/10.1053/j.jrn.2008.04.007

12. Pearl AD, Scanzello CR, George S, et al. Elevated high-sensitivity C-reactive protein levels are associated with local inflammatory findings in patients with osteoarthritis. Osteoarthritis and Cartilage. 2007;15,516–523. http://dx.doi.org/10.1016/j.joca.2006.10.010

13. Lanham-New SA: The balance of bone health: Tipping the scales in favour of potassium-rich bicarbonate-rich foods. J Nutr. 2008;172S–7S.

14. Everitt AW, Hilmer SN, Brand-Miller JC, et al. Dietary approaches that delay age-related diseases. Clin Interv Aging. 2006;(1):1–31. http://dx.doi.org/10.2147/ciia.2006.1.1.11

20

Factors influencing specialist outreach and support services to rural populations in the Eden and Central Karoo districts of the Western Cape

Authors:
Johan Schoevers[1,2]
Louis Jenkins[1,3]

Affiliations:
[1]Division of Family Medicine and Primary Health Care, Faculty of Health Sciences, Stellenbosch University, South Africa

[2]Family Physician, Mossel Bay subdistrict, Western Cape Department of Health, South Africa

[3]George Provincial Hospital, Eden District, Western Cape Department of Health, South Africa

Correspondence to:
Johan Schoevers

Email:
johannes.schoevers@ westerncape.gov.za

Postal address:
Mossel Bay Provincial Hospital, Private Bag X34, Mossel Bay 6500, South Africa

Background: Access to health care often depends on where one lives. Rural populations have significantly poorer health outcomes than their urban counterparts. Specialist outreach to rural communities is one way of improving access to care. A multifaceted style of outreach improves access and health outcomes, whilst a shifted outpatients style only improves access. In principle, stakeholders agree that specialist outreach and support (O&S) to rural populations is necessary. In practice, however, factors influence whether or not O&S reaches its goals, affecting sustainability.

Aim and setting: Our aim was to better understand factors associated with the success or failure of specialist O&S to rural populations in the Eden and Central Karoo districts in the Western Cape.

Methods: An anonymous parallel three-stage Delphi process was followed to obtain consensus in a specialist and district hospital panel.

Results: Twenty eight specialist and 31 district hospital experts were invited, with response rates of 60.7% – 71.4% and 58.1% – 74.2% respectively across the three rounds. Relationships, communication and planning were found to be factors feeding into a service delivery versus capacity building tension, which affects the efficiency of O&S. The success of the O&S programme is dependent on a site-specific model that is acceptable to both the outreaching specialists and the hosting district hospital.

Conclusion: Good communication, constructive feedback and improved planning may improve relationships and efficiency, which might lead to a more sustainable and mutually beneficial O&S system.

Facteurs influençant l'extension des services spécialisés et de soutien aux populations rurales dans les districts d'Eden et du Central Karoo du Western Cape.

Contexte: L'accès aux soins de santé dépend souvent de l'endroit où l'on vit. Les populations rurales ont un bilan de santé plus négatif que leurs homologues urbains. L'extension des services spécialisés aux communautés rurales est une manière d'améliorer l'accès aux soins. Un style de rayonnement à multiples facettes améliore l'accessibilité et l'état de santé, alors que le déplacement des patients externes ne fait qu'améliorer l'accès. En principe, les parties prenantes sont d'accord que l'extension des services spécialisés et de soutien (O&S) aux populations rurales est nécessaire. Cependant, dans la pratique, certains facteurs déterminent si les O&S atteignent ou non leur objectif, et affectent leur durabilité.

Objectif et cadre: Notre but était de mieux comprendre les facteurs qui contribuent au succès ou à l'échec de l'extension des O&S aux populations rurales du districts de l'Eden et du Central Karoo du Western Cape.

Méthodes: On a suivi un processus Delphi anonyme en trois étapes pour obtenir un consensus dans un comité de spécialistes et d'experts d'hôpitaux de district.

Résultats: On a invité huit spécialistes et 31 experts d'hôpitaux de district, avec des taux de réponse de 60.7% – 71.4% et 58.1% – 74.2% respectivement au cours des trois étapes. Ils ont trouvé que les relations, la communication et la planification étaient des facteurs ayant une incidence sur la prestation de service par rapport aux tensions du développement des capacités, qui affecte l'efficacité des O&S. Le succès du programme des O&S dépend d'un modèle adapté au site qui soit acceptable aux spécialistes de l'aide et à l'hôpital de district qui les reçoit.

Conclusion: Une bonne communication, des commentaires constructifs et une meilleure planification pourront améliorer les relations et l'efficacité, qui produiront un système d'O&S plus durable et mutuellement bénéfique.

Background

Access to health care, like childhood survival, often depends on where one lives.[1] The infant mortality rate in rural South Africa (SA) is 52.6 per 1000 births, compared to 32.6 per 1000 births in urban areas.[2] Furthermore, three of the four districts in SA with the highest HIV prevalence are rural.[3] These being two commonly used health indicators, it is clear that rural populations have significantly poorer health outcomes than their urban counterparts.

About half of the world's population lives outside major urban centres, where health services and specialist medical services are concentrated.[4] Rural SA is home to 43.6% of the population, but is served by only 12% of doctors and 19% of nurses.[2] Of the 1200 medical students graduating in SA annually, only about 35 work in rural areas in the long-term.[2] There are 30 generalists and 30 specialists/100 000 people in urban areas, compared to an average of 13 generalists and 2 specialists/100 000 people in rural areas.[5] The question arises whether the poorer access to particularly specialist services is one of the contributing factors towards poorer outcomes.

Stakeholders agree that specialist outreach and support (O&S) to rural communities is necessary, as it improves access to specialised healthcare services, effectiveness, efficiency, and relationships between the different levels of health care.[1,6,7] In practice, however, there are many factors that influence whether or not O&S reaches its goals, which in turn affects the sustainability of O&S projects. Understanding these factors would aid recommendations for a suitable model for O&S.

Shifted outpatient styles of outreach, where the outreaching specialist merely sees patients without focusing on skills transfer and engaging with local health carers, focus only on service delivery and improved access, but do not impact health outcomes.[7] A multifaceted outreach service that focuses on capacity building as well as service delivery improves outcomes and efficiency, whilst reducing use of inpatient services.[7] For the purposes of this study O&S referred to a multifaceted outreach service. Capacity building includes the transfer of knowledge and skills, as well as developing and maintaining codependant support systems between district and regional healthcare systems.

O&S reduces cost to the patient by 19%, and also reduces time wasted by the patient.[7] It increases attendance of booked appointments and patient satisfaction, and leads to more guideline-consistent care. It is unclear whether outreach reduces radiology and laboratory costs, but it reduces outpatient treatment modalities and admissions for inpatient treatment.[7] Although O&S is more costly than hospital-based care, multifaceted outreach interventions improve health outcomes, which justifies its use.[7]

Most research on specialist outreach has been done in urban settings using the shifted outpatients model, where the benefits were few.[7] There is little available research on the effect of specialist outreach to rural communities, where greater benefit is expected.[7]

Specialists' opinion towards outreach differs, some criticising inefficient use of scarce specialist resources, others praising its effectiveness.[7] Many healthcare providers fail to appreciate that health care is delivered within a mutually dependant system. Specialists are dependent on a functional primary care service to protect them from inappropriate problems and to provide a step-down facility in order to allow them to meet their objectives. Developing and strengthening primary care services is a critical step in securing accessible specialist services. A close relationship between components of the health system and a well-functioning referral system with clear referral criteria are the key to achieving equity in access to appropriate levels of care. There also needs to be a shift from a movement of patients to the movement of capacity and resources within the health system.[1]

Outreach that is sustainable, properly organised, relevant to local needs and has an adequate specialist base can integrate and support secondary and primary health care, thus benefitting rural communities.[7] Poorly planned and conducted outreach can draw resources away from primary health care.[7,8]

In the Western Cape the primary objective of outreach is to ensure that patient care is of the highest quality within the available resources.[6] Responsibilities of visiting specialists in SA include ward rounds, outpatient clinics, surgical procedures, morbidity and mortality meetings and other measures to evaluate quality of care, educational meetings, and developing guidelines and protocols with in-service training on these.[6,9,10] Other responsibilities that can be included are professional and/or personal and managerial support.[1,9,10]

In the Eden and Central Karoo districts of the Western Cape of SA there are one level 2 (regional) hospital and 10 level 1 (district) hospitals. All clinical disciplines carry out outreach, with varying frequencies. On average the 4 main district hospitals receive 17 specialist outreach visits per month, whilst the smaller district hospitals receive 3 specialist visits per month, as per interviews with the respective clinical managers. A typical outreach visit includes a problem ward round, outpatient clinic, theatre list for some surgical disciplines, and formal or informal educational sessions.

O&S services in rural SA should focus on empowerment and relationship building with local doctors, rather than service delivery. They should be regular, sustainable and linked to continual professional development.[11] Problems commonly encountered by specialists are poor planning, rapid turnover of district hospital staff, unavailability of essential equipment or drugs, and inadequate preparation of patients for surgery. Resistance to change and limited teaching opportunities due to work pressure or indifference are also problematic.[11] As the district hospital work has to continue despite the specialist visit, O&S can create tension between service and teaching needs. Specialists are sometimes unaware of this disruption and have unreasonable demands.[11]

It has been recommended that specialists doing outreach should have the correct attitude and be able to adapt to rural conditions, without compromising essentials.[11] The same specialist should visit a specific hospital on a regular basis. Teaching should focus on common conditions. Protocols for managing these conditions should be established in consultation with the district hospital management. Surgeons should consider the peri-operative limitations in rural hospitals and confine surgery to what local doctors can be taught to do. Furthermore, a dedicated district hospital doctor should coordinate the local practicalities and follow-up of patients seen. The rural hospital also needs to rearrange its schedule and staff for the day of outreach.[11]

Aim and objectives

There is little research on the attitudes of stakeholders in the Western Cape towards specialist O&S. The aim of this study was to better understand factors associated with the success or failure of specialist O&S services to rural populations in the Western Cape. The objectives included reaching consensus

between outreaching specialists, and between rural district hospital doctors on the major factors influencing O&S services, and making recommendations for provision of O&S services to rural populations.

Research methods and design

Study design

The Delphi method was used to obtain consensus.[12] Specialists and district hospital doctors and nurses were asked to give their opinion on the major factors influencing O&S.

Setting

Figure 1 shows the Eden and Central Karoo districts, which cover an area of 61 573 km^2,with an estimated population of 569 536.[13] They are serviced by one regional hospital in George, and 10 district hospitals of varying sizes. All the hospitals are accessible by tarred road; the furthest from George is Murraysburg Provincial Hospital (327 km).

Study population and sampling strategy

All public service specialists and specialised medical officers currently and previously involved in O&S in the

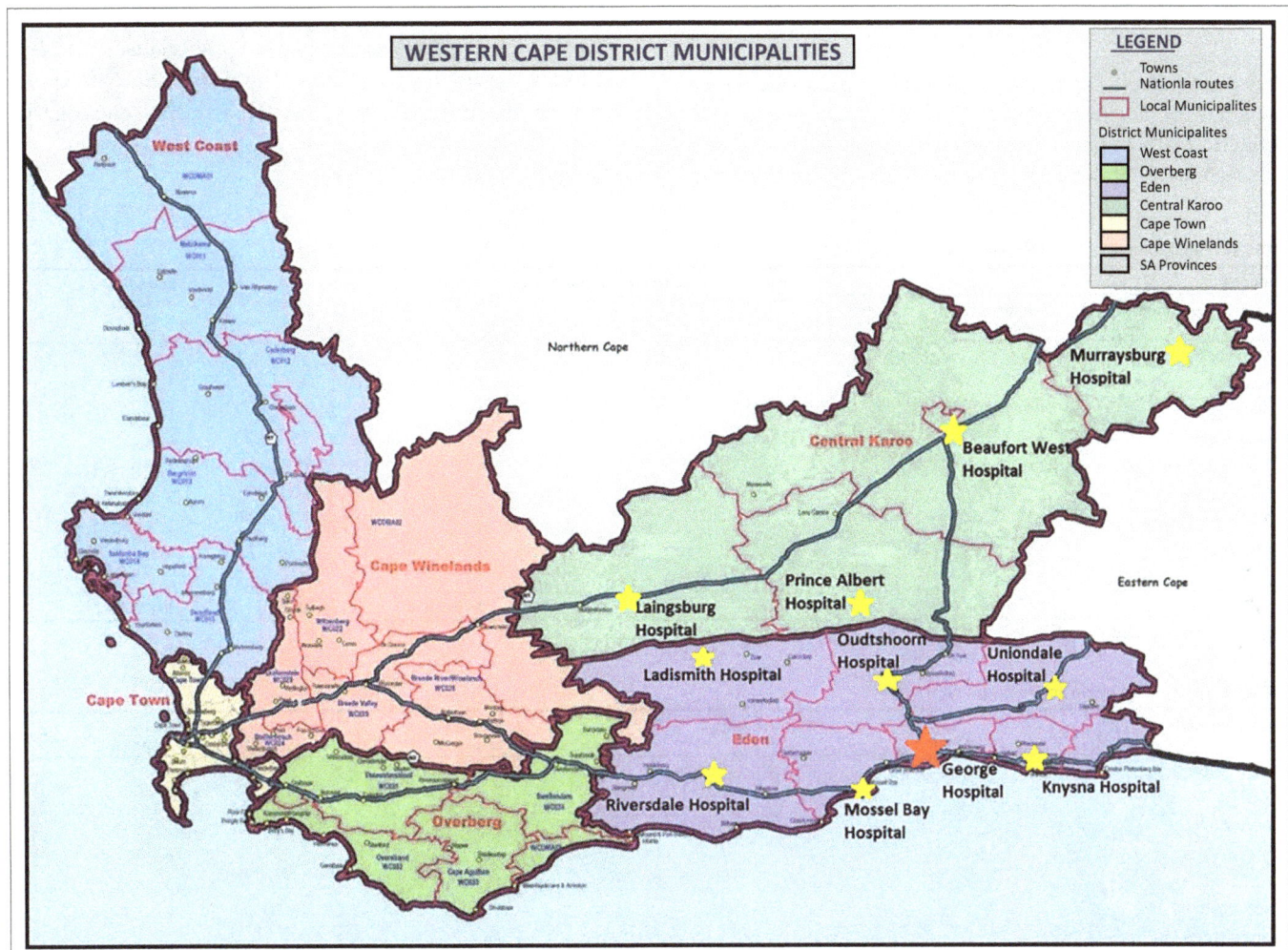

FIGURE 1: Map indicating Eden and Central Karoo districts in the Western Cape.

two districts were invited to participate, comprising the specialist panel. Specialised medical officers refer to career medical officers in a specific department who are trusted by their heads of departments to conduct O&S visits. All hospital medical and clinical managers, as well as some career medical officers or nurses actively involved in O&S at Mossel Bay, Oudtshoorn, Knysna, Riversdale, Ladysmith, Beaufort West and Prince Albert district hospitals were invited to participate, comprising the district hospital panel. Panels bigger than 30 members have not been shown to improve results.[12] Informed consent was obtained from all study participants.

Only O&S from level two to level one was evaluated. Outreach activities from level three to level two, by non-medical personnel, and by private sessional specialists were excluded.

Data collection

Questionnaires were developed from the literature and input from local and national experts, including members of the local O&S service, district healthcare management and academics with a special interest in O&S. Experts were consulted via telephonic interviews or email on the major factors influencing O&S services. An anonymous parallel three-stage Delphi process was followed to obtain consensus.

Data were collected by sending and retrieving questionnaires via email or fax from May to July 2012. Consensus was defined as 70% of panel members giving the same response to a statement. Statements were made regarding O&S and

panel members were asked to respond to these using a Likert scale, with the following options: Agree strongly, Agree, Disagree and Disagree strongly. A neutral middle option was excluded to force panel members to choose either a positive or negative option. Panel members were also given the option to comment on each statement, and to give qualitative feedback regarding other issues affecting O&S that were not covered by the statements. Statements where consensus was reached were removed from subsequent rounds.

Data analysis

Nominal and ordinal data were converted into simple descriptive statistics, in consultation with the University of Stellenbosch's Centre for Statistical Consultation.

Ethical considerations

Ethics approval was granted by the Human Research: Ethics Committee of the University of Stellenbosch (Ref. No.: S11/11/023). Permission was granted by the Research Committee of the Department of Health of the Western Cape, and district hospital management.

Results

Twenty eight experts were invited to the specialist panel, and 31 to the district hospital panel. The distribution of experts between the different specialist departments and district hospitals, as well as the response rates for each round, are shown in Table 1a and Table 1b.

TABLE 1a: Panel composition and response rates.

Composition		Number invited (currently and previously involved in O&S)	Round 1 response	Round 2 response	Round 3 response
Specialist departments	Number currently involved in O&S				
Anaesthetics	2	2	1	1	1
Family Medicine	3	3	3	1	3
General Surgery	3	4	1	1	1
Internal Medicine	4	4	4	4	4
Obstetrics/Gynaecology	3	3	3	3	3
Ophthalmology	3	2	0	0	0
Orthopaedic Surgery	3	3	3	3	3
Paediatrics	4	4	2	2	3
Psychiatry	2	3	2	2	2
Total	27	28	19 (67.9%)	17 (60.7%)	20 (71.4%)

O&S, outreach and support.

TABLE 1b: Panel composition and response rates.

District hospitals	Number invited	Round 1 response	Round 2 response	Round 3 response
Beaufort West	3	1	1	1
Knysna	5	5	4	5
Ladysmith	3	3	3	3
Mossel Bay	7	5	5	6
Oudtshoorn	6	4	2	5
Prince Albert	3	2	1	2
Riversdale	4	2	2	1
Total	31	22 (71.0%)	18 (58.1%)	23 (74.2%)

Round 1

Fifty six and 50 statements were evaluated by the specialist panel and district hospital panel respectively. Consensus was reached on 8 statements in the specialist panel, and on 6 statements in the district hospital panel. These statements were removed from subsequent rounds. Panel members had the opportunity to comment on the statements or to suggest additional issues that needed to be explored. The remaining statements where consensus was not reached, as well as new modified statements, were transferred to round two.

Round 2

The specialist panel evaluated 54 statements during round 2. These included the statements from round one where consensus was not reached, as well as 4 new statements that were based on comments during round one, and 3 confusing statements that were modified and/or expanded to 5 new statements. Consensus was reached on 29 of these statements during round 2.

The district hospital panel evaluated 49 statements during round 2. These included the statements from round one where consensus were not reached, as well as 2 new statements that were based on comments during round one, and 3 confusing statements that were modified/expanded to 5 new statements. Consensus was reached on 33 of these statements during round 2.

Round 3

During round 3 the options on the Likert scale were reduced to only 'Agree' and 'Disagree'. The remaining 25 statements in the specialist panel were evaluated, and consensus was reached on 18 statements. In the district hospital panel 15 statements were evaluated and consensus was reached on 5 statements.

In total consensus was reached on 55 of the 62 statements in the specialist panel and on 44 of the 54 statements in the district hospital panel (Table 2).

No consensus was reached on 7 statements in the specialist panel, and 10 statements in the district hospital panel (Table 3).

Discussion

The key findings, which appear in bold in Tables 2 and 3, can be grouped together in the following themes, and are interconnected to a greater or lesser degree, as shown in Figure 2: relationships; communication; planning; service vs capacity building; and efficiency.

Relationships and communication are central themes in O&S programmes.[1] Comments from the questionnaires that summarised this well were 'It's all about relationships,' and 'Communication is the key'.

Although O&S is part of the job description of regional specialists, it only works in an efficient way if the relational (and emotional) component of this service is recognised and prioritised.[6] O&S generally improves relationships, but O&S that is not properly planned can draw resources away from primary health care and could lead to intense frustration for the specialists or district hospital staff.[7] Specialists and district hospital staff should be equal partners in this relationship. It appears that specialists are generally committed to O&S and are actively involved; however, the commitment of district hospital staff towards O&S is questioned by the specialist group. Without building mutually beneficial and codependant relationships, O&S programmes are bound to fail, paradoxically making specialist care more inaccessible for rural patients. Consensus was reached by both panels on ways to develop healthy relationships and communication: through constructive feedback on referrals, mutual reporting on outreach, mentoring by specialists, and a combined clinical day for specialists and district doctors once or twice a year.

Communication can improve efficiency of O&S in various ways. Both groups agreed that patients should be discussed with the outreaching specialist when an appointment is made for them.[10] Having a specific specialist visiting a specific district hospital makes this a lot easier.[11] The specialists preferred the discussion to be email-based, whilst the district hospital group preferred it to be telephone-based. Reasons mentioned for email-based discussions were to keep medico-legal records and to limit interruptions during consultations. Email-based discussions naturally involve the use of technology (Internet connection or smartphone), and this is not always available; however, fax-to-email is a relatively simple solution to this problem. Reasons mentioned for telephonic discussions included them being easier, quicker, and limiting delayed and/or non-responders.

These discussions serve many purposes. Many of the patients can be managed without the specialist even seeing the patient. It also leads to fewer inappropriate referrals or 'dumping' and to more appropriate work-up of patients, which leads to less overbooked O&S clinics. It also serves as a learning opportunity, and should be seen as part of capacity building. Patients consulted this way are ensured longitudinal care by the doctors involved, whilst the district hospital doctors are given the opportunity to develop capacity and the specialist is given logistical support by the district hospital doctors.

There was consensus that O&S is context- or site-specific. Comments from participants suggest that the same district hospital might have different O&S experiences, depending on the specific specialist or specialty. An exciting prospect is the apparent openness to exchange doctors between district and regional hospitals for a week or two at a time. This will serve the dual purpose of aiding understanding of each other's context, as well as giving doctors the opportunity to learn from each other. This will involve

TABLE 2: Statements where consensus was reached.†

Statements	Specialists	District hospitals
There is enough regional hospital management support for O&S.	Agree	Agree
There is enough district hospital management support for O&S.	Agree	Agree
The planned O&S for the week/month is discussed with all the involved staff in the specialist department.	Agree	-
The planned O&S for the week/month is discussed with all the involved staff at the district hospital.	-	Disagree
Inefficient travel arrangements (like transport, meals, accommodation) are barriers to O&S that happen frequently.	Disagree	-
Travel arrangements (transport, meals and accommodation) are the responsibility of the district hospital.	-	Disagree
O&S visits can be scheduled better to disrupt district hospital less.	Agree	Agree
If O&S visits are cancelled, it is with sufficient warning.	-	Disagree
Both the specialist and district hospital should reflect on O&S encounters in a regular written report.	Agree	Agree
O&S clinics are overbooked.	Disagree	-
Overbooking can be overcome by appropriate referrals and work-up.	Agree	-
Overbooked clinics are due to the number of patients needing specialist care.	-	Agree
There is a need for more O&S visits.	-	Agree
Appropriate patients are seen during O&S.	Agree	-
Patients seen are over-investigated prior to O&S.	Disagree	-
O&S leads to fewer referrals to the regional hospital.	Agree	Strongly agree
A call the day before an O&S visit to inform of the number of booked patients would be helpful.	Agree	-
Patients must be discussed with the specific specialist at booking of the patient.	Agree	Agree
Preferred method.	Email	Telephone
O&S can be more useful with more email/Skype/cell phone/teleconferencing.	Agree	Agree
O&S leads to more efficient patient care.	Strongly agree	Strongly agree
Patients seen on O&S get the same standard of care as at the specialist's base hospital.	Agree	Agree
There are enough district hospital doctors to make O&S work.	Disagree	Disagree
There are enough specialists to make O&S work.	-	Agree
Smaller hospitals generally find it more difficult to live up to the specialist's expectations.	Disagree	-
Sessional specialists should also be involved in O&S.	Agree	Agree
Allied health professionals like specialist nurses, sonographers, etc. should also be involved in O&S.	Agree	Agree
The main focus of O&S currently is service delivery.	Agree	-
The main focus of O&S should be capacity building.	Agree	Agree
A district hospital doctor is present during most consultations.	Disagree	-
Better scheduling of the day's work can allow a district hospital doctor to be present during most consultations.	-	Agree
A district hospital doctor present during consultation will improve O&S.	Strongly agree	Strongly agree
Doctors working in outlying primary health care clinics should also attend O&S sessions, regardless of the logistical challenges.	Agree	-
Logistical support and capacity building should be equally important reasons to have a district hospital doctor present during consultations.	Agree	Agree
It is essential for surgical specialities to do surgery whilst on O&S.	Agree	Agree
Surgery done should be aimed towards what district hospital doctors can be taught to do safely.	Agree	Agree
Anaesthetic and postoperative care are always considered prior to booking patients for surgery.	Agree	Agree
Patients for surgery are properly prepared.	Agree	-
The necessary equipment is available for surgery.	Agree	-
Patients should only be booked for theatre after discussion with the surgeon or being seen by the surgeon.	Agree	-
Most of the expected investigations are available at district hospital level.	Agree	-
Medications prescribed by specialists are generally available at the district hospital.	Agree	Agree
A ward round seeing problem patients as well as random patients will be more helpful than seeing only problem patients.	Agree	Agree
Protocols for the management of common conditions are available.	Agree	Agree
The above protocols are helpful.	-	Agree
Patients seen during O&S are generally sorted out sooner.	Agree	-
Specialists regularly attend morbidity and mortality meetings at district hospital.	Disagree	Disagree
The morbidity and mortality meetings influence quality of care.	Agree	Agree
A specific specialist should be connected to a specific district hospital.	Agree	Agree
Most specialists have the correct personality for O&S (i.e. attitude, motivation, adaptability).	Agree	-
Exchange between district hospital doctors and regional hospital doctors for one/two weeks will aid understanding of each other's context, etc.	Strongly agree	Agree
A district-wide clinical day once or twice a year, for regional and district doctors to interact, will be good to share clinical and operational experiences.	Agree	Agree
O&S leads to easier referral up and down the referral chain due to better relationships.	Strongly agree	Agree
Constructive feedback on the quality of all referrals to specialist care will be helpful.	Agree	Strongly agree
Mentoring district hospital doctors in professional issues is part of O&S.	Agree	Agree
There is a dedicated educational session during O&S.	Agree	Agree
These sessions are well attended.	Agree	-

O&S, outreach and support.

†, Indicate where a statement was not presented to a panel/where consensus was not reached in one of the panels, and the statements in bold were deemed key findings.

Table 2 continues on the next page →

TABLE 2 (Continues...): Statements where consensus was reached.†

Statements	Specialists	District hospitals
Educational sessions are relevant to district hospitals.	-	Agree
Topics for educational sessions are known well in advance.	Disagree	Disagree
District hospital doctors are generally open to advice and change.	Agree	-
District hospital doctors are generally committed to O&S.	Disagree	-
Outreaching specialists are generally committed to O&S.	-	Agree
District hospital doctors have unrealistic expectations of O&S.	Agree	-
Specialists have unrealistic expectations of O&S.	-	Disagree
The success of O&S is context-/site-specific.	Agree	-
O&S is satisfying.	Agree	Agree

O&S, outreach and support.
†, Indicate where a statement was not presented to a panel/where consensus was not reached in one of the panels, and the statements in bold were deemed key findings.

TABLE 3: Statements where consensus was not reached.

Specialists	District hospitals
The main focus of O&S currently is capacity building.	The main focus of O&S currently is capacity building.
The main focus of O&S should be service delivery.	The main focus of O&S should be service delivery.
-	The main focus of O&S currently is service delivery.
There is a dedicated liaison doctor at the district hospital to coordinate the O&S visit.	There is a dedicated liaison doctor at the district hospital to coordinate the O&S visit.
-	District hospitals have a long-term roster of O&S dates.
The referral letters are adequate if no district hospital doctor is present.	Referral letters from regional hospitals to district hospitals are generally adequate.
-	It is almost impossible for doctors working in outlying primary healthcare clinics to attend O&S sessions.
Protocols are generally followed.	Patients are referred according to the protocols without problems.
-	Most specialists have the correct personality for O&S (i.e. attitude, motivation, adaptability).
-	If O&S visits are cancelled, patients are accommodated by an extra visit or during the next O&S.
There are enough specialists at regional hospital to make O&S work.	-
Patients seen during O&S are not worked up appropriately.	-

O&S, outreach and support.

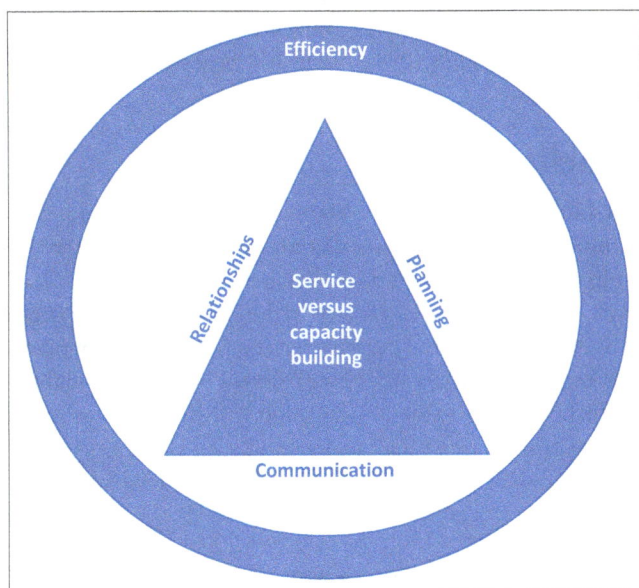

FIGURE 2: Outreach themes.

careful planning by mid-level and senior members of staff from both teams.

Whilst the focus of O&S currently seems to be service delivery, most participants agreed that capacity building should rather be the focus.[11] Many participants commented that the focus should be 50% on service delivery and 50% on capacity building. If the O&S programme in the Eden and Central Karoo districts could make the shift from a service delivery/shifted outpatients model to a multifaceted/capacity building model, the health outcomes of patients in these rural districts could hopefully improve, as suggested in the literature.[7]

Capacity building should not only be limited to traditional lectures, but should be expanded to include bedside teaching, case-based discussions, teaching of procedural skills and mentorship in professional issues.[9,10] In order to do this there needs to be a district hospital doctor present for most of the outreach visit. Both panels agreed that having a district hospital doctor present during consultations would improve O&S. A reason often mentioned for the inability to do this is the other responsibilities that the district hospital doctors have outside of the O&S visits, and the disruption that the O&S visit causes to the routine functioning of the district hospital.[11] One of the participants summarised the counter-argument to this well: 'O&S should be part of the basic core function of a district hospital and therefore cannot be seen as a disruption.'

One should be cognisant of the fact that O&S causes disruption in the regional hospital as well as in the district hospitals, especially when more than one outreaching specialist visits a district hospital on the same day. Both panels agreed that the district hospital doctor presence could be improved by better scheduling of O&S visits, as well as better planning of the day's work at the district hospital.[11]

An alarming fact was that the district hospitals agreed that the planned O&S visits for the week or month are not discussed with the staff involved. This could be due to the fact that there might not be a dedicated liaison doctor at the district hospital to coordinate the visit. With improved planning and/or communication, this could be improved. If there is a long-term programme available for O&S visits and this is adhered to, the workload could be shifted to free up doctors on those days.[11]

O&S visits should preferably be confined to one specialist per hospital per day, to avoid overwhelming the capacity of the district hospital. Human resources or the lack thereof was another reason often mentioned for the lack of a district hospital doctor presence. It seems as if there are not enough district hospital doctors to make O&S work properly. Whilst it was mentioned in the district hospital group that smaller district hospitals often find it more difficult to meet the specialist's expectations, the specialists remarked that some smaller hospitals often perform the best. As it is unlikely that district hospitals will receive extra posts to make O&S work, the old cliché of working smarter instead of harder seems to ring true in this instance.

Recommendations

The success of the O&S programme is dependent on a model that is acceptable to both the outreaching specialists and the hosting district hospital. These two groups should agree on an appropriate model that is well planned, communicated to all involved staff, and adhered to. If O&S visits are seen as a basic function of a district hospital and not as a disruption and/or intrusion, the perceived attitudes towards commitment might change for the better. It is therefore recommended that:

- The main focus of O&S should be capacity building, involving most staff at some stage.
- Both the specialists' and district hospitals' service commitments and constraints should be respected in the scheduling of O&S visits.
- A long-term roster for O&S should be distributed to all involved staff.
- The O&S for the week or month should be discussed with all involved staff in the specialist department and district hospital by a dedicated person.
- A specific specialist should be linked to a specific district hospital for an agreed period.
- Patients should be discussed with the specific specialist prior to making an appointment – preferably via email unless urgent, logistically impossible or agreed beforehand.
- Specialists should respond promptly to these discussions.
- O&S visits should be limited to one specialist per district hospital per day, according to what the district hospital can handle.
- The district hospital workload should be managed to enable doctors to present their patients.
- Logistical support and capacity building should be equally important reasons for district hospital doctor presence.

- Professional relationship building and mentorship should form an integral part of the O&S visit.
- Issues that could be explored in future are:
  - Seeing random inpatients as well as problem patients.
  - Exchange programmes between the district and regional hospitals.
  - Constructive feedback from all referrals to the regional hospital.
  - Involving sessional specialists, and allied health professions that are not available at the district hospital, in O&S.

A report of the results was presented to the two panels and district health and regional hospital management, with a proposed model for O&S.

Limitations

This study was conducted in the Western Cape, which has the highest number of doctors per capita in SA.[14] Human resources influence the way in which O&S happens, and provinces with fewer doctors might struggle to implement the above recommendations.

Due to the relatively small pool of experts available, numerous participants from the different specialist departments and district hospitals were invited. Cross-contamination of ideas were therefore possible, due to close working relationships.

Not all statements were examined by both groups. Statements where the one group directly evaluated an issue regarding the other group were not necessarily evaluated by the latter.

Conclusion

Providing O&S to rural populations remains an integral part of improving access to specialist care for rural populations. A multifaceted style of outreach remains the most effective way of providing O&S services. Due to the complex interpersonal and interprofessional dynamics between the involved parties, it is likely that there will always be the potential for conflict. With good communication, constructive feedback and improved planning, relationships and efficiency may improve, which might lead to a more sustainable and mutually beneficial O&S system.

Acknowledgements

The researchers would like to thank the experts consulted for development of the questionnaires, the members of the panels of experts, as well as the Discovery Fund for funding of the project.

Competing interests

The authors declare that they have no financial or personal relationship(s) that may have inappropriately influenced them in writing this article.

Authors' contributions

J.S. (Stellenbosch University and Western Cape Department of Health) was responsible for conceptualising the research and data collection. Both authors, J.S. and L.J. (Stellenbosch University and Western Cape Department of Health), were responsible for analysis and writing of the article.

References

1. Gaede B, McKerrow NH. Outreach Programme: Consultant visits to rural hospitals. CME. 2011;29(2):54–58.

2. South African National Department of Health. Human resources for health 2030 – Draft human resources strategy for the Health Sector: 2012/13-2016/17. Pretoria: Government Printer; 2011.

3. South African National Department of Health. National Antenatal Sentinel HIV and Syphilis Prevalence Survey in South Africa, 2009. Pretoria: Government Printer; 2020.

4. Gruen RL, Bailie RS, Wang Z, Heard S, O'Rourke I. Specialist outreach to isolated and disadvantaged communities: A population-based study. Lancet. 2006;368(9530):130–138. http://dx.doi.org/10.1016/S0140-6736(06)68812-0

5. Hugo JFM, Couper ID, Thigiti J, Loeliger, S. Equity in health care: Does family medicine have a role? Afr J Prm Health Care Fam Med. 2010;2(1), Art. #243, 3 pages.

6. Department of Health Western Cape. Outreach and support services in the Western Cape. Cape Town: Department of Health Western Cape; 2005.

7. Gruen RL, Weeramanthri TS, Knight SE, Bailie RS. Specialist outreach clinics in primary care and rural hospital settings. In: The Cochrane Library, issue 2, 2004. Oxford: Update Software.

8. Gruen RL, Weeramanthri TS, Bailie RS. Outreach and improved access to specialist services for indigenous people in remote Australia: The requirements for sustainability. J Epidemiol Comm Hlth. 2002;56(7):17–21. http://dx.doi.org/10.1136/jech.56.7.517

9. Department of Family and Internal Medicine, Beaufort West Hospital. Outreach Agreement Circular. Dec 2009;1–2.

10. Jenkins L. Outreach in the Southern Cape/Karoo area – What works and what not – a Family Medicine perspective. September 2006:1–2 (unpublished report).

11. Rural Doctors Association of Southern Africa. Specialist support for rural areas. Rural Doctors Association of South Africa Conference, Empangeni, South Africa, 10–11 August 2006;1-2. (Unpublished consensus statement.)

12. De Villiers MR, De Villiers JT, Kent AP. The Delphi technique in health sciences education research. Medical Teacher. 2005;27(7):639–643. http://dx.doi.org/10.1080/13611260500069947

13. Western Cape Government Provincial Treasury. Working paper - Regional Development Profile 2011, Eden and Central Karoo Districts. Cape Town: Western Cape Government; 2011.

14. Human Sciences Research Council. Doctors in the public service: Too few for too many. HSRC Review; 2010.

21

Adaptation and cross-cultural validation of the United States Primary Care Assessment Tool (expanded version) for use in South Africa

Authors:
Graham Bresick[1]
Abdul-Rauf Sayed[1]
Cynthia le Grange[1]
Susheela Bhagwan[1]
Nayna Manga[1]

Affiliations:
[1]Faculty of Health Sciences, University of Cape Town, South Africa

Correspondence to:
Graham Bresick

Email:
graham.bresick@uct.ac.za

Postal address:
Room 2.20, Level 2, Falmouth Building, Anzio Road, Observatory, South Africa

Background: Measuring primary care is important for health sector reform. The Primary Care Assessment Tool (PCAT) measures performance of elements essential for cost-effective care. Following minor adaptations prior to use in Cape Town in 2011, a few findings indicated a need to improve the content and cross-cultural validity for wider use in South Africa (SA).

Aim: This study aimed to validate the United States of America-developed PCAT before being used in a baseline measure of primary care performance prior to major reform.

Setting: Public sector primary care clinics, users, practitioners and managers in urban and rural districts in the Western Cape Province.

Methods: Face value evaluation of item phrasing and a combination of Delphi and Nominal Group Technique (NGT) methods with an expert panel and user focus group were used to obtain consensus on content relevant to SA. Original and new domains and items with $> = 70\%$ agreement were included in the South African version – ZA PCAT.

Results: All original PCAT domains achieved consensus on inclusion. One new domain, the primary healthcare (PHC) team, was added. Three of 95 original items achieved $< 70\%$ agreement, that is consensus to exclude as not relevant to SA; 19 new items were added. A few items needed minor rephrasing with local healthcare jargon. The demographic section was adapted to local socio-economic conditions. The adult PCAT was translated into isiXhosa and Afrikaans.

Conclusion: The PCAT is a valid measure of primary care performance in SA. The PHC team domain is an important addition, given its emphasis in PHC re-engineering. A combination of Delphi and NGT methods succeeded in obtaining consensus on a multi-domain, multi-item instrument in a resource-constrained environment.

Adaptation et validation de l'Outil d'Evaluation des Soins primaires des Etats-Unis (PCAT version élargie) en vue de son utilisation en Afrique du Sud.

Contexte: Il est important de mesurer les soins primaires pour faire des réformes dans le secteur de la santé. Le PCAT mesure la performance sur des éléments essentiels pour fournir des soins rentables. Après avoir fait de petits changements avant de l'utiliser au Cap en 2011, on a constaté la nécessité d'améliorer le contenu et la validité cross-culturelle pour une utilisation plus large en Afrique du Sud.

Objectif: Cette étude avait pour but de valider le PCAT développé aux Etats-Unis avant de l'utiliser comme mesure de référence de la performance des soins primaires avant de faire des réformes majeures.

Cadre: Les cliniques de soins primaires du secteur public, les utilisateurs, les praticiens et les gestionnaires dans les districts urbains et ruraux de la Province du Western Cape.

Méthode: Evaluation de la valeur nominale de la formulation de l'article et une combinaison des méthodes du Groupe technique nominal et de Delphi avec un panel d'experts et d'un groupe d'utilisateurs pour obtenir un consensus sur le contenu applicable à l'Afrique du Sud. Des domaines et articles nouveaux et originaux avec un consensus de $> = 70\%$ ont été inclus dans le ZA PCAT.

Résultats: Il a été décidé à l'unanimité d'inclure tous les domaines originaux du PCAT. On a ajouté un nouveau domaine, l'équipe de PHC. Trois des 95 articles originaux ont réuni un consensus de $< 70\%$, c.-à-d. de les exclure car ils ne sont pas applicables à l'Afrique du Sud; 19 nouveaux articles ont été ajoutés. Quelques articles ont dû être légèrement reformulés et remplacés par le jargon local des soins de santé. La section démographique a été adaptée aux conditions socioéconomiques locales. Le PCAT pour adultes a été traduit en isiXhosa et Afrikaans.

Conclusion: Le PCAT est une mesure valide de la performance des soins primaires en Afrique du Sud. Le domaine de l'équipe de PHC est une addition importante étant donné son importance dans la reconfiguration du PHC. Une combinaison des méthodes Delphi et NGT a réussi à atteindre un consensus sur un instrument multi-domaine et multipoint dans un environnement aux ressources limitées.

Introduction

Measuring primary care performance

Primary health care (PHC), considered the backbone of a country's health system,[1] is a complex, multifaceted range of activities, a unique integration of knowledge, values and skills drawn from clinical, public health, behavioural and anthropological sciences. In addition to diagnosis, treatment and rehabilitation, the range of skills and activities include person-centred communication, prevention and health promotion applied in a comprehensive family- and community-orientated approach to care. A primary care measurement strategy therefore needs a range of dimensions for it to be a valid measure. Primary care dimensions (e.g. comprehensive care) are themselves multifaceted. Each dimension requires a variety of indicators (items) to describe and measure it (content validity); and item phrasing has to be congruent with the indicator and dimension being measured (face validity).

The Primary Care Assessment Tool (PCAT, http://www.jhsph.edu/pcpc/pca_tools.html) is a multi-dimension, multi-item instrument developed and tested for reliability and validity by Starfield and Shi, Primary Care Policy Center, Johns Hopkins School of Public Health.[2] The PCAT measures primary care organisation and performance on four core dimensions (access, continuity, coordination, comprehensiveness)and three derivative dimensions (community orientation, family-centredness, cultural competence)known as domains defined in the PCAT manual (http://www.jhsph.edu/pcpc/pca_tools.html). They have been shown to be essential for cost-effective primary care in developing and developed contexts.[3,4,5]

When these essential features are available to primary care users and implemented in their care, the outcomes include improved health and satisfaction, reduced cost, and reduced inequity.[5,6] The domains are also in line with the Alma Ata Declaration,[7] universally accepted definitions of primary care,[4,8,9] and the principles of family medicine,[10,11] including principles relevant to sub-Saharan Africa.[12] By surveying the three main primary care stakeholders (users, providers/practitioners and clinic managers) the PCAT measures the extent to which users' experience of primary care approximates what is essential for cost-effective care.

The extent of primary care clinic adherence in each domain is determined by complex summing of participant responses to a range of items (questions) pertinent to that domain. The PCAT is also able to determine the size of differences between the three stakeholders' domain scores when the respective user, provider and manager instruments are used. Whilst the dimensions are considered universal, their generalisability may be limited in different cultural and socio-economic settings. Given the focus on health systems strengthening worldwide, it is not surprising that the PCAT is increasingly being subjected to cross-cultural validation to extend its generalisability to countries wanting to align with

cost-effective care.[13,14,15,16,17] There is also evidence supporting the PCAT's ability to measure the impact of changes to PHC systems.[17,18,19,20]

This article describes the process used to adapt and validate the adult expanded version (PCAT AE) for use in South Africa (SA). Whilst there are other measures of PHC that have been found to be valid in contexts other than that in which they originate,[21] the literature suggests that the PCAT is the most widely used and adapted. Other PHC measures include the Primary Care Assessment Survey (PCAS), the Components of Primary Care Index, the EUROPEP Interpersonal Processes of Care, the Primary Care Evaluation tool (PCET) used mainly in Europe, and the General Practice Assessment Survey (GPAS), all comprising multi-item dimensions.

Study background

In 2011, following an earlier visit by PCAT author, the late Professor Barbara Starfield, a study team in the Division of Family Medicine at the University of Cape Town conducted a pilot audit of primary care in one Cape Town health substructure (two sub-districts) in collaboration with the service provider, Cape Town Metro District Health Services (MDHS). The adult expanded (AE) version of the original United States of America (USA) PCAT was scrutinised by the study team under the supervision of the author to determine whether changes were necessary prior to local use. Adhering to the author's guidelines for changes to the PCAT domains (B-K)[b] only minor adaptations were made.[a] These involved rephrasing some items to improve local comprehension using colloquial phrasing and local healthcare jargon.

Given the high prevalence of tuberculosis (TB) in SA and in the Western Cape in particular, the item screening for lead exposure was replaced with TB screening to improve the content validity of G domain (comprehensiveness – services available). Changes were made to the introduction (A), health insurance (L) and demographic (N) sections to fit the South African context. The adapted version was piloted on 10 patients before the English version was finalised and translated into isiXhosa and Afrikaans to cover the three major languages spoken in Cape Town. Translation included bilingual translators, back translation and piloting with Xhosa- and Afrikaans-speaking users. The translations were further scrutinised by bilingual fieldworkers during their two-day training to administer the PCAT AE. Minor changes were made to the wording of a few items and they were piloted on patients by the fieldworkers as part of their training before the translations were finalised.

---

[a]Edits to item phrasing were made in B2, B3, C3, C6, C8, C9, D7, D12, E1, E2, F1, F3, G2, G3, G10, G12, G13, G14, G15, G18, G20, G21, G22, G23, G25, H2, H8, H12, J1, J2, J3, J18, K2. Local vernacular was used and / or examples added in order to improve user understanding, e.g. 'prenatal' replaced with 'antenatal' (G20), and 'blood or sputum' added to E1 as examples of laboratory tests. In G9, screening for lead exposure was replaced with TB screening. Changes to the introduction and screening (A), insurance (L), and demographic (N) sections were not subject to the guidelines and were made independently by the team to suit the local and SA context. Cross-cultural improvements to demographic and socio-economic sections included adding items on home language, type of housing, sanitation, level of education and household income.

The ZA PCAT (AE) 2011was registered with the Johns Hopkins' Policy Center before starting data collection. All eight clinics in the substructure were sampled. Data from 461 user (patient) PCAT AE questionnaires were entered and analysed. Coding of responses and the analysis was conducted according to the PCAT manual. PCAT Likert scale responses to domain items are coded on a scale of 1 to 4 and 9, with 1 indicating 'Definitely not', 2 indicating 'Probably not', 3 indicating 'Probably', 4 indicating 'Definitely', and 9 indicating 'Not sure/do not remember'. In the analysis 9 is coded as 2 except for comprehensiveness (services provided), where 9 is coded as 0. The score for each domain is calculated by summing all item responses in that domain (with reverse coding where required by the manual) divided by the number of domain items to produce a mean score.

Table 1 shows the results (mean, standard deviation (SD) and range) by domain for the 461 users' data. Users scored community orientation lowest (mean 2.4) and cultural competence highest (mean 3.5).

The distribution of the dimension (domain) scores confirmed what might be expected locally, providing evidence for the PCAT's construct validity in the South African context. This was further supported by service managers and providers generally accepting the results as a reflection of primary care performance in the substructure. The 2013 study team nevertheless wished to strengthen the content and cross-cultural validity of the PCAT before wider use in SA, and to improve its alignment with provincial and national health plans. The 2011 findings suggested that a few domain items may not have been well understood by primary care users. Although none of the items approximated > 50% 'Do not know' responses (requiring adjusted coding and analysis), some were much higher than others. In addition, the users' PCAT score for ongoing care (domain D) was considerably higher than the provider and manager scores and higher than expected by study team members who had years of experience working in the clinics studied.

A European Union grant was obtained to strengthen the PCAT's validity for South African use and to extend the 2011 pilot measure of primary care performance to other health districts in the Western Cape Province prior to major health sector reform. Study objectives to strengthen the relevance of the PCAT content for SA included improving its face, content and cross-cultural validity by (1) reviewing the phrasing of domain items for user comprehension; (2) reviewing the domains and their content for alignment with the healthcare setting in SA, the Western Cape demographic and socio-economic context, local and national healthcare policies; and (3) improving the 2011 translations.

This study is part of a bigger European Union-funded study in the School of Public Health and Family Medicine at the University of Cape Town which is aimed at improving users' experience of primary care.

Research design and method

Approval for the study was obtained from the Human Ethics Research Committee in the University of Cape Town's Faculty of Health Sciences and the Western Cape Provincial Department of Health Research Committee. There were no risks to participants in the study. All data provided were analysed and reported anonymously.

The study was conducted in two parts: (1) an expert panel and a primary care user focus group reviewed the wording of PCAT domain items for their face value; and (2) a combination of modified Delphi and nominal group technique (NGT) methods was used to determine consensus on domain and item relevance for SA. The ZA PCAT was piloted at a primary care clinic before being finalised and translated.

Part 1: Review of item wording for local use
Expert panel (1a)

This panel, consisting of 2011 PCAT study investigators (two family physician researchers, a family physician in charge of clinical governance at a clinic and a fieldworker) had face value evaluation meetings to review the wording of all PCAT items in domains B–K and to rephrase items where necessary to improve comprehension by primary care users in SA. Problematic wording identified in 2011 was given particular attention. Changes were agreed upon by simple consensus. Selected items were referred to the user focus group to assist with improving user comprehension.

User focus group (1b)

Two members of the PCAT study team purposively selected and invited six primary care users from amongst patients attending a clinic in the baseline measure study sampling frame to join a focus group. Six consenting adult patients who had attended the clinic at least four times and who were conversant in two of the three main languages spoken in the Western Cape (namely English and Afrikaans) were selected. A modified form of the NGT method was used to obtain group consensus on the phrasing of items selected in part 1a. The process involves each item in turn being presented to the group on a flipchart in one of the

TABLE 1: Descriptive results of user (patient) scores by subdomain (2011).

Subdomains	Number of items	Mean	s.d.	Range
First contact-access	12	2.5	0.6	1.0–3.8
Ongoing care	15	3.0	0.5	1.3–3.9
Coordination	9	3.4	0.7	1.0–4.0
Coordination (information systems)	3	3.0	0.6	1.0–4.0
Comprehensiveness (services available)	25	3.2	0.5	1.1–4.0
Comprehensiveness (services provided)	11	2.7	0.8	0.0–4.0*
Family-centredness	3	3.2	0.9	1.0–4.0
Community orientation	6	2.4	0.8	1.0–4.0
Culturally competent	3	3.5	0.8	1.0–4.0

s.d., standard deviation.
*, In all subdomains the response code 9 (i.e. not sure/do not remember) was recoded as 2, except for comprehensiveness (services provided) where it was coded as 0 in keeping with the PCAT manual.

two languages. Each participant records her and/or his back translation on a blank sheet without discussion. All responses are recorded anonymously on a flip chart, after which each participant, without discussion, chooses and records the one response that she or he feels most accurately reflects the item presented. Responses (phrasing) achieving > = 70% agreement[22] are accepted. The steps are repeated for each item. The investigators determine whether the phrasing chosen maintains the intention of the original item; if not, investigators rephrase the item to maintain the original intention, taking into account the information obtained from participants by that stage. The above steps are repeated to determine consensus on the item thus phrased.

Part 2: Obtaining consensus on domain and item relevance for South Africa

Delphi process (2a) (steps 1–4 in Appendix 1)

A second expert panel comprising 2 family physicians, 2 clinical nurse practitioners, 2 clinic managers, and 2 family physician educator/researchers were purposively selected by the study team to examine and determine consensus on the relevance of all PCAT domains and domain items (B–K) for the primary care context in SA. The task of each panellist was to determine from her/his own experience, (i) which items were relevant, and (ii) which items, if any, should be added. Background information given to the panellists included a summary of the PCAT, its purpose, and relevance to PHC and family medicine. The panellists were informed of the 2011 PCAT study; that lessons from 2011 were being applied; that rephrasing of some questions might be necessary; and that the process outlined was to validate the ZA PCAT for use in SA by using a combination of the Delphi and NGT methods (Appendix 1). Inviting, consenting and providing information to the panellists were done via email. Panellists were asked to scrutinise all the PCAT domains and their respective items and to score them for relevance on a scale of 0 to 3 (not at all relevant – very relevant). At the end of this stage the emailed data were collated and the percentage agreement calculated for the 9 domains (B–K) and their items. The results together with new items were tabulated.

Nominal Group Technique process (2b) (steps 5–7 in Appendix 1)

The expert panel in 2a was convened by two study investigators and part 2a results presented (items which achieved < 70% agreement; new items generated; and comments) by displaying them verbatim in poster form for panellists to view and to ensure that their items and comments had been recorded. Three questions were provided to guide the selection and scoring of new items generated in part 2a: (i) Is it important and relevant to primary care?; (ii) In which domain does it belong?; and (iii) Can clinic staff do anything about it? The method requires that the meaning of each new item be clarified and similar items merged (step 5) in a facilitated group discussion. Given that the above discussion may stimulate further thinking on domains and items to include, panellists are given a second opportunity on their own (i.e. NGT silent phase repeated) to generate items they wished to include.

All new items thus generated are in turn clarified to ensure they are understood by all participants and that they differ from existing items (step 5 repeated). These were added to a table along with new items generated in the Delphi process (2a) and original PCAT items that achieved < 70% agreement and scored for relevance as in 2a (i.e. items that achieved < 70% agreement in 2a were re-scored), and were recorded independently. Each panellist then verbally submitted her/his scores in round-robin fashion (step 6). The scores were recorded and summed by the investigators, and the summed scores presented in a projected table (step 7). The percentage agreement for each item was calculated to determine which items achieved consensus (step 7), that is > = 70% agreement. Repetition of steps 3–7 above substituted for the usual successive rounds in the Delphi method, which was limited to one round in part 2a. The percentage agreement for each item is calculated, where 100% = the number of panellists x 3, that is the maximum score per item. Only domains and items on which consensus is achieved (i.e. > =70% agreement) are retained (step 8).

Results

Item review and rephrasing (1a and 1b)

Domain and item relevance was not considered at this stage. The phrasing of domain items (questions) considered problematic by the 2011 study teamrequired minimal rephrasing. The team nevertheless wanted user assistance on five questions (D4, F1, G2, J2, K2) to improve user comprehension. These were presented to the six focus group participants for scrutiny as described in 1b of the methods section. Most participants had difficulty understanding the task, especially back translation and its purpose, and preferred to add and discuss questions on problems they encountered with the service. After unsuccessful attempts to explain and guide participants through the planned NGT process, this was abandoned. Instead an open discussion on the phrasing of the questions was conducted to gain as much information from patients as possible for item rephrasing.

The Delphi process (2a)

Results of the Delphi process (2a) revealed that the expert panel considered all the domains as very relevant; median = 92.6%; range = 48.2% – 100.0%; interquartile range 85.2% – 96.3%. Only 3 of the 95 domain items received < 70% agreement (C6: 48.2 %; C7: 48.2%; H9: 51.9%). No new domains but two new items were added (C4NGT, C5NGT) by the end of this stage.

The Nominal Group Technique process (2b)

In the NGT process (2b) a total of 19 new items were generated and scored, as described in methods sections 2a and 2b. The results are presented in Table 2. These items related to the first contact – access (C), ongoing care (D), coordination (E), comprehensiveness (services available [G] and services provided [H]), and culturally competent (K) domains. One new item, the PHC team, emerged during clarification of

TABLE 2: Rescoring of items scored < 100% in part 2a and scoring all new items (parts 2a and 2b).

Item code	Domains and items (questions)	% agreement
C. First contact – access		
C13NGT	Are the signboards (signage/instructions) at your CHC clear?	100
C14NGT	Is the staff friendly and approachable?	100
C15&16NGT	Is it easy to lay a complaint or compliment or make a suggestion at your CHC? (C15) Is there a complaints/suggestion box at your CHC? (C16)	100
C4NGT	Are you able travel safely to your CHC?	67
C5NGT	Is it difficult to get to your CHC? Yes/No. If yes, please explain.	57
C6NGT	How long does it take you to get to your CHC?	Removed by simple consensus
C17NGT	How much does it cost you to get to your CHC?	86
C6*	When your CHC is closed on Saturday and Sunday and you get sick, would someone from there see you the same day?	46
C7*	When your CHC is closed and you get sick during the night, would someone from there see you that night?	54
C5	When your CHC is closed is there a phone number you can call when you get sick?	71
C11bNGT	Is it difficult for you to get a second opinion when necessary?	81
D. Continuity of care (ongoing care)		
D15b&cNGT	If response to D15 is 4 or 3, then: 'Where would you go?' (D15b) If response to D15 is 4 or 3, then: 'Why would you change?' (D15c)	90
D4	If you have a question about your health, can you phone your CHC and talk to the doctor or nurse who treated you before?	83
D14	Can you change your CHC if you want to? (Retained because D15b and c were added)	67
E. Co-ordination		
E9bNGT	How long did it take for you to be given your appointment by your CHC?	95
E9cNGT	From the time that you were given your appointment date, how long before you actually saw the specialist?	90
F. Co-ordination (information systems)		
E14NGT	Would the CHC assist you to get medical-legal or insurance reports if required?	71
G. Comprehensiveness (services available)		
G26NGT	Checking for weight problems?	95
G27NGT	Access to termination of pregnancy services at or via your CHC if required?	100
H. Comprehensiveness (services provided)		
H15NGT	Advice and treatment on sexually transmitted infections	100
H9*	Ask if you have a gun, its storage or its security	10
K. Culturally competent		
K4bNGT	Do you think your CHC understands/respects your culture?	100
K4cNGT	Do you feel comfortable discussing religious or cultural issues that affect your health with the staff at the CHC?	100
P. PHC team (new domain) (items agreed on by simple consensus)		
P1.	Can you see a social worker if you need to? E.g. for help with counselling for a family problem or advice about social services?	-
P2.	Can you see a physiotherapist (and occupational therapist) at your CHC if you need to? E.g. to help with muscle sprains or movement following a stroke.	-
P3.	Can you be visited in your home by a community health worker linked to your CHC if you need it? E.g. for home-based care for TB, HIV or basic care such as wound dressings.	-
P4.	Can you be seen by a health promoter/dietician for advice on these topics?	-
P5.	Can you be seen by a mental health worker at your CHC for help with any mental health problems?	-
P6.	Can you be seen by a dental/oral health worker at/or linked to your CHC if you need it? E.g. any problems with your teeth.	-
P7.	Can a child (under 12 yrs) be seen at your CHC?	-

ZA PCAT validation.
DELPHI-NGT comments and additional questions.
7 Participants; score 0–3; max score per item = 21, that is 100% agreement.
NGT, items added via Delphi-NGT process; CHC, community health centre.
*, Retained in the printed version; explained in discussion section.

newly generated items. The panel felt that it was important to add the PHC team as a domain instead, given the emphasis on the PHC team in SA's district health policies and plans. A list of items to describe the composition of the PHC team in a comprehensive primary care service was generated. PHC team items were agreed on by simple consensus and not subjected to the NGT stepped process due to time constraints.

This was followed by a final round of scoring (individually and without discussion), which included all the original PCAT items which received < 100% agreement in 2a and all new items generated as described above. Whilst rescoring the few original items that achieved < 100% but > 70% in part 2a was not essential, the panel felt that a final round of scoring that included these items should be the final step. Table 2

shows the final percentage agreement for all original items which achieved < 100% agreement, all new items (coded as 'NGT') as well as the PHC team domain.

Following piloting of the ZA PCAT AE 2013 on 10 patients at a clinic in the baseline study sampling frame, minor changes were made to the phrasing of a few items. This completed the ZA PCAT validation process. All domains and items achieving consensus at the end of part 2b constitute the ZA PCAT AE 2013.[b] The rationale for retaining original PCAT items which did not achieve consensus[b] for use if needed is

[b]South African Adult Primary Care Assessment Tool (ZA PCAT AE 2013), adapted from the original PCAT by the South African PCAT Study Team, Division of Family Medicine, School of Public Health and Division of Family Medicine, University of Cape Town, 2013. Original Adult Primary Care Assessment Tool – Expanded Version developed by Barbara Starfield, Primary Care Policy Center, Johns Hopkins University 1998 (for access to the document, please contact corresponding author).

explained in the discussion below. The provider (PE) and manager (FE) instruments were accordingly aligned with the ZA PCAT AE by the study team. The additions to the English AE version were translated and back translated for the isiXhosa and Afrikaans versions and existing items in the 2011 translations were reviewed by bilingual study team members before being finalised.

Discussion

Following lessons from the 2011 pilot study, we sought to validate the PCAT content and cross-cultural applicability for use in SA, that is improve its relevance to primary care in SA and its comprehension in three languages before extending the audit to other health districts. Minimal item rephrasing was necessary following that done in 2011. The fact that no domains were removed, only one new domain was added, only three items achieved < 70% agreement, and a high median percentage agreement on domain and item relevance was achieved, indicates the high content validity of the original PCAT for SA.

The silent phases in parts 2a and 2b ensured that participants were able to generate items and to agree/disagree independently of each other. The discussion during the clarification stage and the range of scores in part 2b suggest that participants were not unduly led by each other's views or scores. The addition of the PHC team domain aligns the PCAT with the emphasis on the PHC team in local and international policy documents and research.[23,24,25,26,27] In a study identifying key principles of family medicine in sub-Saharan Africa, practising as members of a PHC team emerged as important and included nurse practitioners.[12] Including the PHC team as a domain in the ZA PCAT is therefore likely to be supported by primary care physicians in Africa.

Nurse practitioner (CNP) was not generated as a PHC team item. This can be explained by the fact that PHC in SA is a nurse-led service.[23] In most primary care clinics CNPs are the only clinical practitioners. Where there are doctors, CNPs practice as members of the clinical team alongside them.

The PHC team domain uses the same Likert scale for rating responses to items and is analysed in the same way as existing domains. PHC team scores are included in the total primary care score – a summing of all the domain scores. New items which do not use the PCAT Likert scale (patient waiting times, travel costs and patient satisfaction) are included under the relevant domains but are analysed separately. The study team elected to retain original items C6, C7, H9 in the printed version[b] used for the data collection in order to allow for international comparison of results where the original PCAT is used. Analysis of the data will include or exclude these items as required. Cronbach alpha and factor analyses on the ZA PCAT 2013 will be included in the second article reporting the results of the PCAT survey of users, providers and managers.

The method used to improve the wording of domain items for better comprehension by users did not follow the standardised seven-step method described by Sousa and Rojjanasrirat[28] in their review of methodological approaches to translation, adaptation and cross-cultural validation of research instruments; also used in the Korean adaptation of the PCAT.[15] A key component of our cross-cultural method was the user focus group (part 1b). However, most of the participants had difficulty understanding the task, especially back translation and its purpose, which led to the planned NGT process being abandoned. Users' preference for raising and discussing problems they encountered with the service is highlighted in patient satisfaction surveys.

The research team nevertheless constituted an expert panel with years of experience practising and teaching in local primary care services. The same team conducted the 2011 study and included a research assistant with experience in developing and administering questionnaires in other research projects in local primary care services. The combined experience was applied in updating and improving the translations of the English PCAT into the two other main languages spoken in the Western Cape. Edits to the demographic section (N) to align it with Western Cape demographic and socio-economic features were also made. Even though the translation method did not follow all the steps suggested by Sousa and Rojjanasrirat,[28] the bilingualism advised for cross-cultural validation was well represented on the panel and the research assistantwas trilingual.

The pilot conducted on 10 patients before finalising the ZA PCAT AE 2013 will have reduced the impact of our failure to achieve the primary objective of the focus group, by providing another opportunity to identify difficulties with phrasing and administering the PCAT to users. In addition, the 2011 translation conducted by the study team was also scrutinised by the bilingual fieldworkers. Their practical training on patients served as a second pilot of the isiXhosa and Afrikaans translations in 2011.

The focus group experience nevertheless provided important insights, including the depth of feeling amongst users about their frustrations with primary care; the challenges faced by users who are functionally illiterate (which complicated the task of the researchers in this context); the importance of a participatory method when involving user stakeholders and the need for researchers to be flexible. The communication challenge between informant and researcher reflects a common feature of the primary care consultation, namely the potential conflict between patient and practitioner agendas, where 'give and take' is required to achieve a therapeutic partnership.

Combining the Delphi and NGT methods in a two-stage process had the benefit of participants independently generating responses in at least one round before meeting for the NGT, thus reducing the impact of attrition of participants and delayed responses that can bedevil a Delphi process. The combination of the Delphi and NGT methods may be better considered a modification of the NGT.[22] In verbal feedback at the end of part 2b the expert panel reported that, as busy clinicians and managers, they found the combination of Delphi and NGT methods useful in seeking consensus on the content and wording and preferred to meet once-off rather than have a number of iterations as required by the Delphi method. They also preferred the opportunity to interact with each other, especially in the prioritisation and clarification stages of the NGT.

In addition, the modification provided the opportunity for doctors, nurse practitioners and managers to contribute as equals in a key stakeholder group. Modelling such a method that can be used in clinics by managers and practitioners to obtain multi-stakeholder consensus on complex activities and interventions in a time-constrained and limited-resource context may also be useful. Involving these key stakeholders should also increase the likelihood of the ZA PCAT's use in ongoing monitoring, evaluation and quality improvement, also guiding the revitalisation of PHC and assisting health sector reform in SA. Whilst the study did not specifically address aligning the PCAT with provincial and national health policies and plans, it can be argued that including managers, practitioners and educators with years of experience in health services in SA guided the work with these in mind – evidenced by the addition of the PHC team.

As noted above, the findings concur with key principles of family medicine in sub-Saharan Africa and therefore point to the potential for the ZA PCAT to be similarly used in other parts of Africa, as well as to measure the impact of interventions aimed at strengthening PHC systems. This includes measuring the impact of postgraduate training in family medicine (primary care physicians) on person-centred comprehensive, community-based primary care as promoted in the Victoria Falls Statement.[24] Given that primary care in SA is nurse-driven, the finding that the PCAT content is highly relevant to SA suggests that CNPs should also be trained to apply the essential elements of primary care. If the benefits of a PHC team are to be realised, training in the family medicine approach to primary care – currently the preserve of primary care physicians – should be extended to CNPs. Primary care physicians and CNPs should be trained together on the content, application and measurement of the essential dimensions of primary care. Primary care facility and district managers should be aware of the importance of these elements and trained in methods that improve access to them when allocating and managing resources. They should also be trained in the use of the PCAT to monitor the organisation and performance of the primary care services they manage.

Limitations of the cross-cultural validation method used, when compared with those suggested by a scholarly review,[28] are discussed above. This will need to be considered if there are significant differences in scores between the three language groups after the baseline results are analysed. Other study limitations include the expert panel and patient informants being local only. The full Delphi method would

have permitted wider representation on the expert panel and could have included participants in other sub-Saharan countries. The items in the PHC team domain do not describe team functioning or the quality of team-based care and therefore limit the potential value of this measure. Items that describe team function should be developed and added in future studies.

Is the ZA PCAT 2013 suitable for the Western Cape only? Given the diversity across the nine provinces in SA, translation into local languages and some rephrasing will be necessary, along with changes to the demographic section, depending on region or province. However, we think it unlikely that major domain and item changes will be necessary.

These limitations notwithstanding, the findings are in keeping with those of PCAT validation studies in other countries[15,16,17,18,19,20] where the essential features of primary care measured by the PCAT were also found to apply. The Brazilian study[18] kept closely to the original items, whereas other country studies removed a number of domain items, such as in the Chinese PCAT.[17] Haggerty et al.[21] examined the validity of a number of instruments that measure PHC from the user perspective in the Canadian context, including the PCAT, the PCAS, the Components of Primary Care Index, and the EUROPEP Interpersonal Processes of Care – all composed of multi-item dimensions. The study found that these instruments performed similarly in Canada as in their original contexts. The Brazilian PCAT study is of note for SA. It showed that the PCAT also applies in a developing context.[18] The PCET, not included in the Haggerty study, is also of interest.[29] It includes the four core primary care dimensions measured by the PCAT (access, continuity, comprehensiveness and coordination) as well as four health system functions (financing, creating resources, stewardship and delivery services) that are worthy of assessment in a primary care audit. These functions can be included alongside a PCAT audit without having to adapt the PCAT.

Other audit instruments used in SA currently include the National Core Standards (NCS) instrument[26] and the chronic diseases audit tool used in the Western Cape. With respect to possible duplication, whilst the NCS includes items on patient-centred care, they are not used to assess relational continuity (PCAT ongoing care [D]) domain), a multifaceted core primary care dimension. The NCS does not seek to determine performance on the other key dimensions of the primary care process, but focuses instead on infrastructure, equipment and administrative resources required.

Similarly, the chronic diseases audit tool–currently a record audit of selected indicators of common chronic disease care–is not a measure of comprehensive PHC. Regarding patient satisfaction surveys, used as a means to determine patients' views on their health care, there may be some item overlap. However, the PCAT is not a patient satisfaction questionnaire. It is, rather, an evidence-based measure of performance on features of primary care demonstrated to be essential for cost-effective care. Likewise, patient health survey instruments such as the SF-36[30] are limited to evaluation of health and not a measure of the range of dimensions necessary for cost-effective primary care.

Conclusion

This is the first of two articles reporting PCAT studies in Africa. It describes the content and cross-cultural validation of the PCAT for use in SA. The results suggest an important role for the PCAT in the Western Cape Province and nationally, given the South African National Health Policy's imperative of PHC re-engineering and broader health sector reform.[23] Future audits of primary care performance should include private sector services. The findings have implications for the training of primary care doctors and nurse practitioners as well as clinic and district managers.

Further research should include strengthening the PHC team domain to enable assessment of team functioning and performance.

A second article will describe the baseline results of the ZA PCAT 2013 study in the Cape Town MDHS and the Cape Winelands, a rural district.

Acknowledgements

We thank the members of the expert panel and other key informants for their willingness to provide the information necessary to validate the PCAT; the district directors and clinic managers for ready access to the services; other members of the study team, including Prof. Derek Hellenberg, Mr Deon September and Ms Delena Fredericks; Prof. Gregory Hussey for assisting with the structure and editing of this article; and the European Union for funding this study. Deon September (data collection and entry, fieldworker supervision and general research assistance) and Delena Fredericks (administration and management) made a very significant contribution to this study.

Competing interests

The authors declare that they have no financial or personal relationship(s) that may have inappropriately influenced them in writing this article.

Authors' contributions

G.B. (University of Cape Town) is the principal investigator and leader of the PCAT project and assumed primary responsibility for writing the article. A-R.S. (University of Cape Town) provided all the statistical advice and calculations for the study proposal, conducted the data analysis, generated the summary tables, figures and graphs and oversaw reporting of all the statistical elements in the method and results sections. C.I.G. (University of Cape Town) and S.B. (University of Cape Town) were centrally

involved in the data collection and management, advising on the content and structure of the article and ensuring accurate reporting of the method and results sections. N.M. assisted with data collection and management and contributed to general project oversight, coordination and management.

References

1. Bodenheimer T. Primary care – will it survive? NEngl J Med. 2006;355:861-864. http://dx.doi.org/10.1056/NEJMp068155

2. Shi, L, Starfield, B, Xu, J. Validating the Adult Primary Care Assessment Tool. JFamPract. 2001;50(2):161.

3. Starfield B. Primary care tomorrow: Is primary care essential? Lancet. 1994;344:1129–1133. http://dx.doi.org/10.1016/S0140-6736(94)90634-3

4. Starfield B. Primary care: Balancing health needs, services, and technology. New York: Oxford University Press; 1998.

5. Starfield B, Shi L, MacinkoJ. The contribution of primary care to health systems and health. Milbank Quarterly. 2005;83:457–502. http://dx.doi.org/10.1111/j.1468-0009.2005.00409.x

6. Beasley JW, Starfield B, van Weel C, Rosser WW, Haq CL. Global health and primary care research. J Am Board Fam Med. 2007;20(6):518–526. http://dx.doi.org/10.3122/jabfm.2007.06.070172

7. World Health Organization. Declaration of Alma-Ata. 1978. Available from: http://www.who.int/publications/almaata_declaration_en.pdf

8. Molla S, Donaldson K, Yordy D, Lohr K, Vanselow NE. Primary care: America's health in a new era. Report of a study by a Committee of the Institute of Medicine, Division of Health Care Services. Washington, DC: National Academy Press;1996, 395.

9. Institute of Medicine. Defining Primary Care: An Interim Report. Washington, DC: National Academy Press; 1994.

10. Shahady EJ. Principles of family medicine: an overview. Essentials of family medicine. 2nd ed. Baltimore: Williams & Wilkins;1993, pp. 3–8.

11. McWhinney IR. A textbook of family medicine. New York: Oxford University Press; 1997.

12. Mash R, Moosa S. Exploring the key principles of Family Medicine in sub-Saharan Africa - international Delphi consensus process. SA Fam Pract. 2008;50(3):60–65. http://dx.doi.org/10.1080/20786204.2008.10873720

13. Harzheim E, Starfield B, Rajmil L, Alvarez-Dardet C, Stein AT. Internal consistency and reliability of Primary Care Assessment Tool (PCATool-Brasil) for child health services. Cad SaudePublica. 2006;22(8):1649–1659. http://dx.doi.org/10.1590/S0102-311X2006000800013

14. Berra S, Hauser L, Audisio Y, Mantaras J, Nicora V, de Oliveira MM, et al. Validity and reliability of the Argentine version of the PCAT-AE for the evaluation of primary health care. Rev Panam Salud Publica. 2013;33(1):30–39. http://dx.doi.org/10.1590/S1020-49892013000100005

15. Jeon KY. Cross-cultural adaptation of the US consumer form of the short Primary Care Assessment Tool (PCAT): the Korean consumer form of the short PCAT (KC PCAT) and the Korean standard form of the short PCAT (KS PCAT). Qual Prim Care. 2011;19(2):85–103.

16. Haggerty JL, Beaulieu MD, Pineault R, Burge F, Levesque JF, Santor DA, et al. Comprehensiveness of care from the patient perspective: comparison of primary healthcare evaluation instruments. Healthc Policy. 2011;7(Spec Issue):154–166. http://dx.doi.org/10.12927/hcpol.2011.22708

17. Yang H, Shi L, Lebrun LA, Zhou X, Liu J, Wang H. Development of the Chinese primary care assessment tool: data quality and measurement properties. Int J Qual Health Care. 2013;25(1):92–105. http://dx.doi.org/10.1093/intqhc/mzs072

18. Macinko J, Almeida C, Klingelhoefer de Sa P. A rapid assessment methodology for the evaluation of primary care organization and performance in Brazil. Health PolicyPlann.2007;22:167–177. http://dx.doi.org/10.1093/heapol/czm008

19. Haggerty JL, Pineault R, Beaulieu MD, Brunelle Y, Gauthier J, Goulet F, et al. Room for improvement: patients' experiences of primary care in Quebec before major reforms. Can Fam Physician. 2007;53(6):1057, 2001:e.1-6, 1056.

20. Wang W, Shi L, Yin A, Lai Y, Maitland E, Nicholas S. Development and validation of the Tibetan primary care assessment tool. Biomed Res Int. 2014;2014:308739. http://dx.doi.org/10.1155/2014/308739

21. Haggerty JL, Burge F, Beaulieu MD, Pineault R, Beaulieu C, Levesque JF, et al. Validation of instruments to evaluate primary healthcare from the patient perspective: overview of the method. Healthc Policy. 2011;7(Spec Issue):31–46. http://dx.doi.org/10.12927/hcpol.2011.22691

22. Jones J, Hunter D. Consensus methods for medical and health services research. BMJ. 1995; 311(7001): 376–380. http://dx.doi.org/10.1136/bmj.311.7001.376

23. Western Cape Provincial Department of Health. Health Care 2030 - The Road to Wellness. Cape Town: Western Cape Provincial Department of Health; 2014.

24. Primafamed-network. Victoria Falls Vision of the Primafamed-network 20012. [cited 2012 Nov 23]. Available from: http://www.the-networktufh.org/february-2013.

25. Department of Health, South Africa. National Health Insurance in South Africa. Policy (Green) Paper. Pretoria: Department of Health, 2011.

26. Sixty Second World Health Assembly. Primary health care, including health system strengthening. WHA resolution 62.12; Geneva; 2009. Available from: http://www.who.int/hrh/resources/A62_12_EN.pdf?ua=1

27. Van Weel C, de Maeseneer J. Now more than ever: World Health Assembly revisits primary health care. PrimHealthCare ResDev.2010;11;1:1–3. http://dx.doi.org/10.1017/S1463423609990260

28. Sousa VD, Rojjanasrirat W. Translation, adaptation and validation of instruments or scales for use in cross-cultural health care research: A clear and user-friendly guideline. J Eval Clin Pract. 2011;17(2):268–274. http://dx.doi.org/10.1111/j.1365-2753.2010.01434.x

29. World Health Organization, Regional Office for Europe. Primary Care Evaluation Tool (PCET). Available from: http://www.euro.who.int/en/health-topics/Health-systems/primary-health-care/publications/2010/primary-care-evaluation-tool-pcet

30. Brazier JE, Harper R, Jones NM, O'Cathain A, Thomas KJ, Usherwood T, et al. Validating the SF-36 health survey questionnaire: New outcome measure for primary care. BMJ. 1992;18;305(6846):160–164.

Appendix starts on the next page →

APPENDIX 1: Information given to expert panellists (Phase 2).

Consensus method and outline of the process

You are being presented with the user (patient) version of the PCAT only. The same domains and similar questions (items) are asked of clinic practitioners and managers in the practitioner and manager PCAT versions, but from their respective perspectives. Within each domain, a number of questions (domain items) to users of primary care services determine whether that domain is present (accessible) and applied (utilised) in their care. We want to know which questions may not be relevant for determining quality primary care in SA given your understanding of patients' and communities' health needs; your experience managing common presenting problems in their context; and whether any additional questions should be added.

Part 1 (steps 1–3) will be conducted on your own at the end of which you email your responses to the study team.

Part 2 (steps 5–7) will be conducted with the panellists meeting as a group. We envisage that each part can be done in 90mins or less. By the end of step 7 an enhanced ZA PCAT will have been agreed on via the consensus process outlined.

The attached PCAT questionnaire has 9 primary care domains (essential elements) each with a number of items posed as questions to describe the presence and practice of each domain. You are being asked to:

- rate the relevance of domain items on a scale of 0–3.
- add any domains and / or items that you feel are important in the SA context that are missing in the current version.

(comment on italicised text if you wish and have the time)

The ratings of the expert panel will be combined to obtain an overall score for each item; depending on the scores, domains items will be retained, removed or added. Items that receive consistently low scores will be removed at the end of part 1. The remaining and/or additional items will go into round 2 and follow the same process above. Further rounds will follow if necessary until consensus is achieved by the panel on which items should remain, which should be removed and which if any items or domains should be added. Consensus is defined as 70% agreement and will constitute the revised ZA version of the PCAT to be used in the study.

Expert panel: Combined Delphi and Nominal Group Technique method:

PART 2a: Steps 1–4 are conducted independently via email prior to the expert panel convening:

1. Introduction and aim of the exercise
   The purpose and objectives of the consensus method have been explained above.

2. Presentation of the questions and definition
   The domain items (questions) for scoring are as per the attached ZA PCAT Adult Expanded (AE) version along with the definition of each domain. Score the relevance for each domain item in the electronic document.

3. The 'silent' phase – scoring the relevance of each domain and items and generating new domains and items

   3.1 Before you score the domain items, please read the definition of that domain and keep it at hand to refer to as needed.

   3.2 Score the relevance of domain items (questions) from your knowledge and experience of what is required for good comprehensive primary care in SA on a scale of 0–3 where 0 is definitely not relevant, i.e. not at all relevant; and 3 is definitely relevant, i.e. totally relevant.

   3.3 At the end of each domain, add any item(s) not currently in the ZA PCAT that you feel should be included in that domain. You do not need to number them. Please indicate briefly next to any new items, why you would think these should be added.

   3.4 In addition, after scoring all the domains, add any other domain(s) (in the box at the end of the document) that you feel should be included and items that will determine the presence (access to) and utilisation (application) of that domain. Indicate briefly next to any new domain(s), why you think it should be added. You may add a domain even if you do not have items to describe it.

Submit the document with your scores and any additional items (i.e. responses to step 3) to the investigators (Graham Bresick<graham.bresick@uct.ac.za> and Nayna Manga <nayna.manga@uct.ac.za>) via email by 19 April 2013

4. Prioritisation
   All the panellists' responses will be captured, analysed and prioritised by the study team in preparation for Part 2 below.

PART 2b: Expert group convenes

Introduction

Participants and investigators are introduced. A brief overview of the purpose, objectives and process of the consensus method is given and any questions for clarification dealt with.

5. New item presentation, clarification and rationalisation
   Any new items and domains generated in step 3 are presented to the expert panel and their meaning clarified in the group to ensure they are understood by all and how they differ from existing items. New domains and items with similar meanings and intentions will be merged. The relevance of items is not discussed at this

stage. This step ends with a <u>second list of new domains and items</u>.

6. 'Silent' phase rating of new domains and items
    Each participant scores each domain and item in the list generated in step 5 above on his/her own on a sheet of paper as in step 3.2. *(Highlight new items in their respective domains)*. The scores are submitted without discussion and analysed (prioritised) by the investigators to determine which from list will be added.

Presentation of final list to the panel

All domains and items scored as relevant and not relevant in step 3.2 in part 1 and step 6 in part 2 are presented. Any 'borderline' items are noted and can be re-scored - again individually and without discussion.

All the domains and items thus scored as relevant for inclusion will constitute the final content of the ZA PCAT 2013 i.e. <u>> = 70% of the maximum score = consensus</u>

8. Compilation of ZA PCAT v2
    The PCAT study team compile ZA PCAT 2013 according to steps 1–7 in parts 1 and 2 above.

Participants are asked to record two things they found useful and two they did not find useful about the process. Part 2 ends with any general discussion the panel may wish to have.

22

A review of 'medical' knowledge of epilepsy amongst isiZulu-speaking patients at a regional hospital in KwaZulu-Natal

Authors:
Zamir A. Gilani[1]
Kantharuben Naidoo[2]
Andrew Ross[2]

Affiliations:
[1]Department of Family Medicine, Prince Mshiyeni Memorial Hospital, South Africa

[2]Department of Family Medicine, University of KwaZulu-Natal, South Africa

Correspondence to:
Kantharuben Naidoo

Email:
naidook@ukzn.ac.za

Postal address:
Private Bag 07, Congella 4013, South Africa

Background: Epilepsy is a common disorder in South Africa and the literature indicates that many patients do not access treatment. The reasons are complex and include a poor knowledge about causes, symptoms, diagnosis and treatment (medical knowledge). This study aimed to assess the medical knowledge of isiZulu-speaking people with epilepsy (PWE) who attend a combination regional and district hospital in the eThekwini district in KwaZulu-Natal Province.

Method: This was a prospective, cross-sectional, descriptive study. Data were collected using a validated data collection tool for assessing the medical knowledge of PWE and analysed descriptively.

Results: The questionnaires were completed by 199 PWE, with the general level of schooling being low and half being unemployed. Knowledge around causes, symptoms, diagnosis and treatments was good, but there were significant gaps in knowledge that may affect morbidity and mortality.

Discussion: The findings will serve as a useful guide to develop both preventive and educational interventions to enhance knowledge around the causes and treatment of epilepsy in this population. It is important that such interventions also consider family and healthcare providers.

Conclusion: There were considerable gaps in the medical knowledge of isiZulu-speaking PWE's, indicating the need for an educational intervention to improve their understanding of epilepsy. Further research is needed-using a range of tools to ensure that the data is reliable and valid–if the results are to be generalisable to the rest of the province and South Africa.

Examen des connaissances 'médicales' sur l'épilepsie chez les patients de langue zouloue d'un hôpital régional au KwaZulu-Natal.

Contexte: L'épilepsie est un trouble courant en Afrique du Sud et la littérature montre que de nombreux patients n'ont pas accès aux traitements. Les raisons en sont complexes et comprennent une mauvaise connaissance des causes, symptômes, diagnostics et traitements (connaissances médicales). Cette étude avait pour but d'évaluer les connaissances médicales des personnes de langue zouloue atteintes d'épilepsie (PAE) qui fréquentent à la fois les hôpitaux régionaux et de district dans la région d'eThekwini dans la Province du KwaZulu-Natal.

Méthode: C'est une étude prospective, descriptive et transversale. Les données ont été collectées au moyen d'un outil de récolte des données validé pour évaluer les connaissances médicales des PAE, puis analysées de façon descriptive.

Résultats: Les questionnaires ont été remplis par 199 PAE, avec un faible niveau de scolarisation et dont la moitié était au chômage. Les connaissances sur les causes, les symptômes, le diagnostic et les traitements étaient bonnes, mais il y avait des lacunes importantes sur les connaissances affectant la morbidité et la mortalité.

Discussion: Les résultats serviront de guide utile pour mettre au point des interventions à la fois préventives et éducatives afin d'améliorer les connaissances des causes et le traitement de l'épilepsie dans cette population. Il est important que ces interventions examinent aussi la famille et les prestataires de soins de santé.

Conclusion: Il y a des lacunes considérables dans les connaissances médicales des PAE de langue Zouloue, ce qui indique un besoin en matière d'intervention éducative pour améliorer leur compréhension de l'épilepsie. Il faudra pousser les recherches– au moyen de toutes sortes d'outils pour s'assurer que les données sont fiables et valides – si l'on veut généraliser les résultats dans le reste de la province et en Afrique du Sud.

Introduction

Epilepsy is a common, chronic neurological disorder that affects approximately 69 million people worldwide.[1] It affects individuals of all ages, ethnicities, socio-economic class and geographic location.[2] The prevalence is estimated as 1% of the total global population, and there are over 13 million people with epilepsy (PWE) residing in Africa.[1] Epilepsy is particularly common in low-income countries, where the prevalence is more than twice that of high-income countries, possibly due to the higher incidence of risk factors.[3]

The World Health Organization (WHO) estimates that, in Africa, 80% of PWE do not receive treatment, particularly those who are disadvantaged and marginalised, despite effective treatment options being available.[4] Reasons why African patients, in particular, do not access or receive care and treatment are complex and interrelated and include: limited financial resources, poor patient-provider communication, a lack of social support for those with the condition, as well as patient, societal and healthcare provider factors.[5] In addition, patients and their families may lack basic 'medical' knowledge about causes of the disorder, as well as its symptoms, diagnosis and treatment. A lack of 'medical' knowledge was demonstrated in a large door-to-door survey in Senegal amongst 4500 people, where half reported that epilepsy is caused by evil spirits, a third said that it is contagious, and a quarter reported that traditional therapy was better than western treatment.[5] A lack of knowledge, including medical knowledge, underpinned by poor literacy, has been shown to contribute directly to problems associated with poor medicine regimen compliance.[5] As a consequence, PWE often have a lower quality of life than people with other chronic illnesses.[6] A systematic literature review in 2000 reported the mortality rate of PWE in Africa to be 6.2 times greater than that of the general population, with treatment-avoidance behaviour being found to be a significant contributory factor.[6]

Societal beliefs around epilepsy vary from country to country, and may negatively influence health-seeking strategies. For example, people may not seek treatment if epilepsy is not seen as a condition that can be treated by western medicine.[6] In addition, PWE can be socially stigmatized, and may deny their disease when they are described by derogatory labels attached to epilepsy, such as 'mad pig disease.'[7]

A study amongst healthcare workers in Zambia in 2007 found that their poor knowledge about epilepsy and its treatment affected access to appropriate management for PWE.[8] This study recommended that health care workers should receive ongoing education to improve their diagnosis and treatment skills. In addition, educational programmes should address underlying negative attitudes or mistaken knowledge amongst health care workers that may worsen the stigma associated with epilepsy.[8]

In South Africa, although the burden of epilepsy is largely unknown, it is likely to be large, as a 2005 study of children in a large rural community demonstrated a prevalence of 6.7/1000.[9] In another South African study 2341 adults were screened and the prevalence of epilepsy was found to be 13.8/1000, with only 14.7% taking any regular anti-epileptic treatment.[10] The study reported that managing and treating epilepsy were greatly influenced by knowledge, cultural attitudes and beliefs, which varied widely.[10] Participants in both studies were mainly black Africans, which is significant, as many people in this historically disadvantaged population, where there is ongoing stigma around epilepsy, visit traditional healers and respect their opinions.[10]

The high level of epilepsy in South Africa, specifically amongst the African population, highlights the need to establish to what extent this could be affected by their 'medical knowledge', specifically in KwaZulu-Natal (KZN). The aim of this study was therefore to assess the 'medical 'knowledge of isiZulu-speaking PWE receiving treatment at a combination regional and district hospital in the eThekwini District of KZN. Medical knowledge considers issues such as cause, symptoms, diagnostic methods and treatment of epilepsy. This study will provide information about isiZulu-speaking PWE, and will assist in developing a comprehensive, standardised package for medical education around epilepsy.

Method

The study design was prospective, descriptive and cross-sectional, and was conducted at an urban-based epilepsy clinic at a combination regional and district hospital in the eThekwini District of KZN Province. Patients seen at this clinic consist of those referred from Primary Health Care (PHC) clinics when their epilepsy is difficult to control, as well as those who live around the hospital. At the start of this study, the clinic had a total of 2200 registered patients, with an average of 456 being seen on an appointment-basis each month. All patients are reviewed by a doctor at the epilepsy clinic on each visit, and those who are seizure free after three months are referred back to the PHC clinic closest to their home (where such a clinic is available).

The study population included patients 18 years or older attending the clinic, with those affected by mental retardation being excluded. A sample size of 199 patients, which represented 44% of the monthly average number of patients attending the clinic was selected. This sample size was considered adequate for a small descriptive cross-sectional study.[11] To reduce selection bias, every third PWE was invited to participate until the sample size was reached. Files were marked to ensure that patients did not participate more than once. Data collected were from 25 June 2013 to 20 August 2013.

The aim of the study was explained to potential participants by a research assistant who was recruited and supervised by the researcher. The research assistant provided clarity on the questions where required, explained the 'Study Information Sheet', and obtained written consent from all participants (consent forms were available in both English and isiZulu, with isiZulu being the first language of most PWE in this context). Participants were requested to self-complete two questionnaires, and the research assistant was available to help those who required assistance. The first questionnaire (Annexure A)obtained demographic details, including level of education, home language, employment status, duration of epilepsy, and whether they were receiving a social grant from the state.

The second data questionnaire(Annexure B) was based on an internationally-validated questionnaire for assessing medical knowledge of PWE – The Epilepsy Knowledge Profile--General (EKP-G).[12] The EKP-G consists of 55 true/false items (34 medical knowledge items, 21 social knowledge items) that were selected by a range of experts in the field of epilepsy and is considered to be objective, sensitive and unambiguous in its assessment of medical knowledge levels in relation to epilepsy.[12,13] The questionnaire has also been used in international studies and, in 2003, was found to be useful in comparing the medical knowledge of PWE between countries.[13]

In our study, only the questions regarding medical knowledge were presented to participants in both English and isiZulu. The collected data were entered into SPSS (Chicago, Illinois) and analysed descriptively. The EKP-G was piloted by asking the research assistant and five PWE selected from the epilepsy clinic to complete the questionnaire. The resulting analysis indicated that it was understood and instructions to complete it were clear. Having undergone a rigorous process of validation in other contexts and piloted in the KZN context, the EKP-G was considered to be a valid measurement tool for PWEs' medical knowledge.

Approval for the study was given by the hospital management, the KZN Provincial Department of Health and the Biomedical Research Ethics Committee of University of KZN (BE 158/11). Permission to use the EKP-G questionnaire was obtained from the instrument's developer.

Results

A total of 199 PWE completed the questionnaires and the results are presented in two sections: demographic profile and EPK-G results.

Demographic profile

Of the 199 respondents, 86 were male (43%), and the ages ranged from 18 to 69 years. The majority (83%) did not complete their formal school education, 9% never attended school, and only 5.5% attained a post-school qualification. A summary of the findings is presented in Table 1.

Most participants spoke isiZulu as a first language, 2% spoke English and 3.5% spoke another language. Half (53%) reported that they were currently unemployed, 40.7% had never been employed, and 51% were receiving a social grant

TABLE 1: Level of education.

Variable	Number	Percent
No schooling	18	9.0
Grade 1-4	51	25.6
Grade 5-7	26	13.1
Grade 8-11	70	35.2
Matric completed	23	11.6
Higher than Matric	11	5.5
Total	**199**	**100.0**

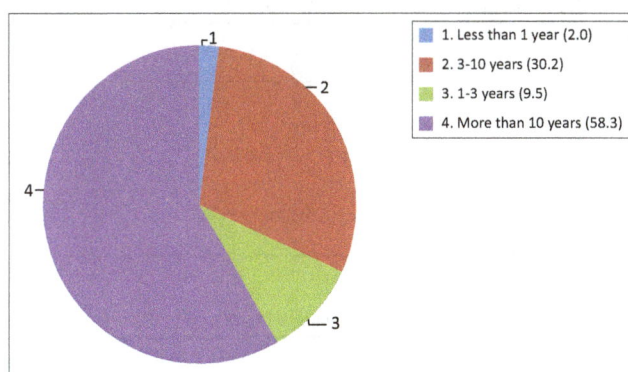

FIGURE 1: Percentage of patients and duration of epilepsy (years).

from the state. Just over half (58%) had been diagnosed with epilepsy for more than 10 years (Figure 1).

A regression equation that considered three variables (highest level of education achieved, duration of epilepsy and highest level of medical knowledge) showed a correlation between level of education and medical knowledge.

Results of EKP-G questionnaire

The following four tables summarize the results of the EPK-G questionnaire (the number of participants and percentage who answered that question correctly). The findings are presented as participants' medical knowledge on: (a) cause of epilepsy (Table 2), (b) symptoms (Table 3), (c) diagnosis (Table 4) and (d) treatment (Table 5).

When asked about the causes of epilepsy (Table 2), responses indicate that the majority of participants (81%) knew that epilepsy is not an infectious disease, and that it can be exacerbated by alcohol (90%) and stress (95%). It was encouraging that the majority (87%) believed epilepsy to be caused by an abnormality in the function of the nerve cells of the brain, as this suggests that they believed there was a medical cause for epilepsy and did not associate it with witchcraft or supernatural causes.

Regarding their knowledge about epilepsy symptoms, a majority (74%) knew that these varied depending on the type and that epilepsy may not always be associated with generalised seizures (e.g., temporal lobe epilepsy may be associated with absence seizures lasting seconds that are not noticed). A significant proportion (83%) knew of the association between an aura and epilepsy, which could

TABLE 2: Knowledge of causes of epilepsy (*n* = 199).

Question	Correct Answer	Correct Responses	
		Number	Percent
Epilepsy is always caused by brain damage	No	67	34
Epilepsy is not infectious	Yes	161	81
Certain forms of brain damage always causes epilepsy	No	13	07
An epileptic seizure can be described as an abnormality in the function of nerve cells of the brain	Yes	174	87
Too much alcohol make seizures more likely	Yes	179	90
Stress may cause some seizures	Yes	189	95

TABLE 3: Knowledge of symptoms of epilepsy (*n* = 199).

Question	Correct Answer	Correct Responses	
		Number	Percent
Epilepsy is a symptom of mental illness	No	70	35
All people with epilepsy have similar symptoms	No	106	53
All people with epilepsy lose consciousness during epilepsy	No	33	17
Some seizures may last a matter of seconds and not be noticed by others	Yes	147	74
Some people get a warning or a feeling just before a seizure	Yes	165	83
Most seizures result in brain damage	No	16	08

TABLE 4: Knowledge of diagnosis of epilepsy (*n* = 199).

Question	Correct Answer	Correct Responses	
		Number	Percent
An EEG can be useful to help diagnose epilepsy	Yes	174	87
If an EEG is abnormal this is a definite sign of epilepsy	No	48	24
An EEG is designed to detect electrical activity from the brain	Yes	175	88
A normal EEG means that you do not have epilepsy	No	93	47

TABLE 5: Knowledge of treatment of epilepsy (*n* = 199).

Question	Correct Answer	Correct Responses	
		Number	Percent
For most people doctors can treat epilepsy effectively with drugs	Yes	126	63
All those who start drugs for their epilepsy have to take them for life	No	8	4
Increasing the dose of anti-epileptic drugs increases the chance of side effects	Yes	164	82
In order for anti-epileptic drugs to be successful, they must be taken regularly	Yes	192	96
If you forget to take anti-epileptic drug for a day, it is usually OK to take two doses together	Yes	22	11
Blood samples can be used to detect the concentration of anti-epileptic drugs in the system	Yes	187	94
People who are taking a combination of anti-epileptic drugs are more likely to have side effects than those taking only one drug	Yes	93	47
Most peoples' seizures are well controlled soon after starting regular drug treatment	Yes	179	90
It is always helpful to take extra doses of anti-epileptic medication when not feeling well	No	177	89
If seizures stop with anti-epileptic drugs, this means that your epilepsy is cured	No	175	88
Few people with a diagnosis of epilepsy are on anti-epileptic drugs	No	139	70
There is no need to continue taking your anti-epileptic drugs if your seizures stop	No	164	82

encourage them to seek help when they felt that a seizure was imminent (Table 3.).

Participants generally had a good knowledge about the use of EEG in epilepsy diagnosis (87%), as indicated in Table 4.

The majority believed that all PWE would have to take drugs for the rest of their lives (96%), whilst a third (37%) did not know that epilepsy can largely be treated and controlled with drugs. However, this latter finding contradicts the answers to two similar questions: in order for anti-epileptic drugs to be successful they must be taken regularly (96%) and most peoples' seizures are well controlled soon after starting drugs (90%).The reasons for this discrepancy in responses need to be investigated further. Most PWE knew they must

continue medication despite an absence of seizures (82%). (Table 5; Figure 2)

Discussion

The 199 participants represented a substantial proportion of the average monthly attendance at the clinic. The majority of participants were black and isiZulu-speaking, which represents the demographics of the population served by this combination hospital. Many participants were unemployed, which may affect their ability to access treatment regularly. Of concern was the over 50% of participants receiving disability grants, despite epilepsy being a managed condition enabling people to work if they take appropriate medication. This suggests that either control is so poor that patients are

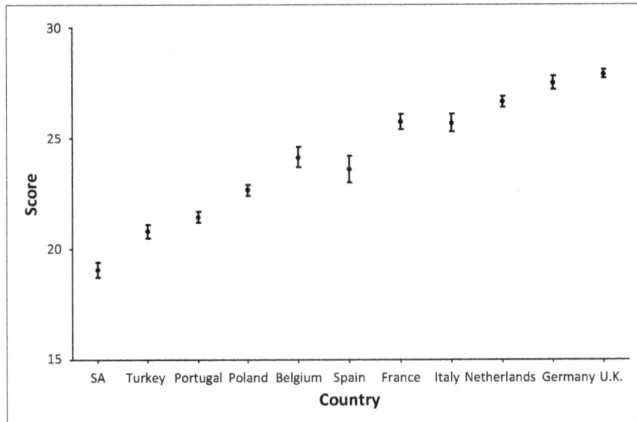

FIGURE 2: Comparison of current study with 2003 European study.

unable to work, that stigma makes it difficult for patients with epilepsy to find work, or that health care practitioners fill in disability grant forms more for social than for medical reasons. With high levels of unemployment in South Africa and the type of work available to PWE often being restricted,[14] obtaining a disability grant may be a more attractive option than looking for work. Future research could explore why so many patients receive social grants, and their effect on adherence, seizure control, and clinic attendance on this vulnerable population.

Education levels were generally low, and whilst the regression model showed a correlation between level of education and medical knowledge, the number of people in this category was small and the type of post-school education unknown. This finding is in contrast to a study amongst black African university students in South Africa, which showed no association between a higher level of education and correct knowledge about epilepsy.[15] The study indicated that the students had limited knowledge regarding epilepsy, with the participants believing that a PWE is a witch or wizard, recommending that they be isolated for the safety of others.[15]

As most participants had suffered with epilepsy for more than a year (98%), their knowledge regarding the condition would be expected to be good, as they would have had access to education about the disease during their regular visits to the epilepsy clinic for follow-up. It was encouraging that most knew that epilepsy is associated with abnormal electrical activity in the brain, which is in contrast to an Ethiopian study where only a quarter of participants had the correct knowledge about the causes of epilepsy.[16] However, it was of concern that most respondents in this study believed that seizures always result in brain damage.

Most participants knew that epilepsy is not an infectious disease, and this knowledge may assist in reducing the stigmatization and social isolation of PWE. However, a difficult concept to explain to PWE may be that some infections do lead to epilepsy, such as neurocysticercosis (NCC), which is a common cause of epilepsy in KZN. A study in the Eastern Cape Province in South Africa illustrated that 100% of participants ($n = 2431$) had no knowledge of NCC,

despite it being a common cause for epilepsy in the area.[17] A literature review did not identify any studies regarding the knowledge of isiZulu PWE about NCC in KZN. A further study amongst this population may indicate whether or not they have any knowledge of NCC, and a prevention campaign based on these findings could be implemented.

It was of concern that two thirds (65%) associated epilepsy with a mental disease, this possibly being due to information provided by health care professionals (HCP's). In a study in Zambia, more than 50% of the HCP's who participated considered epilepsy to be a form of mental illness.[8] This highlights the need for educational interventions to be extended to HCP's to ensure that they have the correct knowledge about the condition and manifest the appropriate attitude towards PWE, which can then be cascaded down to patients and the broader society.

That most participants had knowledge of EEG may reflect the fact that they were diagnosed at a regional hospital where the equipment was available. Any education programme which is developed should, however, consider the general lack of EEG testing equipment in South Africa, particularly at PHC facilities[17] and inform patients of the need to be referred to regional facilities should this test be considered necessary.

It was encouraging to know that most PWE knew that drugs should be continued despite the absence of seizures and that medication must be taken regularly, as prescribed by the healthcare provider. However, it was of concern that the overall levels of medical knowledge compared poorly with PWE in Europe, with low levels of knowledge highlighting the need for urgent educational initiatives to change this situation.

The findings from this study may be of particular interest to healthcare providers who are in a unique and influential position to enhance medical knowledge as well as dispel misconceptions and myths around epilepsy. The findings regarding the gaps in knowledge about epilepsy causes, symptoms, diagnosis and treatment could be used to guide the design of a targeted educational programme for PWE and health care workers. The literature indicates that education is an effective tool that can be used to enhance knowledge about the disease and highlight the importance of adhering to a specific medical and lifestyle regimen.[18]

To validate the findings and to make them more generalisable, additional measures need to be taken to triangulate the findings, namely that data could be collected from other sites using a variety of data collection instruments and methods. Medical knowledge of PWE has been gathered using several other data collection tools such as the Epilepsy Knowledge Questionnaire (EK-Q), which is a ten item questionnaire.[16] Other data collection instruments would be useful to consider other aspects of medical knowledge, for example a family's knowledge regarding what to do when their relative has a seizure. A review of the factors associated with societal and healthcare workers 'knowledge regarding epilepsy would add to the information available to address problems associated with poor 'medical' knowledge of isiZulu-speaking PWE receiving treatment in KZN.

Limitations to the study

A limitation to the study concerns some ambiguity associated with the questions on the data collection instrument, as well as the lack of a 'don't know' option. However, as this was a validated tool used previously in other countries, a decision was taken not to change the questions. A way forward would be to triangulate findings by collecting data on medical knowledge using an alternative data collection instrument. It is also possible that the study was biased towards literate patients, as those unable to read may have been less likely to participate. However, an attempt was made to overcome this by the use of a research assistant to help these patients.

Conclusion and recommendations

This study provided useful information about the medical knowledge of patients with epilepsy who attend the epilepsy clinic at this combination hospital in the eThekwini District of KZN. The results could be used to design an education programme for isiZulu-speaking PWE. In this context, an education programme should consider issues around causes, diagnosis, prevention and treatment, and include enhancing their knowledge about infections, namely NCC and HIV, which can result in epilepsy. Increasing medical knowledge may lead to reduced stigmatization and isolation, and may encourage patients and family to see the condition as a chronic medical disorder.

Acknowledgements

Competing interests

The authors declare that they have no financial or personal relationship(s) that may have inappropriately influenced them in writing this article.

Authors' contributions

Z.A.G. (Prince Mshiyeni Memorial Hospital) conceived the study, conducted the survey, interpreted the data and drafted the manuscript. K.N. (University of KwaZulu-Natal) and A.R. (University of KwaZulu-Natal) critically revised the manuscript for important intellectual content.

All authors read and approved the manuscript for publication.

References

1. Wagner RG, Ngugi AK, Twine R, et al. Prevalence and risk factors for active convulsive epilepsy in rural northeast South Africa. Epilepsy Res [serial online]. 2014;108(4): 782–791. Available from:http://dx.doi.org/10.1016/j.eplepsyres.2014.01.004

2. Ackerman S. Managing first-time seizures and epilepsy in children. A first seizure is a relatively common problem in paediatric general practice. Contin Med Edu. 2012;30(1):17–21.

3. Newton RC, Garcia HH. Epilepsy in poor regions of the world. *Lancet. 2012;*380(9848):1193–1201.

4. World Health Organization. Epilepsy in the WHO African region: Bridging the gap. The global campaign against epilepsy "Out of the shadows" [homepage on the Internet].2004 [cited 2014 Jun 20]. Available from: http://www.globalcampaignagainstepilepsy.org/files/Epilepsy%20in%20the%20African%20Region.pdf

5. Ndoye NF, Sow AD, Diop AG, et al. Prevalence of epilepsy its treatment gap and knowledge, attitude and practice of its population in sub-urban Senegal an ILAE/IBE/WHO study. Seizure [serial online]. 2005;14(2):106–111.

6. Diop AG, Hesdorffer DC, Logroscino G, et al. Epilepsy and mortality in Africa: A review of the Literature. Epilepsia [serial online]. 2005;46(11):33–35. Available from: //http://dx.doi.org/10.1111/j.0013-9580.2005.t01-1-53904.x-i1

7. Tran DS, Odermatt P, Singphuoangphet S, et al. Epilepsy in Laos: Knowledge, attitudes, and practices in the community. Epilepsy Behav [serial online].2007;10(4): 565–570. Available from: http://dx.doi.org/10.1016/j.yeheb.2007.02.018

8. Chombat EN, Haworth A, Atadzhanov M. et al. Zambian health care workers' knowledge, attitudes, beliefs, and practices regarding epilepsy. Epilepsy Behav. 2007;10(1):111–119.

9. Christianson AL, Zwane ME, Manga P, Rosen E, Kromberg JG. Epilepsy in rural South African children - Prevalence, associated disability and management. S Afr Med J. 2000;90(3):262–266.

10. Eastman R. Epilepsy in South Africa. Acta Neurol Scand. 2005;112(s181):8–11.

11. Durrhiem K. Research design chapter 3. In: Terre Blanche M, Durrheim K, Painter D. Research in practice. Cape Town: University of Cape Town Press, 2008: p. 33-60.

12. Jarvie S, Espie CA, Brodie MJ. The development of a questionnaire to assess knowledge of epilepsy: 1- general knowledge of epilepsy. Seizure [serial online]. 1993;2(3):179–185. Available from: http://dx.doi.org/10.1016/s1059-1311(05)80125-6

13. Doughty J, Baker GA, Jacoby A, et al. Cross- cultural differences in levels of knowledge about epilepsy. Epilepsia [serial online]. 2003;44(1):115–123. Available from: http://dx.doi.org/10.1046/j.1528-1157.2003.34402.x

14. Keikelamea MJ, Swartzb L. A lay carer's story about epilepsy in an urban South African context: They call it an illness of falling or an illness of fitting because a person shakes and eventually falls. Epilepsy Behav [serial online]. 2013;28(3): 512–518. Available from: http://dx.doi.org/10.1016/j.yebeh.2013.05.025

15. Pelzer K. Perceptions of epilepsy among black students at a university in South Africa. Curationis. 2001;24(2):62–67.

16. Goldstein LH, Minchin L, Stubbs P, Fenwick PBC. Are what people know about their epilepsy and what they want from an epilepsy service related? Seizure [serial online].1997;6(6):435–442. Available from: http://dx.doi.org/10.1016/S1059131102001504

17. Foyaca-Sibat H, Rio-Romero A, Ibanez- Valdes L. Prevalence of epilepsy and general knowledge about neurocysticercosis at Ngangelizwe Location, South Africa. Int J Neurol. 2005 May;4(1).

18. Bexon M. What needs to change for people with epilepsy? Seizure [serial online].2010;19(10):684–685. Available from: http://dx.doi.org/10.1016/j.seizure. 2010.07.023

23

How far does family physician supply correlate with district health system performance?

Authors:
Robin E. Dyers[1,2]
Robert Mash[3]
Tracey Naledi[2]

Affiliations:
[1]Division of Community Health, Faculty of Medicine and Health Sciences, Department of Interdisciplinary Health Sciences, Stellenbosch University, South Africa

[2]Health Programmes, Western Cape Government: Health, South Africa

[3]Division of Family Medicine and Primary Care, Faculty of Medicine and Health Sciences, Department of Interdisciplinary Health Sciences, Stellenbosch University, South Africa

Correspondence to:
Robin Dyers

Email:
robindyers@me.com

Postal address:
PO Box 19063, Tygerberg
7505, South Africa

Background: Since 2011, a new cadre of family physicians, with 4 years of postgraduate training, was deployed in the district health services of the Western Cape, and tasked with a considerable range of duties aimed at a general improvement in care and health outcomes. There is a need to evaluate the contribution of these family physicians to the district health system.

Aim: To develop a methodology for describing the correlation between family physician supply and district health system performance, clinical processes and outcomes, and to measure this correlation at baseline.

Method: A cross-sectional study was undertaken that analysed data at an ecological level for the period of 01 April 2011 to 31 March 2012. This was a pilot project analysing data from the first year of a 4-year project. The correlations between family physician supply and 18 health system indicators were assessed within a logic model. The supplies of other categories of staff were also measured.

Results: Although most of the correlations with family physicians were positive, the study was unable to demonstrate any strong or statistically significant correlations at baseline. There were significant correlations with other categories of staff.

Conclusions: This study developed a methodology for monitoring the relationship between family physician supply using routinely collected indicators of health system performance, clinical processes and outcomes over time. Additional research will also be needed to investigate the impact of family physicians and triangulate findings as this methodology has many limitations and potential confounding factors.

A quel point le recrutement de médecins de famille va de pair avec la performance du système de santé des districts?

Contexte: Depuis 2011, un nouveau cadre de médecins de famille, avec 4 ans de formation après le Diplôme, ont été déployés dans les services sanitaires des districts du Western Cape, et chargés d'une série de fonctions dans le but d'améliorer les résultats de santé et de soins. Il faut évaluer la contribution de ces médecins de famille au système de santé des districts.

Objectif: Développer une méthodologie pour décrire la corrélation entre le recrutement des médecins de famille et la performance du système sanitaire des districts, les processus et résultats cliniques, et mesurer cette corrélation à la base de référence.

Méthode: Une étude transversale a été effectuée et a analysé les données au niveau écologique pour la période allant du 1er avril 2011 au 31 mars 2012. Ce projet pilote a analysé les données de la première année du projet de 4 ans. Les corrélations entre le recrutement des médecins de famille et les 18 indicateurs de systèmes de santé ont été évalués au sein d'un modèle logique. Le recrutement d'autres catégories de personnel a aussi été mesuré.

Résultats: Bien que la plupart des corrélations avec les médecins de famille étaient positives, l'étude n'a pas pu démontrer de corrélations importantes ou statistiquement significatives à la base de référence. Il y avait des corrélations significatives avec d'autres catégories de personnel.

Conclusion: Cette étude a mis au point une méthodologie pour évaluer la relation entre le recrutement des médecins de famille au moyen d'indicateurs de performance des systèmes sanitaires recueillis systématiquement, les processus et résultats cliniques avec le temps. Il faudra faire des recherches supplémentaires pour évaluer l'impact des médecins de famille et la triangulation des résultats étant donné que cette méthodologie a beaucoup de limitations et des facteurs de confusion potentiels.

Background

Strengthening primary health care and district health systems has been recognised as one of the most important policy objectives for countries trying to improve health outcomes and equity.[1-3] The 2008 World Health Report highlighted the ongoing need for this in its title 'Primary health care: Now more than ever' and also noted that most effective primary health care systems include doctors with a specialisation in either general practice or family medicine.[4] Conversely they noted that many developing countries have developed primary health care in a limited and poorly resourced approach that is unlikely to succeed.

South Africa is seeking strategies to improve primary health care and district health systems with a view to introducing national health insurance in the longer term.[5] The National Department of Health is considering what specialists are needed in the districts to improve the quality of care and health outcomes, especially in relation to maternal and child health.[5]

In South Africa, family medicine was recognised as a new area of specialisation in 2007 and training of family physicians as expert generalists began in 2008, with the first graduates in 2011. The national development plan states that 'family physicians in the district specialist support team will take the primary responsibility for developing a district-specific strategy and an implementation plan for clinical governance'.[6] Family medicine training is aligned with a set of national outcomes aimed at preparing these expert generalists to work independently at district hospitals and in primary care. The six roles of these new family physicians in the district health services (DHS) have been defined as providing clinical care, consulting on patients referred by other members of the health care team, mentoring and training other clinical staff, taking responsibility for clinical governance within the facility or subdistrict, supervising interns and registrars and also contributing to a more community-oriented approach.[7] In general terms family physicians differ from medical officers in that they have 4 years of postgraduate training, have broader roles beyond clinical care and have greater length of experience.

Initial research on the impact of family physicians suggests that they have delivered on their roles as clinicians, consultants and leaders of clinical governance.[8] Usually the family physician is the most senior member of the health care team in primary care or district hospitals and has an influence on the quality of care provided throughout the whole subdistrict. Interviews with district managers also suggest that they are impacting on key clinical processes for important conditions such as human immunodeficiency virus (HIV) infection, tuberculosis (TB), non-communicable diseases and childhood diarrhoea, as well as on the performance of the health services in terms of access to more comprehensive and coordinated care.[9]

Since 2011 the Western Cape has been the only province to employ family physicians at scale in district hospitals and community health centres and therefore provides an opportunity to evaluate the impact of family physicians on the DHS.[10]

Research in the USA and Iran has found a significant correlation between the supply of primary care physicians and better health outcomes, with an inverse relationship to the supply of other specialist doctors.[2,11,12,13,14,15,16,17] This correlation, however, is potentially confounded by many other socio-economic factors such as standard of living, public education, access to information and economic empowerment of people.[15]

The aim of this study was to develop the methodology and to describe the baseline relationship between family physician supply and health system performance, key clinical processes and health outcomes in the DHS of the Western Cape, South Africa. No such work has previously been carried out in an African context. Given that the Western Cape was in the early stages of including family physicians in the DHS, this study focused on developing the methodology to correlate family physician supply with selected indicators from the health information system. Indicators were chosen in terms of the study's conceptual model, which saw the family physicians as a generic intervention that would eventually impact on health outcomes through an initial impact on health system performance and clinical processes. In this baseline study it was not anticipated that an actual impact would be measured.

This new knowledge is particularly relevant to the work currently being carried out by the National Department of Health on re-engineering primary health care, developing district specialist teams and planning for national health insurance.[5] It will also be relevant to Ministries of Health and academic institutions in other African countries that are considering the training of family physicians (e.g. Botswana, Zimbabwe, Namibia, Kenya, Uganda and Rwanda).[18,19,20]

Methods
Study design

This is a cross-sectional ecological study that explores the baseline associations within a broader prospective study that ran from 2011 to 2014. This study focused on the first year from 01 April 2011 to 31 March 2012. The exploratory analysis on the baseline data of the larger study also served as a pilot of the methodology in the South African setting.

Data were collected from the existing health information system used by the Department of Health on the number of family physicians as of 2011, other health workers, key clinical processes, key health system functions, community indicators and health outcomes, and then aggregated to subdistrict and district level. The number of family physicians per 10 000 people was the measure of 'supply'.

Setting

The Western Cape Province is made up of six health districts: Cape Metropole, West Coast, Cape Winelands,

Overberg, Eden and Central Karoo. The Cape Metropole, which represents the city of Cape Town, is further split into four substructures and each substructure is split into two subdistricts.

The Western Cape has 'aligned its Comprehensive Service Plan with the model of having a family physician at each district hospital (> 50 beds) and each community health centre (> 30 000 people served)'.[9,21] Although there were only about 20 family physicians (both old and newly trained) in the province in 2011, the overall perception was that they made a difference.[9] Prior to 2011 family physicians were trained in part-time training programmes, which varied in terms of their learning outcomes and quality. Many of the family physicians employed by 2011 came from these earlier programmes.

As the new family physicians graduate from 2011 onwards, it is expected that the number of family physicians across the province will increase to between 60 and 80 over the next 5 years.[10]

The Western Cape was estimated to have a population of 5 755 607 in 2011 of whom approximately 83% were dependent on public health services. Relative to other provinces, the Western Cape had good access to basic amenities (e.g. 94% of households were electrified), but still had inequities within and between districts.[22,23] The province shared the same quadruple burden of disease as the rest of the country: HIV-related disease and TB, interpersonal violence and trauma, maternal and child health problems and non-communicable chronic diseases.[24]

Sample size

The units of analysis included the five rural districts and the eight Cape Town metropolitan subdistricts in the Western Cape. This mix of a total of 13 organisational units, described in Table 1, provided for similar-sized units for analysis. Whilst this is a small sample size, it is finite in that it includes collated data for the entire Western Cape geographic region for a period of 1 year.

Recruitment

The study included data on the Western Cape population (Table 1) and DHS. Data from central, specialised and regional hospitals were excluded. Private and community-based service data were also excluded.

Inclusion criteria

Data from the following types of facilities within the DHS were included:

- clinics
- community day centres
- community health centres
- dental clinics
- district hospitals
- health posts
- midwife obstetrics units
- mobile services
- reproductive health services
- satellite clinics.

Exclusion criteria

Data from the following types of facilities within the DHS were excluded:

- correctional services
- environmental health offices
- health promotion services
- home-based care
- non-medical sites.

Home-based care services, whilst part of DHS, were excluded because of differential procedures in data collection and resource allocation between the units of analysis in this study.

Measurement tools

Data were collected in respect of the number of family physicians, other health workers, key clinical processes, key health system performance, community indicators and health outcomes.

TABLE 1: Description of units of analysis.

District or subdistrict	Total population	Dependent population	Percentage
Eden District	563 573	485 074	86
Central Karoo District	60 991	55 199	91
Cape Winelands District	768 295	652 148	85
Overberg District	238 086	207 202	87
West Coast District	314 926	270 949	86
Cape Metro Western Subdistrict	429 291	339 332	79
Cape Metro Southern Subdistrict	568 173	413 438	73
Cape Metro Northern Subdistrict	354 446	218 452	62
Cape Metro Eastern Subdistrict	445 037	360 936	81
Cape Metro Khayelitsha Subdistrict	427 157	410 104	96
Cape Metro Klipfontein Subdistrict	456 813	401 163	88
Cape Metro Mitchells Plain Subdistrict	521 966	462 453	89
Cape Metro Tygerberg Subdistrict	606 852	499 127	82

A conceptual model that guided the evaluation and illustrates the inter-relationships between various elements is set out in Figure 1 and elaborated on below.[25] The model, based on a modified Donabedian causal chain, was used to make sense of the complexity of the health system and to provide a rationale for the selection of indicators and identification of confounders. Indicators assessed were grouped according to the following categories:

Policy intervention and structure: Changes in the policy applied to the DHS were monitored qualitatively during the study.

Generic interventions such as human resources impact across a wide range of processes. In this case introducing a new cadre of family physicians was seen as a generic intervention. The study measured the number of family physicians and other practitioners (nurses, doctors and other specialists) in the DHS per 10 000 dependent population.

Targeted interventions were aimed at improving specific clinical processes via training, audit cycles or other clinical governance methods.

Clinical interventions directly impacted clinical processes through the provision of new drugs, devices, procedures or therapies.

Health system performance: Kringos et al. have identified key aspects of the primary care system upon which the family physician can be expected to have some impact.[26] These include access to, continuity of, coordination of, comprehensiveness of, quality of and efficiency of care.

Clinical processes: Family physicians as expert generalists should impact across the full range of clinical processes.

Health outcomes: Key facility-based outcome indicators such as perinatal mortality.

Definitions

Tarimo defines the DHS as a 'well-defined population living within a clearly delineated administrative and geographic area. It includes all the relevant health care activities in the area, whether governmental or otherwise'.[27] However, for this study the DHS definition was restricted to services rendered by the vertical funding programme 2: 'District Health Services' in the annual performance plan, which includes governmental primary health care facilities and district hospitals.[10]

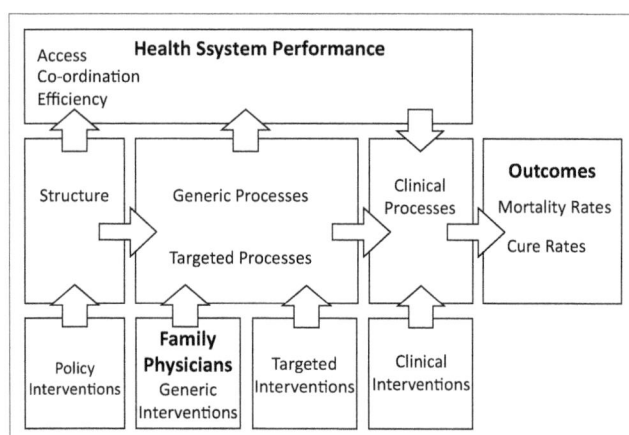

FIGURE 1: Modified Donabedian causal chain – Interventions at structural (policy) and generic service level can achieve effects through intervening variables further down the chain to result in particular health outcomes.[25]

Population-based indicators were expressed per 'dependent population' (Table 1). The dependent population is an estimate of the proportion of the population with insufficient household income to afford private medical care, whether by out-of-pocket payment or by medical insurance. It is therefore different from the 'uninsured population'. Whilst the dependent population provides for a denominator of the population likely to utilise public health services, it can also be used as a proxy for deprivation.[28]

The final set of indicators that had to be collected was defined during the first 6 months of the project through a collaborative process between the researchers, current family physicians, district managers and the directorate for health impact assessment within the Western Cape Department of Health. Indicators were selected according to the conceptual framework (Figure 1) and in terms of their availability, credibility and expected impact by family physicians.

The aforementioned indicators were given shorter names as variables for convenience (Tables 2 and 3). For this study we chose four generic intervention variables (Table 2) and 18 proxy variables for clinical processes, health system performance and health outcomes (Table 3).

Staff numbers were expressed as 'full-time equivalents' (FTE) (Table 4). A FTE is a representation of the time spent by a particular staff category in rendering designated services during the total number of working hours for the financial year.

Data sources

Data were collected from routine health and human resource management information systems as follows:

Persal: human resource management tool, used to establish the numbers of 'generic interventions' such as various categories of staff.

Sinjani: routine monitoring and reporting tool, used to collate all health facility routine data in the province.

ETR.net: electronic TB registers, used to collate and report cohort data of TB patients.

Chronic Diseases Audit: annual provincially coordinated audit on the quality of care for chronic non-communicable diseases in primary health care facilities.

Staff Satisfaction Survey: biennial provincial audit of staff satisfaction.

Statistical analysis

The Centre for Statistical Consultation at Stellenbosch University was consulted to assist with data analysis. Data for the 22 variables were collated using Microsoft Excel™ 2011. Data were then exported to and analysed in Stata™ version 13.1.

The mean and standard deviations (s.d.) were calculated for each of the variables. As this was an ecological study these would be the 'means of means'. The s.d. was preferred to the 95% confidence interval to describe the variance in the data,

TABLE 2: Definitions of independent variables.

Independent variable	Definition
Family physician	Primary health care family physicians per 10 000 dependent population.
Nurse	Primary health care nurses per 10 000 dependent population; includes professional nurses, enrolled nurses and enrolled nursing assistants.
Medical officer	Primary health care medical officers per 10 000 dependent population.
Other specialist	Specialists employed by District Health Services, other than family physicians, per 10 000 dependent population; these include specialists in internal medicine, surgery, paediatrics, obstetrics and gynaecology, anaesthetics and orthopaedics.

TABLE 3: Definitions of dependent variables.

Dependent variable (framework domain)	Definition
PHC utilisation (access)	Rate at which primary health care services are utilised by the target population, represented as the average number of visits per person during the reporting period in the target population.[10]
Access (access)	Average score of questions related to primary health care access in the annual client satisfaction survey (scores ranged from −2 to 2).
Teamwork (coordination)	Average score of the question, 'In my unit/component the staff function well as a team' in the annual staff satisfaction survey (scores ranged from 1 to 5).
Chronic care team (coordination)	Proportion of facilities that have a designated chronic care team.
Hospital expenditure (efficiency)	Average cost (in South African rand) per patient day equivalent in district hospitals. Patient day equivalent is a weighted combination of inpatient days, day patients, and outpatient department and emergency headcounts; all hospital activity is expressed as an equivalent to one inpatient day.[10]
PHC expenditure (efficiency)	Expenditure on primary health care by the provincial Department of Health per dependent population; includes expenditure in primary health care facilities and district hospitals.
Cervical smears (clinical processes)	Proportion of women aged 30 years and older who have screening for cervical cancer.[10]
Isoniazid prophylaxis (clinical processes)	Proportion of HIV-positive patients started on isoniazid prophylaxis.
TB treatment (clinical processes)	Proportion of patients suspected of having TB who have started treatment.
CYPR (clinical processes)	Couple year protection rate: percentage women of reproductive age (15–44 years) who are using (or whose partner is using) a modern contraceptive method; contraceptive methods include female and male sterilisation, injectable and oral hormones, intrauterine devices, diaphragms, spermicides and condoms.[10]
Early antenatal booking (clinical processes)	Percentage of pregnant women who visit a health facility for the primary purpose of receiving antenatal care, often referred to as 'a booking visit', that occurs before 20 weeks after conception.[10]
Immunisation (clinical processes)	Percentage of all children under 1 year who complete their primary course of immunisation during the reporting period; a primary course includes BCG, OPV 0 & 1, DTaP-IPV-Hib 1, 2 & 3, HepB 1, 2 & 3, and first measles at 9 months.[10]
Diabetes score (clinical processes)	Aggregated Annual Chronic Disease Audit score for the questions about the clinical processes and the technical quality of care related to the management of patients with diabetes.
Hypertension score (clinical processes)	Aggregated Annual Chronic Disease Audit score for the questions about the clinical processes and the technical quality of care related to the management of patients with hypertension.
TB cure (outcomes)	Percentage of new smear-positive pulmonary tuberculosis cases cured at first attempt.[10]
Maternal mortality (outcomes)	Number of maternal deaths in facility expressed per 10 000 live births; a maternal death is the death of a woman whilst pregnant or within 42 days of termination of pregnancy, irrespective of the duration and the site of the pregnancy, from any cause related to or aggravated by the pregnancy or its management, but not from accidental or incidental causes (as cited in ICD 10).[10]
Perinatal mortality (outcomes)	Stillbirths plus the number of children who have died in a health facility between birth and 28 days of life, expressed per 10 000 total births in facility.
Under-5 mortality (outcomes)	The number of children who have died in a health facility between birth and their fifth birthday, expressed per 10 000 live births in facility.[10]

PHC, primary health care, TB, tuberculosis.

TABLE 4: Numbers of full-time equivalents per staff category in each district or subdistrict.

District or subdistrict	Family physician	Medical officer	Nurse	Other specialist
Eden District	1.00	54.26	720.17	9.66
Central Karoo District	0.00	12.68	174.89	0.00
Cape Winelands District	3.50	58.27	804.74	5.31
Overberg District	2.00	24.01	317.61	2.69
West Coast District	2.00	35.46	487.91	5.34
Western Cape Town Subdistrict	1.00	45.80	294.40	4.50
Southern Cape Town Subdistrict	1.00	89.05	515.93	22.21
Northern Cape Town Subdistrict	1.00	14.36	84.32	3.50
Eastern Cape Town Subdistrict	2.00	64.37	413.19	15.97
Khayelitsha Subdistrict	2.00	76.97	469.13	3.02
Klipfontein Subdistrict	2.00	89.56	506.88	23.67
Mitchells Plain Subdistrict	2.00	29.93	251.69	4.50
Tygerberg Subdistrict	1.00	91.69	625.43	13.90

rather than the precision of the means, as the results came from a finite data set.[29] The median and interquartile ranges (IQR) were also calculated for each variable.

Simple correlation, Spearman's rho, was used to describe the relationship between the number of family physicians per 10 000 people and key health system performance, clinical processes and health outcomes for 2011. The socio-economic differences between subdistricts and districts were included by expressing population-based data according to 'dependence' (a measure of income inequality).

Data were analysed for all 13 organisational units. The level of significance chosen was $p < 0.05$. We undertook correlation analysis between the family physician supply and the 18 dependant variables listed in Table 3. Correlation values can be interpreted as:[30]

0.90–1.00 (–0.9 to –1.00)	Very high positive (negative) correlation
0.70–0.90 (–0.70 to –0.90)	High positive (negative) correlation
0.50–0.70 (–0.50 to –0.70)	Moderate positive (negative) correlation
0.30–0.50 (–0.30 to –0.50)	Low positive (negative) correlation
0.00–0.30 (0.00 to –0.30)	Negligible correlation.

Graphs were generated using Stata™ version 13.1 to illustrate the relationship between the data points and the correlation (or regression) line. The data points were assigned unique colours and shapes to distinguish rural districts from urban subdistricts.

Ethics considerations

This study was approved by the Health Research Ethics Committee (HREC) at Stellenbosch University, protocol number N11/10/012, and was conducted according to accepted and applicable national and international ethical guidelines and principles, including those of the International Declaration of Helsinki October 2008. Permission was obtained from the Provincial Health Research Committee (PHRC) to conduct the research and to provide the routine data required. Data used in this research were collated at the subdistrict level and did not involve individual patient identifiers.

Results

Tables 5 and 6 present descriptive statistics for the independent and dependent variables, respectively, whilst Table 7 presents the results for the correlations between these variables.

Statistically significant correlations (see Table 7) could not be demonstrated at baseline in 2011 for family physician supply and the 18 dependent variables within the aforementioned framework (Figure 1).

A significant positive correlation was observed between medical officers and hospital expenditure as well as between nurses and primary health care (PHC) expenditure (Table 7). Nurses were significantly correlated with the presence of a chronic care team, isoniazid prophylaxis for TB, higher perinatal and under-5 mortality, as well as lower audit scores for diabetes and hypertension care. The presence of other specialists was significantly correlated with lower access to care.

Figures 2 and 3 illustrate the scatter of data between urban and rural data points and regression lines.

Discussion

The study did not find a strong baseline relationship between the supply of family physicians and the selected indicators of health system performance, clinical processes and outcomes. Whilst most of the correlations between family physicians

TABLE 5: Descriptive statistics of independent variables (number of observations = 13 [organisational units]).

Independent variable	Mean (s.d.)	Median (IQR)	Range: maximum (minimum)
Family physician	0.04 (0.03)	0.05 (0.2–0.54)	0.1 (0)
Nurse	13.13 (6.75)	12.48 (11.44–14.85)	31.68 (3.88)
Medical officer	1.49 (0.58)	1.40 (1.12–1.88)	2.30 (0.65)
Other specialist	0.18 (0.15)	0.16 (0.10–0.28)	0.52 (0)

s.d., standard deviation; IQR, interquartile ranges.

TABLE 6: Descriptive statistics of dependent variables (number of observations = 13 [organisational units]).

Dependent variable (framework domain)	Mean (s.d.)	Median (IQR)	Range: maximum (minimum)
PHC utilisation (access)	3.29 (0.49)	3.37 (2.95–3.70)	4.05 (2.54)
Access (access)	0.20 (0.32)	0.20 (0.03–0.44)	0.70 (–0.43)
Teamwork (coordination)	0.73 (0.18)	0.77 (0.63–0.88)	1.00 (0.41)
Chronic care team (coordination)	0.51 (0.27)	0.54 (0.36–0.67)	1.00 (0)
Hospital expenditure (efficiency)	1475.37 (453.06)	1772.59 (1273.67–1772.59)	2272.16 (728.97)
PHC expenditure (efficiency)	813.17 (360.03)	804.66 (620.24–901.42)	1644.59 (280.62)
Cervical smears (clinical processes)	0.76 (0.17)	0.77 (0.70–0.78)	1.11 (0.46)
Isoniazid prophylaxis (clinical processes)	0.09 (0.10)	0.07 (0.19–0.15)	0.35 (0.01)
TB treatment (clinical processes)	0.88 (0.06)	0.89 (0.84–0.90)	0.95 (0.76)
CYPR (clinical processes)	0.45 (0.09)	0.43 (0.41–0.47)	0.62 (0.32)
Early antenatal booking (clinical processes)	0.57 (0.11)	0.54 (0.49–0.68)	0.71 (0.41)
Immunisation (clinical processes)	0.88 (0.13)	0.87 (0.80–0.91)	1.18 (0.71)
Diabetes score (clinical processes)	0.48 (0.13)	0.49 (0.45–0.54)	0.68 (0.22)
Hypertension score (clinical processes)	0.53 (0.16)	0.55 (0.51–0.59)	0.78 (0.23)
TB cure (outcomes)	0.81 (0.05)	0.85 (0.79–0.86)	0.90 (0.73)
Maternal mortality (outcomes)	3.32 (4.59)	1.73 (0–3.88)	11.38 (0)
Perinatal mortality (outcomes)	140.05 (70.91)	112.61 (91.72–185.66)	272.23 (40.03)
Under-5 mortality (outcomes)	48.83 (52.49)	46.10 (3.65–92.71)	166.05 (0)

s.d., standard deviation; IQR, interquartile ranges; PHC, primary health care, TB, tuberculosis.

TABLE 7: Spearman's rho correlations between independent variables (Table 2) and dependent variables (Table 3).

Dependent variable (framework domain)	Family physician	Medical officer	Nurse	Other specialist
	Correlation coefficient (*p*-value)	Correlation coefficient (*p*-value)	Correlation coefficient (*p*-value)	Correlation coefficient (*p*-value)
PHC utilisation (access)	-0.27 (0.37)	0.18 (0.55)	0.09 (0.76)	-0.27 (0.36)
Access (access)	-0.13 (0.70)	-0.24 (0.46)	-0.19 (0.56)	-0.79* (< 0.01)
Teamwork (coordination)	0.09 (0.76)	0.27 (0.37)	0.47 (0.10)	0.19 (0.54)
Chronic care team (coordination)	0.38 (0.20)	-0.33 (0.27)	-0.83* (< 0.01)	-0.02 (0.94)
Hospital expenditure (efficiency)	-0.13 (0.70)	0.78* (< 0.01)	0.24 (0.44)	0.25 (0.43)
PHC expenditure (efficiency)	0.04 (0.90)	0.45 (0.13)	0.98* (< 0.01)	0.10 (0.73)
Cervical smears (clinical processes)	0.09 (0.76)	-0.33 (0.26)	0.25 (0.42)	-0.54 (0.05)
Isoniazid prophylaxis (clinical processes)	0.13 (0.68)	-0.13 (0.67)	0.56* (0.04)	-0.41 (0.16)
TB treatment (clinical processes)	0.09 (0.77)	-0.17 (0.58)	0.34 (0.25)	-0.10 (0.74)
CYPR (clinical processes)	0.32 (0.28)	0.00 (1.00)	0.45 (0.14)	-0.54 (0.05)
Early antenatal booking (clinical processes)	0.23 (0.45)	-0.47 (0.11)	0.50 (0.08)	-0.20 (0.52)
Immunisation (clinical processes)	0.03 (0.93)	-0.19 (0.53)	-0.08 (0.79)	0.37 (0.20)
Diabetes score (clinical processes)	-0.09 (0.76)	-0.25 (0.41)	-0.95* (< 0.01)	0.01 (0.96)
Hypertension score (clinical processes)	-0.15 (0.65)	-0.24 (0.42)	-0.84* (< 0.01)	0.23 (0.45)
TB cure (outcomes)	0.19 (0.53)	0.09 (0.94)	-0.33 (0.27)	0.24 (0.42)
Maternal mortality (outcomes)	-0.07 (0.83)	-0.08 (0.76)	-0.25 (0.41)	0.28 (0.34)
Perinatal mortality (outcomes)	0.17 (0.58)	-0.06 (0.85)	0.66* (0.01)	-0.26 (0.38)
Under-5 mortality (outcomes)	-0.01 (0.97)	0.06 (0.84)	0.67* (0.01)	-0.37 (0.21)

PHC, primary health care, TB, tuberculosis.
*, Statistically significant correlation (*p* < 0.05)

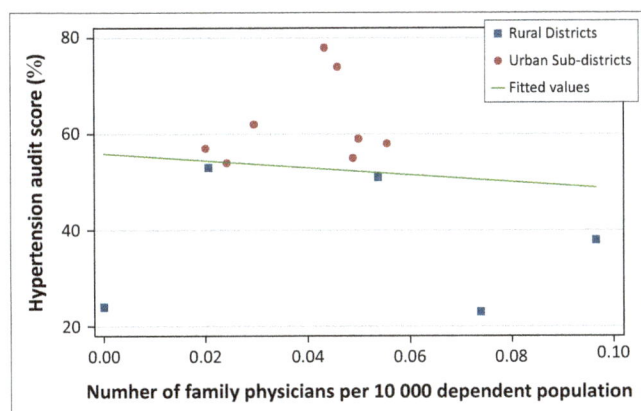

FIGURE 2: Scatter plot and regression line illustrating the correlation between family physician supply and hypertension scores in the annual chronic disease audit of District Health Services facilities.

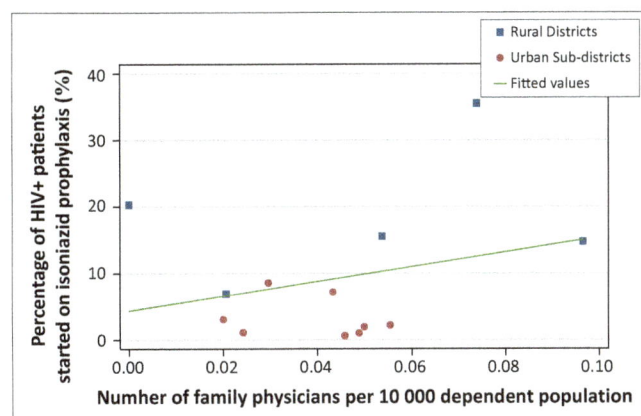

FIGURE 3: Scatter plot and regression line illustrating the correlation between family physician supply and the percentage of HIV-positive patients started on isoniazid prophylaxis for tuberculosis.

and selected indicators within the conceptual framework (Figure 1) were positive, they were weak in magnitude. As this study reports data at baseline, during the first year that specialist family physicians were available to the DHS, it is

not surprising that no strong relationship could be found. In addition, although the study made use of data from the whole province, the small number of units of analysis will have reduced the power of the study to show a statistically significant relationship.

The segregation of data points between rural and urban subdistrict or district in the graphs (Figures 2 and 3) is an indication that there may be confounding factors linked to the degree of rurality. These factors were mentioned in the adjustment models of previous large studies from the USA.[2,11,12] Vogel and Ackerman pointed out that there was significant variation in the population in terms of composition and determinants of health beyond those that were measured and adjusted for in previous research.[14,31]

The correlations in Table 7 may be confounded by known and unknown factors. Access and health outcome variables are particularly prone to confounding by social determinants of health beyond the immediate scope of the family physicians. Given that family physicians' roles include improving clinical governance and teaching junior staff, one would expect districts with higher supplies of family physicians to perform better in audits of clinical processes and in coordination of care.

Limitations of the study design

The issue of temporality is an important limitation of this cross-sectional ecological study. These correlations cannot determine the direction of any underlying cause and effect between the variables. Therefore causality between independent and dependent variables cannot be assumed.

As tempting as it may be, we cannot say that the significant negative association between other specialists and access is in keeping with Shi and Starfield's findings that specialist-dominated health systems have poorer performance.[12,13]

This was an observational study design with no control group. It was merely a 'dose-response' type analysis on an ecological level. This means that any findings, whether positive, negative or inconclusive, cannot be inferred to the level of the individual.

The significance of correlation co-efficient is of limited value with a small sample size.[32] The absence of statistical significance does not necessarily exclude the existence of correlations that could be regarded as important in this policy context.

Given that this study used a finite sample, some may argue that the magnitude of correlations observed can be taken at face value, regardless of the statistical significance. However, those correlations were observed for a period of only 1 year within the province, which limits the validity of non-significant findings beyond that period and beyond the Western Cape borders.

The Spearman's rank correlation test examines correlation between the indicator and the rank of the number of family physicians per population rather than the actual number of family physicians per population. Therefore, it does not factor in dramatic differences in the magnitude of the independent variable.

The selection of indicators was affected by deficiencies in the availability or reliability of data and therefore some indicators which might have been important in terms of the family physicians' impact could not be used.

Recommendations

This study has developed a methodology that can be repeated for subsequent years (2012–2014) to monitor how the relationships evolve over time and with an increasing number of family physicians.

Further research using an experimental or quasi-experimental design is needed to investigate the impact of family physicians on health outcomes. Findings from surveys and qualitative research methods[9] may also be used to determine whether family physicians are performing the envisioned tasks, whilst longitudinal studies may demonstrate their impact on generic, targeted and clinical processes. Cost-effectiveness of family physicians may also be evaluated in future studies.

Conclusion

We were unable to demonstrate strong correlations between family physician supply and clinical processes, health system performance or facility-based outcomes at the baseline of this ongoing study, but we were able to develop the methodology and to illustrate the presence of confounding

factors that were not included in similar research in other settings. Whilst it was arguably too early to show a strong correlation, this study also highlighted the limitations of this study design. Care should be taken not to assume causality within relationships found from such a design. In future it may be necessary to perform additional complementary research in order to triangulate and understand any emerging relationships.

Acknowledgements

We would like to thank the following people at the Western Cape Department of Health for providing us with data for this research: Lesley Shand (Information Management), Enrico Goodman (HAST), Razia Vallie (HAST), Shane Du Plooy (Finance), Michelle Buis (Wellness & Diversity: Transformation Unit). Our thanks also go to Hassan Mahomed (Metro District Health Services) for providing additional public health technical support, to Justin Harvey and Tonya Esterhuizen for statistician support.

Competing interests

The authors declare that they have no financial or personal relationship(s) that may have inappropriately influenced them in writing this article.

Authors' contributions

R.E.D. (University of Stellenbosch, Western Cape Government: Health) was the primary researcher. He coordinated the selection of the health indicators for this study, collected the routine data, performed the analysis and wrote the article. R.M. (University of Stellenbosch) was the study leader. He designed the over-arching bigger study, of which this research work forms a part. He provided appropriate and valuable guidance towards the completion of this work. T.N. (Western Cape Government: Health) was a secondary author and contributed towards the initial design of the study.

References

1. Mash R. Reflections on the development of family medicine in the Western Cape: a 15-year review. S Afr Fam Pract. 2011;53(6):557–562. http://dx.doi.org/10.1080/20786204.2011.10874152

2. Starfield B, Shi L, Macinko J. Contribution of primary care to health systems and health. Milbank Q. 2005;83(3):457–502. http://dx.doi.org/10.1111/j.1468-0009.2005.00409.x

3. The Alma-Ata conference on primary health care. WHO Chron. 1978;32(11):409–430.

4. WHO, Lerberghe W. The World Health Report 2008 – Primary health care (Now more than ever). Geneva: World Health Organization; 2008.

5. National health insurance in South Africa – Policy paper. Government Gazette. 2011;554 (No. 34523).

6. Chapter 10: Promoting Health. National Development Plan 2030. Pretoria: Government Printers; 2012; p. 330–351.

7. Mash R, South African Academy of Family Physicians. The contribution of family physicians to district health services: a position paper for the National Department of Health [homepage on the Internet]. 2014 [cited 2015 Jan 22]. Available from: http://www.saafp.org/index.php/news/48-national-position-paper-on-family-medicine.

8. Pasio KS, Mash R, Naledi T. Development of a family physician impact assessment tool in the district health system of the Western Cape Province, South Africa. BMC Fam Pract. 2014;15(1):204. http://dx.doi.org/10.1186/s12875-014-0204-7

9. Swanepoel M, Mash B, Naledi T. Assessment of the impact of family physicians in the district health system of the Western Cape, South Africa. Afr J Prm Health Care Fam Med. 2014;6(1), Art. #695, 8 pages. http://dx.doi.org/10.4102/phcfm.v6i1.695

10. Househam KC. Annual performance plan 2011/2012. Cape Town: Western Cape Department of Health; 2011.

11. Shi L. The relationship between primary care and life chances. J Health Care Poor Underserved. 1992;3(2):321–335. http://dx.doi.org/10.1353/hpu.2010.0460

12. Shi L. Primary care, specialty care, and life chances. Int J Health Serv. 1994;24(3):431–458. http://dx.doi.org/10.2190/BDUU-J0JD-BVEX-N90B

13. Starfield B, Shi L, Grover A, et al. The effects of specialist supply on populations' health: assessing the evidence. Heal Aff (Millwood). 2005;Suppl Web Exclusives:W5-97-W5-107. http://dx.doi.org/10.1377/hlthaff.w5.97

14. Vogel RL, Ackermann RJ. Is primary care physician supply correlated with health outcomes? Int J Health Serv. 1998;28(1):183–196. http://dx.doi.org/10.2190/3B1X-EE5T-T7GR-KGUD

15. Barati O, Maleki M, Gohari M, et al. The impact of family physician program on health indicators in Iran (2003–2007). Payesh. 2012;11(3):361–363.

16. Shi L, Starfield B, Kennedy B, et al. Income inequality, primary care, and health indicators. J Fam Pract. 1999;48(4):275–284.

17. Macinko J, Starfield B, Shi L. Quantifying the health benefits of primary care physician supply in the United States. Int J Health Serv. 2007;37(1):111–126. http://dx.doi.org/10.2190/3431-G6T7-37M8-P224

18. Mash R, Reid S. Statement of consensus on family medicine in Africa. Afr J Prm Health Care Fam Med. 2010;2(1), Art. #151, 4 pages. http://dx.doi.org/10.4102/phcfm.v2i1.151

19. Mash R. The definition of family medicine in sub-Saharan Africa. S Afr Fam Pract. 2008;50(3):58–59. http://dx.doi.org/10.1080/20786204.2008.10873719

20. Mash R, Moosa S, De Maeseneer J. Exploring the key principles of family medicine in sub-Saharan Africa: international Delphi consensus process. S Afr Fam Pract. 2008;50(3):60–65. http://dx.doi.org/10.1080/20786204.2008.10873720

21. Comprehensive service plan for the implementation of healthcare 2010. Cape Town: Western Cape Department of Health; 2007.

22. Househam C. Official circular H13/2010: Population data. Cape Town: Western Cape Department of Health; 2010.

23. Census 2011 statistical release – P0301.4. Pretoria: Statistics South Africa; 2012.

24. Groenewald P, Berteler M, Bradshaw D, et al. Western Cape mortality 2010. Cape Town: South African Medical Research Council; 2013.

25. Lilford RJ, Chilton PJ, Hemming K, et al. Evaluating policy and service interventions: framework to guide selection and interpretation of study end points. Br Med J (Clin Res Ed). 2010;341:c4413. http://dx.doi.org/10.1136/bmj.c4413

26. Kringos DS, Boerma WG, Hutchinson A, et al. The breadth of primary care: a systematic literature review of its core dimensions. BMC Health Serv Res. 2010;10:65. http://dx.doi.org/10.1186/1472-6963-10-65

27. Tarimo E. Towards a healthy district: organizing and managing district health systems based on primary health care. Geneva: The World Health Organization; 1991.

28. Vallabhjee K, Dettling V. Healthcare 2030: the road to wellness. Cape Town: Western Cape Department of Health; 2013.

29. Altman DG, Bland JM. Standard deviations and standard errors. Br Med J (Clin Res Ed. 2005;331(7521):903. http://dx.doi.org/10.1136/bmj.331.7521.903

30. Mukaka MM. Statistics corner: a guide to appropriate use of correlation coefficient in medical research. Malawi Med J. 2012;24(3):69–71.

31. America's public health report card: a state-by-state report on the health of the public. Washington, DC: American Public Health Association; 1992.

32. Oller, DK. Primer on research: Interpretation of correlation. ASHA Lead. 2006;11(15):24–26.

24

Opinions of South African optometry students about working in rural areas after graduation

Authors:
Khathutshelo P. Mashige[1]
Olalekan A. Oduntan[1]
Rekha Hansraj[1]

Affiliations:
[1]Discipline of Optometry, School of Health Sciences, University of KwaZulu-Natal, South Africa

Correspondence to:
Khathutshelo Mashige

Email:
mashigek@ukzn.ac.za

Postal address:
Private Bag X54001, Durban 4000, South Africa

Background: Eye and vision problems have been reported to be more prevalent in rural than urban areas; and a large proportion of South Africans live in the rural areas.

Aim: To investigate the opinions of South African optometry students about working in rural areas after completion of their training and to identify factors that may influence their decisions.

Method: This was a cross-sectional quantitative study using a survey instrument containing both closed and open-ended, semi-structured questions.

Results: Four hundred and thirty-eight students responded to the questionnaire (85.4% response rate). Overall, many of the respondents did not want to open their first (66%) or second practices (64.6%) in the rural areas. However, most respondents from rural backgrounds reported that they would open their first (77.2%) or second (79.4%) practice in the rural areas. The main reasons cited by the respondents for their unwillingness to work in the rural areas were financial concerns (81.2%), personal safety (80.1%) and poor living conditions (75.3%), with a significantly higher number ($p < 0.05$) being from urban respondents for the latter two issues only.

Conclusion: Many students were not in favour of opening practices in rural areas, but were willing to work for the government or a non-governmental organisation after graduation. Efforts should be made to address financial incentives, safety and living conditions in the rural areas. The results of this study have implications for the future of availability and accessibility of eye care services to those living in the rural and remote areas of the country.

Opinions des étudiants sud-africains en optométrie sur la possibilité de travailler dans les zones rurales après l'obtention de leur diplôme.

Contexte: Les problèmes des yeux et de vision sont plus courants dans les zones rurales qu'en ville; et une forte proportion de Sud-africains vit dans les zones rurales.

Objectif: Examiner les opinions des étudiants sud-africains en optométrie sur la possibilité de travailler dans les zones rurales après avoir terminé leur formation et identifier les facteurs pouvant influencer leur décision.

Méthode: C'est une étude quantitative transversale utilisant un instrument de sondage contenant des questions semi-structurées fermée et ouvertes.

Résultats: Quatre cent trente-huit étudiants ont répondu au questionnaire (un taux de réponse de 85.4%). En général, un grand nombre de répondants ne voulaient pas ouvrir leur premier (66%) ou deuxième cabinet (64.6%) dans les zones rurales. Cependant, la plupart des répondants originaires de la campagne ont répondu qu'ils ouvriraient leur premier cabinet (77.2%) ou leur second (79.4%) dans les zones rurales. Les raisons principales citées par les répondants pour ne pas vouloir travailler dans les zones rurales étaient des préoccupations financières (81.2%), la sécurité personnelle (80.1%) et les mauvaises conditions de vie (75.3%), avec un plus grand nombre ($p < 0.05$) de la part des répondants urbains pour les deux derniers problèmes.

Conclusion: Beaucoup d'étudiants ne voulaient pas ouvrir de cabinet dans les zones rurales, mais étaient prêts à travailler pour le gouvernement ou une organisation non-gouvernementale après l'obtention de leur diplôme. Il faudra s'occuper des incitations financières, de la sécurité et des conditions de vie dans les zones rurales. Les résultats de cette étude ont des implications pour le futur de la disponibilité et de l'accessibilité des services de soins oculaires pour ceux qui vivent dans les zones rurales et les régions reculées du pays.

Introduction

Visual impairment (low vision and blindness) is a major health problem worldwide, the prevalence being likely to increase significantly as the percentage of elderly people increases, as this section of the population is often affected.[1] Whilst most cases of visual impairment are preventable or manageable by surgery and/or refractive error corrections,[2,3,4,5] the prevalence rates remain high in many countries. This is particularly the case in developing nations, for a variety of reasons, including the following:

- **Availability:** Eye care services are not readily available, either because of a lack of trained personnel or because eye care practitioners are concentrated in urban areas.[6,7,8,9] Consequently, people in rural areas with treatable eye conditions are largely unattended to, whilst city facilities remain underutilised.[10,11]
- **Accessibility:** Many people, particularly those in rural areas, do not have access to eye care services. Factors such as lack of funds for transport to eye care facilities may result in poor access to eye care services.[12,13]
- **Affordability:** As eye care services are often provided by private practitioners or on a cost-recovery basis, rather than being freely available through government facilities, many people cannot afford them.[14,15,16,17]

In view of the fact that many causes of visual impairment are preventable, the World Health Organization (WHO) and the International Agency for the Prevention of Blindness (IAPB), with an international membership of non-governmental organisations (NGOs), professional associations, eye care institutions and corporations, developed the global Vision 2020 initiative: the Right to Sight Campaign.[18] This initiative has set goals to eliminate preventable blindness by the year 2020.[18] According to the WHO in 2000,[18] one of the most complex challenges facing policy makers in all countries is ensuring that people living in rural and remote areas have access to trained health workers. Worldwide, a shortage of qualified health workers in remote and rural areas impedes access to healthcare services for a significant percentage of the population, slows progress toward attainment of the Millennium Development Goals (MDGs) and challenges aspirations of achieving the WHO initiative, Health for All.[18]

As with many developing countries, poor access to eye care services is one of the major healthcare challenges facing South Africa.[19] A large proportion of South Africans live in rural areas,[20] where reports indicate poor access to eye care services. For 2014, Statistics South Africa estimated the mid-year South African population to be approximately 54 million, using the cohort-component methodology.[21] Forty-two-and-a-half per cent of the South African population lived in rural areas, according to the latest available data.[22] A recent study by Thivhafuni[23] found poor availability, accessibility and affordability of optometric eye care services in the Mutale Municipality of Vhembe District, Limpopo Province, South Africa. As with many other rural areas, this is because most optometric services in the country are privately owned, making them unaffordable to many citizens, specifically those living in rural areas.[19,24]

No studies were found that explored the reasons for poor eye care services in rural areas, with a number of authors[25,26] having speculated about having access to a sustainable market who can afford their services. This article therefore aims to investigate South African optometry students' opinions about working in the rural areas after graduation, along with factors that may influence such views. Some of the recommendations of the WHO[27] for improving access to healthcare in rural and remote areas will be examined in this study.

Research methods and design
Design

This study followed a quantitative cross-sectional research design in the form of a questionnaire survey of all of the 2013 South African optometry undergraduate students. All the undergraduate optometry students (first year to fourth year) who agreed to participate in the study were included. The study was conducted at all four institutions offering optometry courses in the country: universities of Free State (UFS), Johannesburg (UJ), KwaZulu-Natal (UKZN) and Limpopo (UL). Each department offers a four-year Bachelor of Optometry (BOptom) degree.

Questionnaire

The content and design of the questionnaire was based on a review of other studies,[20,28,29,30] being modified to suit the objectives of the study. The survey took approximately 30 minutes to complete and consisted of 31 questions that explored the following areas:

1. Demographic characteristics: age, gender, marital status, race, institution of learning, year of study, province of origin and place of origin (rural versus urban).
2. Views about practice choice: to establish why they did or did not want to practise in rural areas. This was assessed with questions such as: 'If you were to start a practice, would you establish your first practice in the rural area? – "YES or NO"?'.
3. Possible attractions and incentives: a list of factors was provided and the students indicated whether they were 'very', 'moderately', 'slightly', 'not really' or 'not at all' attractive with regard to the desire to engage in rural optometric practice.

Procedure

All first- to fourth-year South African students were included in this study, with non-South Africans being excluded. A self-administered questionnaire written in English, the official language of the optometry training in South African institutions, was used. Copies of the questionnaire were distributed by hand between June and October 2013 to all optometry students who agreed to participate in the study by staff at each institution.

Data analysis

Data were captured and analysed with the Statistical Programme of Social Sciences (SPSS), version 19.0 (IBM SPSS Inc., Chicago, IL 2010). Responses from the open-ended questions were grouped into common themes and collated. The number of respondents stating a particular response was noted. Descriptive statistics were used to establish values such as means, standard deviation, frequencies and percentages of the collected data. Chi-square tests were used to establish associations between relevant variables. A p-value of < 0.05 was considered statistically significant.

Ethical considerations

Ethical approval to conduct the study was obtained from the Human and Social Sciences Research and Ethics Committee of the University of KwaZulu-Natal (Reference Number: HSS/0067/013). Permission to collect data was obtained from the Head of each Optometry Department at all four universities that offer the programme in South Africa. All those who took part in the study signed the consent form and were provided with the necessary information.

Trustworthiness

The data were collected by an optometric staff member in each of the four institutions. The sample size was high enough to represent the study population. Participants were encouraged to be frank and honest in their responses, with the assurance that their identity will be kept confidential. All literature sources, data and materials utilised and represented by the authors in the paper are credible, dependable and can be verified.

Reliability

Prior to the main study, a pilot study was conducted using 10 students who were not part of the main study to establish the appropriateness of the study procedures, the methods and logistics. These participants were given the questionnaire for completion and retested after four weeks. The responses obtained during the two sessions were similar. All queries that arose from the pilot study were addressed and the questionnaire modified accordingly before the main study was conducted.

Validity

The validity of the findings in this study was ensured by using an adequate sample size and by including all the optometry departments in South African universities. Optometric staff members in each institution distributed and collected the questionnaire, after which a qualified statistician provided expert advice and support with the data analysis.

TABLE 1: Demographics of the 2013 South African optometry students ($n = 438$).

Characteristics	n	%
Age		
17–19	208	47.5
20–21	149	34
>21	81	18.5
Gender		
Male	144	32.9
Female	294	67.1
Race		
Black people	173	39.5
Mixed-race	2	0.5
Indian	118	26.9
White people	145	33.1
Marital status		
Single	425	97
Married	13	3
Place of origin		
Urban	285	65.1
Rural	153	34.9
Province of study		
Eastern Cape	32	7.3
Free State	74	16.9
Gauteng	87	19.9
KwaZulu-Natal	102	23.3
Limpopo	96	21.9
North-West	16	3.7
Mpumalanga	13	3.0
Northern Cape	7	1.6
Western Cape	11	2.5
Training institution		
UFS	75	17.1
UJ	93	21.2
UKZN	145	33.1
UL	125	28.5
Year of study		
1st	133	30.4
2nd	118	26.9
3rd	97	22.1
4th	90	20.5

UFS, University of Free State; UJ, University of Johannesburg; UKZN, University of KwaZulu-Natal; UL, University of Limpopo.

Results

The results are presented with respect to the three categories of the questionnaire: demographic characteristics; their views about working in the rural areas; and possible attractions and incentives.

Demographic characteristics

Of the 513 eligible South African undergraduate optometry students who were registered in 2013, 438 completed the questionnaire, giving a response rate of 85.4%. Their ages ranged from 17 to 35 years, with a mean of 21.1 ± 1.8 years. The majority ($n = 294$; 67.1%) were women, had never married (97%), and were from urban areas ($n = 285$; 65.1%). Slightly less than one-quarter ($n = 145$; 23.3%) of the respondents were from the UKZN, and 133 (30.4%) were in their first year of optometric study (Table 1). The majority of optometry students ($n = 123$; 98%) at University of Limpopo (UL) were black people, whilst there were more white students at

TABLE 2: Respondents' views about working in rural areas.

Variables	Characteristics	Rural		Urban		Total	
		n	%	*n*	%	*n*	%
Establish first practice in the rural area	Yes	115	77.2	34	22.8	149	34.0
	No	53	18.3	236	81.7	289	66.0
Establish second practice in the rural area	Yes	123	79.4	32	20.6	155	35.4
	No	79	27.9	204	72.1	283	64.6
Employed by government	Yes	153	51.5	144	48.5	297	67.8
	No	63	44.7	78	55.3	141	32.2
Employed by non-government organisation	Yes	153	54.6	127	45.4	280	63.9
	No	67	42.4	91	57.6	158	36.1
Reasons not to practise in the rural area	Financial concerns	150	42.1	206	57.9	356	81.3
	Personal safety	122	34.8	229	65.2	351	80.1
	Poor living conditions	99	30	231	70	330	75.3
	Language barrier	74	36.5	129	63.5	203	46.3
Motivation to accept government job in the rural area	Good salary	124	46.4	143	53.6	267	61.0
	Proximity to home	101	100	0	0	101	23.1
	Inability to find a job	33	36.3	58	63.7	91	21.0
	Help the community	113	80.7	27	19.3	140	32.0
Community service for graduates	Yes	82	61.7	51	38.3	133	30.4
	No	39	12.8	266	87.2	305	69.6

TABLE 3: Factors that would influence their decision to engage in rural optometric practice.

Factors	Level of attractiveness					
	Not at all *n* (%)	Not really *n* (%)	Slight *n* (%)	Moderate *n* (%)	Very *n* (%)	Moderate and Very combined
Enhanced profiles of rural health workers	7 (1.6)	27 (6.2)	118 (26.9)	88 (20.1)	198 (45.2)	286 (65.3)
Outreach interaction between the rural and urban health workers	9 (2.1)	14 (3.2)	99 (22.6)	111 (25.3)	205 (46.8)	316 (72.1)
Facilities for knowledge exchange to reduce sense of professional isolation	5 (1.1)	32 (7.3)	81 (18.5)	90 (20.5)	230 (52.5)	320 (73)
Enhance scope of practice	7 (1.6)	20 (4.6)	79 (18)	116 (26.5)	216 (49.3)	332 (75.8)
Facilities for Professional Development	13 (3.0)	19 (4.3)	66 (15.1)	165 (37.7)	175 (39.9)	340 (77.6)
Scholarship and bursary to study	21 (4.8)	27 (6.2)	24 (5.5)	65 (14.8)	302 (68.9)	367 (83.7)
Career ladder for rural health workers	9 (2.1)	17 (3.9)	45 (10.3)	97 (22.1)	270 (61.6)	367 (83.7)
Better living conditions	13 (3.0)	13 (3.0)	32 (7.3)	62 (14.2)	318 (72.6)	380 (86.8)
Financial incentives	8 (1.8)	10 (2.3)	31 (7.1)	59 (13.5)	330 (75.3)	389 (88.8)
Conducive or favourable working environment	3 (0.7)	8 (1.8)	35 (8.0)	67 (15.3)	325 (74.2)	392 (89.5)

the UFS ($n = 64$; 85.7%) and UJ ($n = 57$; 61.1%), respectively. At UKZN, 75 (52%) of the students were black people and 54 (37%) were Indians.

Of the respondents from rural areas ($n = 153$; 34.9%), the majority attended primary ($n = 138$; 90.2%) and high schools ($n = 125$; 81.7%) in the same rural area. Most respondents from rural areas returned home for their holidays ($n = 126$; 82.4%) to visit family members ($n = 148$; 96.7%).

Respondents' views about working in rural areas

Overall, most respondents reported no desire to establish their first ($n = 289$; 66%) or second ($n = 283$; 64.6%) practice in a rural area. However, most respondents from rural backgrounds reported that they would open their first ($n = 115$; 77.2%), or second ($n = 123$; 79.4%) practice in a rural area. There was a significant difference between urban and rural respondents ($p < 0.05$) regarding practice location. Many respondents indicated that they would accept an offer from the government ($n = 297$; 67.8%) or an NGO ($n = 280$; 63.9%) to work in a rural area, with no significant difference between urban and rural respondents ($p > 0.05$). Of those

who did not intend to work in rural areas, most cited finances ($n = 356$; 81.2%) and personal safety ($n = 351$; 80.1%) as being major concerns.

Although there was a significantly higher number ($p < 0.05$) of respondents from urban areas who reported not wanting to work in rural areas, there was no significant difference ($p > 0.05$) between urban and rural respondents regarding 'financial concerns' as an impediment to working in the rural areas. Sixty-one per cent indicated that a good salary would be a motivation for them to accept a government job offer in the rural area, there being no significant difference ($p > 0.05$) between urban and rural respondents. Most respondents ($n = 305$; 69.6%) did not agree with the proposed compulsory community service for graduating optometrists, with a significantly higher number being from urban respondents ($p < 0.05$) (Table 2).

Regarding possible attractions and incentives, the students rated 'financial incentives' ($n = 330$; 75.3%), 'acceptable working conditions' ($n = 325$; 74.2%), 'scholarship and bursary to study' ($n = 302$; 68.9%) and 'career ladder for rural health workers' ($n = 270$; 61.6%) as very attractive factors that would influence them to work in a rural area (Table 3).

A combination of 'Moderate' and 'Very' scores however, indicated that many students would be willing to work in rural areas.

Discussion

Most students studying optometry were relatively young, possibly because the majority apply for admission to the BOptom programme during their matric (final) year. The gender distribution of the respondents indicated that the number of women was similar across all training institutions, with more women (67.1%) than men (32.9%) either seeing optometry as a career option or being accepted into the programme. These findings are similar to those of Mashige and Oduntan[24] in 2011, who reported more female (69.5%) than male (30.5%) students study Optometry in South African institutions. Although the number of black students was on average higher than other race groups, historically white institutions still had the highest number of white students and a traditional black institution had the highest number of black students. Also noteworthy is the significantly low proportion of mixed-race students in all institutions. These racial disparities suggest that optometry departments at these universities should strengthen their efforts to fully effect a change in the student demographics. The majority of the students were from the provinces where institutions with optometry departments are located (Table 1). This again suggests the need for admission policies of training institutions to be re-evaluated and for there to be greater representation of students from provinces where there are no optometry departments. Mashige and Oduntan[24] suggested that such steps could help to change the demographics and distribution of the optometric workforce in the country. The cohort of students surveyed in this study had strong urban representation and contributed a substantial proportion (65.1%) of respondents (Table 1).

In a developing country such as South Africa, rural community residents are at greater risk of having visual impairment because of a scarcity of eye care services. This scarcity is compounded by the poor distribution of the eye care practitioners who are concentrated in the urban areas, leaving the rural areas without services.[11,19,20] In addition, non-availability,[6,7,8,9] poor accessibility[12,13] and non-affordability[14,15,16,17] are barriers to eye care utilisation. These are the major reasons for a greater prevalence of visual impairment amongst residents of rural communities.

Our study also shows that the majority of students from a rural background were willing to return and work in their area of origin. Optometric institutions should attract students from rural areas with academic potential and, if necessary, provide them with academic support or extended curriculum programmes in order to ensure their success. Studies have suggested that graduates from rural areas are more likely to return to their home areas to practise,[31,32,33] providing affordable eye care services and eliminating the costs of transportation to urban areas. It is important to emphasise that these four teaching institutions have no

special admission criteria for rural students, their admission criteria being based on merit and not expected practice location. Efforts should therefore be made to 'use targeted admission policies to enrol students with a rural background, in order to increase the likelihood of graduates choosing to practise in rural areas', as recommended by the WHO.[27] This is further supported in our study by the fact that whilst many respondents reported that they did not want to establish their first or second practice in a rural area, most respondents from rural backgrounds indicated that they would.

As with most health care facilities, the majority of optometric service facilities are located in the urban areas, leaving the majority of the citizens who live in the rural areas without such services. The South African government anticipates that the 'certificate of need' policy would contribute to reversal of this inequality in healthcare services, including optometric services. This policy means that a healthcare professional needs to get a certificate of need from the Director General of Health before establishing, constructing, modifying or acquiring a health establishment.[34] Hence, optometrists who wish to open a private practice or branch(es) will have to apply to the Department of Health for this certificate to give them permission to work in their chosen area. In this study, the majority of respondents, irrespective of origin, indicated that they would gladly accept a government or an NGO offer to work in rural areas. This underscores the value and possible impact of offering sufficient and well-paid employment opportunities in the rural areas. This view is reflected by responses in our study, with 81.3% indicating that financial concerns were an impediment to working in the rural areas (Table 2). Similarly, 61% of the respondents indicated the potential to earn a good income as motivation to accepting a government job in the rural area and 88.8% indicated that this would be a very attractive incentive. These incentives referred to above, together with others discussed below in this article, suggest that less restrictive options (compared to the certificate of need) may attract more optometry graduates to the rural areas where their services are so desperately needed. If the rural community dwellers cannot afford the cost of eye care services, these services may need to be provided as part of public healthcare, with government needing to explore the possibility of providing more eye care services in rural areas.

Sacharowitz[35] indicated that one of the greatest barriers to providing eye care services in South Africa, particularly in the rural areas, is that the previous health policies did not make provision for employing optometrists in government hospitals and clinics. However, Limpopo and KwaZulu-Natal Provinces are now prioritising eye care services as one of the healthcare focus areas, but it is taking a while for the other provinces to do the same. The establishment of posts and budgets for optometrists' salaries in the government or public health sector seem relatively straightforward. However, the financing of the provision of ophthalmic devices would be a major obstacle. It is important to acknowledge the efforts of NGOs, which provide spectacles free of charge in many government or public health sector facilities. It is suggested that the government partner with these NGOs by providing subsidies for spectacles and other assistive visual devices. In addition to ophthalmology clinics, the provincial Departments of Health has optometric services in many provincial hospitals, where they engage mostly in refraction.[36] These government initiatives should be expanded to other provinces. The government's efforts to improve optometric services in rural areas by providing optometry students scholarships annually to attract them to government services following completion of their studies should be expanded.[36] Salary packages for rural optometrists should be adjusted to include incentives such as rural allowances, grants for housing and free transportation. These incentives would attract new optometric graduates to rural areas and would be in line with the WHO[27] recommendation of increasing access to health workers in remote and rural areas.

A notable outcome from the responses from students of a rural background was the desire to serve community eye care needs and a return to their hometown. This reinforces the need for outreach programmes to recruit optometry students from rural areas, as these students enter their professions with an awareness of rural living and the eye care needs of their hometown.

Compulsory community service is an attempt by the government to address the shortage of healthcare professionals, particularly in rural and under-resourced areas.[29] It has been implemented for medical doctors, dentists, pharmacists, physiotherapists, occupational and speech therapists, clinical psychologists, dieticians, radiographers and environmental health officers. However, almost two decades post-apartheid, optometry in South Africa still does not offer community service opportunities.[37] More than two-thirds of the respondents (69.6%) were not in favour of compulsory community service for graduating optometrists, of whom an overwhelming majority were from urban areas. These findings are not surprising, as a previous study has shown that the initial announcement regarding implementing community service for medical doctors was received negatively by the affected students.[29] However, subsequent findings indicated that the majority of those eligible for community service did take up their posts and reported a positive experience.[29]

In this study, the majority of those who agreed with compulsory community service were from the rural areas. This is aligned with a report which indicates that social and personal reasons (the desire to help the community and close proximity to home) influence students' desire to return to and work in their hometown. Community service for graduating optometrists can therefore serve as a platform for urban students to experience the nature of rural clinical settings, lifestyles and sense of community. The WHO[27] recommendations imply that compulsory community service can improve appreciation of rural services and availability of health workers to rural areas. It is, therefore, recommended that the government speed up the implementation of community service for optometrists. This will help to identify the potential barriers to working in, as well as factors that may impede eventual deployment and retention in, rural areas.[38]

Other than economic (financial) incentives alone, personal factors (favourable working environment and better living conditions) were rated by the majority of students influencing their decision not to work in a rural area (Table 3). Studies[28,29] have shown that providing appropriate and adequate infrastructure, such as accommodation, is an important factor that would influence medical professionals to work in the rural areas. Although economic and personal factors were major considerations for students going to practise in the rural areas, it is also noteworthy that crime in the country was a major concern for the students (Table 2). Therefore, the issue of crime needs to be addressed by the government in order to attract and retain optometrists and other healthcare professionals in rural areas. Support and development (in terms of scholarship and bursary and career advancement) were also considered to be attractive options by both urban and rural students. Therefore, besides improving the supply of optometric manpower, training and career issues would also improve the standards of eye care services in the rural areas.

Strengths and limitations of the study

The strength of this study is that it provides information that could improve the availability and accessibility of eye care services in the rural and remote areas of South Africa. This will help to reduce visual impairment in these parts of the country. A limitation of the study is that it did not assess the method of financing their education, which could have influenced the students' responses. Another limitation is its quantitative nature and is therefore subjected to all the shortcomings of a quantitative study, such as limited in-depth understanding and investigation of the students' responses.[39]

Conclusion

This study has shown that few South African optometry students from urban areas have a desire to practise in rural areas after graduation, whilst those with a rural background are more inclined to pursue rural practice. However, many students, irrespective of location background, may opt to work in rural areas for NGOs or in the public sector after their training. Factors such as a conducive working environment, financial incentives, better living conditions and security featured as important factors that would attract graduating optometry students to rural areas, regardless of place of origin. The findings of this study have implications for the future of eye care services in the rural areas of South Africa. It is recommended that South African optometric institutions should accelerate and increase access and support for rural students with academic potential. There is also a need for establishing optometric training facilities in rural areas. It is acknowledged that implementing these recommendations may be challenging as they have serious financial implications for the government. A possible practical suggestion is that the government might have to look into strategies such as increasing health and education budgets in order to provide these needs.

Acknowledgements

The authors are grateful to the departments of Optometry in South Africa for permission to conduct this study and the optometry students for responding to the questionnaires. We thank Ms I. Melwa, Ms P. von Poser and Mr N. Naicker from the disciplines of Optometry at UL, UJ and UFS respectively for assisting with the administration of the questionnaires. We also thank Ms Carrin Martin for commenting on the manuscript.

Competing interests

The authors declare that they have no financial or personal relationship(s) that may have inappropriately influenced them in writing this article.

Authors' contributions

K.P.M. (UKZN) was the project leader who saw to the effective collection of data, write-up and submission. O.A.O. (UKZN) and R.H. (UKZN) were responsible for project execution, analysis of data and write-up. All authors contributed to the conceptualisations and writing of this article.

References

1. Resnikoff S, Pascolini D, Etya'ale D, et al. Global data on visual impairment in the year 2002. Bull World Health Org. 2004;82(11):844–851.

2. Lewallen S, Courtright P. Blindness in Africa: present and future needs. Brit J Ophthalmol. 2001;85(8):897–903. http://dx.doi.org/10.1136/bjo.85.8.897

3. Nwosu SNN. Beliefs and attitude to eye diseases and blindness in rural Anambra State, Nigeria. Nig J Ophthalmol. 2002;10(1):16–20. http://dx.doi.org/10.4314/njo.v10i1.11901

4. Frick KD, Foster A. The magnitude and cost of global blindness: An increasing problem that can be alleviated. Am J Ophthalmol. 2003;135(4):471–476. http://dx.doi.org/10.1016/S0002-9394(02)02110-4

5. Klauss V, Schaller UC. [Tropical Ophthalmology – prevention and therapy. 'Vision 2020' – The right to sight.] German. Ophthalmologe. 2004;101(7):741–765.

6. Buchanan N, Horwitz SM. Health policy and eye care services in Jamaica. Optom Vis Sci. 2000;77(1):51–57. http://dx.doi.org/10.1097/00006324-200001000-00014

7. Khan SA. Setting up low vision services in the developing world. Comm Eye Health. 2004;17(49):17–20.

8. Husainzada R. Situation analysis of human resources in eye care in Afghanistan. Comm Eye Health. 2007;20(61):12.

9. Okoye OI, Aghaji AE, Umeh RE, et al. Barriers to the provision of clinical low-vision services among ophthalmologists in Nigeria. Vis Imp Res. 2007;9(1):11–17. http://dx.doi.org/10.1080/13882350701198702

10. Di Stefano A. World optometry: The challenge of leadership for the new millennium. Optometry. 2002;73(6):339–350.

11. Ashaye A, Ajuwon A, Adeoti C. Perceptions of blindness and blinding eye conditions in rural communities. J Natl Med Assoc. 2006;98(6):887–893.

12. Chandrashekhar TS, Bhat HV, Pai RV, et al. Coverage, utilization and barriers to cataract surgical services in rural South India. Results from a population-based study. Public Health. 2007;121(2):130–136. http://dx.doi.org/10.1016/j.puhe.2006.07.027

13. Dhaliwal U, Gupta S. Barriers to uptake of cataract surgery in patients presenting to a hospital. Indian J Ophthalmol. 2007;55(2):133–136. http://dx.doi.org/10.4103/0301-4738.30708

14. Ndegwa LK, Karimurio J, Okelo RO, et al. Barriers to utilisation of eye care services in Kibera slums of Nairobi. East Afr Med J. 2005;82(10):506–508.

15. Habte D, Gebre T, Zerihun, et al. Determinants of uptake of surgical treatment for trachomatous trichiasis in North Ethiopia. Ophthalmic Epidemiol. 2008;15(5):328–333. http://dx.doi.org/10.1080/09286580801974897

16. Kovai V, Krishnaiah S, Shamanna BR, et al. Barriers to accessing eye care services among visually impaired population in rural Andhra Pradesh, South India. Indian J Ophthalmol. 2007;55(5):365–371. http://dx.doi.org/10.4103/0301-4738.33823

17. Palagyi A, Ramke J, du Toit R, et al. Eye care in Timor-Leste: A population-based study of utilization and barriers. Clin Experiment Ophthalmol. 2008;36(1):47–53. http://dx.doi.org/10.1111/j.1442-9071.2007.01645.x

18. World Health Organization. Elimination of affordable visual disability due to refractive errors: report of an informal planning meeting, Geneva, 03-05 July 2000. (WHO/PBL/00.79). Geneva: World Health Organization; 2000.

19. Mashige KP, Naidoo KS. Optometric practices and practitioners in KwaZulu-Natal, South Africa. S Afr Optom. 2010;69(2):77–85.

20. Oduntan AO, Louw A, Moodley VR, et al. Perceptions, expectations, apprehensions and realities of graduating South African optometry students (PEAR study, 2006). S Afr Optom. 2007;66(3):94–108.

21. Statistics South Africa. Mid-year population estimates 2014. Statistical release P0302 [document on the Internet]. c2014 [cited 2015 Mar 12]. Available from: http://beta2.statssa.gov.za/publications/P0302/P03022014.pdf

22. Statistics South Africa. Census 2001: investigation into appropriate definitions of urban and rural areas for South Africa [document on the Internet]. c2003 [cited 2015 Mar 12]. Available from: https://www.statssa.gov.za/census01/html/C2001urbanrural.asp

23. Thivhafuni G. Availability, accessibility and affordability of optometric services to the rural communities of the Mutale Municipality, Vhembe district, Limpopo Province, South Africa. Unpublished Master's dissertation, University of Limpopo, South Africa; 2011.

24. Mashige KP, Oduntan OA. Factors influencing South African optometry students in choosing their career and institution of learning. S Afr Optom. 2011;70(1):21–28.

25. Mashige KP, Martin C, Cassim B, et al. Utilization of eye care services by elderly persons in the northern Ethekwini district of KwaZulu-Natal province, South Africa. S Afr Optom. 2011;70(4):175–181.

26. Ntsoane MD, Oduntan OA, Mpolokeng BL. Utilisation of public eye care services by the rural community residents in the Capricorn district, Limpopo Province, South Africa. Afr J Prm Health Care Fam Med. 2012; 4(1), Art. #412, 7 pages. http://dx.doi.org/10.4102/phcfm.v4i1.412

27. World Health Organization. Increasing access to health workers in remote and rural areas through improved retention: global policy recommendations [document on the Internet]. c2010 [cited 2013 Feb]. Available from: http://whqlibdoc.who.int/publications/2010/9789241564014_eng.pdf

28. Buykx P, Humphreys J, Wakerman J, et al. Systematic review of effective retention incentives for health workers in rural and remote areas: Towards evidence-based policy. Aus J Rur Health. 2010;18(3):102–109. http://dx.doi.org/10.1111/j.1440-1584.2010.01139.x

29. Reid SJ. Compulsory community service for doctors in South Africa – an evaluation of the first year. S Afr Med J. 2001;91(4):329–336.

30. Jutzi L, Vogt K, Drever E, et al. Recruiting medical students to rural practice: Perspectives of medical students and rural recruiters. Can Fam Physician.2009;55(1):72–73.

31. Anzenberger P, Popov SB, Ostermann H. Factors that motivate young pharmacists to work in rural communities in the Ukraine. Rural Remote Health. 2011;11(4):1509.

32. McAuliffe T, Barnett F. Factors influencing occupational therapy students' perceptions of rural and remote practice. Rural Remote Health. 2009;9(1):1078.

33. Rabinowitz HK, Diamond JJ, Markham FW, et al. Medical school programs to increase the rural physician supply: A systematic review and projected impact of widespread replication. Acad Med. 2008;83(3):235–243. http://dx.doi.org/10.1097/ACM.0b013e318163789b

34. Hassim A, Haywood M, Berger J (editors). Health and Democracy: A guide to human rights, health law and policy in post-apartheid South Africa. Cape Town: Siber Ink; 2007.

35. Sacharowitz HS. Visual impairment in South Africa: Achievements and challenges. S Afr Optom. 2005;64(4):139–149.

36. Oduntan AO, Raliavhegwa M. An evaluation of the impact of the eye care services delivered to the rural communities in the Mankweng Health sub-district of the Northern Province. S Afr Optom. 2001;60(3):71–76.

37. Mashige KP, Rampersad N, Oduntan OA. Perceptions and opinions of graduating South African optometry students on the proposed community service. S Afr Optom. 2013;72(1):11–18.

38. Kaye DK, Mwanika A, Sekimpi P, et al. Perceptions of newly admitted undergraduate medical students on experiential training on community placements and working in rural areas of Uganda. BMC Med Educ. 2010;10:47. http://dx.doi.org/10.1186/1472-6920-10-47

39. Walker W. The strengths and weaknesses of research designs involving quantitative measures. J Res Nurs. 2005;10(5):571–582. http://dx.doi.org/10.1177/13614040960501000505

25

Auditing chronic disease care: Does it make a difference?

Authors:
Vivien Essel[1,2]
Unita van Vuuren[3]
Angela De Sa[4,5]
Srini Govender[5,7]
Katie Murie[4,5]
Arina Schlemmer[5,7]
Colette Gunst[6]
Mosedi Namane[4,5]
Andrew Boulle[2,8]
Elma de Vries[4,5]

Affiliations:
[1]Public Health Registrar, University of Cape Town, South Africa

[2]Western Cape Provincial Health Services, South Africa

[3]Chronic Disease Management, Western Cape Provincial Health Services, South Africa

[4]Family Physician, University of Cape Town, South Africa

[5]Western Cape Metro District Health Services, South Africa

[6]Cape Winelands District Health Services, Western Cape Government: Health, South Africa

[7]Family Physician, Stellenbosch University, South Africa

[8]Public Health Specialist, University of Cape Town, South Africa

Correspondence to:
Vivien Essel

Email:
vabaiden@yahoo.com

Postal address
5th Floor, Norton Rose House, 08 Riebeek Street, South Africa

Background: An integrated audit tool was developed for five chronic diseases, namely diabetes, hypertension, asthma, chronic obstructive pulmonary disease and epilepsy. Annual audits have been done in the Western Cape Metro district since 2009. The year 2012 was the first year that all six districts in South Africa's Western Cape Province participated in the audit process.

Aim: To determine whether clinical audits improve chronic disease care in health districts over time.

Setting: Western Cape Province, South Africa.

Methods: Internal audits were conducted of primary healthcare facility processes and equipment availability as well as a folder review of 10 folders per chronic condition per facility. Random systematic sampling was used to select the 10 folders for the folder review. Combined data for all facilities gave a provincial overview and allowed for comparison between districts. Analysis was done comparing districts that have been participating in the audit process from 2009 to 2010 ('2012 old') to districts that started auditing recently ('2012 new').

Results: The number of facilities audited has steadily increased from 29 in 2009 to 129 in 2012. Improvements between different years have been modest, and the overall provincial average seemed worse in 2012 compared to 2011. However, there was an improvement in the '2012 old' districts compared to the '2012 new' districts for both the facility audit and the folder review, including for eight clinical indicators, with '2012 new' districts being less likely to record clinical processes (OR 0.25, 95% CI 0.21–0.31).

Conclusion: These findings are an indication of the value of audits to improve care processes over the long term. It is hoped that this improvement will lead to improved patient outcomes.

Vérification des soins pour maladies chroniques: Cela fait-il une différence?

Contexte: Un instrument de vérification intégré a été conçu pour cinq maladies chroniques, telles que le diabète, l'hypertension, l'asthme, les maladies pulmonaires obstructives chroniques et l'épilepsie. Des vérifications annuelles ont été effectuées depuis 2009 dans la région métropolitaine du Western Cape. C'est en 2012 que pour la première fois les six districts de la Province du Western Cape en Afrique du Sud ont pris part au processus de vérification.

Objectif: Déterminer si les vérifications cliniques améliorent les soins pour maladies chroniques dans les districts sanitaires avec le temps.

Lieu: Province du Western Cape, Afrique du Sud.

Méthodes: On a fait des vérifications internes des processus et de la disponibilité des équipements dans les établissements de soins primaires, ainsi qu'une vérification de 10 dossiers par condition chronique par établissement. On a utilisé un programme d'échantillonnage aléatoire systématique pour sélectionner les 10 dossiers à vérifier. Les données combinées de tous les établissements ont fourni un aperçu provincial et permis de comparer les districts. On a fait une analyse pour comparer les districts qui ont pris part au processus de vérification de 2009 à 2010 ('2012 anciens') aux districts qui ont commencé la vérification récemment ('2012 nouveaux').

Résultats: Le nombre d'établissements vérifiés a augmenté progressivement de 29 en 2009 à 129 en 2012. Les améliorations entre les différentes années sont modestes et la moyenne générale provinciale semble pire en 2012 qu'en 2011. Cependant, on remarque une amélioration dans les districts "2012 anciens" par rapport aux districts '2012 nouveaux' pour la vérification des établissements et la vérification des dossiers, y compris huit indicateurs cliniques, avec les districts '2012 nouveaux' qui sont moins susceptibles d'enregistrer les processus cliniques (OR 0.25, 95% CI 0.21–0.31).

Conclusion: Ces résultats sont une indication de la valeur des vérifications pour améliorer les processus à long terme. Nous espérons que cette amélioration se traduira par de meilleurs résultats chez les patients.

Introduction

Globally there is a rapidly increasing burden of non-communicable diseases (NCDs). It is expected that by the year 2020, NCDs will account for 57% of the global burden of disease. This will be an increase of 11% from the 2001 figure of 46%.[1] Previously seen as diseases of the wealthy, NCDs are now a significant problem amongst the world's poor, especially in sub-Saharan Africa (SSA).

The age-standardised mortality rate due to NCDs was found to be higher in four SSA countries (Democratic Republic of Congo, Nigeria, Ethiopia and South Africa) compared to wealthier countries with a higher income.[2] South Africa at the moment is characterised by a quadruple burden of communicable, non-communicable, perinatal and maternal diseases, and injury-related disorders with NCDs, specifically cardiovascular diseases, type 2 diabetes, cancer, chronic lung disease and depression are on the rise in both rural and urban settings.[3] In South Africa's Western Cape Province from 2003 to 2006 pooled estimates of causes of death found NCDs to be the main cause of death amongst adults aged 40 years and older.[4]

There is increasing demand for chronic care at health facilities, and this is putting strain on services. Measures are needed to address the growing burden of NCDs in South Africa and in the Western Cape Province; without them it is estimated that NCDs will rise considerably in South Africa over the next decades.[3]

One such measure is the use of clinical audits as part of a surveillance system to improve the quality of care given to patients, especially in primary healthcare (PHC) settings.[5,6] The purpose of a clinical audit is to evaluate and measure one's own practice against a recognised professional standard. It reminds clinicians of the available standards and guidelines that relate to their practice, and identifies training needs.[7,8] Using clinical audits to improve services is not a new concept. Several studies including a meta-analysis have shown significant improvements in health services that were audited compared to those that were not.[9,10,11] Where there were improvements, the effects seen were generally small to moderate.[8,12] An evaluation of diabetic audits done from 2005 to 2009 in Cape Town, Western Cape, South Africa found an improvement in all nine clinical processes. The findings from this study showed that in resource-limited areas quality improvement can be attained by doing clinical audits.[13]

In the Western Cape Province NCDs account for a higher proportion of deaths in adults (58%) than seen nationally in the country (38%).[14] This prompted the Western Cape Department of Health to consider the management of people with NCDs comprehensively. For this reason the annual integrated chronic disease audit was established for five chronic diseases, namely diabetes, hypertension, asthma, chronic obstructive pulmonary disease (COPD) and epilepsy. The Integrated Audit for Chronic Disease Management follows from the work done on the Cardiovascular Risk Factor or Diabetic Audit that has been done in its Metro District since 2005.[13,15]

As part of a quality improvement project, clinical governance structures in the department proposed that an integrated audit be done. An annual integrated chronic disease audit which looks at chronic disease care and management of risk factors enables the Department of Health to identify gaps and strengthen its health systems, specifically PHC. Currently a separate HIV and/or AIDS, sexually transmitted diseases (STIs) and tuberculosis (TB) (HAST) audit is done annually in the province. In future it is envisioned for the Western Cape Province to have a truly integrated audit which will include all chronic conditions such as mental health and HIV infection.

The aim of this study was to assess the effectiveness of clinical audits done for NCD care over time in the Western Cape Province by comparing districts that have being participating in the audit process from 2009 and 2010 compared to districts that started auditing recently (2011 and/or 2012).

Methods
Study design

This cross-sectional study was an internal audit where facility staff members audited themselves. It is believed that by involving them, they will take ownership of the process and use the results to improve services at their own facilities. Staff members included family physicians, senior medical officers or clinical nurse practitioners at each facility. Family physicians, who were the facilitators for the audit process, held an annual teaching seminar prior to the audit where every staff member who was involved in the audit was trained in a standardised manner on the appropriate collection of data.

Setting and sampling

In the Western Cape Province there are six health districts (the Metro, Cape Winelands, Eden, Central Karoo, West Coast and Overberg). Chronic care in these six districts is mainly provided at PHC facilities. In 2012 there were 326 PHC facilities providing services to patients with NCDs. All six districts participated in the audit in 2012 and each district was asked to list the facilities providing chronic care in their district that would participate in the audit. Selection of facilities was based on feasibility to perform the audit.

Two components of the audit were evaluated using a standardised chronic disease audit tool. The two components looked at the facility's process and equipment availability as well as a folder review of five chronic conditions. Facility process and equipment involved auditing patient preparation rooms, consulting rooms, clinical management processes and access to equipment used in chronic care.

For the folder review, in each facility random systematic sampling was used to select 10 folders per chronic condition (diabetes, hypertension, asthma, COPD and epilepsy). It was a pragmatic decision to select 10 folders per chronic condition per facility. This number was considered feasible for facilities and also sufficient to monitor trends in care processes across facilities within a given sub-district. Folders were eligible for selection if the adult patient had been receiving treatment at the PHC facility for at least one year. Folder review per chronic condition looked at a set of fundamental chronic care indicators based on national guidelines for the different conditions, the Standard Treatment guidelines and Essential Medicines List for South Africa[16,17,18,19,20] as well as the criteria set in the Primary Care 101 guidelines, a symptom-based approach to the adult in PHC.[21]

Data were collected in February of each year of 2009 to 2012.

Data analysis

Data were analysed using the statistical programme Stata version 12.1 (StataCorp, College Station, Texas). Data collected were in a binary format where a positive response was given to the presence of specified indicators. With the unit of analysis being the facility, the final score for each district was obtained from the average score for all participating facilities within that district. Pooled district scores gave rise to provincial totals for each year.

Initial exploratory analysis showed that the data were not normally distributed and hence median percentages were used to present the results of facility audit processes and folder review. To determine the effectiveness of audits results for the years from 2009 to 2012 were compared, and for 2012 pooled results for districts that have been auditing since 2009 and 2010 (Metro, Eden and Cape Winelands), referred to as '2012 old', were compared to districts that started auditing recently in 2011 and 2012 (West Coast, Overberg and Central Karoo), referred to as '2012 new'. Descriptive statistics with inter-quartile ranges and bar graphs were used to show the changes in the audit results over the years. To test the statistical significance between '2012 old' and '2012 new' results the Mann-Whitney non-parametric test was used.[22]

For the 2012 audit results data were expanded from percentage scores per question to binary responses by folder, enabling a logistic regression model to be fitted with history of previous audits (new versus old); rural (Eden, Cape Winelands, West Coast, Overberg and Central Karoo) versus the Metro district and comparing selected indicators for the five chronic diseases (HbA_{1C} and foot exam for diabetes; serum creatinine and random total cholesterol for hypertension; control of asthma for asthma; counselling for smokers and counselling on inhaler use for COPD; and number of visits recording seizures for epilepsy). Data were clustered on patient folders to account for where responses to more than one question were from the same folder, ensuring robust standard errors.

Ethical considerations

Ethics approval for the annual audit was granted by the University of Cape Town's Research Ethics Committee in 2009 (HREC Ref.: 181/2009). In order to continue auditing and to publish this evaluation annual extensions have been given.

Results

The number of facilities participating in the audit has increased from 2009 to 2012 and is represented in Table 1.

Improvements in the audit process from 2009 to 2012 were minimal (Table 2 and Figure 1). The overall results may not show evidence of improvement when comparing 2011 to 2012, but if a comparison is made of '2012 old' districts with '2012 new' districts, improvements can be seen (Table 2 and Figure 2). With regard to the facility audit presented in Table 2, the patient preparation room was well stocked.

In the consulting rooms, the availability of blood pressure cuffs for the obese was poor. In 2012 only 45% of audited consulting rooms had cuffs for the obese, with the '2012 old' districts achieving 47% and '2012 new' districts only achieving 39%. The 2012 provincial average achieved 50% of facilities having chronic care teams. However, this was mainly due to what was achieved in the '2012 old' districts (57%) rather than in the '2012 new' districts (25%).

Figure 1 shows the median proportions achieved for certain indicators per chronic disease for the folder review done from 2009 to 2012. Generally proportions achieved for the overall provincial average in 2012 in most of the chronic disease indicators (except serum creatinine and counselling for smokers) were less than 50%. However, higher proportions were achieved in the '2012 old' districts compared to the '2012 new' districts (Table 3 and Figure 2).

Although the provincial average for 2012 showed that HbA_{1C} and foot exam in diabetics were done at poor rates (47% and 28% respectively), '2012 old' districts achieved more than the '2012 new' districts (Table 3). For hypertensive care the number of folders that recorded serum creatinine having been measured was 62% in the '2012 old' districts and only 18% in the '2012 new', with that of random total cholesterol being 62% and 15% in '2012 old' and '2012 new' respectively. Improvements were also seen when '2012 old' districts were compared to '2012' new districts for the folder review of asthma, COPD and epilepsy.

Across all five chronic disease indicators '2012 new' districts were 75% less likely to record clinical processes compared to the '2012 old' districts (Table 4). Similarly, in 2012 rural districts were 68% less likely to record clinical processes compared to the Metro district. Auditing of specific diseases showed that compared to folders on diabetes, those on asthma were 48% less likely to have recorded clinical processes; folders on COPD were 3.47 times more likely to have recorded clinical processes (Table 4).

TABLE 1: Participating facilities per district, 2009–2012.

Year	Metro	Eden	Cape Winelands	Overberg	West Coast	Central Karoo	Total
2009	29	0	0	0	0	0	29
2010	33	2	3	0	0	0	38
2011	43	7	11	0	5	12	78
2012	46	12	14	24	24	9	129

TABLE 2: Facility audit, 2009–2012.

Variable	Median percentage achieved per process					
Year (Number of participating facilities)	2009 (29)	2010 (38)	2011 (78)	2012 (129)	'2012 old' (72)	'2012 new' (57)
Consulting rooms						
Standard BP cuff	88	84	87	92	93	91
Cuff for the obese	49	45	50	45	47	39
Footscreening forms	68	58	73	63	71	38
Peak expiratory flow meter	60	53	59	56	58	51
Patient preparation rooms						
Functioning scale	100	100	96	99	99	100
Height chart	100	90	91	99	100	96
BMI chart or wheel	69	66	74	84	81	93
Urine dipsticks	97	100	98	100	100	99
Glucometer	97	100	96	100	100	100
Access to equipment						
Monofilaments for foot exam	90	73	74	78	84	57
Snellen Chart (normal)	97	100	96	94	95	93
ECG machine	100	96	89	76	88	39
Processes						
Chronic Disease Register	83	83	89	77	84	54
Chronic care team	61	73	63	50	57	25
Group health education	70	90	78	80	84	66
Community support groups	62	70	76	74	80	54

BP, blood pressure; BMI, body mass index; ECG, electrocardiogram.

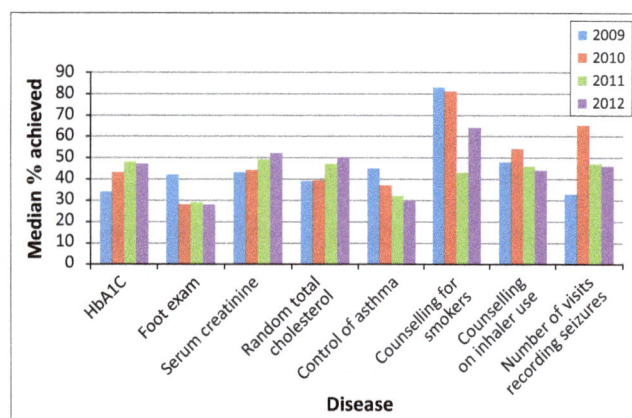

FIGURE 1: Folder audit per chronic disease, 2009–2012.

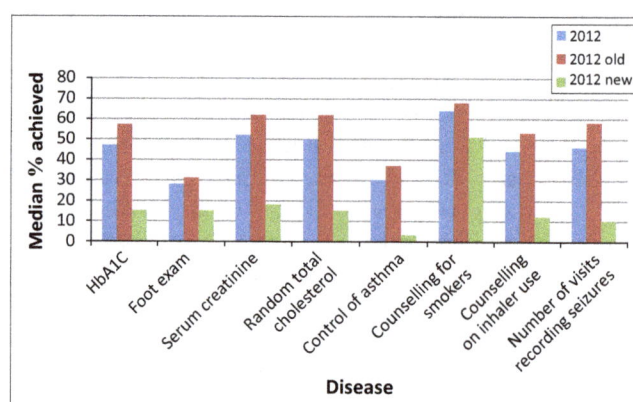

FIGURE 2: Folder audit 2012, comparing '2012 old' and '2012 new' districts.

Discussion

This article describes for the first time the results of a clinical governance initiative on the treatment of NCDs which has been ongoing in the Western Cape for four years. The findings demonstrate clear areas for service improvement, but also improving performance for facilities with a longer history of conducting this audit.

Increasing coverage of the audit with time

More facilities than in previous years (129 in 2012 compared to 29 in 2009) and all six districts in the Western

Cape were involved in the audit in 2012. This shows the willingness of facilities to participate in the audit and to improve services.

Effect of audit on quality of care

The evaluation showed small to moderate improvements in clinical processes from 2009 to 2012. In cases where there was low baseline adherence to what is recommended and accepted as standard practice, audits have been shown to be very effective at improving care; where adherence was already high, there were smaller effects.[8,12] This can partly explain the modest improvements seen over the years. It is

TABLE 3: Folder audit comparing '2012 old' and '2012 new' districts.

Variables	Median percentage achieved (IQR)	2012 total	2012 old	2012 new	Mann-Whitney test/ p-value
Number					
Number of folders audited	-	6450	3600	2850	-
Number of facilities	-	129	72	57	-
Diabetes					
HbA$_{1c}$	47	-	57 (50–63)	15 (7–24)	< 0.001
Foot exam	28	-	31 (19–37)	15 (2–30)	0.029
Hypertension					
Serum creatinine	52	-	62 (55–70)	18 (8–25)	< b0.001
Random total cholesterol	50	-	62 (50–68)	15 (8–23)	< 0.001
Asthma					
Control of asthma	30	-	37 (27–45)	3 (0–4)	< 0.001
COPD					
Counselling for smokers	64	-	68 (64–80)	51 (38–68)	0.016
Counselling on inhaler use	44	-	53 (31–70)	12 (0–20)	< 0.001
Epilepsy					
Number of visits that recorded seizures	46	-	58 (48–63)	10 (3–14)	< 0.001

IQR, interquartile range.

TABLE 4: Associations with positive responses in 2012 audit.

Variable	Univariable OR (95% CI)	Multivariable OR (95% CI)
New districts	0.28 (0.26–0.31)	0.25 (0.21–0.31)
Rural districts	0.35 (0.32–0.38)	0.32 (0.28–0.37)
Disease category		
Diabetes	1.00 (reference)	1.00 (reference)
Hypertension	1.51 (0.82–2.77)	1.57 (0.80–3.06)
Asthma	0.54 (0.26–1.10)	0.52 (0.24–1.10)
Epilepsy	1.19 (0.59–2.42)	1.21 (0.56–2.62)
COPD	3.07 (1.77–5.31)	3.47 (1.90–6.33)

OR, odds ratio; CI, confidence interval.
Total number of folders audited was 6450.

evident from the facility audit that in the case of most of the processes initial adherence was already high in 2009, with some indicators (such as the availability of a functioning scale) being as high as 100%. Where there were no improvements, such as comparing 2011 to 2012, this could be attributed to the 'newer' health districts doing worse ('2012 new') than/ the 'older' health districts ('2012 old').

Overall there were marked improvements in the '2012 old' districts compared to the '2012 new' districts on all eight clinical indicators for the folder review. Irrespective of the disease, 'new' districts had lower odds of recording clinical processes than the 'old' districts. The improvements seen are probably due to changes in practices at health districts where audits have been done for a longer period. This could be seen when the Metro district, the longest participating district in the province, was compared to the rural districts. If clinicians are given feedback about their practices, it will be expected that they will alter what they do if their clinical practice is found to be suboptimal and not according to the accepted standard and guidelines.[8] It has been found that when this feedback was given intensively and regularly to all healthcare professionals and when it came from peers, the effects were greater.[8,23] Such was the case in certain districts where the presence of good managerial support, dedicated champions and regular meetings where feedback was given frequently saw improvements in the audit processes (Van Vuuren U,

Provincial Chronic Diseases programme coordinator, oral communication, 12 August 2013).

Furthermore, district NCD management forums were implemented to monitor improvement plans in the rural districts, and in the Metro district reorganisation of the PHC management meant that there was zero tolerance for the availability of minimum equipment. Patient care was also improved in the Metro through setting up appointment systems and strengthening dedicated days where patients were managed more intensively. It was also found that districts where auditing has been done for longer periods were likely to have permanent staff, and this contributed to stability in knowledge and skills gained and confidence in the clinical care given to patients (Van Vuuren U, oral communication, 12 August 2013).

Room for improvement

Despite the improvements seen, a lot still needs to be done in improving the overall care given to patients with NCDs, especially in the case of asthma, which had 48% lower odds of clinical processes being recorded compared to diabetes. Also evident in the folder review is that the highest proportion achieved in 2012 was 64% for counselling for smokers with COPD, and only 28% for diabetic foot examination. This is not surprising, since previous audits and other studies done in the same context have shown shortfalls in the quality of care given to patients with NCDs, particularly those with hypertension and diabetes.[24,25]

Several barriers need to be overcome in order to improve the overall quality of care provided to patients with NCDs. Apart from health system issues, one of the major barriers to the successful translation of evidence into locally accepted policies lies in leaders and managers being ineffective and unaccountable.[26] Mash et al.[25] make a number of recommendations to improve chronic disease care, including building chronic care teams, involving the community, skills training for healthcare professionals and providing leadership for the chronic disease management teams.

Integration with clinical governance for care of patients with other conditions

There are more and more patients suffering from both NCDs as well as communicable diseases. This is more so in South Africa with its quadruple burden of disease.[3] Although this study analysed audit data for NCDs, audits can be used to improve care in patients with communicable diseases such as HIV and/or AIDS and TB.[27]

In moving forward it may be helpful to develop an integrated audit tool that not only looks at five NCDs (diabetes, hypertension, asthma, COPD and epilepsy), as was done here, but also looks at mental health as well as the communicable diseases for a more inclusive and comprehensive monitoring approach. This will need cross-programme collaboration and strengthening of partnerships with policy makers, healthcare professionals, public health researchers and funding organisations.[28,29]

Limitations

The main limitation in this study was the fact that the audit was done internally by senior health professionals within each facility. This essentially led to the possibility of reporting bias. Furthermore, there was no internal or external validation. In 2011, 24 clinics were not included in the analysis; this was because they were unable to collect 10 folders for each chronic condition due to their small size. Data to differentiate clinics participating in the audit for the first time from those who had audited previously was only available in 2012. The associations between clinics with and without a history of having conducted the audit previously could be confounded by unmeasured factors such as clinic size and stability, which contributed both to their earlier participation in the audit process as well as better clinical care and management. Finally, an audit of this nature is not the best way to assess long-term clinical outcomes because of the sample size. A different research methodology will be required for assessing clinical outcomes such as strokes and amputations.

Conclusion

Audits are done to create awareness about standards of care and for facilities to use their own data to identify areas where quality of care can be improved. Due to the efficiency of audits and quality of the data collected, audits are preferred over routinely collected data. The findings from this study have shown that audits done over time can significantly improve clinical processes in health districts. Even when the improvement is small, it may still be useful based on the context in which it was done.

However, beyond audits much still needs to be done to improve chronic disease care. Emphasis should be placed on facilities to set up multidisciplinary chronic care teams which will take responsibility for improving the chronic care

that they provide. Community participation in the form of Community Health Committees should be part of healthcare service planning. Also, a patient experience questionnaire could be included in future audits to explore patient satisfaction with services.

Given the value of audits in improving care processes over the long term, it is recommended that the audit be extended to all PHC facilities in the Western Cape, and expanded to audit care processes across all chronic diseases. This will require political backing and dedication from health programmes within the Department of Health and from service providers as implementers.

It is anticipated that the improvements seen will translate into improved patient outcomes in the future.

Acknowledgements

Competing interests

The authors declare that they have no financial or personal relationship(s) that may have inappropriately influenced them in writing this article.

Authors' contributions

V.E. (University of Cape Town, Western Cape Provincial Health Services) wrote the manuscript. U.V.V. (Western Cape Provincial Health Services) provided support to the districts. A.D.S. (UCT, Western Cape Metro District Health Services), S.G. (Stellenbosch University, Western Cape Metro District Health Services), K.M. (UCT, Western Cape Metro District Health Services), A.S. (Stellenbosch University, Western Cape Metro District Health Services), C.G. (Cape Winelands District Health Services) and M.N. (UCT, Western Cape Metro District Health Services) were responsible for developing the audit tool and collecting data. E.D.V. (UCT, Western Cape Metro District Health Services) and A.B. (UCT, Western Cape Provincial Health Services) provided technical and statistical assistance.

References

1. World Health Organisation. The global burden of chronic [homepage on the internet]. c2012 [cited 2013 Oct 16]. Available from: http://www.who.int/nutrition/topics/2_background/en/index.html

2. Dalal S, Beunza JJ, Volmink J, et al. Non-communicable diseases in sub-Saharan Africa: What we know now. Int J Epidemiol. 2011;40(4):885–901. http://dx.doi.org/10.1093/ije/dyr050

3. Mayosi BM, Flisher AJ, Lalloo UG, et al. The burden of non-communicable diseases in South Africa. Lancet. 2009;374(9693):934–947. http://dx.doi.org/10.1016/S0140-6736(09)61087-4

4. Puoane TR, Tsolekile L, Sanders D. A case study of community-level interventions for non-communicable diseases in Khayelitsha, Cape Town. Evidence report No.27. Brighton: Institute of Development Studies; 2013.

5. Al-Baho A, Serour M, Al-Weqayyn A, et al. Clinical audits in a postgraduate general practice training program: An evaluation of 8 years' experience. PLoS One. 2012;7(9):e43895. http://dx.doi.org/10.1371/journal.pone.0043895

6. Bailie R, Si D, Connors C, et al. Study protocol: Audit and best practice for chronic disease extension (ABCDE) project. BMC Health Serv Res. 2008;8:184. http://dx.doi.org/10.1186/1472-6963-8-184

7. Patel S. Achieving quality assurance through clinical audit. Nurs Manag. 2010;17(3):28–34. http://dx.doi.org/10.7748/nm2010.06.17.3.28.c7800

8. Jamtvedt G, Young JM, Kristoffersen DT, et al. Audit and feedback: Effects on professional practice and health care outcomes. Cochrane Database Syst Rev. 2006;2:CD000259. http://dx.doi.org/10.1002/14651858.CD000259.pub2

9. Weiss KB, Wagner R. Performance measurement through audit, feedback, and profiling as tools for improving clinical care. Chest. 2000;118(2):53S–58S. http://dx.doi.org/10.1378/chest.118.2_suppl.53S

10. Szecsenyi J, Campbell S, Broge B, et al. Effectiveness of a quality-improvement program in improving management of primary care practices. CMAJ. 2011;183(18):E1326–E1333. http://dx.doi.org/10.1503/cmaj.110412

11. Shojania KG, Ranji SR, McDonald KM, et al. Effects of quality improvement strategies for type 2 diabetes on glycemic control: A meta-regression analysis. JAMA. 2006;296(4):427–440. http://dx.doi.org/10.1001/jama.296.4.427

12. Flottorp SA, Jamtvedt G, Gibis B, et al. Using audit and feedback to health professionals to improve the quality and safety of health care: Policy summary 3. Copenhagen: WHO Regional Office for Europe; 2010.

13. Govender I, Ehrlich R, Van Vuuren U, et al. Clinical audit of diabetes management can improve the quality of care in a resource-limited primary care setting. Int J Qual Health Care. 2012;24(6):612–618. http://dx.doi.org/10.1093/intqhc/mzs063

14. Chopra M, Steyn N, Lambert V. Western Cape burden of disease reduction project, volume 6 of 7: Decreasing the burden of cardiovascular disease [homepage on the internet]. c2007 [cited 2013 Oct 28]. Available from: http://www.westerncape.gov.za/text/2007/6/cd_volume_6_cardiovascular_diseases.pdf

15. Martell R, De Vries E. Audit report on CVS risk factor management. Cape Town: Metro District Health Services; 2005.

16. Department of Health. Standard treatment guidelines and essential medicines list for South Africa: Primary health care level. Pretoria: National Department of Health; 2008.

17. Department of Health. Hypertension: National programme for control and management at primary level. Pretoria: Department of Health; 1998.

18. Department of Health. National guideline on primary prevention of chronic diseases of lifestyle (CDL). Pretoria: Department of Health; 2005.

19. Department of Health. National guideline: Management of asthma in adults in primary care. Pretoria: Department of Health; 2002.

20. Department of Health. National programme for control and management of diabetes type 2 at primary level. Pretoria: Department of Health; 1998.

21. Department of Health. Primary care 101: Symptom-based integrated approach to the adult in primary care 2013/2014. Pretoria: National Department of Health; 2013.

22. Nachar N. The Mann-Whitney U: A test for assessing whether two independent samples come from the same distribution. Tutor Quant Methods Psychol. 2008;4(1):13–20.

23. Bowie P, McKay J, Murray L, et al. Judging the quality of clinical audit by general practitioners: a pilot study comparing the assessments of medical peers and NHS audit specialists. J Eval Clin Pract. 2008;14(6):1038–1043. http://dx.doi.org/10.1111/j.1365-2753.2008.00941.x

24. Steyn K, Levitt NS, Patel M, et al. Hypertension and diabetes: Poor care for patients at community health centres. SAMJ. 2008;98(8):618–622. http://dx.doi.org/10.1080/22201009.2008.10872172

25. Mash R, Levitt NS, Van Vuuren U, et al. Improving the annual review of diabetic patients in primary care: an appreciative inquiry in the Cape Town District Health Services. S Afr Fam Pract. 2008;50(5):50. http://dx.doi.org/10.1080/20786204.2008.10873764

26. Kleinert S, Horton R. South Africa's health: Departing for a better future? Lancet. 2009;374(9692):759–760. http://dx.doi.org/10.1016/S0140-6736(09)61306-4

27. Siddiqi K, Volz A, Armas L, et al. Could clinical audit improve the diagnosis of pulmonary tuberculosis in Cuba, Peru and Bolivia? Trop Med Int Health. 2008;13(4):566–578. http://dx.doi.org/10.1111/j.1365-3156.2008.02035.x

28. Beaglehole R, Epping-Jordan J, Patel V, et al. Improving the prevention and management of chronic disease in low-income and middle-income countries: A priority for primary health care. Lancet. 2008;372(9642):940–949. http://dx.doi.org/10.1016/S0140-6736(08)61404-X

29. Epping-Jordan J, Pruitt SD, Bengoa R, et al. Improving the quality of health care for chronic conditions. Qual Saf Health Care. 2004;13(4):299–305. http://dx.doi.org/10.1136/qshc.2004.010744

26

Antimicrobial susceptibility profile of uropathogens in Maluti Adventist Hospital patients, 2011

Authors:
Phillip Mubanga[1]
Wilhelm J. Steinberg[1]
Francois C. Van Rooyen[2]

Affiliations:
[1]Faculty of Health Sciences, Department of Family Medicine, University of the Free State, South Africa

[2]Faculty of Health Department Sciences, Department of Biostatistics, University of the Free State, South Africa

Correspondence to:
Wilhelm Steinberg

Email:
steinbergwj@ufs.ac.za

Postal address:
PO Box 339, Bloemfontein 9330, South Africa

Background: Urinary tract infections (UTIs) are amongst the most common infections encountered globally and are usually treated empirically based on bacterial resistance to antibiotics for a given region. Unfortunately in Lesotho, no published studies are available to guide doctors in the treatment of UTIs. Treatment protocols for Western countries have been adopted, which may not be applicable for this region.

Aim: To determine the antimicrobial susceptibility profile of uropathogens in outpatients at the Maluti Adventist Hospital.

Setting: The study was conducted at the outpatient department of the Maluti Adventist Hospital in Mapoteng, Lesotho.

Methods: This was a prospective cross-sectional study using consecutive sampling of patients with clinical symptoms of UTI. Midstream urine samples were screened through chemistry and microscopy, then positive urine samples were cultured. The isolated uropathogens underwent antimicrobial susceptibility testing and inclusion continued until 200 culture samples were obtained. Descriptive statistics were used in the data analysis.

Results: The top five cultured uropathogens were *Escherichia coli* (61.5%), *Staphylococcus aureus* (14%), *Pseudomonas* species (6.5%), *Enterococcus faecalis* (5.5%) and *Streptococcus agalactiae* (5%). The isolated uropathogens showed low sensitivity to cotrimoxazole (32.5% – 75.0%) and amoxicillin (33.2% – 87.5%) and high sensitivity to ciprofloxacin (84.0% – 95.1%) and nitrofurantoin (76.9% – 100%)

Conclusion: In the Maluti setting, cotrimoxazole and amoxicillin should be avoided as first-line drugs for the empirical treatment of community-acquired UTI. We recommend the use of nitrofurantoin as first choice.

Profile de risque antimicrobien d'uropathogènes chez les patients du Maluti Adventist Hospital, 2011.

Contexte: Les infections urinaires (UTI) sont les infections les plus courantes dans le monde et sont traitées en général de façon empirique en se basant sur la résistance bactérielle aux antibiotiques dans une certaines région. Malheureusement il n'y a pas au Lesotho d'études publiées pour aider les médecins à traiter les UTI. On a adopté les programmes de traitement des pays occidentaux, ce qui n'est pas forcément applicable à cette région.

Objectif: Déterminer le profile de risque antimicrobien d'uropathogènes chez les patients externes du Maluti Adventist Hospital.

Lieu: L'étude a été faite au service de consultation externe du Maluti Adventist Hospital à Mapoteng, Lesotho.

Méthodes: C'était une étude prospective transversale au moyen d'échantillons consécutifs des patients présentant des symptômes cliniques d'UTI. Les échantillons d'urine prélevés à mi-miction ont été testés chimiquement et au microscope, puis les échantillons d'urine positifs ont été cultivés. Les uropathogènes isolés ont été testés pour risques antimicrobiens et l'inclusion a été poursuivie jusqu'à l'obtention de 200 échantillons de cultures. On a utilisé les statistiques descriptives dans l'analyse des données.

Résultats: Les cinq uropathogènes principaux cultivés étaient les espèces *Escherichia coli* (61.5%), *Staphylococcus aureus* (14%), *Pseudomonas* (6.5%), *Enterococcus faecalis* (5.5%) et *Streptococcus agalactiae* (5%). Les uropathogènes isolés ont montré une faible sensibilité au cotrimoxazole (32.5% – 75.0%) et à l'amoxicilline (33.2% – 87.5%) et une forte sensibilité à la ciprofloxacine (84.0% – 95.1%) et nitrofurantoine (76.9% – 100%)

Conclusion: Dans le contexte du Maluti, il faut éviter le cotrimoxazole et l'amoxicilline comme médicaments de première intention pour le traitement empirique de l'UTI communautaire. Nous recommandons l'utilisation de la nitrofurantoine en premier choix.

Introduction

Urinary tract infections (UTIs) are a major cause of morbidity worldwide. In a study done in Turkey on outpatient infections, UTIs were the second most common diagnosis after upper respiratory tract infections.[1] A UTI occurs when there is the presence of pathogenic microorganisms along the urinary tract, involving one or more of the following: urethra, prostate, bladder and/or kidneys.[2] Bacteria are by far the most common causative microorganisms of UTIs.

Escherichia coli is the leading bacterial uropathogen in the world.[3] In a study on community-acquired infections, E. coli accounted for 68% of all the positive cultures for UTIs.[4] This was followed by Proteus mirabilis (12%), Staphylococcus aureus (10%), Enterococcus faecalis (6%) and Klebsiella aerogenes (4%).[4] These percentages and order of uropathogens after E. coli will vary from region to region, between men and women and between children and adults. For instance, in a study done at a tertiary hospital in South Africa, E. coli was also found to be the most cultured microorganism but it represented only 39% of all the uropathogens isolated. Klebsiella spp. followed at 20.8% and then Enterococcus faecalis at 8.2%.[5] These differences highlight the importance of regional and institutional audits of antimicrobial susceptibility profiles.

Uncomplicated community-acquired UTIs are usually managed by the empirical prescription of antibiotics based on the bacterial resistance profile. This is done in order to avoid the unnecessary cost of doing a urine culture for every patient who presents with UTI symptoms. Guidelines recommend the empirical use of antibiotics if the bacterial resistance is less than 20%.[6,7]

The Ministry of Health and Social Welfare in Lesotho published the Standard Treatment Guidelines for Lesotho for the management of medical conditions in the country in 2006.[8] For UTIs, the guidelines stipulate the use of cotrimoxazole, 80 mg or 400 mg, twice a day for seven days, as the first-line therapy for uncomplicated adult UTIs.

The use of amoxicillin is the other alternative recommended in the guideline. In severe cases, ampicillin by intravenous route is recommended and if patients do not respond, then ofloxacin or ciprofloxacin may be used.

Aim and objectives

This study sought to determine the antimicrobial susceptibility profile of uropathogens responsible for community-acquired UTI in patients at the Maluti Adventist Hospital outpatient department, Lesotho. This information may be used to formulate a protocol for the appropriate and cost-effective empirical antibiotic treatment of uncomplicated UTIs in this resource-constrained setting.

The objectives of this study included:

- To establish the current profile of uropathogens responsible for community-acquired UTIs in patients at the Maluti Adventist Hospital outpatient department, Lesotho.
- To determine the antimicrobial susceptibility of these organisms.
- To formulate a suitable protocol for empirical antibiotic treatment of uncomplicated UTIs in this setting that is also cost-effective.

Significance of the study

In the light of worldwide growing resistance of uropathogens to antibiotics, the variability in bacterial sensitivity profiles from region to region and the cost of re-treatment with its associated morbidity, it becomes imperative to establish a baseline and do periodic audits of the susceptibility profile of these pathogens so that treatment can be appropriate. Unfortunately for Lesotho, there are no published studies available to guide doctors in the treatment of UTIs. Empirical treatment protocols of other regions have been adopted, which may not be applicable.

Research methods and design
Study design

This was a prospective cross-sectional study on adult patients presenting with community-acquired uncomplicated UTIs, to the outpatient department of Maluti Adventist Hospital in Lesotho. A prospective study was chosen in order to eliminate the selection bias of a retrospective design done on past laboratory results only.

Setting

The study was conducted in 2011 at the outpatient department of the Maluti Adventist Hospital in Mapoteng, Lesotho. This hospital is situated in the rural Berea District of Lesotho, about 70 km north of Maseru, the capital of Lesotho. Between July 2007 to June 2008, 29 125 outpatient visits were recorded. In the same period, 1298 patients were diagnosed with UTI based on clinical history and urine chemistry or microscopy. At Maluti Adventist Hospital's outpatient department, most UTIs are treated empirically with cotrimoxazole, amoxicillin or ciprofloxacin.

Sample population and sampling strategy

Patients attending the outpatient department of Maluti Adventist Hospital with symptoms of UTI were eligible for recruitment. These included men and women older than 18 years who gave written consent for themselves and their urine samples to be used for the study.

Patients who had been hospitalised or had taken a course of antibiotics within the month prior to the study were excluded. Patients too ill to give consent, those with indwelling catheters and patients younger than 18 years of age were also excluded.

Sample size

A sample size of 200 urine samples that were culture positives for UTI-causing microorganisms was thought to be sufficient to meet the objectives for this study. Each month, approximately 100 to 110 patients are seen at Maluti Adventist Hospital who have a positive urine microscopy or urinalysis suggestive of UTI. It was expected that more than 50% of these would give significant culture isolates. It was estimated that within a four- to six-month period, the needed 200 cultures would be obtained.

Sample selection

Consecutive sampling was used. Patients qualifying for the study were selected for participation based on a clinical assessment for UTI. The symptoms included one or more of the following: dysuria, frequency, urgency and suprapubic pain. Potential candidates were informed about the study and asked to sign voluntarily consent. Thereafter, a thorough medical history and examination was done. They were then asked to give a midstream urine sample after a briefing on the technique.

This sequential recruitment of patients was done until the required number of culture-positive urine samples was obtained. Only one urine sample was obtained per patient.

Intervention

Routine treatment procedures were initially followed at the outpatient department. But those participants whose culture samples showed that the antibiotics they had received where not effective, were changed to a susceptible antibiotic regime on follow-up.

Data collection

Demographic data, including age, gender and UTI symptoms, results of microscopy and chemistry analyses and susceptibility testing, were captured on a data sheet.

Midstream urine samples from patients with UTI symptoms were collected in sterile containers and sent to the laboratory on the grounds of Maluti Adventist Hospital. Urine microscopy and chemistry were initially done to identify the urine samples for culture. Urine samples that qualified presented with one or more of the following: pyuria (> 4 white blood cells per ml) by microscopy, a positive leukocyte esterase result by chemistry and/or a positive nitrite result by chemistry.

The qualifying urine samples were inoculated on blood agar and MacConkey agar plates using a 0.001 mL inoculation loop. The inoculants were incubated aerobically at 37 °C for 24 hours. The presence of colony-forming units (CFUs), after incubation, greater than 10^5 per mL was considered as significant bacteriuria, as per Kass criteria.[9]

For growths between 10^3 to 10^5 CFUs per mL, in which the source of the urine sample was a young woman with symptoms of cystitis or pyuria, the culture was also accepted as significant bacteriuria based on the Stamm criteria.[10] The selected isolates were processed further for identification and antimicrobial susceptibility testing.

Identification was done on the basis of gram stains, morphology and biochemical features. The testing of the isolates for antimicrobial susceptibility was performed by means of the disc diffusion technique, according to the Clinical and Laboratory Standards Institute guidelines.[11]

The following four antibiotics were selected based on availability and cost implications: cotrimoxazole, amoxicillin, nitrofurantoin, and ciprofloxacin.

Methodological and measurement errors

Potential methodological and measurement errors that could negatively affect data collection, analysis and interpretation of results were identified and remedial measures implemented:

- Improper urine collection technique leading to microbial contaminants and a subsequent false picture of the microbial profile was prevented by clearly instructing the patients on how to collect midstream urine.
- Inter-observer errors were minimised by using one microbiologist to perform the urinalysis, culture and antibiogram interpretation of the samples.

Data analysis

Data collected during the study were analysed by the Department of Biostatistics at the Faculty of Health Sciences, University of the Free State. Descriptive statistics, namely means and standard deviations or medians and percentages, were used to calculate continuous data. Frequencies and percentages were used to calculate categorical data. The sensitivity of each uropathogen to the named antibiotics was determined in percentages. Charts and tables were used for clarity.

Ethical considerations

Patients were asked to sign voluntary consent forms which were available in both English and Sesotho (the main language of Lesotho). Patients with positive urine culture results were informed and appropriate antibiotics prescribed by the treating doctor, if the empirical antibiotics had been inadequate.

Assurance was given to all patients that strict confidentiality would be maintained and that it would not prejudice their treatment if consent was denied.

Permission was obtained from the hospital management before going ahead with the study. The protocol was approved by the Ethics Committee of the Faculty of Health Science, University of the Free State (ETOVS number 21/07).

Each patient was assigned a study number and this was recorded on the datasheet.

Results

Urine samples collected from 609 patients with symptoms of UTI were sent to the laboratory for urine microscopy and chemistry testing. Of the 452 samples that qualified for culture, 200 samples yielded cultures and were further subjected to antibiotic sensitivity tests. The remaining 252 samples did not grow sufficient colonies or grew contaminants.

The patients of these 200 samples were between the ages of 18 to 84 years. Almost half (49.5%) were in the 20–29 year age group. The majority of patients were women (87.0%), of whom 28.3% were pregnant.

The pick-up ratio for UTI by symptom was as follows: dysuria 86.8%, suprapubic pain 63.1%, frequency 53.0%, urgency 41.9% and other symptoms 6.2%. The pick-ratio for UTI from urinalysis was urine microscopy 94.9%, urine leucocyte esterase 74.4% and urine nitrite 19.6%.

Isolated uropathogens from cultured urine samples

More than two-thirds (61.5%) of the uropathogens isolated from the 200 cultured urine samples were identified as *E. coli* (Table 1).

The uropathogens showed high resistance (low sensitivity) to cotrimoxazole and amoxicillin. A much better susceptibility profile was seen for ciprofloxacin, but the uropathogens were most sensitive to nitrofurantoin (Table 2).

TABLE 1: Uropathogens isolated from the cultured samples collected from patients with community-acquired urinary tract infections at the Maluti Adventist Hospital, Lesotho.

Uropathogens isolated	Variable	
	n	(%)
Total number of urine samples	609	100.0
Total number of urine samples with uropathogens	200	32.8
Uropathogens isolated (*n* = 200)		
Escherichia coli	123	61.5
Staphylococcus aureus	28	14.0
Pseudomonas spp.	13	6.5
Enterococcus faecalis	11	5.5
Streptococcus agalactiae	9	4.5
Proteus mirabilis	8	4.0
Staphylococcus epidermidis	5	2.5
Klebsiella aerogenes	3	1.5
Other	10	5.0

The sensitivity profile of this sample showed poor susceptibility to the commonly-used antibiotics, with acceptable susceptibility of the cultured microorganisms to ciprofloxacin and nitrofurantoin. The highest sensitivity was found for nitrofurantoin.

Discussion

Community-acquired UTIs are usually treated empirically with antibiotics.[12] Given this background, many doctors will send urine samples to the laboratory only after initial empirical treatment failure or for a complicated UTI, which may produce a bias in the laboratory records for urine culture and sensitivity. To avoid this bias, a prospective study, instead of a retrospective study, was done on past laboratory results.

E. coli was the most common uropathogen (61.5%) isolated from the cultured urine samples of this study population. This is similar to findings from studies done in other developing countries such as India (59%, 68%)[13,14] and Madagascar (67%).[15] A study done in South Africa reported the presence of *E. coli* in 75% of uncomplicated and 59% of complicated UTIs.[16]

E. coli had very low sensitivity levels to cotrimoxazole and amoxicillin. This may be a result of their widespread use in Lesotho. For example, cotrimoxazole is used for long-term infection prophylaxis in people with HIV.[8]

On the other hand, *E. coli* and the other uropathogens of this region had a high sensitivity to nitrofurantoin and ciprofloxacin. These antibiotics are not used as commonly in Lesotho compared with cotrimoxazole and amoxicillin. According to the *Standard Treatment Guidelines for Lesotho*,[8] nitrofurantoin is not amongst the drugs listed for the treatment of community-acquired UTI and may be one of the reasons it is not commonly prescribed. *E. coli* sensitivity to ciprofloxacin and nitrofurantoin is less than 10% and therefore falls within the recommended guidelines for use in the empirical treatment of community-acquired UTI.[6,7] However, there are concerns with the routine use of ciprofloxacin and other quinolones as first-line drugs, as resistance to these drugs may develop easily.[17,18] Nitrofurantoin is also much cheaper than ciprofloxacin in terms of cost of treatment.[19]

It needs to be considered whether the antimicrobial susceptibility profile of uropathogens identified in this study can be used as representative of the general situation in Lesotho. Many patients at the Maluti Adventist Hospital outpatient department originate from outside the hospital catchment area, which can reach to Maseru and beyond.

TABLE 2: Susceptibility profiles of the top five uropathogens isolated from patients with community-acquired urinary tract infections at the Maluti Adventist Hospital, Lesotho.

Top five uropathogens	% isolated from urine samples	Cotrimoxazole		Amoxicillin		Ciprofloxacin		Nitrofurantoin	
		n	% sensitivity	*n*	% sensitivity	*n*	% sensitivity	*n*	% sensitivity
Escherichia coli	61.5	40	32.5	41	33.3	117	95.1	117	95.1
Staphylococcus aureus	14.0	10	40.0	20	80.0	21	84.0	20	80.0
Pseudomonas spp.	6.5	4	30.8	6	46.2	11	84.6	10	76.9
Enterococcus faecalis	5.5	5	45.5	7	63.6	7	63.6	11	100.0
Streptococcus agalactiae	4.5	6	75.0	7	87.5	7	87.5	7	87.5

Limitations

Financial constraints limited the number of antibiotics used in testing the isolates for antimicrobial susceptibility.

In addition, the microbiologist was not available at all times and other laboratory staff had to stand in. This may have influenced inter-observer errors.

Recommendations

For the Maluti Adventist Hospital catchment area, we recommend that cotrimoxazole and amoxicillin no longer be used as first-line drugs in the empirical treatment of adult community-acquired uncomplicated UTI. Nitrofurantoin should be the first choice of treatment, if there are no contraindications. It is also advised that the above recommendation be adopted for Lesotho in general until further evidence-based studies indicate otherwise. More studies need to be done in different parts of Lesotho to determine the overall antimicrobial susceptibility profile of uropathogens in the country and to keep tract of the uropathogen profile of this region.

Conclusion

Bacteria causing community-acquired UTIs seen in patients at the Maluti Adventist Hospital outpatient department, show high resistance to cotrimoxazole and amoxicillin. This makes these antibiotics unsuitable as first-line treatment drugs. Bacterial resistance to nitrofurantoin and ciprofloxacin is very low, making them the preferable drugs. Yet costs make nitrofurantoin more favourable as a first-line drug in the empiric treatment of community-acquired UTI in adults.

Acknowledgements

The authors would like to acknowledge Mr Sam Sinkoto, head of Maluti Hospital Laboratory services, for his support and for allowing the study to be conducted; and Ms Matsepo T. Mofokeng (microbiologist) for her valuable time and commitment in the laboratory. The Maluti outpatient department medical staff is thanked for their assistance in selecting and processing patients for urine collection to the laboratory. In addition, the authors would like to acknowledge Mrs T. Mulder, medical writer, School of Medicine, University of the Free State, for technical and editorial preparation of the manuscript.

Competing interests

The authors declare that they have no financial or personal relationship(s) that may have inappropriately influenced them in writing this article.

Authors' contributions

P.M. (Registrar, Department of Family Medicine, University of the Free State) had the idea, developed the protocol and performed the data collection of this study. W.J.S. (Department of Family Medicine, University of the Free State) was the supervisor in this study, assisting with the development, analysis and write up of this study. F.C.v.R. (Department of Biostatistics, University of the Free State) assisted with the planning and data analysis.

References

1. Avci IY, Kilic S, Acikel CH, et al. Outpatient prescription of oral antibiotics in a training hospital in Turkey: Trends in the last decade. J Infect. 2006;52(1):9–14. http://dx.doi.org/10.1016/j.jinf.2005.07.007, PMid:16181680

2. Stamm WE. Urinary tract infections, pyelonephritis, and prostatitis. In: Fauci AS, Braunwald E, Kasper DL, et al., editors. Harrison's principles of internal medicine. 17th ed. New York: McGraw-Hill, 2008; pp. 1821–1826.

3. Miragliotta G, Di Pierro MN, Miragliotta L, et al. Antimicrobial resistance among uropathogens responsible for community-acquired urinary tract infections in an Italian community. J Chemother. 2008;20(6):721–727. http://dx.doi.org/10.1179/joc.2008.20.6.721, PMid:19129070

4. Kumar P, Clark M, editors. Clinical medicine. 6th ed. London: Elsevier Saunders; 2005.

5. Habte TM, Dube S, Ismail N, et al. Hospital and community isolates of uropathogens at a tertiary hospital in South Africa. S Afr Med J. 2009;99(8):584–587. PMid:19908617

6. Sanford PJ, Gilbert DN, Moellering Jr. RC, et al., editors. The Sanford guide to antimicrobial therapy. 38th ed. Sperryville, VA: Antimicrobial Therapy, Inc, 2008; p. 27 (Table 1), 30.

7. Grabe M, Bjerklund-Johansen TE, Botto H, et al. Guidelines on urological infections [document on the Internet]. c2009 [cited 2014 Apr 07]. Available from: http://www.uroweb.org/fileadmin/tx_eauguidelines/2009/Full/Urological_Infections.pdf [updated URL cited 2014 Apr 04, available from: http://uroweb.org/wp-content/uploads/18_Urological-infections_LR.pdf]

8. Ministry of Health and Social Welfare. Standard Treatment Guidelines for Lesotho, 2006. Lesotho: Ministry of Health and Social Welfare, 2006; p. 58–59.

9. Kass EH. Asymptomatic infections of the urinary tract. J Urol. 2002;167(2 Pt 2):1016–1020. http://dx.doi.org/10.1016/S0022-5347(02)80328-7, PMid:11905871

10. Stamm WE, Counts GW, Running KR, et al. Diagnosis of coliform infection in acutely dysuric women. N Engl J Med. 1982;307(8):463–468. http://dx.doi.org/10.1056/NEJM198208193070802, PMid:7099208

11. Clinical Laboratory Standards Institute. Performance standards for antimicrobial susceptibility testing; 15th informational supplement. NCCLS/CLSI M100-S15. Clinical Laboratory Standards Institute, Wayne, PA; 2005.

12. Keah SH, Wee EC, Chng KS, et al. Antimicrobial susceptibility of community-acquired uropathogens in general practice. Malays Fam Physician. 2007;2(2):64–69.

13. Tambekar DH, Dhanorkar DV, Gulhane SR, et al. Antibacterial susceptibility of some urinary tract pathogens to commonly used antibiotics. Afr J Biotechnol. 2006;5(17):1562–1565.

14. Kothari A, Sagar V. Antibiotic resistance in pathogens causing community-acquired urinary tract infections in India: A multicenter study. J Infect Dev Ctries. 2008;2(5):354–358. http://dx.doi.org/10.3855/jidc.196, PMid:19745502

15. Randrianirina F, Soares JL, Carod JF, et al. Antimicrobial resistance among uropathogens that cause community-acquired urinary tract infections in Antananarivo, Madagascar. J Antimicrob Chemother. 2007;59(2):309–312. http://dx.doi.org/ 10.1093/jac/dkl466, PMid:17138569

16. Bosch FJ, van Vuuren C, Joubert G. Antimicrobial resistance patterns in outpatient urinary tract infections – the constant need to revise prescribing habits. S Afr Med J. 2011;101(5):328–331. PMid:21837876

17. Nicolle L, Anderson PA, Conly J, et al. Uncomplicated urinary tract infection in women. Current practice and the effect of antibiotic resistance on empiric treatment. Can Fam Physician. 2006;52:612–618. PMid:16739835, PMCid:PMC1531733

18. Scottish Intercollegiate Guidelines Network (SIGN). SIGN guideline 88: Management of suspected bacterial urinary tract infection in adults. A national clinical guideline [document on the Internet]. c2006 [cited 2011 Dec 12]. Available from: http://www.sign.ac.uk/guidelines/fulltext/88/index.html

19. McKinnell JA, Stollenwerk NS, Jung CW, et al. Nitrofurantoin compares favorably to recommended agents as empirical treatment of uncomplicated urinary tract infections in a decision and cost analysis. Mayo Clin Proc. 2011;86(6):480–488. http://dx.doi.org/10.4065/mcp.2010.0800, PMid:21576512, PMCid:PMC3104907

27

Healthcare provider and patient perspectives on diagnostic imaging investigations

Authors:
Chandra R. Makanjee[1]
Anne-Marie Bergh[2]
Willem A. Hoffmann[3]

Affiliations:
[1]Faculty of Health Sciences, Department of Radiography, University of Pretoria, South Africa

[2]MRC Unit for Maternal and Infant Health Care Strategies, Faculty of Health Sciences, University of Pretoria, South Africa

[3]Department of Biomedical Sciences, Tshwane University of Technology, South Africa

Correspondence to:
Chandra Makanjee

Email:
chandra.makanjee@up.ac.za

Postal address:
Private Bag X323, Arcadia 0007, South Africa

Background: Much has been written about the patient-centred approach in doctor–patient consultations. Little is known about interactions and communication processes regarding healthcare providers' and patients' perspectives on expectations and experiences of diagnostic imaging investigations within the medical encounter. Patients journey through the health system from the point of referral to the imaging investigation itself and then to the post-imaging consultation.

Aim and setting: To explore healthcare provider and patient perspectives on interaction and communication processes during diagnostic imaging investigations as part of their clinical journey through a healthcare complex.

Methods: A qualitative study was conducted, with two phases of data collection. Twenty-four patients were conveniently selected at a public district hospital complex and were followed throughout their journey in the hospital system, from admission to discharge. The second phase entailed focus group interviews conducted with providers in the district hospital and adjacent academic hospital (medical officers and family physicians, nurses, radiographers, radiology consultants and registrars).

Results: Two main themes guided our analysis: (1) provider perspectives; and (2) patient dispositions and reactions. Golden threads that cut across these themes are interactions and communication processes in the context of expectations, experiences of the imaging investigations and the outcomes thereof.

Conclusion: Insights from this study provide a better understanding of the complexity of the processes and interactions between providers and patients during the imaging investigations conducted as part of their clinical pathway. The interactions and communication processes are provider–patient centred when a referral for a diagnostic imaging investigation is included.

Perspectives des prestataires de soins et des patients sur les examens d'imagerie diagnostique dans un complexe hospitalier sud-africain: une étude qualitative.

Contexte: Beaucoup d'encre a coulé sur l'approche centrée sur le patient dans les consultations du docteur avec son patient. On sait très peu sur les interactions et les processus de communication en ce qui concerne les perspectives des prestataires de soins et des patients sur les attentes et expériences des examens d'imagerie diagnostique pendant la rencontre médicale. Les patients parcourent le système de santé du point de référence à l'examen d'imagerie même, puis à la consultation post-imagerie.

Objectif et lieu: Examiner les perspectives des prestataires de soins et des patients sur l'interaction et les processus de communication pendant les examens d'imagerie diagnostique dans le cadre de leur parcours clinique dans un complexe sanitaire.

Méthodes: Une étude qualitative a été menée avec une collecte de données en deux phases. On a sélectionné aisément vingt-quatre patients dans un complexe hospitalier public de district, puis on les a suivi tout au long de leur parcours dans le système hospitalier, depuis l'admission jusqu'à la sortie de l'hôpital. La seconde phase consistait en entrevues avec un groupe cible menées avec les prestataires de soins dans l'hôpital de district et l'hôpital universitaire voisin (agents médicaux et les médecins de famille, infirmières, radiographe, les consultants en radiologie et les registraires).

Résultats: Deux thèmes principaux ont guidé notre analyse: (1) perspectives du prestataire; et (2) dispositions et réactions du patient. Les fils conducteurs qui recoupent ces thèmes sont les interactions et les processus de communication dans le contexte des attentes, des expériences des examens d'imagerie et le résultat de ceci.

Conclusion: Les éclairages apportés par cette étude offrent une meilleure compréhension de la complexité des processus et interactions entre les prestataires et les patients au cours des examens d'imagerie effectués dans le cadre de leur parcours clinique. Les interactions et processus de communication sont centrés autour de la relation du prestataire avec le patient quand un examen d'imagerie diagnostique est inclus.

Introduction

Referral for a diagnostic imaging investigation is not an isolated event but is rather an integral part of a complex medical encounter that often involves interaction with multiple healthcare providers and technologies. A patient-centred approach to justifying a referral for and conducting a diagnostic imaging investigation entails knowing the patient as a person, engaging with and listening to the patient as an active participant and providing quality professional services.[1] Diagnostic reasoning not only comprises an analytic process, but also involves an affective component.[2]

The demand for greater patient-initiated access to medical[3] and imaging[4,5] services has grown, especially as a result of the consumerist movement.[6,7] Failure to meet patient needs or requests impacts on visit satisfaction and patients' health-related anxiety increases when the desired diagnostic intervention is not received.[8] However, patient centredness does not imply giving a patient what he or she wants;[9] uncritical compliance with such requests is both unprofessional and unethical.[8] Therefore, effective communication is essential in patient-centred medical practice in order to be able to give the necessary priority to patient safety.[10]

Referral for a test could increase patient concern and fears that the symptoms indicate a serious illness.[11,12] Patients referred for a diagnostic imaging investigation are often in a vulnerable state[13] and their anxiety and discomfort may contribute to poor patient satisfaction.[14]

There are numerous research reports on patient participation in clinical decision making. However, not much has been written on interactions and communication processes between healthcare providers and patients and amongst different providers regarding diagnostic imaging investigations, nor have these processes been positioned within the broader context of the medical journey from admission to referral and discharge.

Aims and objectives

The aims of this study were to explore how patients expressed and positioned themselves and how they changed their perceptions in the period between pre- and post-diagnostic imaging; and how healthcare providers perceived patient expectations and their ability to participate in a medical encounter.

Research methods and design

This study represents one of the first attempts to explore multi-perspective decision making and interactions in diagnostic imaging investigations. A qualitative research design with two consecutive phases was used. The first phase entailed shadowing patients from admission to discharge, whereas the second phase consisted of focus group interviews with healthcare providers.

Study design

The study was conceptualised around the metaphor of a patient's journey through the hospital system (admission through to discharge), in the context of accessibility of diagnostic imaging investigations. The various healthcare providers with whom the patient interacts along the journey form part of the organisational culture of the healthcare institution. Upon arriving at the hospital, the patient connects with nurses and doctors. During the medical consultation, the doctor makes a decision regarding a diagnostic investigation referral. At the imaging department, the patient then interacts with radiographers and/or radiologists before returning to the referring medical practitioner or specialist.

Setting

This study was conducted at an urban South African district hospital that is part of an academic complex including a primary healthcare (PHC) clinic, a provincial tertiary hospital and a central hospital. The complex provided the whole spectrum of imaging services with a system of upward and downward referral according to choice of imaging modalities provided at the different levels of care. Patient journeys started at a PHC clinic or at the casualty or outpatient (OPD) departments of the district hospital.

Sampling

Twenty-four patients were recruited for phase one through convenience sampling. The inclusion criteria were the ability to give consent, as well as a willingness to communicate with the researchers in English or through an interpreter and to spend an extra half hour after completion of the last medical consultation. Under-18 and critically-ill patients were excluded. Patient participants came mostly from poor socioeconomic communities. Table 1 provides an overview of these participants.

TABLE 1: Overview of patient participants.

Characteristic	Breakdown	n
Hospital entry route	Direct	15
	Referral	9
Origin of referral	Self	15
	Clinic	3
	Casualties	1
	Private	4
	Follow-up	1
Admission department	Casualties	14
	Outpatients	10
Referral for diagnostic imaging	Yes*	18
	No	6
Gender	Male	7
	Female	17
Age (years)	Mean	40
	Median	45
	Range	18–83

*, General x-rays only (n = 12); General x-ray and CT (n = 2); Stereotactic breast biopsy and mammography (n = 1); Diagnostic ultrasound (n = 2); Gynaecological ultrasound conducted by medical practitioner (n = 1).

TABLE 2a: Data collection process and methods - Phase I: Data sources for each patient.

Steps	Patients (*n* = 24)	The journey	Providers (*n* = 62)
Step 1: Pre-consultation	Entry interviews (*n* = 24) (audio-recordings)	-	-
Step 2: Medical encounter	-	Doctor–patient consultations (*n* = 19) (observations, audio-recordings, medical files & field notes)	-
Step 3: Diagnostic imaging	-	Radiographer–patient interactions (*n* = 17) (observations, request forms and field notes)	-
Step 4: Post-imaging	-	Doctor–patient consultations (*n* = 17) (observations, audio-recordings, medical files & field notes)	-
Step 5: Discharge	Exit interviews (*n* = 22) (audio-recordings)	-	-
Step 6: Provider interviews	-	-	Medical practitioners (*n* = 20) Radiographers (*n* = 18) Radiologists and registrars (*n* = 17) Other specialties (*n* = 4) Nurses (*n* = 3) (audio-recordings)

TABLE 2b: Data collection process and methods - Phase 2: Provider focus groups (audio-recordings and field notes).

Profession	Focus groups (*n* = 12)	Participants (*n* = 53)
Medical practitioners and family physicians	3	13
Radiographers	3	15
Radiologists and radiology registrars	2	8
Nurses	4	17

Healthcare providers were recruited for both phases of the study. In the first phase, they were interviewed individually following the medical consultations. The providers included: nurses; radiographers; medical students; interns; community service doctors; medical officers; family physicians; radiology consultants and registrars; and specialist consultants and registrars.

For the second phase, a purposive sample of healthcare providers was recruited to participate in focus group interviews. Some providers participated in both phases of the study, whereas others only participated in either phase one or phase two.

Data collection methods

Table 2a and Table 2b provide details of the data collection process and methods used in the two study phases. The study design for phase one included researcher observations of the patient-provider interactions at all points of medical and imaging care services. Most inter-actions were accompanied by an audio-recording and the attending researcher made field notes.

We conducted individual, semi-structured interviews with patients at the entry and exit points, as well as individual interviews with healthcare providers involved with each of the patient participants. Most interviews were held in English, with interpretation for two patients. Entry interviews with patients were conducted before consultation with the medical practitioner. The interviews probed patients' reasons for their visit, their expectations and their specific knowledge of diagnostic imaging. Exit interviews were conducted after they had received a treatment plan from the attending medical practitioner or specialist. These interviews focused on whether their expectations had been fulfilled regarding the care they had received during their hospital journey.

The individual interviews with healthcare providers probed the following aspects of the specific patient consultation and interaction: referral decision and justification; outcome(s) of the diagnostic imaging investigation(s); and approach to engaging with the patient. Although the ideal was to follow (shadow) all patients at all times, in two cases the medical providers changed their referral decisions, resulting in those patients being taken for x-rays without the presence of a researcher. Because of the unpredictability of discharge dates and admission times, follow-up exit interviews with two patients could not be conducted.

The phase two focus group interviews were conducted with 53 participants from different healthcare provider categories: medical practitioners and family physicians; nurses; radiographers; and radiologists and radiology registrars (Table 2a and Table 2b). Issues addressed in the focus groups included patient expectations and experiences of referrals, as well as provider experience of accessibility to diagnostic imaging services.

Data analysis

All audio-recordings were transcribed. One researcher (C.R.M.) conducted the first round of data analysis manually. This was followed by several consensus discussions by the research team. Figure 1 illustrates the data analysis process. The phase one data analysis followed a 'bottom up' (p. 38)[15] approach in which the data from each patient case (including observations and provider interviews) were analysed by coding for categories. Data were organised into four components. Data from the entry and exit interviews and observations were grouped together and analysed concurrently to inform the patient's journey, whereas the providers' individual interview data informed the provider perspective. Emergent codes for each patient case were compared, consolidated and expanded with the analysis of each subsequent patient case. At the next level of analysis, categories emerging from the patients' journeys and those from the provider

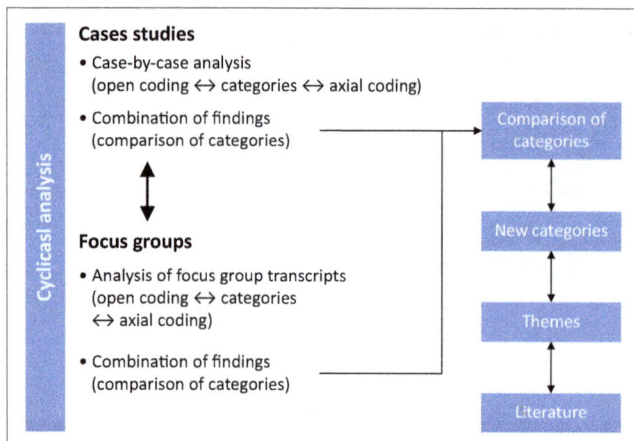

FIGURE 1: The data-analysis process.

perspectives were compared and ultimately integrated in a comprehensive provisional structure of categories, subthemes and themes.

The phase one findings informed the content and structure of the focus group interviews. Data analysis of the transcripts of the focus groups followed the interviews. Member checking was performed by eliciting feedback from healthcare providers, but not from all patient participants because of the recurrent change in contact details or non-availability of participants after the exit interviews.

Trustworthiness

The principles of confirmability, credibility, transferability and dependability were followed to ensure the trustworthiness of this study.[16] The three researchers had different roles regarding their 'insider'–'outsider' relationship with the research setting.[17] Two researchers were outsiders (A.M.B., W.A.H.) and the third researcher (C.R.M.) was familiar with the setting and knew some of the radiographer participants but was not employed in the setting. This provided sufficient distance to allow the researchers to appreciate the patients' journeys and the providers' perspectives without jeopardising the confirmability of the study.

The credibility of the findings was enhanced by the active participation of all three researchers in data analysis and interpretation. At times they served as peer reviewers for each other with regard to the identification and integration of categories, subthemes and themes. Study findings were submitted for scrutiny to two independent healthcare experts familiar with the research setting, a radiologist and a family physician.

With regard to transferability, thick descriptions with verbatim accounts are used to enable readers to discern whether the findings are applicable to similar settings. To ensure dependability, the accounts of each patient case and the focus group data for the different healthcare provider categories were included in the data analysis process; deviant cases were also noted and taken into account.

TABLE 3: Summary of main themes, subthemes and categories.

Themes	Subthemes	Categories
Provider perspective	Perceptions of patient expectations	-
	Patterns of communication and consultations	Medical practitioners Nurses Radiographers Radiologists Communication of results
Patient dispositions and reactions	Expectations and reluctance to communicate	Unfamiliarity with x-ray investigations Wait-and-see
	Experiences of imaging investigation process	From anxiety/fear to relief The whole story

Data collection triangulation in the form of individual interviews, observations of consultation sessions and focus groups ensured that the voices of patients and various healthcare provider categories were integrated in the study findings.

Ethical considerations

This study formed part of a qualitative project on decision making and interactions in diagnostic imaging investigations. Ethics approval was granted by the Research Ethics Committee, Faculty of Health Sciences, University of Pretoria, South Africa (170/2008) and health managers gave written permission for access to the research sites. Signed informed consent was obtained from all research participants, which included strict assurances of voluntary participation and confidentiality. Five provider participants declined audio-recording of the patient-doctor consultation. All, except one of these, gave permission for the field researcher to be present and taking written notes during the consultation. Three of these providers chose not to be interviewed individually after the consultations.

Results

The analysis centred around two main themes: (1) provider perspectives; and (2) patient dispositions and reactions. Table 3 provides a summary of subthemes and categories associated with each main theme. Direct quotations from the individual interviews and focus group interviews are provided, where appropriate, as supportive evidence for each subtheme. The following codes are used to refer to the different participant groups: [FG] = focus group; [II] = individual interview; [PI] = patient interview; [MP] = medical practitioner or family physician; [RADL] = radiologist or radiology registrar; [RAD] = radiographer; and [NP] = nurse. Where applicable, a number refers to the number of a particular patient participant.

Provider perspective

The two main emerging subthemes for providers are their perceptions of patient expectations and communication patterns with patients.

Providers' perceptions of patient expectations

Medical provider participants often referred to the so-called 'demand' by patients created by the nature of some patients' injuries, by observing other patients being referred for diagnostic imaging investigations, or by expectations raised by the referring centre. The following quote is illustrative:

'There are two groups of patients ... those who accept whatever the doctor says. They have come here for diagnosis. And those who made up their mind, they're coming to confirm their suspicion. Those are the patients that will demand diagnostic investigations, even if they don't need it. They demand and these are from the good socioeconomic status, the ones that are educated.' (II: Neurosurgery registrar, Patient 7)

Another provider perception was that patients thought that pathology would be missed if they were not referred for diagnostic imaging investigations:

'The problem is that the patient sometimes has funny ideas about what is wrong with them. ... For instance, if the patient experiences a cough for a long time or for a week; it might just be a cold but [the patient] might think it's cancer. ... So for them not to be sent for x-rays ... they don't understand it, because we are going to miss their possible cancer. That's what makes it difficult for patients.' (FG:MP)

Medical practitioners were of the opinion that patients 'think we can see everything on x-ray' and expected to be healed by 'this magical thing' that is 'going to change my life now forever' (FG:MP), 'like a treatment they're going through' (FG:RAD).

Healthcare providers' perceptions that patients expected referrals for diagnostic imaging investigations resulted in them favouring the use of technology as a pacifier and a 'quick fix' to prevent 'come backs' (FG:MP):

'But then they still go away thinking that lousy doctor did not send them for x-rays. Doctors are not doctors until they have done x-rays, given an injection and big fat packet of medicine and then they feel good. You think the patient is fine, but they think you actually look into their problems when you have an x-ray. It is actually psychological that you do something, even if it's not 100% indicated. The patient feels you're doing something, because the patient is worried. To prevent more visits.' (FG:MP)

Other medical providers justified referrals for diagnostic imaging investigations out of moral obligation: 'Some of them [patients] claim from the road accident funds' (FG:MP). Others were concerned about failing to make the correct diagnosis:

'I think you can take a lot of x-rays ... a little bit over-treating the patient. ... I feel more comfortable doing ... everything. I think there could be a possible fracture, more just purely on clinical [grounds], so if you're doing one side, then you can miss something. Often when it comes to comparing, it is when you can see it.' (II:MP, Patient 24)

Patterns of communication and consultations with patients

One of the communication challenges and concerns high-lighted by different providers was language comprehension and/or the less-than-ideal provision for language diversity between providers and patients:

'Things get lost in translation. ... I worry sometimes that maybe I ask a question, they don't quite get the proper clinical picture. And maybe when I give the information, they don't quite understand everything that I am saying.' (II:MP, Patient 16)

Medical practitioners: The observation data collected during the initial provider-patient consultations indicated that medical practitioners tended to take the patient histories in the form of rapid question-and-answer sessions without offering patients sufficient time to elaborate on their responses. Similarly, decisions to refer patients for diagnostic imaging investigations mostly involved one-way, non-negotiated communication, without any significant discussion regarding the risks and benefits or what could be expected of the investigation. One practitioner admitted that 'sometimes we forget to really talk to the patient' (FG:MP).

Others assumed that patients were knowledgeable about x-rays:

'That is where the doctors are lacking a lot. Because we don't talk to the patients about it, the risk and it is dangerous and things like that.' (FG:MP)

In most cases, patients were merely informed that they were going to be 'sent for x-rays' (PI:1), without seeking their approval or disapproval. Nurses and medical practitioners also alluded to system pressures and organisation of patient care encroaching on time available for patient interactions:

'This is not a quiet clinic. I have seen 69 patients. I have got six clinics running ... x-ray department closes at three. ... Chemist close at quarter to four; if they're not there they have to also return the next day. So it's all time constraints that you're working with.' (II: NP, Patient 17)

Patients also observed the 'time constraints' medical practitioners referred to, saying that 'the doctors do not give us the chance to talk to them; they are already on the move' (PI:13).

Interprofessional blaming emerged during the study, specifically with regard to who should be responsible for providing patients with information regarding diagnostic imaging procedures. Radiographers and radiologists often blamed medical practitioners because 'they don't inform the patients what they're going to do and who's going to do it' (FG:RAD).

Nurses: Nurses indicated that patients viewed them as a source of information at various points of contact, whereas the actual need for information varied from person to person:

'Some [patients] don't even know what x-ray [is]. They ask you, "What is x-ray? What are we going to do there? Is there any big machines? Am I going to feel the pain when they're going to do this?" And then I try to explain to them ... "You are going to stand there and they have got a big light and a big machine and they are going to take a photo of you. But this photo take of your inside, not your outside appearance.'" (FG:NP)

'Some of them don't even ask. They just take the [x-ray] envelope, open it and start looking like this and they want you to start explaining to them.' (FG:NP)

Radiographers: The observation data indicate that the imaging process resembled a production-chain setup. One radiographer admitted: 'Sometimes I do not check … [*with*] the patient what's going on' (II:RAD, Patient 1). This is how one patient described her experience:

'I just gave her [*radiographer*] the paper [*request form*] the doctor gave me. She took the paper. She took me next door [*to the x-ray room*]. She took the x-ray and after that she said I must sit on the bench. She came; she gave me the x-rays. "Go back to the nurses to give it there."' (PI:24)

There were, however, also patients who expressed appreciation for the radiographers' interpersonal interactions, saying that 'they were good; I observed how their attitude was and how they handled me' (PI:5).

Radiologists: The interaction between radiologists and patients can mostly be described as a non-relationship:

'We don't have much contact with the patient on sort of day-to-day running of plain x-rays to see the patient.' (FG:RADL)

This was also the case of our observations of patients referred for computerised tomography (CT) and ultrasound investigations. Patient 8, who shared her fear of losing her leg with the field researcher, had a very impersonal experience, with minimum interaction during her ultrasound investigation. The radiology registrar looked at the screen – not visible to her – without explaining anything and merely instructing her occasionally to elevate her leg.

Communication of results: In addition to the above lack of significant communication interactions, the researchers observed information download during post-imaging consultations where the patient was not afforded sufficient time to fully comprehend what had been said. In the majority of instances, healthcare providers did not involve the patients in the interpretation process, despite some patients showing interest in viewing their radiographs and wanting to be part of this. At this point, the issue of the 'big secret' (FG:RADL) arises. When Patient 21 tried to get a look at her x-rays the medical practitioner grabbed the x-rays and envelope, saying, 'This is mine!'

Patients frequently expected information about their outcomes at the imaging site: 'I would have liked to know whilst I was at the x-ray department' (PI:10). On the other hand, providers also seemingly expected patients to initiate the information-seeking process:

'That's if the patient wants to see the investigation or the films then and they should have the right to ask. The referring clinician has to have a look at the films as well and I think it's at that point that the patient should be shown the images.' (FG:RADL)

Patient dispositions and reactions

Patient expectations and reluctance to communicate, as well as patient experiences of the imaging investigation process are the two main subthemes that emerged from the analysis.

Patient expectations and reluctance to communicate

Unfamiliarity with x-ray investigations: Unfamiliarity could be one of the reasons for patients' reluctance to communicate with the healthcare providers. Although most participants knew about x-rays, only a few had a good understanding of radiation and its effects on the human body. This is how a patient with acute right hypochondriac pain expressed his understanding:

'No, you don't have x-rays too often, maybe once every six years. You don't have it a lot. X-rays are harmful because they're radioactive. But cell phones are just as harmful.' (IP:7)

The same patient was the only participant who explicitly verbalised a need for x-ray referral: 'Well, just take x-rays of my [*abdomen*] … Show what's up and what is going on' (IP:7). Other patients were less vocal and expressed their expectations in more general terms such as 'I want them to help me' (IP:4). They often relied on or complied with the medical practitioner's opinion – 'If they [*the doctors*] say for an x-ray, I know I must go' (IP:16).

Wait-and-see: During the doctor–patient consultation, patients tended to adopt an approach of 'one looks at the situation before you can ask' (IP:13). Most patients were reluctant to ask the medical practitioner for information as they did not feel comfortable with that or with divulging detailed information during history taking. In addition, hardly any opportunities were created for patients to ask for clarification or to express concerns – in a metaphorical sense, the patients' voices were silenced.

'The doctors don't talk to you so much … but sometimes the doctor … was a harsh somebody … It might frighten me sometimes if I don't know my story … I keep quiet about it. … Sometimes even before you give him the answer, he already answers it for you.' (IP:17)

The inadequate sharing of information and referral decisions by medical practitioners with patients regarding the purpose of the referral and/or potential alternative diagnostic options was highlighted when those patients interacted with radiographers at the imaging department. One radiographer shared the following:

'I had this experience where this patient came in for an [*barium*] enema. "Did they explain to you?" Then she said, no, she doesn't want it; are there any alternatives? And then I said, "Maybe you could get a scope or a scan." Then she wanted to go back to the doctor to get another second investigation. She refused the enema because she didn't understand what she made that appointment [*for*].' (FG:RAD)

Patient experiences of the imaging investigation process

One shared experience of patients journeying through the health system was the oscillation between fear or anxiety and feelings of relief. By the end of their journey, very few patients had adequate communication experiences.

From fear and anxiety to relief: Patient reactions during the exit interviews succinctly illustrated their fear or anxiety during the journey, as well as the ultimate relief experienced. On the one hand, they experienced fear of technology – the 'cold environment' (FG:NP) – at the diagnostic imaging department, whereas on the other hand, they experienced anxiety about the possible diagnosis.

Fear was clearly illustrated by a patient who had received inadequate information regarding what to expect from a stereotactic breast biopsy performed with imaging techniques. She was also frightened by the interactions that took place between the radiology registrars, radiographers and a nurse during the image-guided biopsy, but her journey had a good end:

> 'I was feeling scared. ... How are they going to do this thing? They say they are going to cut a piece of meat. It's where my imagination started to make me scared because I thought they were going just to cut me like that. ... They told me that they are going to inject me with a needle and they are going to cut me. ... I was not sure [*how*] they were going to do that. Maybe they [*wanted to*] make me not to be scared. ... I was not expecting it to be like this. It horrified me. ... I didn't even see the doctor [*radiology registrar*] that was doing the biopsy. ... I thought those nurses are going to do it. ... I know that in my family there is a cancer problem. ... I was so scared until now ... when they did do the results. ... But today at the end I am very happy.' (IP:13)

Inadequate preparation could lead to anxiety-provoking experiences for some patients and persons accompanying them when they had their first overwhelming encounter with 'the big machine':

> 'The minute we got into the x-ray room, we saw these big machines, ... [*my daughter*] started to cry. ... I did not really prepare [*her*] for this psychologically, because she is three years old. ... Everything is okay until we got to this cold room. ... There was no talking. She [*the radiographer*] said, "Come in"; "Okay, hold her arm"; and that was it. ... I felt neglected; you are not important. Just do this, that's all. They don't care. They just have to do their job. ... You know, when you work with kids ... that [*reassuring*] voice of yours. But there was nothing. "Okay, we're finished. Okay, go. Bye."' (FG:NP, on her own experience)

At the conclusion of the diagnostic imaging examination, some patients expressed a sense of relief, even if it was based on a seemingly incorrect understanding of the aim and/or outcome of the actual examination:

> 'Some patients really, they don't understand what x-rays are all about. Because the patient comes in and you ask him if he can stand, he says, "No, I can't stand." And you go to the room and then the patient stands up, you do the PA [*postero-anterior projection*], you do the lateral. And so, "I feel much better now." So he doesn't even know what the x-ray is all about. He just thinks we've done this big thing on him, now he is feeling lighter than before or "I am feeling much better now."' (FG:RAD)

'The whole, whole story': One may reasonably expect that patients at the end of their journeys would have a good idea of the underlying causes and/or explanations of their symptoms, the ultimate diagnosis and implications of their conditions, and the treatment plans that they should follow. Medical practitioners were of the opinion that it was 'the duty of the attending physician to put everything together, tell the patient the whole story' (FG:MP).

However, by not engaging in effective communication with patients and not confirming their comprehension level, patients can get lost in their journey and end up with inadequate information and understanding of their condition:

> 'I have seen patients; they have been through the whole system. They come back and you ask them ... "Have you got a fracture?" "No, I don't know. They never told me."' (FG:MP)

Only two patients reported getting the 'whole story'; one of them expressed it as follows:

> 'It was really a benefit to me because even on the x-rays the doctor showed me. I like also the fact that the doctor showed me ... in the book ... how the whole thing started and it helped me as well. So I think the x-rays are a very good thing and what I like from that, I just know that I have sinus. Before when I go to the doctor, then they check. ... They say my sinuses are blocked inside. So it's the first time that I experience that they show me the x-rays; how even my eyes, I didn't know that, the x-rays will take it out as well, as it's part of the sinus, the infection of the eye. I know now the whole, whole story of the problem that I have. And then for that I know I will be more careful. For sometimes you know you mustn't be in the place where people smoke, but still you are there. So now I know exactly that I must really strictly avoid those types of things ... That is how it must go. The doctor must explain to you the cause of the sickness and show how the parts happen and what happens.' (IP:12)

Discussion

This study explored the expectations and experiences of patients regarding diagnostic imaging investigations from the point of consultation and referral up to the reporting of the results and outcomes of the imaging investigations within the medical encounter. The study also explored the various healthcare providers' perceptions of patient expectations and patterns of communication and interaction.

The perceived patient expectations by medical providers are sometimes based in the providers' own uncertainty, cautiousness and desire to confirm or exclude a diagnosis.[18] In other cases, patients may demand referrals for diagnostic imaging investigations, as was found in a study by Baker et al.[19] in which medical practitioners were under pressure to refer patients for spinal x-rays. Some medical practitioners in our study also reported similar demands, whereas some conceded to using technology as a pacifier – a 'quick fix' approach – to prevent come-backs. System pressures were sometimes experienced as a dominant factor in referrals; the emphasis was on throughput of relatively large numbers of patients per day. Similar to the study by Jayadevappa and

Chattre,[20] the current study found that patient satisfaction was not so much linked to their specific expectations but rather with the effective management of the condition and/or situation.

Communication gaps identified during the provider-patient interaction were limited two-way communication and low patient participation in the decision-making process at the time of the referral for a diagnostic imaging investigation, during the actual investigation and during the post-investigation consultation. A clear advantage of informing patients about the potential risks of imaging would enable them to make informed decisions at that moment and in the future regarding complex issues concerning their healthcare.[7] Similar to Malone et al.'s findings,[3] this study found hardly any evidence that information on radiation risks was mentioned or explained in the doctor–patient consultations or radiographer-patient interactions. Some of the medical practitioners in our study seemingly assumed that patients had an adequate knowledge of the radiation risks and benefits associated with diagnostic imaging investigations. Radiographers focused on possible risks during pregnancy and with the procedure task at hand. Reeves and Decker[21] describe the image and not the patient as being the centre of the diagnostic radiography practice; the images distance the radiographer from the patients and their suffering. Murphy[22] suggests that radiographers merely act as operators of equipment in a patient-unfriendly environment that leaves little room to actually listen and respond to patients' information and support needs.

Patient participants' general unfamiliarity with diagnostic imaging investigations and their reservations about initiating information-seeking dialogue with healthcare providers are reflected in their wait-and-see attitude. The reason for this 'passive partner role' (p. 578) is aptly described by Mabuza and colleagues,[23] who refer to the trust patients have in the South African public health sector with regard to healthcare providers' decisions. Furthermore, some patients prefer to not be involved in decision making and rather rely on the providers as the only authority.[24]

The 'silence' of patients can be explained from a sociological and organisational perspective in that their voices are not always duly respected and recognised by healthcare providers,[25] leaving little room for meaningful information-seeking discussions. Longtin et al.[26] contend that the nature of patient participation is a reflection of societal norms and the culture of an organisation, in our case a public hospital complex. In a context where there is a cultural expectation that patients should play a passive role, it is not surprising that they will be more reluctant to initiate active participation. The organisational and system pressures on healthcare providers evident in this study did not support opportunities for sufficient interaction, despite patients' rights to information on diagnosis, treatment options, benefits, risk and costs and to participation in decisions pertaining to their health, as set out by the South African Patients' Charter[27] and the *National Health Act* 61 of 2003.[28]

Another factor affecting patient participation is potential language barriers within multilingual settings. However, in our study we did not explicitly interrogate the role and extent of the actual and/or perceived language barriers. According to Dauer et al.,[29] it is important to evaluate a patient's level of understanding during a consultation. This was rarely observed in our study. It is difficult to change established communication patterns,[26] as consultations often focus on moving towards closure.[30] With diagnostic imaging, communication patterns are even more complex. Where technology forms part of the interaction process, there is a tendency toward 'objectification of a patient's body' (p. 172)[31] that may limit the social interaction between patients and the radiographers and radiologists performing the procedures.

Much has been reported on patient experiences of diagnostic imaging investigations, including their anxiety regarding an uncertain future.[32,33] Our study found that the absence of appropriate information often resulted in patient uncertainty and anxiety about the imaging investigation itself and the role of the investigation in the treatment of their condition. According to Van Ravesteijn et al.,[11] the quality and amount of information given to patients before ordering the diagnostic investigation is likely to have a reassuring effect.

In the current study, patients were often kept in suspense about the imaging results. They were unsure who would communicate the results and at which point the communication should take place. Furthermore, the patients' journeys through the health system exhibited several points of disjointed communication, even lack of communication, which may have significantly contributed to their fears and anxieties.

There should be a balance and an interdependence between healthcare-provider responsibilities and the responsibility of patients to seek information and clarification where they have not understood.[23,34] Such interrelatedness and interdependence should also characterise the interactions amongst healthcare providers within the organisation itself. Technical interconnectedness in the diagnostic imaging context is an essential attribute of any quest to achieve the desired outcomes. Therefore, we propose that the communication and interaction processes where diagnostic imaging investigations are involved should be based on a provider–patient-centred approach mediated through (and in some instances shaped by) technology.

Recommendations

Because of the complex nature of interactions and communication processes, more feasibility studies are needed, using interventions at various points of contact. Recommendations and interventions to improve patient communication regarding diagnostic imaging investigations are the following:

- More effort by healthcare providers to probe patients' level of understanding of important information.[29,35]

The teach-back method is an evidence-based method often used in health education.[36,37]

- Pamphlets and visual aids, such as posters and videos, on what to expect from diagnostic imaging investigations in general (routine referrals) or from a specialised investigation.[38]
- Special efforts to ensure that patients and parents understand the implications of specialised investigations for which signed consent is required.[38] An appropriate information leaflet or video explaining the specific investigation – benefits, risks, procedures and process – is essential. Healthcare providers may need training in adequate counselling techniques for obtaining signed consent.
- Short questionnaire to patients prior to a consultation or an imaging investigation to explore their desires and preferences for participation or to ensure that their concerns have been covered.[39]
- Availability of a radiographer to answer questions of patients waiting for an investigation to improve patients' comprehension of procedures and relieve anxiety and fear.
- More emphasis in undergraduate training of doctors, radiographers and nurses in explaining diagnostic imaging investigations and elicit patient participation, for example, including appropriate scenarios in practical training and in examinations.

Limitations

This study had a number of limitations. It was conducted in only one public healthcare setting, where a small number of patients were shadowed along their journey through the healthcare system. The findings are therefore not generalisable, although the supportive verbatim accounts provided in the above sections may enhance transferability to similar settings. Patient exit interviews were less informative than expected; once the patients' healthcare concern had been solved or attended to they were less willing to commit additional interview time to the field researcher. Some of the logistical and language constraints have already been alluded to in earlier sections.

Conclusion

Several studies have been conducted on doctor–patient consultations and interactions at specific points of contact within the health system. The unique contribution of the current study is that it followed individual patients through various points of contact in healthcare provision, from admission to ultimate discharge or ward admission. To the best of our knowledge, this was the first study with diagnostic imaging investigations as its focal point, with the casualty and outpatient departments as point of departure.

This study could serve as a basic framework to facilitate the interactional coherence between the medical consultation, a referral for a diagnostic imaging investigation, the imaging investigation itself, the decision-making process

and interactive communication of information from a South African perspective. This could contribute to a better understanding of the broader medical encounter that expands beyond the dyadic doctor-patient consultation. The referral for a diagnostic imaging investigation and the encounter with providers and technology at the imaging department necessitates an appreciation of the complexity of patient participation and interaction with multiple healthcare providers. An awareness of the expectations and experiences of patients beyond the doctor-patient consultation as they journey through the health system is essential to achieving quality provider-patient-centred care.

Acknowledgements

The authors wish to thank all the colleagues and patients who contributed to the study.

Competing interests

The authors declare that they have no financial or personal relationship(s) that may have inappropriately influenced them in writing this article.

Authors' contributions

All authors, namely, C.R.M. (Department of Radiography, University of Pretoria), A.-M.B. (MRC Unit for Maternal and Infant Health Care Strategies, University of Pretoria) and W.A.H. (Department of Biomedical Sciences, Tshwane University of Technology) were involved the design of the study. C.R.M. did most of the data collection. All authors contributed to the data analysis and interpretation. C.R.M. drafted the first version of the manuscript on which the other two authors gave inputs and approved the final version.

References

1. Bairstow P, Persaud J, Mendelson R, et al. Reducing inappropriate diagnostic practice through education and decision support. Int J Qual Health Care. 2010;22(3):194–200. http://dx.doi.org/10.1093/intqhc/mzq016

2. Patel VL, Kaufman DR, Arocha JF. Methodological review: Emerging paradigms of cognition in medical decision-making. J Biomed Inform. 2002;35(1):52–75. http://dx.doi.org/10.1016/S1532-0464(02)00009-6

3. Malone J, Guleria R, Craven C, et al. Justification of diagnostic medical exposures: Some practical issues. Report of an International Atomic Energy Agency Consultation. Brit J Radiol. 2012;85(1013):523–538. http://dx.doi.org/10.1259/bjr/42893576

4. Hofmann B, Lysdahl K. Moral principles and medical practice: The role of patient autonomy in the extensive use of radiological services. J Med Ethics. 2008;34(6):446–449. http://dx.doi.org/10.1136/jme.2006.019307

5. Larsson W, Lundberg N, Hillergård K. Use your good judgement – radiographers' knowledge in image production work. Radiography. 2009;15(3):e11–e21.

6. Kenen RH. The at-risk health status and technology: A diagnostic invitation and the 'gift' of knowing. Soc Sci Med. 1996;42(11):1545–1553. http://dx.doi.org/10.1016/0277-9536(95)00248-0

7. Gray V. Reducing radiation exposure in diagnostic imaging [document on the Internet]. c2010 [cited 2011 Apr 10]. Available from: http://www.sagehms.com/Reducing%20Radiation%20Exposure.pdf

8. Kravitz RL, Callahan EJ. Patient's perceptions of omitted examinations and tests: A qualitative analysis. J Gen Intern Med. 2000;15(1):38–45. http://dx.doi.org/10.1046/j.1525-1497.2000.12058.x

9. Epstein RM, Fiscella K, Lesser CS, et al. Why the nation needs a policy push on patient-centered health care. Health Aff (Millwood). 2010;29(8):1489–1495. http://dx.doi.org/10.1377/hlthaff.2009.0888

10. Jordan JL, Ellis SJ, Chambers R. Defining shared decision making and concordance: Are they one and the same? Postgrad Med J. 2002;78(921):383–384. http://dx.doi.org/10.1136/pmj.78.921.383

11. Van Ravesteijn H, Van Dijk I, Darmon D, et al. The reassuring value of diagnostic tests: A systematic review. Patient Educ Couns. 2012;86(1):3–8. http://dx.doi.org/10.1016/j.pec.2011.02.003

12. Kravitz R. The physician-patient relationship: Measuring patients' expectations and requests. Ann Intern Med. 2001;134(9 Pt 2):881–888.

13. Munn Z, Jordan Z. The patient experience of high technology medical imaging: A systematic review of the qualitative evidence. Radiography. 2011;17(4):323–331. http://dx.doi.org/10.1016/j.radi.2011.06.004

14. Nightingale J, Murphy F, Blakeley C. 'I thought it was just an x-ray': A qualitative investigation of patient experiences in cardiac SPECT-CT imaging. Nucl Med Commun. 2012;33(3):246–254. http://dx.doi.org/10.1097/MNM.0b013e32834f90c6

15. Creswell J. Qualitative inquiry and research design: choosing among five approaches. 2nd ed. Thousand Oaks, CA: Sage; 2007.

16. Ng CKC, White P. Qualitative research design and approaches in radiography. Radiography. 2005;11(3):217–225. http://dx.doi.org/10.1016/j.radi.2005.03.006

17. Leigh J. A tale of the unexpected: Managing an insider dilemma by adopting the role of outsider in another setting. Qual Res. 2014;14(4):428–441. http://dx.doi.org/10.1177/1468794113481794

18. Espeland A, Baerheim A. Factors affecting general practitioners' decisions about plain radiography for back pain: Implications for classification of guideline barriers – a qualitative study. BMC Health Serv Res. 2003;3:8. http://dx.doi.org/10.1186/1472-6963-3-8

19. Baker R, Lecouturier J, Bond S. Explaining variation in GP referral rates for x-rays for back pain. Implement Sci. 2006;1:15. http://dx.doi.org/10.1186/1748-5908-1-15

20. Jayadevappa R, Chattre S. Patient centred care – a conceptual model and review of the state of art. Open Health Serv Policy J. 2011;4:15–25. http://dx.doi.org/10.2174/1874924001104010015

21. Reeves PJ, Decker S. Diagnostic radiography: A study in distancing. Radiography. 2012;18(2):78–83. http://dx.doi.org/10.1016/j.radi.2012.01.001

22. Murphy F. Understanding the humanistic interaction with medical imaging technology. Radiography. 2001;7(3):193–201. http://dx.doi.org/10.1053/radi.2001.0328

23. Mabuza L, Omole OB, Govender I, et al. Reasons for inpatients not to seek clarity at Dr George Mukhari Academic Hospital, Pretoria. Afr J Prm Health Care Fam Med. 2014;6(1):Art. #576, 8 pages.

24. Kiesler DJ, Auerbach SM. Optimal matches of patient preferences for information, decision-making and interpersonal behavior: Evidence, models and interventions. Patient Educ Couns. 2006;61(3):319–341. http://dx.doi.org/10.1016/j.pec.2005.08.002

25. Malterud K, Taksdal A. Shared spaces for reflection: Approaching medically unexplained disorders. Junctures. 2007;9:27–38.

26. Longtin Y, Sax H, Leape L, et al. Patient participation: Current knowledge and applicability to patient safety. Mayo Clin Proc. 2010;85(1):53–62. http://dx.doi.org/10.4065/mcp.2009.0248

27. Health Professions Council of South Africa. Guidelines for good practice in the health care professions. National Patients' Rights Charter. Booklet 3. Pretoria: Health Professions Council of South Africa; 2008.

28. Republic of South Africa. National Health Act, 2003 (Act No. 61 of 2003) (Chapter 2, p. 11–30). Government Gazette. 2004;No 26595.

29. Dauer LT, Thornton RH, Hay JL, et al. Fears, feelings, and facts: Interactively communicating benefits and risks of medical radiation with patients. Am J Roentgenol. 2011;196(4):756–761. http://dx.doi.org/10.2214/AJR.10.5956

30. Barry CA, Bradley C, Britten N, et al. Patients' unvoiced agendas in general practice consultations. BMJ. 2001;320:1246–1250. http://dx.doi.org/10.1136/bmj.320.7244.1246

31. Murphy FJ. The paradox of imaging technology: A review of the literature. Radiography. 2006;12(2):169–174. http://dx.doi.org/10.1016/j.radi.2005.03.011

32. Olivier L, Leclère J, Dolbeault S, et al. Doctor-patient relationship in oncologic radiology. Cancer Imaging. 2005;11(5):S83–S88.

33. Undeland M, Malterud K. Diagnostic work in general practice: More than naming a disease. Scand J Prim Health Care. 2002;20(3):145–150. http://dx.doi.org/10.1080/028134302760234582

34. Kasper J, Légaré F, Scheibler F, et al. Turning signals into meanings – 'shared decision making' meets communication theory. Health Expect. 2011;15(1):3–11. http://dx.doi.org/10.1111/j.1369-7625.2011.00657.x

35. Giroldi E, Veldhuizen W, Mannaerts A, et al. 'Doctor, please tell me it's nothing serious': An exploration of patients' worrying and reassuring cognitions using simulated recall interviews. BMC Fam Pract. 2014;15:73. http://dx.doi.org/10.1186/1471-2296-15-73

36. Tamura-Lis W. Teach-back for quality education and patient safety. Urol Nurs. 2013;33(6):267–271, 298.

37. DeWalt DA, Broucksou KA, Hawk V, et al. Developing and testing the health literacy universal precautions toolkit. Nurs Outlook. 2011;59(2):85–94. http://dx.doi.org/10.1016/j.outlook.2010.12.002

38. Farrell EH, Whistance RN, Phillips K, et al. Systematic review and meta-analysis of audio-visual information aids for informed consent for invasive healthcare procedures in clinical practice. Patient Educ Couns. 2014;94(1):20–32. http://dx.doi.org/10.1016/j.pec.2013.08.019

39. Middleton JF, McKinley RK, Gillies CL. Effect of patient completed agenda forms and doctors' education about agenda on the outcome of consultations: randomised controlled trial. BMJ. 2006;332(7552):1238–1242. http://dx.doi.org/10.1136/bmj.38841.444861.7C

28

Development of a training programme for primary care providers to counsel patients with risky lifestyle behaviours in South Africa

Authors:
Zelra Malan[1]
Bob Mash[1]
Katherine Everett-Murphy[2]

Affiliations:
[1]Family Medicine and Primary Care, Stellenbosch University, South Africa

[2]Chronic Diseases Initiative in Africa (CDIA), Faculty of Health Sciences, University of Cape Town, South Africa

Correspondence to:
Zelra Malan

Email:
zmalan@sun.ac.za

Postal address:
PO Box 241, Cape Town 8000, South Africa

Background: We are facing a global epidemic of non-communicable disease (NCDs), which has been linked with four risky lifestyle behaviours. It is recommended that primary care providers (PCPs) provide individual brief behaviour change counselling (BBCC) as part of everyday primary care, however currently training is required to build capacity. Local training programmes are not sufficient to achieve competence.

Aim: This study aimed to redesign the current training for PCPs in South Africa, around a new model for BBCC that would offer a standardised approach to addressing patients' risky lifestyle behaviours.

Setting: The study population included clinical nurse practitioners and primary care doctors in the Western Cape Province.

Methods: The analyse, design, develop, implement and evaluate (ADDIE) model provided a systematic approach to the analysis of learning needs, the design and development of the training programme, its implementation and initial evaluation.

Results: This study designed a new training programme for PCPs in BBCC, which was based on a conceptual model that combined the 5As (ask, alert, assess, assist and arrange) with a guiding style derived from motivational interviewing. The programme was developed as an eight-hour training programme that combined theory, modelling and simulated practice with feedback, for either clinical nurse practitioners or primary care doctors.

Conclusion: This was the first attempt at developing and implementing a best practice BBCC training programme in our context, targeting a variety of PCPs, and addressing different risk factors.

Développement d'un programme de formation pour prestataires de soins primaires pour leur permettre de conseiller les patients à comportement à risque en Afrique du Sud.

Contexte: Nous sommes confrontés à une épidémie globale de maladies non transmissibles (MNT), liées à quatre comportements à risque. Nous recommandons que les prestataires de soins primaires (PSP) offrent des consultations individuelles visant à modifier les comportements (CIMC) dans le cadre des soins de santé primaire; cependant, il faudra organiser des formations pour renforcer les capacités. Les programmes de formation locaux ne suffisent pas pour développer les compétences.

Objectif: Cette étude avait pour but de remanier la formation actuelle des PSP en Afrique du Sud, autour d'un nouveau modèle pour la CIMC qui offrirait une approche normalisée pour s'occuper des comportements à risque des patients.

Lieu: La population de l'étude comprenait des infirmières cliniques et des médecins de soins primaires dans la province du Western Cape.

Méthodes: Le modèle ADDIE a offert une approche systématique à l'analyse des besoins d'apprentissage, à la conception et au développement du programme de formation, à sa mise en œuvre et à son évaluation initiale

Résultats: Cette étude a conçu un nouveau programme de formation pour les PSP en CIMC, basé sur un modèle conceptuel combinant 5 processus (demander, alerter, évaluer, assister et organiser) avec un style directeur fondé sur l'entrevue motivationnelle. Le programme a été conçu comme un programme de formation de huit heures combinant la théorie, la modélisation et la simulation avec des feedback, pour les infirmières cliniciennes ou les médecins de soins primaires.

Conclusion: C'était la première fois qu'on élaborait et mettait en œuvre un programme de formation de meilleure pratique en CIMC dans notre contexte, qui ciblait une variété de PSP, et abordait les différents facteurs de risques.

Introduction

Many countries, including South Africa, are reporting an increase in the prevalence of non-communicable diseases (NCDs) such as hypertension and diabetes. These NCDs have been linked to underlying risky lifestyle behaviours such as tobacco smoking, unhealthy diet, alcohol abuse and physical inactivity.[1,2] Brief behaviour change counselling (BBCC), which is integrated into routine primary care, can be effective in helping patients change these risky behaviours.[3,4,5] The importance of this has been recognised by the South African Department of Health in its National Strategic Plan for the Prevention and Control of NCDs.[6] Capacitating primary care providers (PCPs) to deliver BBCC in primary care settings is recommended for all four risk factors.

It is feasible for BBCC to be effectively delivered by PCPs, who have both the opportunity and credibility to do so.[3,4,5] Training can enhance PCPs efficiency and capacity to provide this counselling, provided adequate resources and support are available in the workplace.[5,7] Most of the research that explores training interventions for PCPs to deliver this counselling is from developed countries, such as the USA, Australia and Canada.[7,8,9] The few studies that have been undertaken locally suggest that such training is currently inadequate.[10,11,12]

PCPs face a difficult task in helping patients to change their risky lifestyle behaviours. In South Africa the experience of counselling in practice tends to be discouraging, because of the poor response of patients, and challenging because of numerous barriers. These include language barriers, lack of time, poor knowledge of lifestyle modification, inadequate counselling skills, lack of self-efficacy, and poor continuity of care. PCPs reported lack of confidence in their ability to help patients change and their scepticism about the effectiveness of lifestyle counselling may partly be a reflection of inadequate training in this area.[10,11]

Recent situational analyses in the Western Cape showed that current training programmes on behaviour change counselling for PCPs are not sufficient to achieve competence in clinical practice.[10,11] Training programmes were mostly theoretical and without the opportunity to practise key skills, and receive constructive feedback on performance. PCPs therefore were not confident to perform BBCC. Due to time constraints, training was not integrated throughout the curriculum and there was no reinforcement afterwards. The training outcomes were not assessed, and even lecturers were unaware of the evidence in support of BBCC and had low confidence in the effectiveness of their training.[11] Therefore trainers, and not just students, needed training in BBCC.

Traditionally PCPs rely mostly on the directive style when counselling patients on behaviour change, resulting in resistance from the patient, and frustration for the PCPs.[13] Changing the PCPs current style of communication could be challenging, and we realised that the training should focus not only on teaching PCPs a structure for BBCC and

evidence-based knowledge of lifestyle modification, but also to transform their style of communication.

Capacitating PCPs to deliver BBCC in a skilful way that is integrated within the consultation is essential.[3,4,14] This study aimed to address this need by redesigning the current training around a new model for BBCC that would offer a standardised approach to addressing different NCD risk behaviours, be realistic in terms of training time and resources, be feasible to perform in clinical practice, as well as evidence-based and effective.

Aims and objectives

The aim of this study was to develop a training programme for PCPs that delivered a best practice BBCC method for patients with risky lifestyle behaviours and evidence-based information on NCDs. This paper focuses on the development of the training intervention; the evaluation of it in clinical practice will be reported on at a later date. Specific objectives were to:

- Design a best practice BBCC training programme to meet the needs of PCPs.
- Develop the structure and content of the training intervention, as well as the skills and resources needed to deliver this programme.
- Implement the training programme.
- Evaluate and revise the training programme.

Research methods and design
Study design

Most approaches to instructional systems design reflect the ADDIE (analyse, design, develop, implement and evaluate) model, which uses a systemic problem solving approach to develop new training programmes.[15] The ADDIE model may be particularly useful if the main focus of the new training programme is changing the behaviour of participants.[15] The objectives above were based on the ADDIE model, which is also shown in Figure 1. The ADDIE model provided a systematic approach to the analysis of learning needs, the design and development of the training programme, its implementation and initial evaluation.[15] The ADDIE process had also been previously used in local educational research and development of training programmes.[16,17] The methods used to complete each step of the model are described below.

Setting

Eighty percent of the South African population make use of public sector health care facilities, particularly those with NCDs, which are amongst the commonest conditions seen in primary care.[18] The majority of patients are seen by clinical nurse practitioners in either small clinics or larger health centres. Clinical nurse practitioners only receive an additional one year of training to cope with the wide range of problems seen in primary care. Clinical nurse practitioners are supported by primary care doctors, who usually have no additional postgraduate training. Therefore, the PCPs

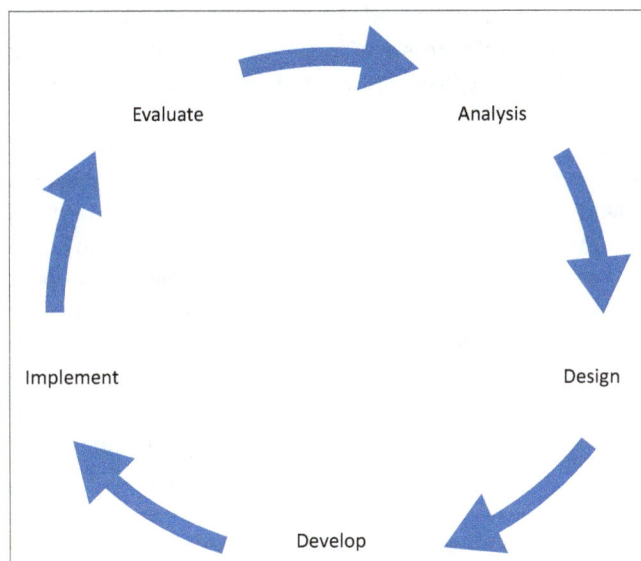

FIGURE 1: The ADDIE model for design of training programmes.

targeted by this training programme were clinical nurse practitioners and primary care doctors.

The training programme was developed with the intention of initially implementing and evaluating it as part of the one-year Diploma course (Diploma in Clinical Nursing Science, Health Assessment, Treatment and Care) at Stellenbosch University, which focused on training clinical nurse practitioners, and the four-year postgraduate training programme in family medicine, which was aimed at doctors, at both the University of Cape Town and Stellenbosch.

Educational team

An educational team was created to collaborate on the ADDIE process and consisted of the three authors. The team combined expertise in motivational interviewing, adult education, NCDs, primary care research and brief behaviour change counselling (BBCC).[16,17,18,19,20,21,22]

ADDIE process
Step 1 Analysis

The situational analysis of current training and clinical practice for the target audience has been summarised in the introduction and published elsewhere.[11] This article reports on the remaining ADDIE process.

Step 2 Design

In the design stage the educational team developed a conceptual model and learning outcomes that were derived from the findings of the situational analysis and a literature review. The literature review searched PubMed, Google Scholar and local African journals for evidence on effective models of BBCC, as well as approaches to the design and implementation of training programmes.

Step 3 Development

The educational team then developed the structure and content of the training programme, learning activities and strategies, as well as the educational resources required. Care was taken to ensure that all of these elements were aligned with the design of the learning outcomes and conceptual model.

The educational team then prepared the actual content, for instance power point slides, instructions for role plays and practical exercises, by drawing on existing materials and previous experiences in training motivational interviewing. This process also helped the team to determine which resources were available and which needed to be developed, or obtained.

The training programme that emerged from the design and development phases was presented to a group of programme managers, clinicians and trainers of family medicine and primary care at Stellenbosch University to obtain further input from experts in primary health care.

Step 4 Implementation

During 2012–2013 three groups of nurses and three groups of primary care doctors completed the training programme at Stellenbosch University.

Step 5 Evaluation

Feedback forms from the training courses during 2012–2013 were used to obtain the participants' opinions on how to improve the model, content or approach to teaching. The trainers analysed the information, and used it to revise the training programme accordingly. Revisions were also made based on the reflections of the educational team on their training experience.

Ethical considerations

This study was approved by the Health Research Ethics Committees (HREC) at Stellenbosch University (Reference number: N11/11/321), on 27 February 2012.

Results
Design

The Canadian Task Force on Preventative Health, the Royal Australian College of General Practitioners, the National Health Service in the UK, the Department of Health and Aging in the Australian government and the Kinect consortium, all recommend the use of the 5 A construct in BBCC and promote its integration into primary care.[3,4,7,8] The 5A construct consists of five steps: ask, advise, assess, assist and arrange. It provides PCPs with a broad framework for BBCC, which is simple to understand, applicable to different settings, and can be used by PCPs from different disciplines and levels of expertise.

Motivational interviewing (MI) is a flexible, evidence-based, clinical skill that can be used when talking to patients about how and why they might change their behaviour.[13,23] MI provides an alternative approach to the usual more authoritarian approaches and outperforms traditional advice-giving in 80% of studies.[22] PCPs, who have little time with patients, can expect a 10% – 15% improvement in patients changing their risky lifestyle behaviours after counselling based on motivational interviewing (MI).[23] At the core of MI lies the guiding style, which promotes collaboration, empathy, evocation, respect for choice and control, and a clear focus.

A guiding style communicates an approach of 'I can help you solve this for yourself' as opposed to 'This is what you must do'. To accomplish this, PCPs need to be able to switch from their traditional role as directive, expert advice givers, to guides that can skilfully assist the patient to make difficult decisions about change.

Training practitioners to be competent in MI is not easy, and in our context unlikely to be achievable with the majority of PCPs in a short training course.[19,24] The decision was taken therefore to rather focus on the characteristics of a guiding style derived from MI and the essential underlying communication skills.[19,22,25] The recommended approaches to completing each of the steps in the 5A model were rewritten to adopt this guiding style. The title of the second step, which was 'advise' in the original model, was changed to 'alert' as unsolicited advice-giving is seen as incongruent with a guiding style. The concept of alerting someone to a potential risk and evoking their response was, however, seen as more congruent with a guiding style.

The underlying spirit of the guiding style was based on three elements, which were collaboration vs. confrontation between the provider and the patient, evoking or drawing out the patient's ideas about change rather than imposing ideas, and emphasising the patient's autonomy versus being authoritative.[13,14,22] Core key communication skills that support the guiding style were defined as asking open-ended questions, reflective listening, affirmations and summaries (OARS).[13] Reflective listening and summarisation are perhaps the most crucial skills, which demonstrate empathy and encourage the patients to elaborate, whilst the use of open-ended questions invites patients to consider how and why they might change. Offering affirmations helps the patient to recognise their own strengths.

Therefore, in our model of BBCC the key principles of a guiding style were integrated into each step of the 5As structure as shown in Table 1. This approach to BBCC was supported by a local quasi-experimental study that demonstrated its effectiveness in helping pregnant women reduce, or stop, tobacco smoking when delivered by nurse midwives and lay counsellors.[20]

Based on this conceptual model, the results of the situational analysis and learning outcomes identified from the literature, as well as the educational team's own expertise in MI, the following learning outcomes were developed. At the end of the training programme participants would be able to:

1. Use a guiding style of counselling.
2. Practice reflective listening.
3. Recognise, elicit, and respond to change talk.
4. Exchange information.
5. Assess readiness to change.
6. Use the 5A steps (Ask, Alert, Assess, Assist, Arrange).
7. Counsel patients regarding the four key risk factors.

TABLE 1: Model of brief behaviour change counselling.

Step in the 5 As	Tasks in a guiding style
Ask	Ask about and document behavioural risks: Identify risk behaviour and document in record. Ask the patient what he/she already knows about the risks associated with the behaviour or would like to know. Respectfully affirm what he/she knows. Request permission to provide further information.
Alert	Provide relevant information in a neutral manner: Before giving information, emphasise that your role is to assist the patient in making informed choices, not to compel them to a particular course of action. Offer information on the health risks or benefits of change in a neutral way. Provide information using the 'E-P-E' method which is to elicit what the patient already knows and wants to know, provide relevant information, and elicit the patients understanding of this. If there is already a health problem related to the risk behaviour, clearly link the two.
Assess	Assess readiness to change: Ask the patient how they feel about the information provided and the possibility of making a change at this time. Assess how important change is for the patient and how confident he/she feels about change. Recognise and respond to 'change talk', which are statements by the patient revealing a desire, ability, reason, need or commitment to change. Offer support and assistance, but respect the patient's decision.
Assist	If response is 'Not ready to change': Ask about and acknowledge patient's concerns with empathy, avoiding any arguments. Offer help if he/she comes to a decision to change in the future. Request permission to give patient materials (if available), which could assist in them making a decision in the future. If response is 'Yes, am ready to change' then provide practical assistance to change such as: Positively reinforce any intentions to change which the patient expressed, no matter how small they may be. Express confidence in their capacity to achieve their health goal. Offer materials which teach behavioural change strategies and skills and express confidence that they will help. Prompt the patient to anticipate problems and barriers and to consider how to overcome these. Prompt patient to seek social support in their social environment. Prescribe medication, if appropriate.
Arrange	Arrange for follow up and/or referral: Document decisions made and materials given in the clinic record, add a reminder to discuss progress during the next visit and schedule follow up contact. Reiterate your and clinic staff's commitment to provide further information and support during behavioural change process. Refer patient to other health care providers for more intensive counselling if possible or to community based resources.

Development

A key principle of this stage was to develop an educational process that itself resonated with the guiding style. In essence we recognised that we were asking PCPs to change their own behaviour regarding how they counselled other people about behaviour change. Therefore, the principles being recommended for BBCC should also be embodied in the course itself regarding its structure and process.

These principles needed not only to be embodied in the structure and process of the course, but also modelled by the trainers themselves. In other words, the trainer's style of training needed to be congruent with the style of counselling being taught.[26]

Behaviourist learning theory is particularly useful when a change in behaviour is the desired outcome of a training intervention.[27] This approach recognises three key areas: namely, that the desired behaviour is the clear focus of the learning, that participants can practice the behaviour in a controlled and safe environment and that the training reinforces the behaviour by providing feedback on performance. Typically, the teacher demonstrates the specific behaviours, whilst participants observe, and then they practice and receive feedback on their own performance under controlled circumstances.[27]

The training was designed to give participants time to create a safe, supportive and reflective group environment.[26] Group discussions provide an essential component of training, and to ensure participation from every participant, group size should be limited to 20 or less. For this training programme, a ratio of one trainer to 12 students was thought to be possible, but ideally one trainer to eight participants was seen as the ideal.

Traditional didactic teaching methods were not considered effective in changing behaviour.[26] Although the training included some brief sharing of theory using didactic methods, these were combined with other approaches, such as the jig-saw method, in which members of a small group collectively master a piece of the whole theory and then share this piece with others in a new small group that includes peer-experts in all the other pieces. After information was given in a didactic manner the participants were also encouraged to reflect as a group, or individually, and consider their response to the theory or ideas presented.[26] The programme included information on the specific risk factors, as this improves participant content knowledge and confidence in delivering effective interventions.[26,28]

Based on best evidence from the literature review, the following principles were used in the development of the training course:[26,28,29]

- Provide evidence of the current deficiencies in counselling, the reasons for them, and the consequences for patients and doctors.

- Offer an evidence base for the skills needed to overcome these deficiencies.
- Demonstrate the skills to be learned.
- Provide the opportunity to practice these skills.
- Give constructive feedback on performance.

Based on the time that could reasonably be made available for the training within the selected curricula for nurses and doctors, the training was designed as an eight-hour workshop, with four two-hour sessions. The final training programme that was developed is summarised in Table 2.

A checklist of all the educational resources required was developed. This included the PowerPoint slides needed for the talks, the DVD material, the instructions for the small group exercises, the course manual with information on risk factors, and the equipment needed. From this list the team decided which resources could be accessed from already available materials, and which resources needed to be developed.

The international Motivational Interviewing Network of Trainers (MINT) operates a website with extensive information about the clinical method and training of MI.[30] This website has a manual containing a menu of exercises that MINT trainers use for various skills training. Practical exercises were chosen from the MINT manual, adapted for our setting, and used as practical exercises after a skill had been modelled.[30]

A training manual that summarised the model of BBCC and the underlying evidence, as well as applying the model practically to each risk factor, was printed for each participant. In addition each participant received, on each risk factor, patient educational material that was designed to dovetail with the approach to BBCC. All of these printed materials can be accessed via the web at www.ichange4health.co.za.

Both the researcher and Dr Katherine Everett-Murphy were trained internationally as MI trainers during the development of the course and became members of MINT.[30] This experience was useful to improve their embodiment of the guiding style in the teaching approach, to update the practical exercises, and to incorporate the latest theory of MI.[13]

Implementation

Twelve family medicine registrars, two general practitioners in private practice, and four family physicians were trained. Twenty three nurses on the one year Diploma course (Diploma in Clinical Nursing Science, Health Assessment, Treatment and Care) at the University of Stellenbosch were trained.

Evaluation

Overall feedback on the conceptual model and content was positive. Doctors reported that the 5As framework was a

TABLE 2: Summary of the training programme.

Session	Time (minutes)	Purpose of session	Activities for session
1.1	15	Introductions and overview of programme and learning outcomes	Introduce the training programme in terms of the people involved, the intended learning outcomes and the process to be followed.
1.2	30	Understand participant's own prior experience of the challenges and successes of BBCC	Invite students to reflect in pairs and then share with the whole group on their prior experience with BBCC. This step was thought to be important in terms of building rapport between the trainers and participants, understanding the participant's context, allowing them to express their ambivalence and frustrations and have these recognised, and helping to focus attention on behaviour change counselling.
1.3	45	Evidence for BBCC	Provide evidence of the current deficiencies in counselling, the reasons for them, the consequences for patients and health care providers. Provide evidence for the model of BBCC and its effectiveness. Allow time for discussion / questions.
1.4	30	Understand the guiding style	Identify the key characteristics of the guiding style by contrasting two DVD clips of BBCC – the one in a directing style and the other in a guiding style. Ask students to identify the key characteristics of each style, record and compare on newsprint.
2.1	40	Reflective listening	Talk: Give a brief overview of the theory of reflective listening. Modelling: Demonstrate using DVD. Practice: Using small group interactive exercises.
2.2	40	Recognise, elicit and respond to change talk	Talk: Brief overview of theory from motivational interviewing. Practical: Trainers read out a list of statements and students drum on tables if they recognise change talk.
2.3	40	Introduction to the 5 As	Talk: Overview of the 5 A steps, the purpose of each step and communication skills involved. Allow time for discussion / questions.
3.1	80	Applying the 5 As to each risk factor	Form 4 groups: Each group looks at the training manual (5A steps and patient education material) for one behavioural risk factor. Form 4 new groups with one person from each of the previous groups. Each person teaches the others about their risk factor. Elicit feedback / discussion in whole group.
3.2	40	Exchanging information	Talk: Brief overview of theory from motivational interviewing. Modelling: Demonstrate elicit-provide-elicit with DVD. Practice: Small group interactive exercises.
4.1	30	Assess readiness to change	Talk: Brief overview of theory from motivational interviewing and application to the assess stage. Modelling: Demonstrate in role play or DVD. Practice: Small group interactive exercises.
4.2	60	Practice integrated BBCC	Groups of 4: Allocate one different risk factor per person. Each person thinks of a patient to role play. Role play BBCC. Observe, give feedback and discuss. Facilitator to rotate to each group.
4.3	25	Planning integration into real world	Interview each other in pairs: Assess how ready your partner is to implement BBCC. Assist the person appropriately to plan change. Each person briefly gives feedback on their way forward to whole group. Discuss ways of ongoing learning with group.
4.4	5	Closure and evaluation of workshop	Complete end of workshop with feedback form.

useful structure, and that the patient information materials could help them save time during counselling. Nurses felt that reflective listening skills could help them feel less frustrated when counselling patients, as they conceptualised their potential roles as expert guides, rather than expert advice givers. Nurses found the course materials useful, not only as a source of information on NCDs, but also as resource when arranging for referral. Whilst participants found the interactive sessions (role-playing, group discussions and practical exercises) to be valuable in practicing new skills, they also identified the need for clearer instructions from trainers before exercises. Participants valued feedback from trainers during practical sessions, as they felt this improved their confidence in trying out new skills.

The training programme was adapted by the team using the participant's feedback, as well as their individual experiences during training. The team realised that, ideally, two trainers were needed during clinical skills training sessions to ensure individual feedback from a trainer. The need to encourage and strengthen the value of peer reviews was identified, therefore trainers purposefully selected group members to combine stronger and weaker members.

To improve individual participation and save time, trainers provided clearer instructions before practical exercises.

Discussion

This study has led to the design, development and implementation of a training programme for BBCC aimed at primary care providers (PCPs) in the South African context. The training programme incorporated best practice from both international and local studies and was tailored to the needs of local PCPs and their context. To our knowledge, this training programme is the first attempt at developing and implementing best practice BBCC training in our context, targeting a variety of PCPs, and addressing all four NCD risk factors.

The adaptation of the 5 A approach with a guiding style derived from MI was an innovation in the African context, and there are only a few other published examples internationally.[4,25,31,32] Although approaches to training elsewhere include combinations of e-learning, with face-to-face training as well as ongoing support and feedback, they all aim to teach the underlying spirit of the guiding style of MI.[25,26,28,31,32] Training as part of continuing professional development through GP networks showed incomplete uptake, which could imply the need to integrate BBCC training into undergraduate and postgraduate programmes.[25] One training programme which measured patient level outcomes was found ineffective, and interestingly did not train clinicians in listening skills, but focused more on the value of the guiding style, rather than achieving clinical competence.[32]

Training interventions for BBCC are not always clearly described and the terminology used is inconsistent.[33] In an attempt to address this a review of BBCC and training resulted in a best practice checklist for training programmes.[26,28] In line with the checklist our programme includes: clear information about the evidence base and theoretical underpinning of the model, tools for assessing readiness to change, reflective listening skills, provides tailored made information for patients, and topic specific training, whilst focussing on the development of essential communication skills by providing time for demonstrations, practice of skills and feedback. Our programme, however, does not include training on tailoring information specifically for different patient groups, such as the young, those with cultural differences, or minority ethnic groups.

The best practice checklist suggests that the individual context of participants, the trainer's attributes, as well as the process of delivery influence effectiveness. In our programme the participants were from a variety of linguistic, cultural, and professional contexts. In order to improve the trainer's understanding of their context, the programme always started with a session to elicit participant's prior experience, attitudes and expectations. Our trainers had completed training both in MI and in how to train MI, which enabled them to embody and evoke the guiding style during the training. We believe that trainers should have this level of proficiency, which may limit the immediate scaling up of training. If trainers with less proficiency are used then this may reduce the effectiveness of the training. Regarding the process of delivery, the workshop style used is supported by the checklist.[28] However, ongoing support and feedback was not provided. Booster sessions to provide feedback and continuous support is regarded as important to maintain and develop skills over time.[28,34] On-line support and feedback with the use of formative assessment of audiotapes is currently being developed to supplement this course.

The WIDER recommendations were developed to improve reporting of behaviour change interventions in clinical trials.[35] This article is consistent with the WIDER recommendations in giving a detailed description of the intervention, which includes the characteristics of the trainers, the recipients, the setting, the mode of delivery, the intensity and duration of delivery, and a detailed description of the content. Likewise, the findings have described how the intervention was designed and developed, the techniques used to elicit change and the underlying conceptual model. A detailed manual has also been made available as a supplementary

file. As this is not yet being assessed as part of a clinical trial the characteristics of a control group are not relevant here and the fidelity of the trainers to the design was not formally assessed.

A possible limitation of the ADDIE process is that there was less engagement with nurses, compared to doctors, in the design and development stages. For example, the design was presented mainly to expert doctors in primary care, and the educational team consisted of two family physicians and a social scientist. Nevertheless we did consult extensively with nurses during the situational analysis. During the implementation phase, the training was offered as an optional extra to nurses on the diploma programme as the time required was too much for the formal curriculum, and this could have selected a more motivated group. The majority of doctors were registrars in family medicine and their motivation and experience could also be different from other primary care doctors working in the public and private sector.

The study was conducted in the Western Cape, where the health system and human resources for health are generally better developed than elsewhere in the country. Additional contextual challenges might have been encountered if the programme had been developed in another province.

Evaluating the effect of training is good practice, and future research is focussing on evaluating the effectiveness of this training programme. The results of this evaluation will be published elsewhere. Evaluation should make it possible to determine the impact on clinical practice amongst the target groups, measure the degree to which the learning outcomes were met, and might also indicate which PCPs are best to train.[9,10,28] Exploring the application of this programme to other PCPs, such as community health workers and lay counsellors, is also recommended for future research. Ultimately evaluation should measure the effect on patient behaviour and risk factors.

Although the training programme has not yet been fully evaluated, the need for it in our context has been immediately recognised and embraced. The Chronic Diseases Initiative for Africa, through a programme entitled ichange4health, helped to further develop the materials and train trainers from Departments of Family Medicine and Primary Care throughout South Africa. These trainers are now training medical students, general practitioners and other family physicians in their respective areas. A strength of this training intervention is its feasibility to train PCPs to train others in BBCC, and future research could evaluate the effectiveness of training the trainers. The authors have also presented the training programme in other countries such as Botswana and Namibia.

Conclusion

This study designed a new approach to BBCC, which was based on a conceptual model that combined the 5As (ask, alert, assess, assist and arrange) with a guiding style derived from MI. The study then developed an eight-hour training programme that combined theory, modelling and simulated practice with feedback, delivered also in a guiding style, for either clinical nurse practitioners or primary care doctors in South Africa. The programme was implemented and revised based on initial feedback. The programme has already been widely adopted, but also requires further evaluation in our context.

Acknowledgements

The research is supported by the Chronic Disease Initiative in Africa and Stellenbosch University. We would like to acknowledge the Cancer Association of SA for their funding contribution towards the time spent on the project by Dr Everett-Murphy.

Competing interests

The authors declare that they have no financial or personal relationship(s) that may have inappropriately influenced them in writing this article.

Authors' contributions

All three authors (Z.M. [Stellenbosch University], R.M. [Stellenbosch University] and K.E.-M. [University of Cape Town]) were involved in the design and development stages, as well as the implementation of the pilot training. The rest of the training sessions, and evaluation of feedback, was mostly done by Z.M., and overseen by R.M. and K.E.-M. All the authors contributed to the article, and approved the final manuscript.

References

1. Mayosi BM, Flisher AJ, Lalloo UG. The burden of non-communicable diseases in South Africa. Lancet. 2009;374:934–947. http://dx.doi.org/10.1016/S0140-6736(09)61087-4

2. Bradshaw D, Steyn K, Levitt N, et al. Non communicable diseases: A race against time [homepage on the Internet]. Medical Research Council; 2011. Available from: http://www.mrc.ac.za/policybriefs/raceagainst.pdf.

3. Goldstein MG, Whitlock E, De Pue MPH. Multiple behaviour risk factor interventions in primary care. Summary of research evidence. Am J Prev Med. 2004;27:61–79. http://dx.doi.org/10.1016/j.amepre.2004.04.023

4. Royal Australian College of General Practitioners. Smoking, nutrition, alcohol and physical inactivity (SNAP): A population health guide to behavioural risk factors in general practice [homepage on the Internet]. 2004. Available from: http://www.racgp.org.au/document.asp?id=?14803.

5. Beaglehole R, Epping-Jordan J, Patel V. Improving the prevention and management of chronic disease in low and middle income countries, priority for primary health care. Lancet 2008;372:940–949. http://dx.doi.org/10.1016/S0140-6736(08)61404-X

6. Department of Health, Republic of South Africa. Strategic plan for the prevention and control of non-communicable diseases, 2012–2016.

7. Spanou C, Simpson SA, Hood K. Preventing disease through opportunistic, rapid engagement by primary care teams using behaviour change counseling (PRE-EMPT): Protocol for a general practice-based cluster randomized trial [serial on the Internet]. BMC Fam Pract. 2010. Available from: http://www.biomedcentral.com/1471-2296/11/69.

8. Sim M, Wain T, Khong E. Influencing behaviour change in general practice. Aust Fam Physician. 2009;38:885–888.

9. Strayer S, Martindale J, Pelletier S. Development and evaluation of an instrument for assessing brief behavioural change interventions. Patient Educ Couns. 2011;83:99–105. http://dx.doi.org/10.1016/j.pec.2010.04.012

10. Parker W, Steyn NP, Levitt NS. They think they know but do they? Misalignment of perceptions of lifestyle modification knowledge among health professionals. Public Health Nutr. 2010;14:1429–1438. http://dx.doi.org/10.1017/S1368980009993272

11. Malan JE, Mash R, Everett-Murphy K. A situational analysis of the current training and approaches to behaviour change counselling amongst primary health care nurses, doctors and key stakeholders in the Western Cape, South Africa. PHCFM Article. 2015.

12. Everett–Murphy K, Odendaal H, Steyn K. Doctor's attitudes and practices regarding smoking cessation during pregnancy. S Afr Med J. 2005;95:350–354.

13. Miller WR, Rollnick S. Motivational interviewing: Helping people change. 3rd ed. New York, NY: Guildford Press, 2013; p. 392–393.

14. Emmons K, Rollnick S. Motivational interviewing in health care settings. Am J of Prev Med. 2001;20:68–74. http://dx.doi.org/10.1016/S0749-3797(00)00254-3

15. Allen WC. Overview and evolution of the ADDIE Training System. Advances in Developing Human Resources [serial on the Internet]. 2006;8:430–441. Available from: http://adh.sagepub.com/content/8/4/430 http://dx.doi.org/10.1177/1523422306292942

16. Mash R. Development of the programme Mental Disorders in Primary Care as internet-based distance education in South Africa. Med Educ [serial on the Internet]. 2001;35:996–999. http://dx.doi.org/10.1111/j.1365-2923.2001.01031.

17. Mash RM. Diabetes education in primary care: A practical approach using the Addie model. CME. 2010;28:485–487.

18. Mash R, Fairall L, Adejayan O, et al. A morbidity survey of South African primary care. Plos One [serial on the Internet]. 2012;7(3):e32358. http://dx.doi.org/10.1371/journal.pone0032358.

19. Mash R, Baldassini G, Mkhatshwa H. Reflections on the training of counsellors in motivational interviewing for programmes for the prevention of mother to child transmission of HIV in sub-Saharan Africa. SA Fam Pract. 2008;50:53–59. http://dx.doi.org/10.1080/20786204.2008.10873697

20. Everett-Murphy K, Steyn K, Matthews C, et al. The effectiveness of adapted, best practice guidelines for smoking cessation counselling with pregnant smokers attending public sector antenatal clinics in Cape Town, South Africa. Acta Obstet et Gynecol Scand. 2010;89:478–490. http://dx.doi.org/10.3109/00016341003605701

21. Malan Z. The influence of information given on general practitioners' management of overweight patients. Pretoria: University of Pretoria, Department of Family Medicine; 2008.

22. Rollnick S, Butler CC, Kinnersly P, et al. Competent novice motivational interviewing. Brit Med J. 2010;340:1242–1245. http://dx.doi.org/10.1136/bmj.c1900

23. Lundahl B, Moleni T, Burke L, et al. Motivational interviewing in medical settings: A systematic review and meta-analysis of randomised controlled trials. Patient Educ Couns. 2013;93:157–168. http://dx.doi.org/10.1016/j.pec.2013.07.012

24. Miller W, Mount KA. A small study of training in MI: Does one workshop change clinician and client behaviour? Behav Cogn Psychother. 2001;29:457–471. http://dx.doi.org/10.1017/S1352465801004064

25. Butler CC, Simpson SA, Hood K, et al. Training practitioners to deliver opportunistic multiple behaviour change counselling in primary care: A cluster randomised trial. Brit Med J. 2013;346:1–25. http://dx.doi.org/10.1136/bmj.f1191

26. Powell K, Thurston M. Commissioning training for behaviour change interventions: Guidelines for best practice [document on the Internet]. 2008. Available from: http://hdl.handle.net//10034/46839.

27. Torre DM, Daley BJ, Sebastian JL. Overview of current learning theories for medical educators. Am J Med. 2006;119:903–907. http://dx.doi.org/10.1016/j.amjmed.2006.06.037

28. Stredder K, Sumnall H, Lyons M. Behaviour change training delivered across Cheshire and Merseyside. A report mapping programmes and exploring processes [document on the Internet]. 2009. Available from: www.champs-for-health.net.

29. Maguire P, Pitceathly P. Clinical review: Key communication skills and how to acquire them. Brit Med J. 2002;325:697–700. http://dx.doi.org/10.1136/bmj.325.7366.697

30. Motivational Interviewing Network of Trainers (MINT) [document on the Internet]. Available from: http://www.motivationalinterviewing.org

31. Neuner-Jehle S, Schmid M, Gruninger U. The health coaching programme: A new patient-centred and visually supported approach for health behaviour change in primary care [serial on the Internet]. BMC Fam Prac. 2013;14:1–8. Available from: http://www.biomedcentral.com/1471-2296/14/100

32. Achra A. Health promotion in Australian general practice: A gap in GP training. Aus Fam Physician. 2009;38:605–608.

33. Michie S, Van Stralen MM, West R. The behaviour change wheel: A new method for characterising and designing behaviour change interventions [serial on the Internet]. Implement Sci. 2011;6:42. Available from: http://www.implementationscience.com/content/6/1/42. http://dx.doi.org/10.1186/1748-5908-6-42

34. Schwalbe CS, Oh Hy, Zweben A. Sustaining motivational interviewing: A meta-analysis of training studies. Addiction. 2014;109(8):1287–1294. http://dx.doi.org/10.1111/add.12558

35. Albrecht L, Archibald M, Arseneau D, et al. Development of a checklist to assess the quality of reporting of knowledge translation interventions using the Workgroup for Intervention Development and Evaluation Research (WIDER) recommendations. Implement Sci. 2013;8:52. http://dx.doi.org/10.1186/1748-5908-8-52

29

The impact of health service variables on healthcare access in a low resourced urban setting in the Western Cape, South Africa

Authors:
Elsje Scheffler[1,2]
Surona Visagie[1,2]
Marguerite Schneider[2,3]

Affiliations:
[1]Centre for Rehabilitation Studies, Stellenbosch University, South Africa

[2]Psychology Department, Stellenbosch University, South Africa

[3]Centre for Public Mental Health, Department of Psychiatry and Mental Health, University of Cape Town, South Africa

Correspondence to:
Elsje Scheffler

Email:
elsje@dareconsult.co.za

Postal address:
20 Kleinvallei Street, Stellenbosch 7600, South Africa

Background: Health care access is complex and multi-faceted and, as a basic right, equitable access and services should be available to all user groups.

Objectives: The aim of this article is to explore how service delivery impacts on access to healthcare for vulnerable groups in an urban primary health care setting in South Africa.

Methods: A descriptive qualitative study design was used. Data were collected through semi-structured interviews with purposively sampled participants and analysed through thematic content analysis.

Results: Service delivery factors are presented against five dimensions of access according to the ACCESS Framework. From a supplier perspective, the organisation of care in the study setting resulted in available, accessible, affordable and adequate services as measured against the District Health System policies and guidelines. However, service providers experienced significant barriers in provision of services, which impacted on the quality of care, resulting in poor client and provider satisfaction and ultimately compromising acceptability of service delivery. Although users found services to be accessible, the organisation of services presented them with challenges in the domains of availability, affordability and adequacy, resulting in unmet needs, low levels of satisfaction and loss of trust. These challenges fuelled perceptions of unacceptable services.

Conclusion: Well developed systems and organisation of services can create accessible, affordable and available primary healthcare services, but do not automatically translate into adequate and acceptable services. Focussing attention on how services are delivered might restore the balance between supply (services) and demand (user needs) and promote universal and equitable access.

L'impact des variables des services de santé sur l'accès aux soins dans un cadre urbain à faibles revenus dans le Western Cape, Afrique du Sud.

Contexte: L'accès aux soins est complexe et polyvalent, et étant un droit fondamental, tous les groupes d'utilisateurs devraient avoir également accès à ses services.

Objectifs: Le but de cet article est d'examiner l'impact de la prestation de services sur l'accès aux soins pour les groupes vulnérables dans un cadre urbain de soins primaires en Afrique du Sud.

Méthodes: On a utilisé un modèle d'étude qualitative. On a recueilli les données au moyen d'entrevue semi-structurées avec des participants préalablement sélectionnés, puis on les a analysées au moyen d'une analyse thématique du contenu.

Résultats: Les facteurs de prestation de services sont présentés par rapport à cinq aspects d'accès selon le Cadre ACCESS. Du point de vue du fournisseur, l'organisation des soins dans le cadre de l'étude a eu pour résultat des services disponibles, accessibles, raisonnables et adéquats par rapport aux politiques et directives du Système de santé de district. Cependant, les prestataires de service se sont heurtés à des obstacles considérables dans la prestation de services qui ont eu un effet sur la qualité des soins, et ont mal répondu aux besoins des clients et des prestataires, et ont fini par compromettre l'admissibilité des prestations de service. Bien que les utilisateurs aient trouvé que les services étaient accessible, l'organisation des services présentait des défis dans les domaines de la disponibilité, de la rentabilité et du caractère adéquat, ce qui a eu pour effet des besoins non satisfaits, peu de satisfaction et une perte de confiance. Ces défis ont nourri des sentiments de rejet des services.

Conclusion: Les systèmes et l'organisation de services bien développés peuvent créer des services sanitaires primaires accessibles, abordables et disponibles, mais ne se traduisent pas automatiquement en services adéquats et acceptables. L'attention accordée à la façon dont sont fournis les services pourrait rétablir l'équilibre entre la fourniture (services) et la demande (besoins de l'utilisateur) et promouvoir un accès universel et équitable.

Introduction

Access to healthcare is a basic human right,[1] and governments should aim to provide universal and equitable access to high quality health care services.[2] A feature of vulnerable populations may be the risk of less health care access and poorer health care outcomes than the general population.[3] An exploration of the experiences of vulnerable groups can provide information on their access to, and satisfaction with, health care services.

A number of authors have tried to capture the complexity and multi-faceted nature of health care access through different frameworks.[2,4,5,6,7,8] The more comprehensive of these frameworks, such as the Health Access Livelihood Framework (ACCESS) described below, acknowledges a dynamic interaction between demand (user) and supply (service).[2,5,6,8,9,10] For instance, an accessible service will attempt to structure hours of operation (supply) in accordance with the schedule of users (demand).

In this article, ACCESS[2,9,10] is used to explore health care access for vulnerable groups in a specific setting. According to this framework, healthcare access constitutes five dimensions: availability, accessibility, affordability, adequacy and acceptability, as defined in Table 1. These are influenced by a dynamic interaction with user livelihood assets (the human, social, physical, financial and natural assets, or capital, a person has access to)[11] on the one hand, and policies, institutions, organisation and processes on the other.[2,6,8,9,10]

As set out by Flaskeru and Winslow[12] (p. 70), 'vulnerable populations are defined as social groups who have an increased relative risk (of-) or susceptibility to adverse health outcomes'. Typically, these include poor people and groups who experience stigma, discrimination and intolerance, and/ or political marginalisation,[12] and those whose human rights are violated. Understanding the experiences of vulnerable groups in relation to the five components of ACCESS can assist in changing the provision of health care to enhance health outcomes.

The focus of this article is on the impact of these five dimensions on the health care access of a group of vulnerable users, including people living in poverty, people living with HIV and/or AIDS or chronic conditions such as diabetes mellitus, people with disabilities (PWD), women, all members of women-headed households, youths, elderly people, members of minority cultures and persons with low levels of education and literacy.

Research methods and design
Study design

This article is based on the results from a large international study entitled 'Enabling universal and equitable access to healthcare for vulnerable people in resource poor settings in Africa'.[13] This article presents the results of one component of that study: the qualitative phase from one of the four South African (SA) sites. The larger study had three phases and was conducted concurrently in four countries in Africa and four sites in each country.[13,14,15] The site for the study component reported in this article, an urban township in Cape Town, was purposively selected because it is a small, densely populated and impoverished urban community.

Setting

Gugulethu, a small township (less than 10 km²) in the Klipfontein subdistrict of the Klipfontein and Mitchells Plain substructure of the City of Cape Town Metro health district, has a population density of 15 161.7 persons per km².[2,16] The population comprises mainly black Africans (98.58%)[16] with only 3.6% being 65 years or older.[17] Whilst 2.2% of the population is illiterate, 60% have not completed high school.[17] Almost 40% of this poverty-stricken community was unemployed[16] and 71.4% of households (average size of 3.33) had an income of R3200.00 (approx. $300.00) or less per month in 2011.[17]

Study population and sampling strategy

The study population comprised the community and service providers in the public, traditional and private health care services in Gugulethu. Purposive and snowball sampling techniques were employed to identify a participant group with a wide diversity of experience and views.[18]

Eight public health care users, and four persons who stopped using public health care (non-users) were selected from various vulnerable groups in consultation with community leaders and non-governmental organisations. Table 2 provides an overview of the vulnerability profile of these participants. The numbers in the table total more than 12 as some participants fall into more than one group. The identification of vulnerable groups is described and

TABLE 1: The dimensions of access to healthcare services according to the ACCESS Framework.[2]

Dimension	Definition[2p1586]	Aspects to consider[22]
Availability	'The existing health services and goods meet clients' needs.'	Adequate supply of services, goods and facilities, including types of services, sufficient skilled human resources
Accessibility	'The location of supply is in line with the location of clients.'	Proximity, means of transportation and travel time
Affordability	'The prices of services fit the clients' income and ability to pay.'	Direct and indirect costs of accessing health care
Adequacy	'The organization of health care meets the clients' expectations.'	Organisation of services, including the standard of the facilities and meeting user expectations
Acceptability	'The characteristics of providers match with those of the clients.'	Ethical standards and the appropriateness of services, goods and facilities to address cultural and gender differences and life-cycle requirements; to improve outcomes; and to ensure confidentiality, effective communication and facilitating attitudes

TABLE 2: Vulnerability profile of health care users and non-users.

Vulnerability factor present	Non-users	Users
Poverty	4	8
HIV and AIDS	0	3
Chronic conditions, excluding HIV and AIDS	2	4
Physical disability	3	5
Women	3	4
Women-headed household	1	3
Aged	1	0
Youth	0	1
Minority groups (subculture)	0	1
Low level of education (Illiterate or education level of less than grade 7)	1	2

TABLE 3: Occupational profile of providers interviewed at the Primary Health Care facilities.

Post/category of provider	Number
Security staff	1
Cleaning staff	1
HIV and/or AIDS Counsellor	1
Health promoter	1
Administrative clerk	2
Enrolled nurse	2
Orthopaedic aftercare professional nurse	1
Community liaison officer	1
Clinical nurse care practitioner	1
Professional nurse	3
Physiotherapist	1
Family physician	1
Operation manager (professional nurse)	1
Orthotist-prosthetist	1
Social worker	1

defined by Mannan, Amin, MacLachlan and the EquitAble Consortium (2014)[19] and Eide, Amin, MacLachlan, Mannan and Schneider (2013).[20]

Health care providers were purposively sampled from the Community Health Centre (CHC) and two clinics. The first author used her knowledge of the health care system to identify the clinics, one east and the other west of the more centrally located CHC. One clinic was near an informal housing area, whilst the other in a slightly more resourced area with formal housing close to a shopping centre. The public healthcare providers interviewed included professional service providers, community health care workers, support staff (e.g. administrative, cleaning, security) and a community liaison officer. Table 3 sets out the occupational profile of the service providers at the public primary health care (PHC) facilities. One general practitioner and 12 traditional healers were also interviewed. However, as this article focuses on the public health care sector, these interviews were not included in the results presented in this article.

Data collection

Data were collected through 44 semi-structured interviews between April and November, 2010. Fourteen interviews (private general practitioner and traditional healers) were excluded in the results presented in this article since the

data did not add any insights to the PHC service delivery process, which is the focus of this study. As an adjunct to the interviews, direct observation[18] was done at the facilities, and institutional process and policy documents were perused by the primary author. Data on services provided, equipment, access and resources were captured on specifically designed data capture sheets.

The interviews were divided between research team members according to language proficiency and were conducted by the primary author (14 interviews), a co-researcher (2 interviews) and three research assistants (28 interviews). This might have added bias, since the primary author and co-researcher, unlike the research assistants, are graduates with experience in the fields of research and health care service delivery. The team was trained by the core research group. Additional training sessions for the research assistants were held by the primary author.

Interviews were conducted at venues determined by the participants and included the participants' homes, places of work and public places such as community centres. The study was explained to each participant, and informed consent and permission to digitally record the interviews was obtained. Interviews lasted between 45 and 90 minutes.

Data analysis

Data management and analysis

All interviews were transcribed verbatim and the isiXhosa and Afrikaans interviews translated into English. The one Afrikaans translation was verified by the primary author, an Afrikaans first language speaker; the isiXhosa translations were verified by an independent person employed in the public health care service, whose duties included interpreting, and who was not part of the EquitAble research team. Data were analysed using thematic content analysis to identify emerging and recurring themes. Individual experiences and factors relating to health care access were identified and coded from each transcript. Codes were then grouped together into themes. Some themes were predetermined based on the interview schedule, whilst new themes were identified as experiences were explored. Recurring themes were grouped together to eventually form three main themes, as set out in the results section.

Verification

Data coding was developed and verified, through discussion in the research team, to allow for comparative coding for the four SA sites.

Triangulation of data was done by comparing experiences of participant groups with one another and was augmented by direct observations and perusal of policy and procedure documents. Presentation of the results to the wider community provided a further opportunity to verify and triangulate the findings.

Ethical considerations

The study was registered and approved by the Committee for Human Research of Stellenbosch University (reference number N09/10/270), and permission to perform the study was granted by the Western Cape Department of Health for the CHC and the City of Cape Town for the two clinics.

Identifiable information was depersonalised by means of coding along the guidelines developed for the EquitAble framework. All digital data were stored and backed up electronically using password protected entry to both the folders and files. Paper records were archived with Stellenbosch University.

Results

Three main themes, namely service factors, personal factors and environmental considerations were identified. This article presents the findings on the service factors according to the five dimensions of access as defined by the ACCESS Framework:

- availability
- accessibility
- affordability
- adequacy
- acceptability.

Quotes from the interviews are provided as examples of common themes.

Availability

Availability refers to the type of services offered, whether human and other resources are sufficient to meet the demand, and to the knowledge and skills of service providers.

Type of services

Public healthcare services in Gugulethu are provided by a CHC and four clinics. Table 4 presents information on the services offered, staff complement and service hours of these facilities.

Although the services offered at the CHC and clinics are in line with District Health System (DHS) requirements

(as noted in the process and policy documents perused), users expressed dissatisfaction as services were not always what they expected. For instance, the CHC had both emergency and rehabilitation services, but the clinics did not (see Table 4), a situation that users found unsatisfactory:

'And they [clinic] don't have an emergency [section] – no matter how serious your situation.' (Non-user, female, 35–49 years, single parent)

'It's not right because I must see the physiotherapist every now and then. I sometimes don't have money but I'm forced to get it [privately] because there's nothing that I can get from clinic. Their service is very poor for me and if the condition doesn't change some people will always ignore to go there.' (Non-user, female, 50–64 years, arthritis)

Observation showed that rehabilitation services were offered at the CHC only and was facility-based with a focus on treating acute conditions through individual sessions weekly, twice monthly, or monthly. Frequency of sessions is often determined by time constraints rather than the norm for specific conditions.

Human resources

Providers complained that, although they had full staff complements in accordance with the approved post lists (APL), they were not sufficient for the number of patients. Service delivery was further compromised by absenteeism, leave and compulsory training:

'We do have a high absenteeism rate – that's part of the problem. So you've got ... 15 nurses on the staff but there's only seven of them on duty because two of them are on a course, two are on leave and three are off sick, you know. So actually on paper our staff is enough, but maybe on the floor we don't have enough because of absenteeism.' (Healthcare professional, female, 34–49 years)

Rehabilitation services were provided by one specialised professional nurse and one physiotherapist who also served the larger district. The physiotherapist was based at the CHC whilst the professional nurse was based outside the study area:

'. . . sometimes I only get to see a patient every two weeks which is not ideal but that is the best that I can come up with . . . some

TABLE 4: Summary of the public health care services in Gugulethu.

Summary	Community health Centre ($n = 1$)	Clinics ($n = 4$)
Hours	7.30 am until 4.30 pm weekdays 24 hours emergency and maternity services Extended hours (Saturday and after hours clinics) for services such as women's health clinics, children and baby clinics to accommodate people who work.	7.30 am until 4.30 pm weekdays
Health care staff	Medical officer Family physician Professional nurses Clinical nurse care practitioners Other levels of nursing staff Social workers Physiotherapists Community health workers Counsellors Health care promoters Outreach visits by the sub district occupational therapist and prosthetist from the provincial orthotic and prosthetic workshop	Professional nurse Clinical nurse care practitioners Other levels of nursing staff Weekly consultant visits by clinical specialists Community health workers Counsellors Health care promoters
Services offered	Full primary health care package	Health promotion Various preventative and curative care services

patients they require it [*treatment*] immediately and I'll try and see to those patients, but otherwise it is really difficult ... And I would try and give them an exercise program to follow in that time ...' (Healthcare professional, female, < 34 years)

Provider's knowledge

Providers felt that they lacked the necessary knowledge and skills to manage health care for PWD and that the support systems were inadequate:

'We're just loaded with everything. I would say that the Department of Health is just loading us because it wants us to do everything yet we don't have the skills or the facilities to refer to.' (Health care professional, female, 50–64 years)

Users with disabilities concurred with this view:

'They [*the staff*] do not have ... the right understanding ... our disabilities are different, therefore, also the approach is supposed to be different.' (User, male, 35–49 years, ankylosing spondylitis)

'I thought if they communicate with people or patients, for instance in my case they should have approached my special doctor [*clinical consultant at tertiary hospital*] for advice ... but they did not listen to me.' (User, male, 35-49 years, ankylosing spondylitis)

Users in need of comprehensive rehabilitation or medical management of impairments underlying their disabilities are referred to services outside of the area but service providers did not appear well informed of these referral pathways:

'I think it is more difficult now for the people to get what they need, because there are just so few people who really know what is going on. It takes a long time before the patients are being directed in the proper channels.' (Healthcare professional, disability-specific services, female, 34–49)

According to the providers many referral services had backlogs, with waiting periods as long as two years.

Equipment, resources and assistive devices

Periodic shortages of equipment and resources were experienced, particularly in the trauma unit of the CHC:

'This month it could be gloves. Next month it could be oxygen masks ...' (Health care professional, female, 50–64 years)

In addition, administrative delays were reported with the purchasing of consumables and the replacement of condemned equipment. Equipment was reportedly shared between departments and consultation rooms in the CHC and clinics, leading to time wasted searching for it:

'... your practitioners are spending most of their time running around to borrow this or to find that. That is not a system that can work, you know.' (Health care professional, female, 50–64 years)

Whilst some providers found creative solutions, others were unable to deliver services without all available equipment:

'I mean, we sometimes run out of a certain size of bandages; I just saw [*name removed*] cutting a bandage in half for

cost-effectiveness. So some people will be creative because we really do have the patients' needs as a priority.' (Health care professional, female, 50–64 years)

There was an ample supply of assistive devices, such as basic folding frame wheelchairs, walking sticks and crutches at the CHC. However, periodic shortages of consumables like catheters and stoma bags were reported, and although users are notified and supplied immediately when consumables are again available, they may be without these necessary health supplies for short periods.

In summary, providers and users agreed that service availability was challenged by a lack of equipment and consumables and too few service providers. Services to PWD specifically were further hampered by a lack of disability-specific knowledge, not enough human resources and the way in which services were delivered.

Accessibility

In the context of accessibility within the ACCESS Framework,[2] participants were positive about the proximity of the health care facilities to their homes. They lived within a 3 km radius of the services and most accessed the facilities on foot. The accessibility of the facilities was overall good for PWD.

Affordability

Affordability refers to the direct costs of care as well as indirect costs such as travel costs, lost time and loss of income.[2] All PHC services were delivered free of charge.

According to the liaison officer, long waiting times was the most common complaint received from users. Waiting times varied between two hours for those with scheduled appointments and four hours or longer for those without appointments.

Users employed strategies to decrease waiting times such as asking staff or other users to take their registration cards to the facility ahead of their arrival:

'Some of them in the neighbourhood ask us, which makes things difficult for us. An old person knocking at your door in the morning – "please can you take my card in there". You can't say no to an older person ...' (Health care services staff, non-professional services, female, 50–64 years)

Adequacy
Organisation of services

In accordance with DHS guidelines users had to access the facility (CHC or clinic) that provided services to the geographic service area (GSA) in which they live. However, some users preferred to access the CHC instead of the clinic in their GSA. They accessed the CHC after normal clinic hours knowing that, in accordance with policy, they would not be turned away:

'I think they're [*the patients*] running away from their clinics ... So they will wait until their clinic is closed and then definitely we must admit everybody ...' (Health care professional, female, 50–64 years)

In addition, according to set referral pathways, users are not allowed to access secondary or tertiary level services without a referral from primary level:

'I don't have a problem to go to hospital. But the road to hospital is via the clinic ... I can't go there.' (Non-user, female, 35–49 years, single parent)

As reported by providers and documents reviewed, in excess of 1500 patients are seen daily at the CHC and at the two clinics investigated. Systems such as appointments and 6-monthly prescriptions for chronic medications were introduced to reduce overcrowding, improve patient management and flow and to contribute to patient-focussed care. Extended service hours and outreach services further improve both access and patient flow. Triage systems at all entry points screen and prioritise unscheduled users. The elderly and PWD receive preferential services. Service delivery is divided into dedicated service streams such as diabetes, hypertension, psychiatric and HIV clinics. These clinics are open on specific days and at specific times (see Table 4). This can create access barriers as, for instance, early morning appointments may be difficult for those with disabilities:

'But I don't always make it (to appointments) when they give me the time and maybe the afternoon can be better for me to attend.' (User, female, 35–49 years, wheelchair user and partially sighted)

'In my case, a disability person, I send someone in the morning to stand [in the queue] for me ... Due to the fact that I am crippled it takes too long for me to reach the clinic early.' (User, female, 35–49 years, post-polio, HIV and/or AIDS, psychiatric condition)

In the past, users were seen on a first come, first serve basis, which resulted in long waiting times and people queuing hours before opening time, often in the dark, with concomitant safety risks of traveling from home in the dark. Despite significant positive changes to improve patient flow, negative perceptions continued to dominate the decision of non-users:

'No, I stopped (going to the clinic). I almost got killed ... one of them had a gun against me ...' (Non-user, female, 80 + years, arthritis)

'... I can't go to clinic – wake up by 4 am while I'm sick – it's a huge risk to my life.' (Non-user, female, 35–49 years, single parent)

Similarly, the past lack of systematic management of the patient load causing backlogs and frustration still continues to influence decisions of non-users to not use PHC services:

'I was the first one in and put my medical card on the nurse's desk but as other people came in, their cards piled up on top of mine and I ended up being the last one. I got so upset and ended up slapping one of the nurses.' (Non-user, female, 80 + years, arthritis)

Users cannot request a specific health care provider, and follow-up appointments are not made with the same provider. In addition, students and community service providers rotate through the services, often on a monthly

basis. These practices impacted negatively on continuity of care and led to poor follow up:

'Last year I went to the clinic to collect the test results of my father with a letter that shows to them what was done, but each and every one sent me to someone else ... They show the signs of lack of understanding and incompetence.' (User, female, 20–34 years, post-polio, HIV and/or AIDS, single parent)

Meeting user expectations

The second most common complaint the community liaison officer at the CHC dealt with was unmet user expectations:

'... they complain that the doctor did not treat them according to their specifications.' (Health care support staff, male, 34–49)

'I was the one expecting them to take an X-ray for my chest pain but they never did that.' (User, female, 20–34, post-polio, HIV and/or AIDS, single parent)

'At [name of tertiary hospital] I was given a letter to give to [name removed] clinic for my treatment. When I go there they give me totally different medication. I do not know if that medication is going to help ...' (User, female, 35–49 years, post-polio, HIV and/or AIDS, psychiatric condition)

'Like sometimes they [nursing staff] write you a prescription and then you ask to see a doctor, then they will shout at you and ask why ... They are not doctors ... In my case I told them I'm the one who is sick here. I want to see a doctor or I will phone Manta, [previous] Minister of Health and tell her that you do your [swear word] here.' (User, female, 35–49 years, post-polio, HIV and/or AIDS, psychiatric condition)

In summary, despite efforts to improve adequacy, defined as the organisation of care, and the extent to which services met the expectations of users, such as the introduction of GSA referral systems, the number of clinics and diversity of services provided, extended hours, outreach services, triage systems, preferential treatment for the elderly and PWD, six monthly prescriptions and organising the services into disease specific clinics, users felt that services did not adequately meet their needs.

Acceptability
Attitudes

Some users found providers to be caring, positive, committed and professional and felt that they were treated in an acceptable manner:

'Some of the staff are very organised and committed to serve people. They treat us equally and they keep your matters confidentially. So far I'm still satisfied about the way they treated me.' (User, male, 20–34 years, diagnosis unknown)

'I use the clinic because they give my treatment and explain to me the direction to use and if I cheat [on] my medication they also tell me what is going to happen ...' (User, male, 20–34 years, epilepsy)

Other users experienced the services as unacceptable. They felt providers were disrespectful, rude, uncaring and rushed:

'... the nurses treat them with no respect.' (User, female, 20–34 years, post-polio, HIV and/or AIDS, single parent)

'And you end up sacrificing your last money to go to the private doctor to avoid humiliation because of the behaviour of the staff.' (User, male, 35–49, amputee)

'When they [the nurses] give directions [about taking medication] they talk so fast. As a result you get lost when you are at home. You ended up taking a wrong medication because that person never checked your understanding by that time because she is in a hurry.' (User, female, 20–34 years, post-polio, HIV and/or AIDS, single parent)

'... when you tell the doctor what you have like headache, swollen feet and thrush, the doctor response will say, 'Do not mention everything! You did not come here to do some grocery shopping.' (User, female, single parent, 15–19 years, HIV and/or AIDS)

Providers had been accused of favouritism and nepotism:

'... there is favouritism – they treat better their families and friends. When their friends come, they give them folders before us and they finish sooner than those of us who were there from early in the morning.' (User, female, 20–34 years, post-polio, HIV and/or AIDS, single parent)

When asked about these user comments, providers acknowledged negative attitudes:

'It is difficult. Let me see. That's a tricky one because in any environment you've got good potatoes and rotten ones so the truth is that you'll find those that will really not work well with the patients, you see. But obviously from time to time I will reprimand them you see? Yes, [the complaints are usually] from the same person or the same department. There are those cases – it is an open secret that we cannot hide.' (Health care support staff, male, 34–49 years)

Stringent confidentiality policies and practices inadvertently place the health care support staff in a dilemma and portray them as unhelpful or uncaring:

'... at times a patient might come out the doctor's consulting room, they will come to you – 'Where must I go now'? The doctor has told the patient to go to a certain place, but as soon as they come out of this door, the first person they meet they ask, 'Where must I go to now'. And I as a worker here, I do not have the right to open that folder to guide me where is this person supposed to go. I do not have that right. For that person it must be strange for not knowing where must they go, so my answer to that person will be, 'Go back to the doctor and ask him where you must go to.' (Health care services staff, non-professional services, female, 50–64 years)

Yet, at the same time, confidentiality is unintentionally breached by the organisation of services:

'There is no confidentiality because if you are HIV and/or AIDS or diabetic there are different sides for those diseases. I felt that is wrong because if diagnosed with HIV most of the time you are not ready to be known by other people. They embarrass us because they will call loudly saying: 'Those who came for antiretroviral drugs that side and the result of HIV that side.' (User, female, single parent, 15–19 years, HIV and/or AIDS)

User behaviour and low morale amongst providers contributes to negative attitudes:

'So even patients themselves ... they can be very bad. You see? Sometimes some of them come drunk ... But sometimes you try to understand their problems because this person is hungry, he is coming from poverty he is vulnerable and he is sick ... yes, and that person will take it out on the staff. And they even do it to me sometimes ... These behaviours are normally seen over weekends and after four ... They come smoking, drinking and all those problems ... Or they come during gang fights ... some of the gangs will be bringing in their friend they will demand that everything stops ... that this is the patient that needs to be seen ... Yes, that person must be prioritised and others will just drink and shout and swear, you see?' (Health care support staff, male, 34–49 years)

'You will find that in terms of caring for them [providers] and supporting them and acknowledging the hostile environment that they are working in and the situation and the long hours that we work there isn't much of an appreciation. So the morale is not that high. Sometimes they will complain that when they work overtime it will take 4 to 5 months for their overtime to be paid.' (Health care support staff, male, 34–49 years, tertiary education)

Furthermore, assumptions and stereotyping exclude PWD from general healthcare practices and access:

'Even the HIV and/or AIDS diseases nurse will say: 'Hee-hee! Where did you get it?' It does not register to them that you are sexual active and you have blood. Even if you ... are pregnant they will asked why are you pregnant, how this person make you pregnant ... by saying how many children do you have and when you tell them they make a joke of you and the other patients will laugh at you and you became frustrated and angry, all of that.' (User, female, 20–34 years, post-polio, HIV and/or AIDS, single parent)

Similar examples of stigma and discrimination included not giving pamphlets on sexually transmitted infections (STI) to a physically disabled person but to others, giving a room number to a partially sighted patient to find unassisted, and disability accessible toilets being used as storage rooms and kept locked.

Language

Language barriers existed. The majority of the nursing, administrative and support staff spoke isiXhosa, compared to only one of the rest of the professional staff and interns. Although users did not report language to be a barrier, providers frequently did. Since there are no formally trained interpreters, bilingual staff act as interpreters and inadvertently increase their own and other staff-members' workloads:

'Sometimes the issue of the language. Maybe the doctor ... they [the doctor and the user] did not understand each other properly, you see? ... but we did try and address it and said there must be an assistant nurse to interpret for the doctor, but sometimes you don't have enough staff to do such things. There are other core businesses and a nurse will sit there and just interpret for the doctor ...' (Health care support staff, male, 34–49 years)

In general, many users experienced barriers with regards to the acceptability of services, particularly in the form of provider attitudes and the impact of diagnoses-based organisation of services on confidentiality and poor communication. Acceptability of service delivery was compromised for service providers through negative user behaviour, language as barriers, short contact sessions and fragmentation of services.

Discussion

Considering the historical context of a fragmented and inefficient healthcare system with poor capacity,[8] remarkable achievements in health care service delivery were observed in the PHC health care facilities of Gugulethu. From a service provider's perspective the results demonstrate available, accessible, affordable and adequate services in the study setting through efficient organisation of services according to the DHS guidelines and policies. However, user perspectives differed. Although services were accessible, challenges were experienced with regard to affordability, availability and adequacy. The discussion will show how challenges in health care service delivery created conflict between users and providers, contributed to unacceptable behaviour from both groups, eroded trust, and led to decreased satisfaction and quality of care and, ultimately, resulted in unacceptable services for both groups.

Despite full staff complements according to DHS guidelines, daily availability was compromised by a lack of human resources, with providers seemingly under pressure. Care was punctuated by rushed consultations, long waiting times, fragmentation and poor continuity, which together with limited time for patient education culminated in errors and perceptions of poor quality care and a lack of satisfaction amongst users and providers.

Long waiting times seem to be characteristic of the SA healthcare system.[4,14,21,22] Strategies by users to decrease waiting times may put providers in a difficult position. Refusing assistance was perceived as uncaring and assisting their actions was perceived as favouritism. These perceptions, in conjunction with impatience and frustration at long waiting times, may negatively influence user attitudes and lead to impatience and rudeness.

PHC services are largely nurse-driven, but for many users this impacts on adequacy and acceptability of services. Previous studies on nurse-driven services[23,24] found high patient satisfaction rates as nurses spent more time and provided more information and counselling than doctors. Unfortunately the demand on the services might have prevented a similar finding in this study setting. In addition, it seems that, for some users, the traditional picture of the doctor as the PHC provider was strongly embedded and thus a key expectation, as described by Branson et al.[24] Users might view treatment by a nurse as a compromise in quality of care[25] especially in an urban context where expectations of care from a medical doctor are high and not unreasonable.

Large numbers of patients are effectively managed and waiting times reduced through organising services into diagnostic clinics such as HIV, diabetes, hypertension and arthritis clinics. However, such organisation impacted negatively on user privacy and confidentiality and the acceptability of the services. Merely attending a specific clinic or unit robbed the user of confidentiality as their health status was publically displayed. Such unintentional breaches in confidentiality may act as powerful deterrents to accessing public health care services. In addition, this constitutes an impairment-oriented approach that depersonalises the user,[26,27] compromises holistic, patient-centred care,[27,28] as well as continuity and coordination of care.[28] Whilst promoting standardised care and protecting providers from full personal contact with users, it also limits provider work satisfaction and fuels stress and anxiety.[27]

Acceptability of the services was limited as users were disempowered through lack of choice, thus affecting quality of care and satisfaction.[28] They could not choose which facility to use, the service provider they would like see, nor the day or time of their appointment. There was no trust relationship to explore user expectations.

Unmet expectations fuelled perceptions of inadequacy and unacceptability. According to Dixon-Woods and colleagues,[7] unmet needs exist as a result of the conflict between health services seeking to constitute and define the appropriate objects of medical care versus what the user defines as the focus of care. The outcome of this continuous reinforcing of conflict dynamically shapes access[7] and perceptions of the quality of care.[28,29] For example, the user expectation of the availability of an emergency service at the clinics may not be that of health providers. Setlhare and colleagues[30] emphasised the need for context-specific patient-provider models which are sensitive to cultural and regional constructs. In the current study, some users asserted themselves by accessing the CHC after hours. However, such a strategy can impact negatively on planning, services and resources.[31] In addition, providers felt taken advantage of, which may have resulted in negative attitudes towards users.

Past studies[4,32,33,34,35] have demonstrated how working conditions lead to poor staff morale and negative attitudes and affect user satisfaction and quality of care. Staff morale in this study was eroded by inadequate numbers of service providers, high turnover of providers and interns, periodic shortages of equipment and/or consumables, language barriers and the absence of interpreters, time pressures, working in an unsafe community and with users who may be rude, abusive and violent. Together these factors may result in already tenuous interpersonal relations culminating in negative attitudes and behaviours.

Overall the behaviour of both providers and users in this study demonstrated little mutual respect, empathy and tolerance. Unfortunately negative attitudes and unprofessional behaviour of providers noted in this study have all too often been documented within the SA health care literature.[4,21,22,31,36,37,38] Although limited to certain individuals, these attitudinal barriers may well end the user's relationship with the facility,[4,37,39] as was evident in this study. The impatient, rude and abusive behaviour of users may demonstrate their lack of trust in and respect for the provider-patient relationship. On the other hand, such behaviours result in providers feeling negative towards users. Expanding the human resource component of service provision will improve capacity of services and might result in an improvement in attitudinal challenges, as demonstrated in previous research.[31] Although many strategies were already implemented to improve efficiency, flow management and referral procedures, potential to improve leadership and the quality of management within facilities should also be explored.

Ongoing trust relationships form the foundation of client centred healthcare[39] and are especially important in the management of chronic diseases.[28] PWDs often suffer from chronic conditions or require ongoing healthcare due to the nature of their impairments,[40,41] but are twice as likely than their non-disabled peers to experience inadequate care at health facilities.[42,43,44,45,46] PWDs in this study were no exception with both healthcare providers and users alluding to this fact. Their healthcare was compromised by a lack of rehabilitation service providers, stereotyping and a lack of skills and knowledge. They often faced delayed referral and long waiting times to access these referral services. Waiting times can lead to a deterioration of the health condition and impairment and can aggravate the disability or turn a temporary disability into a permanent one.[41] Stereotyping, from lack of knowledge, caused discrimination, rudeness and exclusion from important services. The need for more training and support for primary care providers in the comprehensive management of chronic and more complex conditions has been recognised before.[14,47] In the climate of re-engineering of PHC[48,49,50] and provision of a continuum of all four dimensions of care at primary level (promotive, preventive, curative and rehabilitation services), the poor availability of rehabilitation-specific services on the PHC platform in Gugulethu was concerning.

In summary, providers experience significant stressors in their efforts at providing satisfactory heath care, despite many positive features and favourable impressions of the services reported by users. These were, however, quickly overshadowed by negative experiences and perceptions, leaving users feeling disempowered and voiceless, victimised and betrayed by the very system that is supposed to enhance their well-being. Their desperation can be summarised by the lament of this user who responded as follows when her health care needs were not met:

> 'My heart is becoming broken.' (User, female, single parent, 15–19, HIV and/or AIDS)

Limitations

The qualitative nature of this study limits the generalisability of the results to a wider context.

The language and cultural barrier between the primary researcher and the participants may have affected the depth of experiences explored, especially where an interpreter was used or both parties conversed in their second language.

Implication and recommendations

Considering the limitations of this study and the multi-dimensional facets of health care access, recommendations pertain to the study site only. Some of the recommendations may be applied in other settings after careful consideration of contextual differences and similarities.[51]

Whilst the recommendations are based on the service dimension only, the authors second the need for research in the development of context-specific patient-provider models[30] where the emphasis is on user constructs. These should include holistic health care provider models with a focus on personal continuity and choice, as well as the management and inclusion of PWD and disability-specific services.

In particular, the lack of communication about the service structure and function seems to be an important factor which perpetuates negative perceptions of the services. Community information strategies[52] must therefore be employed to inform and educate[24] the community on the scope and structure of health care services and to market positive changes in services.

Codes of conduct for users (Patient Rights Charter)[53] and providers (the Public Servants Code of Conduct[54] and the principles of the Batho Pele [People first] initiative[55]) are systems measures aimed at achieving service acceptability. However, the failure of these strategies to effect change indicates the need for innovative strategies which consider both the user and the service.

Conclusion

The study showed that efficient administrative and logistical organisation of health care service and systems does not automatically translate into adequate and acceptable services from a user's perspective. The balance can be restored by changing how services are delivered and how users are informed. Service delivery should include a patient-centred approach with consideration of aspects such as choice, comprehensive individualised care, continuity of care, shared consultation and participative decision making, non-discrimination, as well as good communication with a focus on mutual respect and courtesy.

Restoring the balance between service provision and user demands should facilitate universal access and equitable health care service delivery, particularly for vulnerable groups, and ensure that the public PHC services become the key to the management of health, as was stated by one of the participants:

> 'The clinic is a very most important place to be because it is the key to any health centre or doctor.' (Non-user, female, 35-49, single parent)

Acknowledgements

This research was funded by the European Commission Framework Programme 7: Project Title: Enabling universal access to healthcare for vulnerable people in resource poor setting in Africa; Grant agreement No. 223501. With gratitude to all the participants and service providers who willingly shared their experiences.

Competing interests

The authors declare that they have no financial or personal relationship(s) that may have inappropriately influenced them in writing this article.

Authors' contributions

E.S. (University of Stellenbosch) did the data collection and analysis and drafted the article. S.V. (University of Stellenbosch) was involved in project design and made conceptual contributions to the article and M.S. (University of Cape Town) was involved in project design and made conceptual contributions to the article.

References

1. World Health Organization. Human rights, health and poverty reduction strategies. Geneva: WHO; 2008.

2. Obrist B, Iteba N, Lengeler C, et al. Access to healthcare in contexts of livelihood insecurity: A framework for analysis and action. PLOS Med. 2007;10(4):1584–1588.

3. World Health Organization. Poverty reduction strategy papers. Their significance for health: second synthesis report. WHO: Geneva, Switzerland; 2004.

4. Harris B, Eyles J, et al. Adverse or acceptable: Negotiating access to a post-apartheid healthcare contract. Globalization and Health [serial online]. 2014 [cited 2014 June 13];10:35. Available from: http://www.globalizationandhealth.com/content/10/1/35.

5. Levesque JF, Harris MF, Russel G. Patient-centred access to health care: Conceptualising access at the interface of health systems and populations. Int J Equity Health [serial online]. 2013;12:18. Available from: http://www.equityhealthj.com/content/12/1/18. http://dx.doi.org/10.1186/1475-9276-12-18

6. Gilson L, Schneider H. Understanding health service access: Concepts and experience. Global Forum Update Research Health. 2007;4:28–32.

7. Dixon-Woods M, Cavers D, Agarwal S, et al. Conducting a critical interpretive synthesis of the literature on access to healthcare by vulnerable groups [serial online]. 2006 [cited 2014 June 13];6:35. doi:10.1186/1471-2288-6-35. Available from: http://www.biomedcentral.com/1471-2288/6/35.

8. Oliver A, Mossialos E. Equity of access to healthcare: Outlining the foundations for action. J Epidemiol Community Health. 2004;58:655–658. http://dx.doi.org/10.1136/jech.2003.017731

9. Balen J, Liu Z-C, McManus DP, et al. Health access livelihood framework reveals potential barriers in the control of Schistosomiasis in the Dongting Lake area of Hunana Province, China. PLOS Negl Trop Dis [serial online]. 2013 [cited 2014 June 12];7(8):e2350. doi:10.1371/journal.pntd.0002350

10. Bakeera SK, Galea S, Pariyo GW, et al. Community perceptions and factors influencing utilization of health services in Uganda. Int J Equity Health [serial online]. 2009 [cited 2014 June 12];8:25. doi:10.11861475-9276-8-25. Available from: http://www.equityhealthj.com/content/8/1/25.

11. Department for International Development. Sustainable livelihoods guidance sheets: Chapter 2 Framework [homepage on the Internet]. No date [cited 2009 Oct 19]. Available: http://www.livelihoods.org/info/info_guidancesheets.html.

12. Flaskerud JH, Winslow BJ. Conceptualizing vulnerable populations health-related research. Nurs Res. 1998;47(2):69–78. http://dx.doi.org/10.1097/00006199-199803000-00005

13. EquitAble. Enabling universal and equitable access to healthcare for vulnerable people in resource poor setting in Africa [homepage on the Internet]. No date [cited 2014 May 28]. Available from: http://www.equitableproject.org.

14. Visagie S, Schneider M. Implementation of the principles of primary healthcare in a rural area of South Africa. Afr J Prm Healthcare Fam Med [serial online]. 2014 [cited 2014 May 29];6(1). Available from: http://dx.doi.org/10.4102/phcfm.v6i1.562

15. Braathen SH, Vergunst R, Mji G, et al. Understanding the local context for the application of global mental health: A rural South African experience. Int Health [serial online]. 2013;5(1):38–42. doi:10.1093/inthealth/ihs016

16. Frith, A. Census 2012: Gugu1ethu [homepage on the Internet]. No date [cited 2014 May 29]. Available from: http://census2011.adrianfrith.com/place/199030.

17. City of Cape Town. 2011 census suburb Gugulethu [homepage on the Internet]. July 2013 [cited 2014 May 29]. Available from: http://www.capetown.gov.za/en/stats/2011CensusSuburbs/2011_Census_CT_Suburb_Gugulethu_Profile.pdf.

18. Domholt E. Rehabilitation research. Principles and applications. 3rd ed. Elsevier: Missouri; 2005.

19. Mannan H, Amin M, MacLachlan M, EquitAble Consortium. The EquiFrame manual: a tool for evaluating and promoting the inclusion of vulnerable groups and core concepts of human rights in health policy documents. 2nd ed. Dublin: Global Health Press; 2014.

20. Eide AH, Amin M, MacLachlan M, et al. Addressing equitable health of vulnerable groups in international health documents. ALTER, Eur J Disability Res [serial online]. 2013;7:153–162. doi:10.1016/j.alter.2013.04.004

21. Hasumi T, Jacobsen KH. Healthcare service problems reported in a national survey of South Africans. Int J Qual Health Care [serial online]. 2014 [cited 2014 June 1]. Available from: http://intqhc.oxfordjournals.org/.

22. Day C, Gray A. Health and related indicators. In: Barron P, Roma-Reardon J, editors. South African Health Review 2008. Durban: Health Systems Trust; 2008. p. 239–396.

23. Delamaire M, Lafortune G. Nurses in advanced roles: A description and evaluation of experiences in 12 developed countries. OECD Health Working Papers No 54, OECD Publishing [homepage on the Internet]. 2010 [cited 2014 June 12]. doi:10.1787/5kmbrcfms5g7-en. http://dx.doi.org/10.1787/5kmbrcfms5g7-en

24. Branson C, Badger B, Dobbs F. Patient satisfaction with skill mix in primary care: A review of the literature. Primary Healthcare Res Dev. 2003;4:329–339. http://dx.doi.org/10.1191/1463423603pc162oa

25. Kapp R, Mash RJ. Perceptions of the role of the clinical nurse practitioner in the Cape Metropolitan doctor-driven community health centres. SA Fam Pract. 2004;46(10):21–25. http://dx.doi.org/10.1080/20786204.2004.10873150

26. Mosadeghrad AM. Healthcare service quality: Towards a broad definition. Int J Health Care Qual Assur [serial online]. 2013 [cited 2014 June 12];26(3):203–219. doi:10.1108/09526861311311409. Available from: http://www.emeraldinsight.com/0952-6862.htm

27. Van der Walt H, Swartz L. Isabel Mensies Lyth revisited. Institutional defences in public health nursing in South Africa during the 1990s. Psychodyn Couns. 1999;5:483–495. http://dx.doi.org/10.1080/13533339908404985

28. Sofaer S, Firminger K. Patient perceptions of the quality of health services. Annu Rev Public Health. [serial online]. 2005 [cited 2014 June 9];26:513–559. http://dx.doi.org/10.1146/annurev.publhealth.25.050503.153958

29. Bell R, Kravitz RL, Thom D, et al. Unmet expectations for care and the patient-physician relationship. J Gen Intern Med. 2002;17:817–824. http://dx.doi.org/10.1046/j.1525-1497.2002.10319.x

30. Setlhare V, Couper I, Wright A. Patient-centredness: Meaning and propriety in the Botswana, African and non-Western contexts. Afr J Prm Health Care Fam Med [serial online]. 2014 [cited 2014 June 22];6(1). doi:10.4102/phcfm.v6i1:554.

31. Masango-Makgobela A, Govender I, Ndimande JV. Reasons patients leave their nearest healthcare service to attend Karen Park Clinic, Pretoria North. Afr J Prm Healthcare Fam Med [serial online]. 2013 [cited 2014 June 16];5(1). doi:10.4102/phcfm.v5i1.559.

32. Tshitangano TG. Factors that contribute to public sector nurses' turnover in Limpopo province of South Africa. Afr J Prm Health Care Fam Med [serial online]. 2013 [cited 2014 June 22]. 5(1). doi:10.4102/phcfm.v5i1.479

33. Gross K, Pfeiffer C, Obrist B. "Workhood" – a useful concept for the analysis of health workers'resources? An evaluation from Tanzania. BMC Health Serv Res [serial online]. 2012 [cited 2014 May 28];12:55. Available from: http://www.biomedcentral.com/1472-6963/12/55.

34. Karliner LS, Jacobs EA, et al. Do professional interpreters improve clinical care for patients with limited English proficiency? A systematic review of the literature. Health Serv Res [serial online]. 2007 [cited 2014 June 16];42(2):727–754. doi:10.1111/j.1475-6773.2006.00629.x

35. Newman K, Maylor U. Empirical evidence for "the nurse satisfaction, quality of care and patient satisfaction chain". Int J Health Care Qual Assur [serial online]. 2002 [cited 2014 June 13];15(2):80–88. Available from: http://www.emeraldinsight.com/0952-6862.htm.

36. Lotika AA, Mabuza LH, Okonta HI. Reasons given by hypertensive patients for concurrently using traditional and Western medicine at Natalspruit Hospital in the Gauteng Province, South Africa. Afr J Prm Health Care Fam Med [serial online]. 2013 [cited 2014 June 22];5(1). http://dx.doi.org/10.4102/phcfm.v5i1.458

37. Schneider H, le Marcis F, Grard J, et al. Negotiating care: patient tactics at an urban South African hospital. J Health Serv Res Policy. 2010;15(3):137–142. http://dx.doi.org/10.1258/jhsrp.2010.008174

38. Jewkes R, Abrahams N, Mvo Z. Why do nurses abuse patients? Reflections from South African obstetric services. Soc Sci Med. 1998;47(11):1781–1795. http://dx.doi.org/10.1016/S0277-9536(98)00240-8

39. Logie DE, Rowson M, Jugisha NM, et al. Affordable primary health care in low-income countries: Can it be achieved? Afr J Prm Health Care Fam Medn [serial online]. 2010 [cited 2014 June 22];2(1). doi:10.4102/phcfm.v2i1.246. http://dx.doi.org/10.4236/health.2014.65058

40. Park JM. Disability and health service utilization among old Koreans. Health [serial online]. 2014;6(5):404–409. doi:10.4236/health.2014.65058. http://dx.doi.org/10.4236/health.2014.65058

41. Shakespeare, T. Disability rights and wrongs revisited. 2nd ed. London: Routledge; 2014.

42. Story MF, Kailes JI, Mac Donald C. The ADA in action at healthcare facilities. Disabil Health J. 2010;3:245–252. http://dx.doi.org/10.1016/j.dhjo.2010.07.005

43. Yee S, Breslin ML. Achieving accessible healthcare for people with disabilities: Why the ADA is only part of the solution. Disabil Health J. 2010;3:253–261. http://dx.doi.org/10.1016/j.dhjo.2010.07.006

44. Story MF, Schwier E, Kailes JI. Perspective of patients with disabilities on the accessibility of medical equipment: Examination tables, imaging equipment, medical chairs, and weight scales. Disabil Health J. 2009;2:169–179. http://dx.doi.org/10.1016/j.dhjo.2009.05.003

45. Graham CL, Mann JR. Accessibility of primary care physician practice sites in South Carolina for people with disabilities. Disabil Health J. 2008;1:209–214. http://dx.doi.org/10.1016/j.dhjo.2008.06.001

46. Gulley SP, Altman BM. Disability in two healthcare systems: access, quality, satisfaction, and physician contacts among work-age Canadians and Americans with disabilities. Disabil Health J. 2008;1:196–208. http://dx.doi.org/10.1016/j.dhjo.2008.07.006

47. Mash B, Fairall L, Adejayan O, et al. A morbidity survey of South African primary care. PLOS ONE [serial online]. 2012 [cited 2014 June 19];7(3):e32358. http://dx.doi.org/10.1371/journal.pone.0032358

48. Naledi T, Barron P, Schneider H. Primary Healthcare in SA since 1994 and implications of the new vision for PHC re-engineering. South African Health Review. In: Padarath A, English R, editors. South African Health Review 2011. Durban: Health Systems Trust, 2011; p. 17–28.

49. Western Cape Government: Health. Annual performance plan 2012/13. Cape Town: Department of Health; 2012 Available from: https://www.westerncape.gov.za/text/2012/3/doh_app_20122013.pdf.

50. Western Cape Government: Health. 2020: The future of health care in the Western Cape: A draft framework for dialogue. Cape Town: Department of Health, South Africa; 2011. Available at: https://www.westerncape.gov.za/other/2011/12/healthcare_2020_-_9_december_2020.pdf. http://dx.doi.org/10.1002/casp.2124

51. Hodgetts DJ, Stolte OEE. Case-based research in community and social psychology: Introduction to the special issue. J Community Appl Soc Psychol. 2012;22(5):379–389.

52. Ensor T, Cooper S. Overcoming barriers to health service access: Influencing the demand side. Health Policy Plan [serial online]. 2006 [cited 2014 June 12];19(2):69–79. Available from: http://heapol.oxfordjournals.org.

53. South Africa. Department of Health. Patient rights charter [homepage on the Internet]. 2007 [cited 2014 May 30]. Available from: http://222.doh.gov.za/docs/legislation/patientsright/chartere.html.

54. South Africa. Public Service Commission. Code of conduct for public servants [homepage on the Internet]. 1997 [cited 2014 May 30]. Available from: http://www.psc.gov.za/documents/code.asp.

55. South Africa. Department of Public Service and Administration. Batho Pele handbook [homepage on the Internet]. No date [cited 2014 May 30]. Available from: http://www.dpsa.gov.za/batho-pele/docs/BP_HB_optimised.pdf.

30

Student perspectives on the value of rural electives

Author:
Ian Couper[1]

Affiliation:
[1]Centre for Rural Health, Faculty of Health Sciences, University of the Witwatersrand, South Africa

Correspondence to:
Ian Couper

Email:
ian.couper@wits.ac.za

Postal address:
PO Box 1368, Hartbeespoort 2016, South Africa

Background: Medical students in the Faculty of Health Sciences at the University of the Witwatersrand (Wits) in Johannesburg have the opportunity to do electives at the end of the first and third years of a four-year graduate-entry medical programme. Upon their return they are required to write a short portfolio report. Over the period 2005 to 2011, 402 students chose to do rural electives.

Aim and setting: To understand the value of rural electives from the perspective of medical students in the Faculty of Health Sciences at Wits, as derived from their assessment reports.

Methods: A review was conducted of 402 elective reports. Common themes were identified through repeated reading of the reports, and then content analysis was undertaken using these themes.

Results: Major themes identified were the reasons for choosing a rural facility for the elective, including going to a home community; benefits of the elective, especially in terms of clinical skills and personal growth; relationship issues; the multiple roles of the rural doctor, who is often a role model working in difficult conditions; and the challenges of rural electives.

Conclusion: The electives were overwhelmingly positive and affirming experiences for students, who developed clinical skills and also learnt about both themselves and their chosen career.

Les points de vue des étudiants sur la valeur des stages ruraux.

Contexte: Les étudiants en médecine de la Faculté des Sciences de la Santé de l'Université du Witwatersrand (Wits) à Johannesburg peuvent choisir de faire un stage électif à la fin de la première et troisième année du programme de quatre ans d'accès aux études médicales. A leur retour ils doivent rédiger un court rapport de portefeuille. De 2005 à 2011, 402 étudiants ont choisi de faire un stage en zone rurale.

Objectif et cadre: Comprendre la valeur des stages en zone rurale du point de vue des étudiants en médecine de la faculté des Sciences de la Santé de Wits, à partir de leurs rapports d'évaluation.

Méthodes: On a étudié les 402 rapports électifs. On a identifié des thèmes communs en relisant les rapports, suivis d'une analyse du contenu conformément à ces thèmes.

Résultats: Les thèmes clés identifiés étaient les raisons du choix d'un établissement en milieu rural pour le stage électif, y compris la communauté d'origine; les avantages du stage électif, surtout du point de vue des compétences cliniques et du développement personnel; les problèmes relationnels; les rôles multiples du médecin de campagne qui est souvent un modèle travaillant dans des conditions difficiles; et le défi des stages électifs en zone rurale.

Conclusion: Les stages électifs ont été des expériences très positives et mémorables pour les étudiants qui ont développé leurs compétences cliniques, et ces stages leur ont aussi enseigné des choses sur eux-mêmes et leur future carrière

Introduction

Exposure of undergraduate medical students to rural health care during their training is recognised to be an essential strategy in the eventual recruitment of doctors to rural areas.[1-3] Various models exist for this exposure, which include both compulsory and voluntary placements in rural health facilities and practices. The role that rural electives can play in encouraging students to consider rural practice, as well as in their general educational development, has not been explored in the literature.

The University of the Witwatersrand (Wits) in Johannesburg introduced a new medical curriculum in 2003, in the form of a four-year graduate-entry medical programme (GEMP). GEMP years 1 and 2 focus on problem-based learning in systems blocks, with weekly clinical skills and hospital exposure. GEMP years 3 and 4 consist of a series of clinical rotations in all major disciplines. Two elective periods are included in the programme: the first is a two-week period at the end of the first GEMP year, which may be undertaken anywhere in Southern Africa, whilst the second is a four-week exposure (that may be split into two two-week periods) at the end of GEMP third year, which may be undertaken anywhere in the world. Students are required to submit a two-page portfolio report reflecting on their elective experience, based on objectives set prior to the elective in consultation with a faculty supervisor, in order to sit the final examinations in the second and fourth GEMP years.

As part of its strategic goals, the Centre for Rural Health in the Wits Faculty of Health Sciences aims to recruit, educate and support human resources for rural health care. Through the academic division of Rural Health it offers the opportunity for students doing electives to gain rural experience, mainly in rural district hospitals, all over South Africa and even in other countries.

A steadily increasing number of students signed on for rural electives between 2003 (when GEMP 1 rolled out) and 2008, increasing from 5 (2.3% of the GEMP 1 class) to 85 (19.8% of the combined GEMP 1 and 3 classes), with a current steady state of 60–80 students (about 12% – 18%) signing up for rural electives. The initial increase in numbers, which occurred largely due to interpersonal communication, and the ongoing level of interest suggests that students were gaining something important through the rural elective experience.

Aim and objectives

It was decided to ascertain what the value of these rural electives is in the eyes of the students themselves. A review was conducted of the student elective reports received over seven years from 2005 to 2011.

Methods

A qualitative review was conducted of the portfolio reports submitted by students completing rural electives over the period 2005–2011. A total of 402 electives were undertaken. Of these, 371 were undertaken in rural public health facilities in South Africa, in all of the nine provinces, and 3 in urban district hospitals (due to last-minute difficulties encountered by students, such as lack of finances to travel); 13 were completed with rural private general practitioners in South Africa. Twelve students completed their electives in rural areas outside of South Africa, 11 of these in other African countries and one in the Northern Territory of Australia. Three students worked in non-governmental organisations, one of which was in Swaziland.

The majority of students (72%) completed these electives at the end of GEMP 1.

All 402 reports submitted over the seven years were included in the review. Common themes were identified through careful reading of the reports over the first five years. A content analysis of each report was then undertaken using these themes, to ensure that all major issues mentioned by students were covered, and copies of the reports were divided into the themes using cut and paste. The reports for the latter two years were reviewed in the light of the above themes; no additional themes were found, but relevant comments by students were added to the database.

Students are required in their portfolio reports to explain why they chose the particular site, what learning occurred and how this related to the objectives set with the internal (faculty) supervisor. These reports are assessed by this supervisor, and therefore reflections were likely to be more positive in nature, creating an inherent bias. However, this is mitigated by the fact that the mark has a negligible impact on overall grading – the main requirement is to submit a report. Furthermore, the reports are not seen by the external (host) supervisors, so honesty about the experience is also promoted.

Ethical considerations

Prior ethical approval was obtained from the Human Research Ethics Committee of Wits. Reports were only reviewed after students had, at a minimum, completed their assessment process for the year subsequent to their elective, and therefore there was no possible influence on student outcomes.

Results

The major themes identified in the reports are listed in Table 1. Quotations from the reports are used below to illustrate these themes.

TABLE 1: Themes that emerged from the reports of students who completed the rural elective.

Theme	Sub-themes
1. Reasons for choosing a rural hospital	a. Going home
	b. Experience of different culture
	c. Visiting beautiful places
	d. Gaining broad clinical experience
	e. Experience of less-resourced/poor area
2. Benefits of the elective	a. Clinical skills
	b. Personal growth
	c. Confirmation of chosen career
3. Relationship issues	a. Communication
	b. Teamwork
4. The rural doctor	a. Generalists
	b. Role models
	c. Negative examples
	d. Differences
	e. Working conditions
5. Challenges of the rural elective	a. Language barriers
	b. Cultural differences
6. Reflections	a. On rural medicine

Reasons for choosing a rural hospital

Students offered a variety of reasons for choosing rural sites for their electives. For a number of these who came from rural areas, they were returning home, to the health facility closest to where they lived:

> 'I did my elective at [A] Hospital. ... Since it is my home hospital, I did not realise how "rural" it is because I am used to such an environment.'

> 'I chose it because it is very close to my home [*about 20 min drive*] and from previous experience I knew that I would be able to do a lot of practical work.'

Even within the motivation of going home there were nuances illustrating different student needs and interests:

> 'I thought it would be a good opportunity to get away from it all. I am from a small town in Mpumalanga. The city lights and all it has to offer holds no attraction for me. I miss home a lot, not only the veld or the simplicity of it all, but especially the people. The further you move out of the city the warmer the people become, when they ask you how you are, they really care.'

> 'I actually wanted to have an exposure to the kind of service my family and my community gets.'

> 'I spent the entire four weeks of my elective at the [B] Hospital, being my hometown, and also the place where I intend spending my future career. Just being able to treat patients who remembered me as a little boy growing up in front of them brought about a feeling not matched in my five years of training so far.'

Some students specifically saw the elective as part of the process of giving back to the community that supported them:

> 'I wanted to know the health problems that my community was facing. It is a hospital that I have grown to love and I hope to find myself serving the community in that hospital one day. I was born in that community hospital and I plan to give the people in my community the best health care they need.'

> 'I felt it necessary to give back to the rural community who had supported me during my high school years.'

For a few students there was an opposite reason – to get away from home:

> 'I wish I could say that the reasoning behind choosing to do a rural elective was altruistic ... The truth behind it is that choosing to do to a rural hospital meant a two-week holiday, away from home, all under the guise of "community service at a rural hospital".'

Some students wanted to experience a different cultural milieu.

> 'An elective in rural medicine in South Africa was a way for me to understand rural poverty and the pertinent issues at play in public health in developing areas.'

> 'This was a chance for me to enhance my personal and professional development by understanding my culture better, then I could understand my patient's culture ...'

Whatever other reasons there were, the opportunity to gain hands-on clinical experience was very important:

> 'My main objective ... was to do as many practical things as possible in order to prepare for my clinical years.'

> 'I felt that I needed exposure to working in communities and dealing with common conditions.'

> 'The reason for my choice was because I wanted to experience total medicine as well as go to a hospital where I would learn a lot. I think I made the correct choice because at the end of my two-week elective I felt as though I had learnt so much more than I expected to and was more passionate about wanting to be a doctor and work in South Africa than I have ever been before.'

Students recognised that this practical learning was different from what they were experiencing in the tertiary academic hospitals:

> 'I also thought that it would be a great opportunity for me to learn new things as well as practice the skills and theory that I have been taught, since there wouldn't be situations where a consultant, three registrars, two interns and four medical students are all crowding around one patient, as is sometimes the case at the hospitals we attend in Johannesburg.'

> 'I chose [C *hospital*] because of the opportunity of non-competitive learning. Students are the most curious creatures and get tremendously fascinated by the new environment of medicine they find themselves in – filled with the abundant amenity of learning about the human being. Deliveries, lumbar puncture, pleural taps, anything, we jump at the opportunity to be the ones performing the procedures. But how often do you get to do these on a daily basis in a teaching hospital like [Z] Hospital, hardly.'

Part of the broader experience was also seen to be gaining an understanding of less-resourced or poorer areas

> 'I had heard many stories about the facilities at rural hospital being inadequate, and living conditions being nearly as bad, thus it was with trepidation that I decided to step away from the comforts of urban life, and actually understand what the majority of South Africans deal with on a daily basis.'

> 'I truly wanted to experience and understand the difficulties rural health practitioners face on a day-to-day basis, away from the busy and bustling resource-rich urban areas of South Africa.'

This included a desire to compare rural and urban hospitals:

> 'to see the difference existing between rural and urban settings.'

> 'I needed to understand the community better and also be exposed to the rural health setting that is so prevalent in this country. It would be naïve of me to assume that work environment in the big city hospitals is a reflection of the many smaller hospitals serving the bulk of the nation.'

Benefits of the elective

Improvement in clinical skills

Students identified a range of important benefits from doing a rural elective. Most significantly, all students reported improvements in their clinical skills. A number of reasons were given for this. Firstly, there was greater independence and responsibility:

'I was following up patients, not just any random patients but "my own patients".'

'Due to the massive doctor shortage, I was able to get heavily involved in a wide range of activities at the hospital that most third-year students of medicine would never be able to participate in.'

There was the opportunity to put theory into practice, which was valued especially because it allowed students to realise how much they had learnt:

'Though initially nervous, I surprised myself with my own ability as I became more confident in applying the theoretical knowledge and clinical skills I had acquired at Wits through the year.'

'It was so encouraging to realise that we have learnt a great amount this year, as we could start to ignite our own reasoning processes using the facts that we have accumulated through GEMP 1. Being able to pull the basic sciences, clinical skills and patient doctor and community doctor themes all together into one reality of practicing medicine was very stimulating.'

Students developed a wide range of clinical skills as a result of 'learning by doing':

'This elective gave us the unique opportunity to *do* rather than observe.' [*Student's emphasis*]

'It was a wonderful opportunity to hear different heart and chest sounds and practice the clinical skill we have learnt through the year. … Now I finally know what crackles are meant to sound like!'

'We got hands-on experience that every medical student craves from the first day of registration.'

This was enhanced by local supervising doctors who 'were also very helpful when it came to my learning':

'I appreciated the care and time the doctors took in explaining and teaching different theory and skills to me.'

'We could experience all the challenges of dealing with a wide spectrum of patients, from first encounter to discharge, but all the time we had a safety net – we could always ask for help or advice if we were uncertain what to do.'

For some the process gave them a new appreciation of their medical school training:

'Another important thing I realised is that the GEMP programme is not as bad as I thought. It is actually a good programme compared to the programmes offered in other universities. I realised this when I met medical students from other medical schools who seemed not to know a lot and had no idea of some of the models.'

However, they also discovered gaps in what they are learning:

'You learn a lot about yourself and you learn an approach to disease unlike what is taught in the syllabus …'

Personal growth

Personal growth was identified as another major benefit of the rural elective experience, and was described in a multitude of ways. Much of this was about learning aspects of medicine outside of the curriculum:

'I came to realise that getting 90% in the exams won't make me a good doctor but will make me pass and get promotion. But the real world out there in the hospitals is all about helping patients, saving lives, handling sensitive issues and understanding all your patients and their needs. This elective made me to consider my own fears, likes, dislikes, this will help me in choosing my area of specialisation in future as a doctor.'

'One of the most profound realisations that I had whilst on my rural elective, was the need for inward reflection. Throughout the academic GEMP 1 year, it becomes easy to place all one's focus on the theoretical studies, and forget about analysing how certain experiences affects one as a doctor and an individual. I never thought that my feelings and beliefs could be influenced by interacting in the consultation, believing that I could focus only on my skills and knowledge.'

'I did not expect to come out of the elective with a better understanding of who I am, and a large amount of personal growth.'

Aspects of professional life and coping with being a doctor were important:

'I learnt how to handle pressure at work and also to discuss sensitive issues. I then realised that you don't need books to study how to handle pressure at work. This comes from you as an individual.'

'I came to realise, and I hope that I never forget this, that as a doctor it will never be my place to judge people for anything they do, but rather act compassionately and professionally no matter the circumstance.'

'My elective revived my faith in medicine. It made me think. It made me re-evaluate my reasons for studying medicine. It made me realise that in a cold world and an icy profession there is still love and the warmth in caring.'

Some students described the experience as life-changing:

'It started out as a challenge of surviving two weeks in a rural setting and ended up a life-changing experience.'

'I was not the same I was before I went and I will be forever changed by it.'

'I believe I learnt the most important lessons in life, of which one of them is the fact that we need to see "people" before we see "patients".'

'Somewhere in the middle of rural KZN [*KwaZulu-Natal province*], when I thought I had lost everything, I found myself. I found who it is I'm meant to be. I found who I truly am. For that, I will be forever grateful.'

Being alone and outside of their comfort zone was certainly a factor in this growth:

'Sure everyone says you "grow" on electives, but I had first-hand experience of growth. I firmly believe that being alone strengthened me tremendously. I found I could work alone, ask as many questions as I wanted to, go anywhere.'

'Having entered medical school in my sixth year of tertiary study, I quickly realised that professional and indeed personal development only occur by continuously seeking alien situations, which provide opportunities to challenge oneself.'

For some students personal growth occurred in facing the reality of medical practice in South Africa for the first time:

> 'I have been well aware of how big a problem TB [*tuberculosis*] and HIV [*infection*] present but being confronted with the human face of the disease every day in the volumes we were, really brought home the magnitude of the problem. The feeling of helplessness weighs heavy, but on this background the moments of hope, painted in such stark relief, stand out most boldly.'

> 'I realised that as a doctor I will have to face crises and deal with losing patients and I needed to have adequate coping mechanisms to get me through these dark times and prevent burnout.'

> '… by the end of two weeks, I was accepting limitations (power cuts, limited time with patients, etc.) such as these far more easily and focusing on the solutions to the problems, rather than on the problems themselves.'

> 'This was the first time, I feel, that I was truly exposed to the personal lives of people who visit the hospitals. I have never felt such anger as I felt when I saw a nine year old girl who had been abused and actually prostituted by her family.'

Confirmation of their chosen career

Another benefit expressed by many students was a sense of confirmation of their chosen career:

> 'Not only has this elective experience confirmed my aspiration to become a doctor but it also has opened my eyes to other hospitals in this country and how they work.'

> 'My enthusiasm [*was*] rekindled in the exciting medical field, not only by all the practical experiences I have had but also by the spirit of the wonderful people and patients I have met.'

> 'I learnt a lot in so many ways, clinically, culturally, personally and spiritually. It definitely also encouraged me as a medical student, [*to*] study hard, not necessarily only for myself, but also for the patients that I will one day have as a qualified doctor.'

Relationship issues

Students learnt a lot through working together with doctors and other health professionals, particularly in terms of communication and team work.

Need for good communication

Good communication and positive working relationships were frequently noted as important:

> 'It made me realise that having good relationships with other people is very important.'

> 'My elective was a positive experience that taught me the value of working with the people in the community including the staff of the hospital who were part of that community.'

This included good communication with patients:

> 'For the first time I felt as though I had the opportunity to truly understand the doctor-patient relationship and its significance in assuring quality health care.'

> 'Even though I tend to be shy and battle to talk to people I do not know, I started really enjoying listening and talking to patients

and even tried to speak some Zulu, which made them feel much more comfortable and willing to share their experiences.'

Sometimes the lessons were learnt from poor examples:

> 'In the consultation the doctor could make the person feel like a nuisance or better for just being there, simply by virtue of their attitudes. I saw patients being dismissed and ignored and not listened to.'

> 'It is evidently clear that poor relationship between health care workers and patient has a detrimental effect on the general services delivered by the hospital.'

Importance of teamwork

Many lessons on the importance of teamwork were presented:

> 'One of the most valuable lessons I learned is how important teamwork is in the hospital setting. As one nurse told me: "We work hard in this hospital because we all care for each other".'

> 'It was here that I learned the value of teamwork as doctors of various departments, physios, nurses and counsellors worked hand in hand in the management of patients.'

> 'Team work is vital … I came to realise that as a doctor I would be incapable of fulfilling all the patient's health care requirements and depend on other disciplines for their expertise.'

Students came to realise that it is people that make the difference to health care:

> '… my biggest lesson: Infrastructure and equipment is important, but they don't define a health facility, nor do they predict the success of that facility. Success is determined by the *people* who work in that facility.' [*Student's emphasis*]

The multiple roles of the rural doctor

The opportunity to work very closely alongside rural doctors provided insight into their roles. Rural doctors were seen to be capable generalists, who need to deal with a wide range of problems:

> 'To put it bluntly, rural doctors are just generally more capable and in control than urban doctors.'

> 'It amazed me that a rural doctor is able to treat all the signs and symptoms so effectively and treat every system of the body, even though he is just a general practitioner.'

> 'They walk in each morning and their job description is not "the surgeon" or "the physician". They are doctors who just have to deal with whatever gets thrown in their face.'

> 'It's not just about working in the hospital, but it is also about being an active member of the community.'

Rural doctors were also seen to be role models and mentors for the students:

> 'One of the doctors practises medicine in a way that I would like to be able to do one day soon – with knowledge, skill, compassion, and love while at all times respecting the patient and being realistic about my own limitations.'

> 'One ward round stood out particularly in my mind, with Dr [*M*], who was a caring, gentle, humble man. The mutual respect and the dynamic working relationship between the Dr and the nurses were awe-inspiring. Dr [*M*] greeted each patient by name,

asked her how she was and inquired if their families had been to visit them the previous day. At the end of his instructions to the nurse, he added "Also, give a liberal dose of TLC". The genuine interest and care of Dr [M] for his patients set an example for me as to what kind of doctor I would like to be one day.'

Even with their imperfections, doctors could still inspire students:

'This was the most inspiring of the elective, that the doctors, although overworked and underpaid and sometimes lost it with the non-complaint patient, they put patients as top priority.'

However, a number of students also encountered negative examples:

'I do not ever want to be a Dr like the Dr that was on call that night. Imagine – he caused a baby to die because he did not show up when he was on call. If I ever become a Dr like that, I would want to be shot … how can a person call him or herself a Dr and then be so negligent?'

'One of the two doctors assigned to work once a week at the clinic … has a mega attitude, does not exam patients, does not talk to the nurses and chooses who he wants to work with.'

Students learnt that all doctors are different, and that they need to choose what kind of doctor to be:

'I found [E] Hospital to be a place of great compassion, dedication and excellence, but also a place of apathy and desolation … There are those individuals who approach situations seeking excellence, those individuals who are always challenging themselves to do better and those who choose a path of apathy and discontent that ultimately results in poor service. I … will use my experience as the basis to continually evaluate the effort I put into and quality of my service to patients.'

The working conditions of rural doctors

The working conditions of rural doctors made a great impression on students. Multiple challenges faced in terms of resources were described:

'The biggest barrier is the lack of a transport system for patients. We referred to hospitals that were hundreds of kilometres away and there were no arrangements made for patients to be picked up or dropped off.'

'At this under-resourced, understaffed and overburdened hospital, patients have gotten used to waiting an average of 12 hours to be seen. Walking past the waiting room, I saw people with broken limbs and chronic illnesses almost cussing at the arrival of the paramedics because they know that an emergency meant that they will have to wait a few more hours.'

Facilities were, however, noted to be variable:

'From a resource allocation point of view I was very very impressed: the hospital had supplies in abundance; the supply cupboards were always fully stocked with a variety of items, so treatment of a patient was never compromised because a needle was too big, or the plaster of Paris was too small.'

'Patient care was seriously being affected by this poor infrastructure. Patients couldn't be admitted in the correct wards because of a lack of space and beds. The doctors were under too much pressure and overworked also decreasing quality patient care.'

'The most striking thing about the hospital's impression was how clean and organised it was. It almost seemed like a private hospital. It gave me hope that it really wasn't impossible to keep a hospital clean. It takes dedication, good management and team work, but it sure is possible.'

Challenges of the rural elective

Students highlighted particular challenges, in addition to those mentioned above. Language barriers were often raised as an issue:

'Communication was an enormous predicament. It was very difficult to come across a person who could actually speak English, so most consultations were done with a nurse on hand.'

'Out in the community I realised the absolute barrier that language could be. Many times I sat like an idiot nervously smiling at the patient when the doctor and translator had gone. From this I realise that I desperately need to make a plan to learn an African language if I ever hope to serve in a community like this.'

'It was a challenge for me to work with an interpreter. I often felt that my questions were not asked sufficiently and the interpreters were having private conversations unrelated to the topic at hand.'

Students also noted cultural differences as potential barriers:

'I learnt a lot about the history, cultures and way of life in Africa's Eden.'

'The cultural barriers were as frustrating as ever.'

However, these were also great opportunities for learning:

'As well as diagnostic and clinical skills learnt, there were many other lessons that I learnt … Some of these included valuable lessons on the Xhosa culture. The Transkei is very much dominated by the Xhosa people of South Africa which has its own culture very different to my Western ways. Some of these lessons included not [to] look/stare at patients directly in the eyes and that you should always greet people!'

'This inspired me to learn some Zulu and I picked up practical phrases on my elective.'

Reflections on rural health care

Students expressed their opinions about a number of issues, but in particular about rural medicine, and rural hospitals. Students argued for the value of rural exposure, for themselves and others:

'I think that as a future doctor it is important to experience rural medicine as it forms an integral part of our country's medical need. We need to be able to interact with people of different cultures and different perceptions of health. This will allow us to see the challenges faced by rural doctors so that we may become adequate doctors who are better equipped at providing holistic and effective treatment to our patients.'

'I did learn a lot but my question is that what do I (we) do to improve the health service of our rural hospitals? I think that I am the answer of this question. If we mobilised government to provide adequate resources and enough staff and create jobs, empowering people with education that might help.'

> 'I am so glad that I decided to go rural for my elective and really think that every student should at least consider it for maximum return from their elective.'

Nearly all the students came away with a very positive feeling about rural health care, despite the problems encountered:

> 'I really did find it amazing that despite the setbacks, the doctors were coping and the hospital was running smoothly. It is fantastic to see how much can be done with so little.'

> 'If I were to sum up my time in Lesotho in one sentence it would be: "The happiest 10 days of my life".'

> 'After working [*in a rural hospital*], a doctor will be able to handle any other hospital setting.'

> 'Rural health is amazing and my two weeks elective just made me realise the need of health practitioners in my hometown.'

Discussion

Medical students at Wits have the opportunity to do a rural elective placement, an option chosen by a substantial minority of students. The reports of those students who chose to do the rural elective offer a fascinating perspective on the importance of this experience. Whilst these reports were submitted for assessment, which introduces bias, they do indicate the value of the rural elective experience.

The term 'elective' refers to a range of different curricular elements, with a common factor of student choice;[4] in fact, in the United Kingdom the only essential requirement of a period of study defined as an elective is that students choose the clinical experience they have and set their own learning objectives,[5] which is how electives are also viewed in the Wits programme. Usually electives involve short attachments outside of their immediate study environment, and most have a clinical focus.[4]

The range of reasons for choosing an elective site suggest that, whilst maintaining a clinical focus, diversity and complexity should be welcomed. It is very encouraging that many students go back home, as this portends well for future practice, according to international literature on retention,[1] confirmed by local research.[6,7,8,9] The fact that students are open to persuasion indicates an opportunity to use electives as a recruitment tool for rural practice. Whilst it is recognised that electives may be seen as tourist opportunities by some students, which will have negative influences on learning outcomes and on students' attitudes,[4] there was no evidence to suggest that this was the case amongst the reports reviewed, even in cases where students frankly described a beautiful environment as a key factor in their choice.

Rural training placements are frequently described as positive learning experiences by students and preceptors.[10] Such rural experiences not only impact on student learning and the development of clinical skills, but there is also evidence of that rural training influences future practice site and career choice.[10] Whilst this study cannot offer any evidence of this,

the impact described by students and the personal growth reflected in their portfolio entries is indicative of a significant effect, and electives in international health – many of which are in rural and underserved areas – have been shown to influence career choices.[11,12] Whether or not it influences future practice location, the electives motivate students with regard to medicine as a career in general.

Students' willingness to explore and learn about issues such as rural health care, working in under-resourced areas, and the challenges of poverty is encouraging. This opportunity for students to explore the possibility of a future career in rural medicine in a relatively low-stress situation fairly early on in their clinical careers is important.

Developing clinical skills was noted as the most significant benefit of the elective reported by students. This is commonly described as a key positive feature of rural training[13] and of international electives.[11,12] What is clear is that this broad clinical experience and personal growth, which was obviously also critical for many students, occur side-by-side, making the learning more holistic than usually experienced in traditional rotations. The clinical skills development is a major pull factor in students seeking to do rural electives, but the enthusiasm of their colleagues in preceding years arising from the personal growth reported is no doubt also a motivator. Whilst there were students who encountered negative examples and were distressed by individual experiences, it seems these did not detract from their overall learning and development. These factors alone make a strong case for extending this experience.

Students spontaneously wrote about personal growth and reflected on their experiences in relation to their present and future situations; such reflection may be important in developing social accountability amongst students.[4] The level of reflection also demonstrates the connection students were able to make between theory and practice, which is often not possible to achieve within a classroom environment or even a pressurised academic hospital rotation.

A literature review of international health electives, most of which are not dissimilar from the Wits rural electives, indicates that these provide opportunities for medical students to strengthen existing skills or learn new diagnostic skills, with a focus on history-taking and clinical reasoning, and to practice medicine with fewer resources,[11] which is what our students also report. This review also found that participants in such electives were generally more likely than non-participants to report attitudinal changes, such as greater appreciation of the importance of cross-cultural communication, public health interventions, and providing care to the underserved,[11] which also accords with this study. In addition to these features, another study in the United States of America (USA) found students (like ours) also reported heightened awareness of social determinants of health, increased self-awareness and greater insight into the human side of medicine.[14]

Students express an interest in becoming rural doctors and doing rural medicine. How much this is presented for the sake of the report and in the emotion of the moment is unclear. Long-term follow-up would be needed to determine this. No doubt further nurturing of this interest would be required to make a difference. Preceptors are often important role models, and have been shown to have a very strong influence on future career choices.[15] However, simply having a strongly positive attitude towards rural health care, regardless of future practice location, is already an important movement. For a few perhaps the elective was the life-changing moment that some claimed it to be. If the elective did nothing other than affirm students in their choice of career and rekindle their determination to succeed in their studies, as expressed by many, then it surely still had an important role.

It is encouraging for Wits that students felt that the GEMP programme gave them a good preparation for the practical work in a rural hospital, and that they felt better prepared compared to students from other universities. However, many students suggested the need for an African language course to facilitate doctor-patient communication.

The limitation of this study is the use of reports that have been submitted for grading and assessment, which does bias the kind of input that students give, as noted earlier. However, the numbers involved and the consistency of the information obtained from students in many different sites, over two curricular years and seven calendar years, suggests that the themes do in fact closely represent the reality of the rural elective experience for our students.

Possible future research includes interviews and skills audits with students after rural electives (immediately and after a year or more), as well as interviews with host supervisors.

Conclusion

Whilst it is important continually to review the value of electives, it is clear that students completing rural electives at Wits are benefitting greatly from the experience. A review of the fourth-year curriculum across medical schools in the USA indicated that elective experiences commonly duplicated other experiences and did not enhance student education;[16] the evidence from these student reports is in stark contrast to that.

In conclusion, the rural elective was overwhelmingly a positive experience for the students. They learnt a great deal about themselves as well as developing their clinical skills. The elective was an affirming experience for most, which gave them confidence in their clinical skills and their chosen career.

Who can argue with a student's perspective that 'the most important lesson I have learnt is to love what I am doing'? This would argue for consideration to be given to making a rural elective a required component of the curriculum, which also has the potential to address the ongoing medical workforce shortage in rural South Africa.

Acknowledgements
Competing interests

The author declares that no financial or personal relationship(s) have inappropriately influenced the writing of this article.

References

1. Wilson NW, Couper ID, De Vries E, Reid S, Fish T, Marais BJ. A critical review of interventions to redress the inequitable distribution of healthcare professionals to rural and remote areas. Rural Remote Health. 2009;9(2):1060.

2. Grobler L, Marais BJ, Mabunda SA, Marindi PN, Reuter H, Volmink J. Interventions for increasing the proportion of health professionals practising in rural and other underserved areas. Cochrane Database Syst Rev. 2009(1):CD005314.

3. World Health Organization. Increasing access to health workers in remote and rural areas through improved retention. Geneva: World Health Organization; 2010.

4. Murdoch-Eaton D, Green A. The contribution and challenges of electives in the development of social accountability in medical students. Med Teach. 2011;33(8):643–648.

5. Hastings A, Dowell J, Eliasz MK. Medical student electives and learning outcomes for global health: A commentary on behalf of the UK Medical Schools Elective Council. Med Teach. 2014; 36(4):355–7. http://dx.doi.org/10.3109/0142159X.2013.849330

6. De Vries E, Reid S. Do South African medical students of rural origin return to rural practice? S Afr Med J. 2003;93(10):789–793.

7. Couper ID, Hugo JF, Conradie H, Mfenyana K. Influences on the choice of health professionals to practice in rural areas. S Afr Med J. 2007;97(11):1082–1086.

8. De Vries E, Irlam J, Couper I, Kornik S. Career plans of final-year medical students in South Africa. S Afr Med J. 2010;100(4):227–228.

9. Reid SJ, Couper ID, Volmink J. Educational factors that influence the urban-rural distribution of health professionals in South Africa: A case-control study. S Afr Med J. 2011;101(1):29–33.

10. Barrett FA, Lipsky MS, Lutfiyya MN. The impact of rural training experiences on medical students: A critical review. Acad Med. 2011;86(2):259–263. http://dx.doi.org/10.1097/ACM.0b013e3182046387

11. Jeffrey J, Dumont RA, Kim GY, Kuo T. Effects of international health electives on medical student learning and career choice: Results of a systematic literature review. Fam Med. 2011;43(1):21–28.

12. Thompson MJ, Huntington MK, Hunt DD, Pinsky LE, Brodie JJ. Educational effects of international health electives on U.S. and Canadian medical students and residents: A literature review. Acad Med. 2003;78(3):342–47. http://dx.doi.org/10.1097/00001888-200303000-00023

13. Tesson G, Curran V, Pong R, Strasser R. Advances in rural medical education in three countries: Canada, the United States and Australia. Educ Health (Abingdon). 2005;18(3):405–415. http://dx.doi.org/10.1080/13576280500289728

14. Smith JK, Weaver DB. Capturing medical students' idealism. Ann Fam Med. 2006; 4 Suppl 1:S32–37; discussion S58–60.

15. Stagg P, Prideaux D, Greenhill J, Sweet L. Are medical students influenced by preceptors in making career choices, and if so how? A systematic review. Rural Remote Health. 2012;12:1832.

16. Walling A, Merando A. The fourth year of medical education: A literature review. Acad Med. 2010;85(11):1698–704. http://dx.doi.org/10.1097/ACM.0b013e3181f52dc6

31

Diabetic patients' perspectives on the challenges of glycaemic control

Authors:
Oladele V. Adeniyi[1]
Parimalane Yogeswaran[1]
Graham Wright[2]
Benjamin Longo-Mbenza[1]

Affiliations:
[1]Department of Family Medicine, Faculty of Health Sciences, Walter Sisulu University, Mthatha, South Africa

[2]Centre for Health Informatics Research and Development (CHIRAD), University of Fort Hare, South Africa

Correspondence to:
Oladele Adeniyi

Email:
vincoladele@gmail.com

Postal address:
Private Bag X 9047, East London 5200, South Africa

Introduction: The factors affecting the control of diabetes are complex and varied. However, little is documented in the literature on the overall knowledge of diabetic patients about glycaemic control. This study explored the patients' perspectives on the challenges of glycaemic control.

Methods: In this qualitative study, semi-structured interviews were conducted with seventeen purposively selected diabetic patients with HBA1c ≥ 9% at Mthatha General Hospital, South Africa. The interviews were conducted in the isiXhosa language and were audiotaped. Two experienced qualitative researchers independently transcribed and translated the interviews. Thematic content analysis was conducted.

Results: Three main themes emerged: overall knowledge of diabetes and treatment targets, factors affecting the control of diabetes and how glycaemic control could be improved.
The majority of the participants demonstrated poor knowledge of treatment targets for diabetes. The majority of the participants reported that lack of money affected their control of diabetes. Some of the participants reported that the nearest clinics do not have doctors; hence, they are compelled to travel long distances to see doctors.

Conclusion: Poverty, lack of knowledge and access to doctors affect the control of diabetes in the rural communities of Mthatha, South Africa. The government should address recruitment and retention of doctors in primary health care.

Perspectives des patients diabétiques sur les défis du contrôle de la glycémie.

Introduction: Les facteurs affectant le contrôle des diabétiques sont complexes et variés. Cependant, il y a peu de choses dans la littérature sur les connaissances générales des patients diabétiques sur le contrôle de la glycémie. Cette étude a examiné les perspectives des patients sur les défis du contrôle de la glycémie.

Méthodes: Pour cette étude qualitative, on a mené des entrevues semi-structurées avec 17 diabétiques choisis expressément avec le HBA1c ≥ 9% à l'hôpital général de Mthatha, en Afrique du Sud. Les entrevues ont été effectuées en langue Xhosa et enregistrées. Deux chercheurs qualitatifs expérimentés ont transcrit et traduit séparément les entrevues. Puis une analyse du contenu thématique a été effectuée.

Résultats: Trois thèmes principaux sont apparus: la connaissance générale sur le diabète et les objectifs à atteindre en matière de traitement, les facteurs affectant le contrôle du diabète et comment améliorer le contrôle de la glycémie.
La majorité des participants avait peu de connaissances des objectifs à atteindre pour le traitement du diabète. La majorité des participants a déclaré que le manque d'argent affectait leur contrôle du diabète. Certains participants ont déclaré que les cliniques les plus proches n'avaient pas de médecins; aussi, étaient-ils obligés de se déplacer loin pour consulter des médecins.

Conclusion: La pauvreté, le manque de connaissances et l'accès aux médecins affectent le contrôle du diabète dans les communautés rurales de Mthatha, en Afrique du Sud. Le gouvernement devrait s'occuper du recrutement et du maintien en poste des médecins dans le domaine de la santé primaire.

Introduction

Diabetes mellitus is a chronic non-communicable disease that affects about 2 million people in South Africa.[1] According to the International Diabetes Federation, an estimated 63 061 South

Africans died from diabetic-related complications in 2012.[2] The increase in the prevalence of diabetes mellitus (predominantly type 2) in the population is the cause of the rise in complications: non-traumatic amputation, cardiovascular diseases, blindness, end-stage renal failure, and many others.[3,4,5,6,7] Poor glycaemic control amongst patients with diabetes mellitus constitutes a major public health problem.[8] The progression of diabetes complications occurs due to poor glycaemic control, which can be managed by quality healthcare services.[9]

Diabetic patients should be empowered with knowledge to manage themselves.[10,11] Basic knowledge of diabetes is considered a prerequisite for self-care management.[11] Diabetes self-care management has been linked with diabetes education and knowledge acquisition.[10,12] Self-care management is associated with a reduction of complications and improvement in the quality of life of diabetic patients.[13]

The depth of diabetic information that would lead to better glycaemic control is not documented in the literature. However, patients should know about the nature of diabetes, complications, medication and side-effects, role of dietary adjustment, exercises, self-monitoring of blood sugar, treatment targets and many others. This should start at the time of diagnosis and be updated at regular intervals. The benefits of maintaining normal body mass index must be explained. Patients need to understand the deleterious association of cigarette smoking and cardiovascular risks. Patients should be taught how to take care of their feet, inject insulin, recognise complications and skills required to cope with living with diabetes.[5]

Diabetes education should be evidence-based and structured according to the socio-demographic characteristics of each patient.[10] According to Kumar and Clark, if health care workers fail to provide appropriate information, then friends and family members give patients all sorts of inaccurate information.[5] Diabetic educators are crucial to the successful implementation of diabetic education programmes.[8] However, very few public health care facilities in South Africa can boast of diabetic educators;[10] therefore, time to educate patients is limited given the vast numbers of patients and shortage of health personnel.

The importance of the knowledge of diabetes to glycaemic control has been evaluated in a number of studies.[14,15,16,17,18] There have been mixed reports in the literature: whilst some studies reported that an improvement of knowledge of diabetes might predict good glycaemic control,[8,19] others demonstrated no significant association with glycaemic control.[11,16,20] Earlier studies suggested that patients with chronic diseases (T2DM inclusive) who are active participants in their health care have better health outcomes.[14,15] Heisler et al. highlighted the American Diabetes Association's position to launch a campaign to urge diabetic patients to be aware of their treatment target and actual values of HBA1c, blood pressure and cholesterol levels (their ABCs).[16]

A number of studies have examined the relationship between knowledge of treatment target and glycaemic control.[16,17,18] The majority of the participants in these studies had no knowledge of their recent HBA1c.

Heisler et al. concluded that knowledge of HBA1c alone was not sufficient to translate increased understanding of diabetes care into improvement in self-management of diabetes.[16] Santos et al. reported that glycaemic control did not correlate with knowledge of diabetes amongst the participants in their study.[11] They suggested that theoretical or practical understanding of diabetes is not by itself significantly associated with appropriate glycaemic control.

Iqbal et al. examined the impact of improving the knowledge of diabetic patients on glycaemic control.[19] The baseline measurement of the knowledge of the participants showed that the majority were not familiar with HBA1c. Knowledge of glycaemic control was generally poor amongst the participants. Intervention with diabetic education yielded improvement in glycaemic control amongst poorly controlled T2DM, who were in the unfamiliar group (10.7% versus 9.5%, $p = 0.04$). Knowledgeable diabetic patients tend to have a good attitude, which is linked to improvement in glycaemic control.[8]

A few studies found no significant association between the level of knowledge of diabetes and glycaemic control.[11,20] Notwithstanding, there is overwhelming evidence that diabetes education is central to self-care management and ultimately, improvement in glycaemic control.[5,10,19,21] Hence, the Joint Task Force of American Diabetes Association, the European Association on the Study of Diabetes, (2012)[21] and the Society of Endocrinology Metabolism and Diabetes of South Africa Guideline, (2012)[10] recommended diabetic education as a major component of the care for diabetic patients.

Many studies examined the association and magnitude of the relationships between health literacy and diabetes outcomes. However, qualitative exploration of the depth of knowledge of patients about glycaemic control appears to be neglected in the literature. Such information might influence the structure of patient education by clinicians. The feedback from patients provides valuable inputs into quality improvement of health care services, policy formulation and guideline development.

Method
Operational definitions

Good glycaemic control: According to the Society of Endocrinology, Metabolism and Diabetes of South Africa, the majority of patients with a glycosylated haemoglobin level < 7% will be considered as having achieved good glycaemic control. This is also supported by the recommendation of the American Diabetes Association.[21] HBA1c levels above 7% will be regarded as poor glycaemic control in the study.

Critically poor glycaemic control: Levels of glycosylated haemoglobin ≥ 9% is considered to be critically poor in this study.

Rural versus semi-urban community: there is no consistency in the definitions. However, South African government policies refer to rural areas as those that are non-metropolitan.[22] They are characterised by inferior infrastructure, low income, poor site conditions, unreliable water availability and poor access to health facilities.[23] Rural areas in South Africa have been defined in relation to poverty, underdevelopment and low habitation.[24] The place of residence of participants, other than Mthatha, is classified as rural in this study.

Semi-urban community: based on the pace of urban population growth of rural communities, semi-urban areas share the characteristics of rural-urban communities. Mthatha is considered to be semi-urban in this study.

Aim

The aim of this study was to explore the overall knowledge of diabetic patients about diabetes and glycaemic control. It was the second component of a bigger study on diabetes in rural South Africa.

Setting of the study

The study was conducted at Mthatha General Hospital, Mthatha, Eastern Cape Province, South Africa. This is a 258-bed district hospital serving a predominantly Xhosa-speaking population of about 1.5 million people.

Study design

In order to gain an in-depth understanding of the patients' perspectives of diabetes and glycaemic control; a qualitative study was conducted using semi-structured open-ended interviews with prompts.

Period of study

The study was conducted in October and November 2013.

Research methods and design
Sampling and procedure of the study

Seventeen purposively selected participants were drawn from the follow-up review of results of participants who took part in the first component, which was a quantitative study. Critical case sampling was employed to track down patients with the worst control of diabetes and high risks for diabetes complications. Participants were selected if their recent glycosylated haemoglobin was ≥ 9%, they were willing to participate in the interview, age ≥ 30 years at diagnosis of DM and had been on treatment for diabetes for a minimum period of at least one year. Participants were excluded from the interview if they were receiving treatment for less than one year or acutely ill at the time of the study.

The interview explored the following key areas of diabetes and glycaemic control: nature of diabetes, complications, treatment targets, medication and access, adherence to treatment and self-care efforts to achieving control.

A trained interviewer used open-ended techniques to elicit in-depth information from the participants. An interview guide was used to ensure that the key questions were asked if they did not arise spontaneously. The interviews were conducted in the local language of the participants (isiXhosa) to ensure that participants were free and confident in their responses. The interviews were audiotaped and the interviewer also kept notes of the process. Recruitment continued until no new information emerged during the interviews (data saturation).

Data analysis: Two experienced qualitative researchers transcribed the audiotaped interviews independently and translated them verbatim. Notes were then compared to ensure accuracy of transcription and translation. Field notes were reviewed for additional information. Thematic analysis technique was used for data analysis. Line numbers were used to identify questions asked by the interviewer and responses made by the participants. Themes were developed from the participants' responses on different questions and various issues. Participants' responses were categorised according to themes. Themes were colour-coded and those colours were used to shade any response relating to specific themes in the interviews. Content theme analysis was employed to maximise the chance that all relevant information was grouped and coded appropriately. The notes were cross-checked to ensure responses of participants were coded appropriately.

Ethical considerations

Institutional approval: the researchers obtained ethical approval from the Walter Sisulu Higher Degrees and Biosafety and Ethical Committee (Protocol number: 031/2013; Dated on 09/10/2013), Nelson Mandela Hospital Complex Ethics committee and the Eastern Cape Department of Health Epidemiological Research and Surveillance Management. Consent of the Chief Executive Officer of Mthatha General Hospital was sought and obtained. Each participant provided written informed consent after obtaining relevant information on the process of the research. They were each given a participant's information sheet detailing the purpose, process, who to contact and dissemination of research output.

Results

Characteristics of Participants (Table 1): according to the gender, age, residence, employment status, duration of diabetes and glycosylated haemoglobin. The majority of participants were women (11/17), unemployed (10/17) and lived in rural communities (14/17). Four participants were pensioners (4/17) and 3 participants were employed. The ages of the participants ranged from 45–72 years. The duration of type 2 diabetes mellitus amongst the participants were: 2–5

TABLE 1: Characteristics of participants.

Participants	Gender	Age (years)	Residence	Employment status	T2DM duration (years)	HbA1c (%)
P01	F	56	Rural	Unemployed	7	10.8
P02	F	65	Rural	Unemployed	15	9.4
P03	F	70	Rural	Pensioner	> 20	12.4
P04	M	53	Semi-urban	Employed	7	9.6
P05	F	48	Rural	Unemployed	3	12.8
P06	F	54	Rural	Unemployed	2	11.0
P07	M	66	Rural	Unemployed	> 10	13.6
P08	F	45	Rural	Employed	3	10.4
P09	M	51	Semi-urban	Unemployed	5	10.8
P10	F	68	Rural	Pensioner	> 15	9.4
P11	F	63	Rural	Unemployed	8	12.6
P12	M	50	Rural	Unemployed	5	13.2
P13	F	42	Rural	Unemployed	2	11.2
P14	M	55	Rural	Employed	4	9.8
P15	M	62	Rural	Pensioner	> 10	10.5
P16	F	72	Semi-urban	Pensioner	> 20	13.6
P17	F	54	Rural	Unemployed	3	12.4

P, participants; M, males; F, females; T2DM, Type 2 Diabetes Mellitus; HbA1c, Glycosylated haemoglobin.

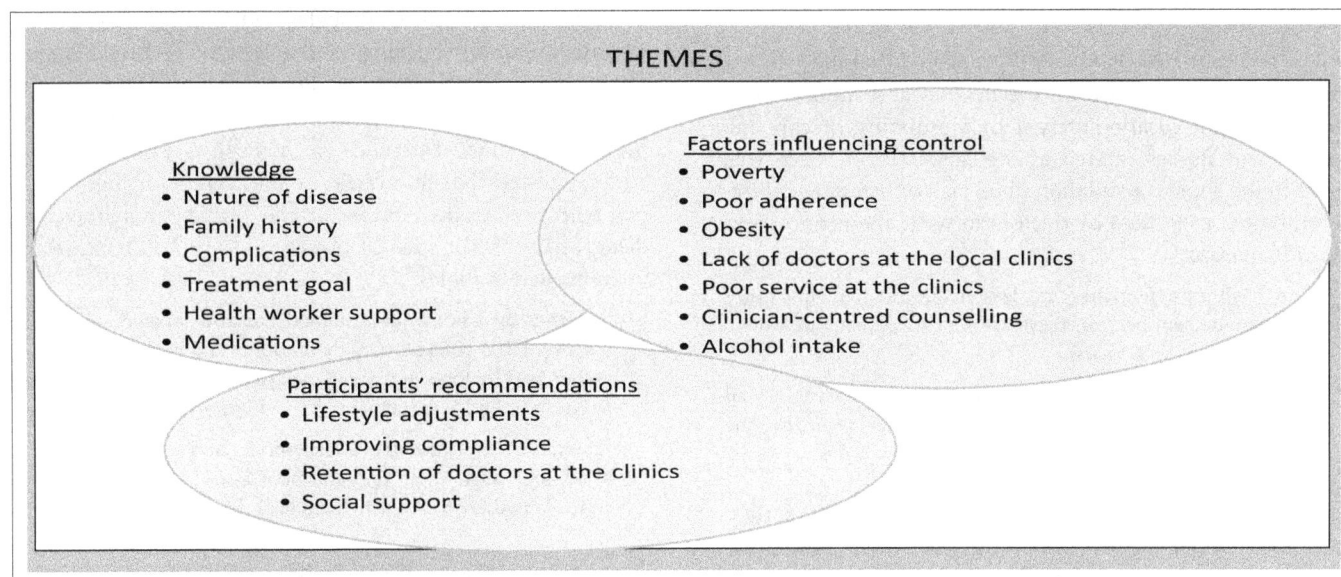

FIGURE 1: Pictorial analysis of the themes and sub-themes.

years (8/17), 6–10 years (3/17) and > 10 years (6/17). The levels of control of diabetes amongst the participants were critically poor (HBA1c ≥ 9%) with a range of 9.4%–13.6% and mean HBA1c of 11.4%.

Themes

Three main themes emerged from the interviews: knowledge of diabetes and glycaemic control amongst participants, factors influencing the control of diabetes and perspective of participants on how to improve glycaemic control. The themes and sub-themes are presented in Figure 1.

Theme 1: Knowledge of diabetes and glycaemic control amongst participants

All the participants understood the nature of the disease: incurable but manageable. The majority of the participants ($n = 15/17$) had at least one family member already diagnosed

with diabetes. They confirmed that diabetes could affect family members:

'My mother was living with diabetes and it affected her eyes. I was diagnosed of diabetes about three years ago.' (Participant 05; F, 48 years)

There was a good level of awareness of diabetes complications amongst the participants:

'I developed stinking wounds, filthy lump under my foot and spread to the leg, the doctor told me that I have few days to live before I die, if the leg is not amputated.' (Participant 07; M, 66 years)

'Not dating any woman because of this diabetes, my body is not responding anymore, I used to be strong but has lost my spark, I went to the pharmacy to buy boosters but they are not helping.' (Participant 12; M, 50 years)

'I have something that developed few weeks ago, my feet are feeling hot and painful, and when asleep I take them out of the blankets.' (Participant 16; F, 72 years)

The majority of the participants ($n = 13/17$) had no knowledge of what is considered to be good glycaemic control or the desired treatment target for using diabetic medication. The minority ($n = 4/17$) who had some idea about the control of blood sugar reported that they were not sure if blood sugar levels should be less than 8 or 10:

> 'My blood sugar fluctuates between 20, 17 and 18, only last month; I saw a change when it was 6.8. I am not sure what the level is supposed to be.' (Participant 08; F, 45 years)

> 'My sugar is not controlled because I faint regularly and wake up in the hospital then feel better. The doctor placed me on insulin injection. I think the sugar should be less than 10 if it is normal.' (Participant 17; F, 54 years)

The majority of the participants ($n = 14/17$) get help and support from family members. The doctors and nurses also provide assistance to the diabetic patients:

> 'I always get a good service at the hospital because I make sure that I get to the clinic first and I always meet the health care workers in good mood.' (Participant 10; F, 68 years)

Only a few participants ($n = 7/17$) reported that they do not get the help they need from the doctors and nurses. They expressed their disappointment in the quality of care the doctors and nurses offered at the hospital; reference was made to the short consultation time, lack of listening during consultation, eagerness by doctors to write medication and the long queues:

> 'The healthcare workers care less about the patients but I understand them because they care for 200 patients in a day.' (Participant 11; F, 63 years)

> 'People are not the same, other health care workers treat us well and others don't. I never received any advice regarding the control of my diabetes.' (Participant 02; F, 65 years)

All the participants remembered the type of medication they were using and some of them brought out their clinic cards for the interviewer to check the name of the medication. All of them were either on oral medication (metformin, glibenclamide or gliclazide) alone or a combination of oral medication and injections (insulin).

Theme 2: Factors influencing the control of diabetes

All the participants considered poverty as an important reason why blood sugar is not controlled. Some of the participants explained how lack of money was contributing to poor control of their blood sugar:

> 'No money for taxi, hence, cannot keep clinic appointments and cannot go to clinic to fetch my pills.' (Participants 06; F, 54 years and 08; F, 45 years)

> 'I don't eat breakfast and I cannot drink pills on an empty stomach, sometimes, no money to buy food at home.' (Participant 02; F, 65 years)

Lack of money is linked to the dietary adjustment required for the control of their blood sugar, which seemed impossible because the majority of the diabetic patients were very poor.

They had no money to buy a glucometer to monitor blood sugar at home.

Adherence to medication was explored: thirteen participants ($n = 13/17$) acknowledged that they miss some doses of their medication when they travel away from their home. Six participants reported poor adherence to treatment. Some of the reasons for non-adherence included: forgetfulness in taking medication, not collecting medication from the clinics, fear of taking medication on an empty stomach, being tired of using drugs every day, too many pills to take every day, side-effects of the medication and lack of information:

> 'I do not take my medications when going away from home.' (Participant 16; F, 72 years)

> 'I do not think I should used the medication every single day though I sometimes feel weak when not taking them.' (Participant 07; M, 66 years)

The relationship between diabetes and obesity was explored to gain an understanding of the control of blood sugar. Fifteen participants acknowledged that there is a definite relationship between diabetes and obesity. Some of the participants made reference to themselves as being obese and suggested that that could be the reason for their sugar not being controlled. Some of the participants however, disagreed with the idea of obesity as a probable cause for uncontrolled diabetes.

> 'Diabetes does not want fatty food and now when one is obese, it's a sign that you eat more than normal and you also take fatty and unhealthy food so that can make it difficult for your diabetes to be controlled.' (Participant 10; F, 68 years)

> 'There is no relationship between obesity and control of diabetes at all, look at me how tiny and poor I am and it is difficult to control my diabetes.' (Participant 02; F, 65 years)

Assessment of the quality of diabetes education at the clinics was explored; this generated mixed results. Eight participants were appreciative of the diabetic education provided by the doctors and nurses whilst some were disappointed that doctors were always in a hurry to prescribe medication for the patients. Some of the participants, who reported that health care workers do counsel them about control of their diabetes, felt that the advice was not practical. They were often told to eat healthy, avoid fatty meals, and eat fruit and vegetables, all of which require money to buy, and they are poor. But all of the participants were in agreement that alcohol and cigarette smoking were not good for diabetic patients:

> 'No advice from the health care workers, sometimes, they are too much hurrying.' (Participant 06; F, 54 years)

> 'No advice from the health care workers regarding the control of my sugar, I only hear from other people outside who have experience in living with diabetes.' (Participant 11; F, 63 years)

> 'I once visited a private doctor who told me that the combination of the pills is not correct for me but the nurses at the clinic kept on giving the wrong pills.' (participant 16; F, 72 years)

Fifteen of the participants (*n* = 15/17) reported that their nearest clinics usually do not have doctors; they are compelled to travel to Mthatha to see doctors, which requires money for transport fares. They usually get to the hospital by 06:00 to join the queue for doctors, who would arrive at the consulting rooms at 09:00. Four participants reported that they sometimes see doctors who do outreach programmes at their local clinics:

> 'I am dependent on the doctor who visits from the hospital. Absence of doctors at the local clinics creates complications for me, I feel weak when I am exposed to the sun.' (Participant 07; M, 66 years)

Theme 3: Perspective of participants on how to improve glycaemic control

All the participants were certain about healthy eating: avoidance of fatty meals, eating small amounts of food at a time and eating fruit and vegetables. Ten participants understood that exercise is beneficial. Six of them would recommend exercise to other diabetic patients. Fourteen participants suggested that diabetic patients must keep their clinic appointments for check-ups. Thirteen participants emphasised that taking medication as directed by the health care workers is crucial for control of blood sugar.

Twelve participants were certain that if people could take their treatment and avoid starvation, their blood sugar would be controlled. Ten of the respondents recognised that diabetic patients need to heed the advice of the health care workers and other people who are living with diabetes. Nearly all the participants (*n* = 16/17) recommended that health centres need to be upgraded to provide quality diabetes care services.

Doctors were needed at each of the local clinics close to their communities; this would relieve the burden of traveling to town to attend hospitals. Dedicated nurses at the clinics should provide diabetes education:

> 'No seminars or health educational classes are taking place at the clinics. Government only focuses on HIV/AIDS and other conditions like diabetes are ignored.' (Participant 01, F, 56 years)

Eleven respondents were convinced that if more attention was diverted towards diabetes care at the various health facilities, patients would achieve better control. The participants reiterated that increased awareness and communication are crucial for improvement in the control of diabetes:

> 'Government should try means exactly the way they do with HIV/AIDS. People with HIV/AIDS used to take many pills and now they are only taking one pill.' (Participant 09; M, 51 years)

Ten participants were of the opinion that government needs to provide money and food supplements to diabetic patients:

> 'The government can also try and have a way of identifying those people who are struggling financially and support them with food parcels because sometimes they default as a result of not having food in time so that they can take their medications.' (Participant 04; M, 53 years)

Fifteen participants thought that by monitoring the blood sugar at home, they would achieve better control, hence suggesting that government should provide glucometers. Some participants also suggested that health facilities must keep a stock of medication for diabetes to prevent running out.

Discussion

There have been mixed reports[8,14,15,16,17,18,20] from previous research studies: whilst some reports showed that improvement of knowledge of diabetes care might predict good glycaemic control,[8,14,15] others did not link with improvements.[11,16,20] Our study reported that the majority of the respondents (*n* = 15/17) had some knowledge of diabetes and its complications despite their critically poor glycaemic control. Most of the participants (*n* = 14/17) understood what is necessary for good glycaemic control but had little idea about the treatment target for such control. This is an aspect of the diabetes care that clinicians could improve during consultations.

Diabetic patients should have basic knowledge of the treatment goal and what is necessary to achieve this. Basic knowledge of diabetes is considered a prerequisite for self-care management.[11] Every diabetic patient should, at a minimum, know about the disease condition, complications, treatment options and dietary adjustment. This concept is supported by earlier studies, which suggested that patients with chronic diseases who are engaged and are active participants in their health care have better health outcomes.[14,15]

The finding of poor glycaemic control amongst the participants, despite their good awareness of diabetes and its complications, suggests gaps in translating knowledge to actions. Santos et al.[11] reported that glycaemic control does not correlate with knowledge of diabetes. They suggested that theoretical understanding of diabetes is not by itself significantly associated with appropriate glycaemic control. Also, Heisler et al.[16] concluded that the knowledge of HBA1c alone was not sufficient to translate increased understanding of diabetes care into improvement in self-management of diabetes.

Thirteen participants in the study demonstrated poor knowledge of the treatment target for their diabetes. The study by Iqbal et al.[19] found that the majority (59.5%) were unfamiliar with HBA1c. Knowledge of glycaemic control was generally poor amongst the participants, especially T2DM patients. Intervention with diabetic education, however, yielded improvement in glycaemic control amongst the poorly controlled T2DM, who were in the unfamiliar group. Whether diabetes education would lead to improvement in glycaemic control in this study population requires another research study.

The glycosylated haemoglobin of 9.4% – 13.6% in this study may suggest a poor relationship between diabetes knowledge and glycaemic control. A number of studies have found no significant association between the level of knowledge of diabetes and glycaemic control.[11,20] However, the evidence for the benefits of patient education on diabetes is overwhelming.[8,10,12,14,15,21] Hence, national and international bodies continue to emphasise in their recommendations that diabetic education should be provided at all levels of care.[10,21]

Diabetes education of patients should address adherence issues and the other factors of glycaemic control in each patient. Successes from adherence counselling provided to HIV positive individuals[25,26] might lead to improvement in the key performance indicators of diabetes care. As reported by some of the participants, reasons for poor adherence are many and varied; therefore, adherence counselling of diabetic patients may produce similar results as seen in HIV care. The participants highlighted a number of barriers to achieving good glycaemic control: poverty and its impact on the dietary requirements of diabetes, poor treatment adherence, lack of knowledge of treatment targets and lack of doctors at the primary health care centres in the rural areas. These are in keeping with the determinants of glycaemic control documented in the literature.[27,28,29,30,31,32]

The challenges faced by the study population reflect the level of unemployment, rural dwelling and lack of knowledge of glycaemic control in South Africa. The demand for food parcels and financial support by participants in the study reflects the current economic situation in most rural communities. Patients need money to take taxis, buy food and provide the basic needs of life.

Limitations

This study is limited by the fact that qualitative study findings cannot be generalised. The selection of more than one health facility for the study might shed more light on the issues of poor glycaemic control in different areas in the country. Future studies should explore the perspectives of health care workers and health managers on glycaemic control.

Conclusion

The understanding of the patients' perspectives on the challenges of poor glycaemic control is relevant. Useful data on the overall knowledge of diabetic patients were obtained, as well as the barriers to achieving good glycaemic control. Participants in the study highlighted some of the shortcomings of consultations with clinicians: not spending quality time with patients and not paying proper attention to the particularities of each patient. Availability of doctors in the rural health facilities remains a challenge to equitable health service delivery in South Africa. The re-engineering of primary health care in the country should prioritise health service delivery to the rural communities. The participants in the study provided insight into the probability of an association between poverty and poor glycaemic control.

However, the qualitative nature of the study does not allow for such a conclusion to be drawn, hence a prospective study is proposed to test this hypothesis.

Acknowledgements

The authors thank the staff of Mthatha General Hospital and the National Health Laboratory Services, Mthatha. They also thank Ms Phelo Sithole-Tetani for her assistance with data collection and Dr Helen Betts (Chirad-thesis.co.za) for proof reading the article.

We gave oral presentation of the result of this research at the 17th National Family Practitioners' Conference, Pretoria, South Africa on 21 June 2014.

Competing interests

The authors declare that they have no financial or personal relationship(s) that may have inappropriately influenced them in writing this article.

Authors' contributions

O.V.A. (Walter Sisulu University), P.Y. (Walter Sisulu University) and G.W. (University of Fort Hare) made significant contributions in the conceptualisation, protocol write-up, and interpretation of data and draft of the final manuscript. B.L. (Walter Sisulu University) analysed the data and helped in drafting the manuscript.

References

1. Guariguata L. By the numbers: New estimates from the IDF diabetes atlas update for 2012. Diabetes Res Clin Pract. 2012;98:524–525. http://dx.doi.org/10.1016/j.diabres.2012.11.006

2. Whiting D, Guariguata L, Weil C, Shaw J. IDF diabetes atlas: Global estimates of prevalence of diabetes for 2011 and 2030. Diabetes Res Clin Pract. 2011;94:311–321. http://dx.doi.org/10.1016/j.diabres.2011.10.029

3. Sanal T, Nair N, Adhikari P. Factors associated with poor control of type 2 diabetes mellitus: A systematic review and meta-analysis. J Diabetol 2011;3:1–10.

4. Molleuze W, Levitt N. Diabetes mellitus and impaired glucose tolerance in South Africa. Chronic Diseases of Lifestyle in South Africa. 2006:109–121.

5. Kumar P, Clark M. Kumar and Clark's clinical medicine. 7th ed. London, UK: Elsevier Health Sciences; 2009.

6. Herman W, Zimmet P. Type 2 diabetes: An epidemic requiring global attention and urgent action. Diabetes Care. 2012;35:943–944. http://dx.doi.org/10.2337/dc12-0298

7. Tesfaye S, Gill G. Chronic diabetic complications in Africa. Afr J Diabetes. Med. 2011;19(1):4-8.

8. Khattab M, Khader Y, Al-Khawaldeh A, Ajlouni K. Factors associated with poor glycemic control among patients with type 2 diabetes. J Diabetes Complications. 2010;24(2):84–89. http://dx.doi.org/10.1016/j.jdiacomp.2008.12.008

9. Mayosi B, Flisher A, Lalloo U, Sitas F, Tollman S, Bradshaw D. The burden of non-communicable diseases in South Africa. Lancet. 2009;374(9693):934–937. http://dx.doi.org/10.1016/S0140-6736(09)61087-4

10. Amod A, Motala A, Levitt N, et al. The 2012 SEMDSA guideline for the management of type 2 diabetes. JEMDSA. 2012;17(2Suppl 1):1–95. http://dx.doi.org/10.1080/22201009.2012.10872276

11. Santos F, Bernardo V, Gabbay M, Dib S, Sigulem D. The impact of knowledge about diabetes, resilience and depression on glycaemic control: A cross-sectional study among adolescents and young adults with type 1 diabetes. Diabetol Metab Syndr. 2013;5(1):55. http://dx.doi.org/10.1186/1758-5996-5-55

12. Suzuki-Saito T, Yokokawa H, Shimada K, Yasumura, S. Self-perception of glycaemic control among Japanese type 2 diabetic patients: Accuracy of patient perception and characteristics of patients with misperception. J Diabetes Investig 2013;4(2):206–13. http://dx.doi.org/10.1111/jdi.12002

13. Shrivastava S, Shrivastava P, Ramasamy J. Role of self-care in management of diabetes mellitus. J Diabetes Metabol Disord. 2013;12(1):14. http://dx.doi.org/10.1186/2251-6581-12-14

14. Von Korff M, Gruman J, Schaefer J, Curry S, Wagner E. Collaborative management of chronic illness. Ann Intern Med. 1997;127:1097–102. http://dx.doi.org/10.7326/0003-4819-127-12-199712150-00008

15. Anderson R, Funnel M, Butler P, Arnold M, Fitzgerald J, Feste C. Patient empowerment: Results of a randonmised controlled trial. Diabetes Care. 1995;18:943–949. http://dx.doi.org/10.2337/diacare.18.7.943

16. Heisler M, Piette J, Spencer M, Kieffer E, Vijan S. The relationship between knowledge of recent HBA1c values and diabetes care understanding and self-management. Diabetes Care. 2005;28(4):816–822. http://dx.doi.org/10.2337/diacare.28.4.816

17. Fisher L, Skaff M, Chelsea C, et al. Disease management advice provided to African-American and Chinese-American patients with type 2 diabetes. Diabetes Care. 2004;27:2249–2250. http://dx.doi.org/10.2337/diacare.27.9.2249

18. Harwell T, Dettori N, McDowall J, et al. Do persons with diabetes know their HBA1c number? Diabetes Educ. 2002;28:99–105. http://dx.doi.org/10.1177/014572170202800111

19. Iqbal N, Morgan C, Maksoud H, Idris I. Improving patient's knowledge on the relationship between HBA1c and mean plasma glucose improves glycaemic control among persons with poorly controlled diabetes mellitus. Ann Clin Biochem. 2008;45(5):504–507. http://dx.doi.org/10.1258/acb.2008.008034

20. Beebey L, Dunn S. Knowledge improvement and metabolic control in diabetes education: Approaching the limits? Patient Educ Couns. 1990;16(3):217–229. http://dx.doi.org/10.1016/0738-3991(90)90071-R

21. Inzucchi S, Bergenstal R, Buse J, et al. Management of hyperglycemia in type 2 diabetes: A patient-centered approach position statement of the American Diabetes Association (ADA) and the European Association for the Study of Diabetes (EASD). Diabetes Care. 2012;35:1364–1379. http://dx.doi.org/10.2337/dc12-0413

22. Diab P, Flack P, Mabuza L, Reid S. Qualitative exploration of the career aspirations of rural health science students in South Africa. Rural Remote Health [serial on the Internet]. 2012;12:2251. Available from: http://www.rrh.org.au

23. Consultancy Africa Intelligence. Rural areas in the Eastern Cape Province, South Africa: The right to access safe drinking water and sanitation denied? [homepage on the Intenet]. 2013 [cited 2014 Jul 21]. Available from: http://consultancyafrica.com

24. Gopaul M. The significance of rural areas in South Africa for tourism development through community participation with special reference to Umgababa, a rural area located in the province of Kwazulu-Natal. 2006 [unpublished dissertation; cited 2014 Jul 21]. Available from: http://umkn-dspol.unisa.ac.za

25. Paterson D, Swindells S, Mohr J, et al. Adherence to protease inhibitor therapy and outcomes in patients with HIV infection. Ann Intern Med. 2000;133(1):21-30. http://dx.doi.org/10.7326/0003-4819-133-1-200007040-00004

26. Bajunirwe F, Arts E, Tisch D, King C, Debanne S, Sethi A. Adherence and treatment response among HIV-1-infected adults receiving antiretroviral therapy in a rural government hospital in southwestern Uganda. J Int Assoc Physicians AIDS Care. 2009;8(2):139–147. http://dx.doi.org/10.1177/1545109709332470

27. Chan J, Gagliardino J, Baik S, et al. Multifaceted determinants for achieving glycemic control: the International Diabetes Management Practice Study (IDMPS). Diabetes Care. 2009;32:227–233. http://dx.doi.org/10.2337/dc08-0435

28. Khunti K. Use of multiple methods to determine factors affecting quality of care of patients with diabetes. Fam Pract. 1999;16:489–494. http://dx.doi.org/10.1093/fampra/16.5.489

29. Longo-Mbenza B, Muaka M, Mbenza G, et al. Risk factors of poor control of HBAlc and diabetic retinopathy: Paradox with insulin therapy and high values of HDL in African diabetic patients. Int J Diabetes Metab. 2008;6:69–78.

30. Nagrebetsky A, Griffin S, Kinmonth A, Sutton S, Craven A, Farmer A. Predictors of suboptimal glycaemic control in type 2 diabetes patients: The role of medication adherence and body mass index in the relationship between glycaemia and age. Diabetes Res Clin Pract. 2012;96:119–128. http://dx.doi.org/10.1016/j.diabres.2011.12.003

31. Spann S, Nutting P, Galliher J, et al. Management of type 2 diabetes in the primary care setting: A practice-based research network study. Ann Fam Med. 2006;4:23–31. http://dx.doi.org/10.1370/afm.420

32. Teoh H, Braga M, Casanova A, et al. Patient age, ethnicity, medical history, and risk factor profile, but not drug insurance coverage, predict successful attainment of glycemic targets: Time 2 do more quality enhancement research initiative (T2DM QUERI). Diabetes Care. 2010;33:2558–2560. http://dx.doi.org/10.2337/dc10-0440

32

School environment, socioeconomic status and weight of children in Bloemfontein, South Africa

Authors:
Lucia N.M. Meko[1]
Marthinette Slabber-Stretch[1]
Corinna M. Walsh[1]
Salome H. Kruger[2]
Mariette Nel[3]

Affiliations:
[1]Nutrition and Dietetics, University of the Free State, South Africa

[2]School of Physiology and Nutrition, North-West University, Potchefstroom Campus, South Africa

[3]Biostatistics, Faculty of Health Sciences, University of the Free State, South Africa

Correspondence to:
Lucia Meko

Email:
mekonml@ufs.ac.za

Postal address:
PO Box 339, Bloemfontein 9300, South Africa

Background: The continued existence of undernutrition, associated with a steady increase in the prevalence of overweight and obesity in children and adolescents, necessitates identification of factors contributing to this double burden of disease, in order for effective treatment and prevention programmes to be planned.

Aim: To determine the nutritional status of 13–15-year-old children in Bloemfontein and its association with socioeconomic factors.

Setting: Bloemfontein, Free State Province, South Africa (2006).

Methods: This was a cross-sectional analytical study. Randomly selected children (n = 415) completed structured questionnaires on socioeconomic status. The children's weight and height were measured and body mass index-for-age and height-for-age z-scores were computed according to World Health Organization growth standards in order to determine the prevalence of underweight, overweight, obesity and stunting. Waist circumference was measured to classify the children as having a high or very high risk for metabolic disease.

Results: Of the 415 children who consented to participate in the study, 14.9% were wasted and 3.4% were severely wasted. Only 6% of the children were overweight/obese. Significantly more boys (23.0%) were wasted than girls (10%) and severe stunting was also significantly higher in boys than in girls (10.3% and 4.2%, respectively). Children whose parents had graduate occupations were significantly more overweight/obese than those with parents working in skilled occupations. Stunting was significantly higher in low (31.4%) and medium (30.4%) socioeconomic groups compared to the high socioeconomic group (18.1%).

Conclusion: A coexistence of underweight and overweight was found and gender and parental occupation were identified as being predictors of nutritional status.

Environnement scolaire, Statut socioéconomique et poids des enfants à Bloemfontein, Afrique du Sud.

Contexte: La permanence de la sous-alimentation, associée à l'augmentation graduelle de l'obésité et du surpoids chez les enfants et les adolescents, nécessite d'identifier les facteurs qui contribuent à ce double fardeau de maladie, afin de mettre en place des programmes de prévention et de traitement.

Objectif: Déterminer l'état nutritionnel des enfants de 13 à 15 ans à Bloemfontein et son rapport avec des facteurs socioéconomiques.

Cadre: Bloemfontein, Province du Free State, Afrique du Sud (2006).

Méthodes: C'était une étude analytique transversale. Des enfants sélectionnés au hasard (n=415) ont rempli des questionnaires structurés sur leur état socioéconomique. On a mesuré le poids et la taille des enfants ainsi que l'indice de masse corporelle pour leur âge et le rapport taille-âge. Les résultats-z ont été saisis selon les normes de croissance de l'Organisation mondiale de la Santé afin de déterminer la fréquence de sous-poids, surpoids, obésité et retard de croissance. Le tour de taille des enfants a été mesuré pour les classer selon leurs risques élevés ou très élevés de maladies métaboliques, respectivement.

Résultats: Parmi les 415 enfants qui ont accepté de participer à l'étude, 14.9% étaient malingres et 3.4% étaient décharnés. Seuls 6% des enfants étaient en surpoids/obèses. Il est significatif que plus de garçons (23.0%) étaient malingres que de filles (10%) et le retard de croissance étaient beaucoup plus élevé chez les garçons que chez les filles (10.3% et 4.2%, respectivement). Les enfants dont les parents étaient diplômés étaient beaucoup plus en surpoids/obèses que ceux des parents peu qualifiés. Le retard de croissance était plus élevé chez les groupes socio-économiquement faibles (31.4%) et moyens (30.4%) que dans le groupe socio-économiquement élevé (18.1%).

Conclusion: On a remarqué la coexistence des enfants en sous-poids et en surpoids et le sexe et la profession des parents étaient des indicateurs de leur état nutritionnel.

Introduction

The prevalence of obesity amongst children in developing countries is increasing and childhood obesity has become a serious public health challenge of the 21st century. Countries undergoing rapid economic development, such as Brazil, China and South Africa, are experiencing a double burden of both under- and overnutrition.[1,2,3] Although undernutrition, which is caused by energy and micronutrient deficiencies, shows a decline in many parts of the world, it is still increasing in most parts of Africa.[4] The prevalence rates of overweight and obesity in African countries, on the other hand, are showing a pattern similar to that of developed countries.[4] It is estimated that by the year 2015, non-communicable diseases resulting from overnutrition will overtake undernutrition as a leading cause of death in developing countries.[5,6]

Both undernutrition and overnutrition are known to have undesirable health effects. Malnutrition in childhood and adolescence can lead to growth retardation and delays in sexual maturation, amongst others,[7] whilst overweight and obesity may lead to a number of chronic illnesses such as hyperlipidaemia, hyperinsulinaemia, hypertension and early atherosclerosis emerging in childhood rather than in adulthood.[8,9]

'South Africa has a complex mix of developed areas in terms of its population and economy. The gap in income distribution between the poor majority and wealthy minority is huge'.[10] This unequal distribution is reflected by the high prevalence of stunting in black children, especially in rural areas, accompanied by a high prevalence of overweight and obesity in all ethnic groups residing in urban areas.[10]

In developed countries, the prevalence of childhood obesity is associated inversely with socioeconomic status (SES).[11,12] In contrast, wealthier children in most developing countries are at a greater risk of obesity.[13] This trend is referred to as the 'social drift' phenomenon.[10] The main sociodemographic factors known to be associated with body weight regulation (including malnutrition as well as overweight and obesity) in children include gender, age, race, parents' education levels and occupation, household size, residential density and geographical region.[14] The need to assess factors that impact on the nutritional status of South African adolescents of all ethnicities and social backgrounds is necessary so that effective intervention programmes can be implemented at an early stage.[15]

Few studies in South Africa have investigated the impact of sociodemographic factors on the nutritional status of adolescents.[3,16] The aim of this article is to report on the nutritional status of children aged 13–15 years and to indicate the association between the children's nutritional status and their sociodemographic characteristics.

Significance of the study

Studies on the prevalence of malnutrition and overweight and obesity have always focused on children, particularly under the age of five years. There is, however, a steady increase in the investigation of the nutritional status of adolescents and factors contributing to their being either malnourished or overweight. The current study aims to make a contribution to this body of evidence in a South African setting.

Research methods and design
Population and setting

The study population comprised learners aged 13–15 years old ($N = 640$) who attended public comprehensive secondary schools in Bloemfontein and represented all the socioeconomic groups. A cross-sectional study of learners from 26 public secondary schools in Bloemfontein was performed.

Data collection methods

Approval to conduct the study was obtained from the Free State Department of Health. Thereafter, the school principals were contacted and the aim of the study was explained to them. The sample size of 640 children was determined based on relevant literature as well as the amount of time allocated by the school principals compared to the number of interviewers (five, including the principal researcher) available to conduct the research. A proportionally representative number of children to participate in the study was determined using quota sampling for each school. Alphabetical lists of all learners aged 13–15 years were then obtained from the schools' principals and a random sample of children was selected from these lists.

Before the study commenced, four fieldworkers were trained on standardised anthropometric methods, interviewing of children and completion of the questionnaire. A pilot study was carried out before commencement of the main study in order to test the questionnaire. Ten children from one of the schools were interviewed and measured and, where necessary, adaptations and changes were made to the questionnaire. These children were not included in the final sample.

A research room was identified at each school and the researcher and field workers used structured interviews to obtain sociodemographic data from the learners. The interviews were conducted in the children's language of choice – English, Afrikaans, Sesotho or Setswana. The structured sociodemographic questionnaire included information on gender, language, household composition, type and size of dwelling, available cooking and storage facilities, as well as information on the main economic contributor of the household with regard to level of education and occupation. The main contributors were defined as individuals in the household who contributed the most income and were classified as specialist professionals (e.g. doctors, professors, company directors), graduate professionals (e.g. teachers, nurses, managers), skilled individuals (clerks, secretaries, retail workers) or unskilled individuals (cleaners, domestic workers, gardeners). Based on the occupation and highest education level of the main contributor to the household, the children were classified as having a high, middle or low SES.

Standardised methods and techniques[17] were used by the researcher and field workers for anthropometric measurements. Weight was measured on a Seca beam balance to the nearest 0.1 kg with the children wearing minimal clothing and no shoes. Height was measured using a stadiometer (Seca 214) to the nearest 0.5 cm.[17]

The children's body mass index (BMI)-for-age z-scores (BAZ) and height-for-age z-scores (HAZ) were generated using the World Health Organization's (WHO) Anthro 2005 program, Beta version.[18] Nutritional status was classified as follows:[18]

- underweight/stunted if BAZ and HAZ, respectively, were less than two standard deviations below the median reference.
- at risk of underweight/stunting if BAZ and HAZ, respectively, were less than one but more than two standard deviations below the median reference.
- at risk of overweight if BAZ was more than one but less than two standard deviations above the median reference.
- overweight if BAZ was more than two but less than three standard deviations above the median.
- obese if BAZ was more than three standard deviations above the median.

Waist circumference tends to be a better predictor of risk for metabolic disease than BMI.[19] Ethnic-specific percentiles of waist circumference-for-age and gender were used to classify children according to waist circumference-associated risk. Waist circumferences ≥ 75th and ≥ 90th percentiles indicated a high and a very high risk for comorbidities, respectively.[20]

To ensure reliability, 10% of the sampled children were re-interviewed by the researcher two weeks after the initial interview. Anthropometric measurements were obtained in triplicate on the same day in order to ensure reliability and accuracy. Where it was found that an answer to a question differed by more than 10% between the first and second interview, the question was considered unreliable.

Statistical analysis

Descriptive statistics, namely medians and percentiles for continuous data and frequencies and percentages for categorical data, were calculated per group. Differences between groups were compared by means of p-values using the chi-square test. Stepwise logistic regression analysis was performed and the odds ratios, 95% CI and p-values were calculated for each risk factor in the final model. A p-value of < 0.05 was considered to be of statistical significance.

Ethical considerations

The study was approved by the Ethics Committee of the Faculty of Health Sciences, University of the Free State (ETOVS NR. 245/05). The Free State Department of Education and the schools' principals gave permission for the study to be conducted in schools. The learners' parents/guardians had to give written consent for the learners to participate in the study and the learners themselves had to give written assent to indicate their willingness to participate. Confidentiality and anonymity were ensured throughout the duration of the study.

Results

A response rate of 67% was achieved, with 415 children (175 boys and 240 girls) giving consent to participate in the study.

Sociodemographic data

Results of the participants' sociodemographic data are presented in Table 1. Most of the children were black (n = 339; 81.7%), followed by white children (n = 52; 12.5%). The children's median age was 14.3 years and most were in grade 8 (n = 363; 87.5%).

Most children stayed in brick houses (n = 372; 89.7%) and electricity (n = 374; 90.4%) was used as the main type of fuel for cooking in most households. Household appliances, including a working stove (gas, coal or electricity: n = 386; 93.0%) and a working refrigerator (n = 367; 88.7%), were available in most of the households.

For approximately half of the children (n = 192; 46.3%), the father was indicated as the one contributing most income to the household, followed by the mother (n = 152; 36.3%). Most of the main contributors to the household were skilled workers (n = 151; 36.4%) (clerks, office assistants, sales persons), followed by unskilled workers (n = 135; 32.5%) (domestic workers, cleaners, gardeners and contract workers). Only 47 (11.3%) of the children's parents who were contributors had post-matric education. Based on the parent's highest level of education and occupation, 204 (49.2%) of the children were categorised to be of medium socioeconomic status.

Table 2 shows the results of the children's anthropometric measurements. Based on BMI-for-age, 244 (56.7%) of the children could be categorised as having a normal weight. Significantly more girls (n = 18; 7.5%) were overweight and obese than boys (n = 7; 4.0%) (p = 0.0002), whilst on the other hand, significantly more boys (n = 40; 23.0%) were wasted than girls (n = 24; 10.0%) (p = 0.0003). Similar to BMI-for-age, most of the children had a normal height-for-age (n = 273; 65.7%). Another significant difference between genders was that 18 (10.3%) of the boys were more severely stunted, compared to 10 (4.2%) of the girls (p = 0.01).

TABLE 1: Sociodemographic variables of children 13–15 years of age.

Variable	Boys n (%)	Girls n (%)	Total n (%)
School grade			
Grade 8	160 (91.4)	203 (84.6)	363 (87.5)
Grade 9	15 (18.6)	37 (15.4)	52 (12.5)
Race			
Black	140 (80)	199 (82.9)	339 (81.7)
Coloured	8 (4.6)	13 (5.4)	21 (5.1)
Indian	0 (0)	1 (0.4)	1 (0.24)
White	26 (14.9)	26 (10.8)	52 (12.5)
Other (Chinese)	1 (0.6)	1 (0.4)	2 (0.48)
Home language			
Afrikaans	33 (18.9)	31 (12.9)	64 (15.4)
English	5 (2.9)	10 (4.2)	15 (3.6)
Sesotho	72 (41.1)	99 (41.3)	171 (41.2)
Setswana	38 (21.7)	63 (26.3)	101 (24.3)
isiXhosa	26 (14.9)	35 (14.6)	61 (14.7)
Chinese	1 (0.6)	2 (0.8)	3 (0.72)
Type of dwelling			
Brick or concrete	158 (90.3)	214 (89.2)	372 (89.7)
Traditional mud	2 (1.1)	0 (0)	2 (0.48)
Corrugated iron	13 (7.4)	19 (7.9)	32 (7.7)
Apartment	2 (1.1)	6 (2.5)	8 (1.9)
Wood	0 (0)	1 (0.4)	1 (0.24)
Type of toilet			
Flush	154 (88)	209 (87.1)	363 (87.5)
Pit	4 (2.3)	8 (3.3)	12 (2.9)
Bucket	16 (9.1)	20 (8.3)	36 (8.7)
Mobile toilet	1 (0.6)	3 (1.3)	4 (0.96)
Fuel mostly used for cooking			
Electric	158 (90.3)	217 (90.4)	375 (90.4)
Gas	6 (3.4)	4 (1.7)	10 (2.4)
Paraffin	9 (5.1)	19 (7.9)	28 (6.8)
Wood, coal	2 (1.1)	-	2 (0.48)
Working refrigerator in household			
Yes	159 (90.9)	209 (87.1)	368 (88.7)
No	16 (9.1)	31 (12.9)	47 (11.3)
Working stove in household			
Yes	164 (93.7)	222 (92.5)	386 (93.0)
No	11 (6.3)	18 (7.5)	29 (6.99)
Working microwave oven in household			
Yes	118 (67.4)	143 (59.6)	261 (62.9)
No	57 (32.6)	97 (40.4)	154 (37.1)
Working radio and/or television in household			
Yes	173 (98.9)	236 (98.3)	409 (98.6)
No	2 (1.1)	4 (1.7)	6 (1.4)
Main contributor to the household			
Mother	66 (37.7)	86 (35.8)	152 (36.3)
Father	82 (46.9)	110 (45.8)	192 (46.3)
Sister/brother	9 (5.14)	12 (5.0)	21 (5.1)
Grandparent	9 (5.14)	20 (8.3)	29 (6.99)
Uncle/aunt	9 (5.14)	12 (5.0)	21 (5.1)
Occupation of main contributor of income in household			
Unskilled	48 (27.4)	87 (36.3)	135 (32.5)
Skilled	69 (39.4)	82 (34.2)	151 (36.4)
Graduate	48 (27.4)	63 (26.2)	111 (26.8)
Specialist	10 (5.8)	8 (3.3)	18 (4.3)
Main contributor's highest level of education			
Primary	12 (6.9)	35 (14.6)	129 (31.1)
High school	48 (27.4)	7 (30.0)	119 (28.7)
Matric	53 (30.3)	66 (27.5)	120 (28.9)
Post-matric	62 (35.4)	67 (27.9)	47 (11.3)
Socioeconomic status category			
Low	32 (18.3)	74 (30.8)	106 (25.5)
Medium	95 (54.3)	109 (45.4)	204 (49.2)
High	48 (27.4)	57 (23.8)	105 (25.3)

TABLE 2: Anthropometric data of children 13–15 years of age.

Variable	Boys n (%)	Girls n (%)	Total n (%)
Body mass index-for-age z score category (BAZ)	n = 174	n = 240	n = 414
Severely wasted	8 (4.6)	6 (2.5)	14 (3.4)
Wasted	40 (23.0)*	24 (10)	64 (14.9)
Normal weight	103 (59.2)	141 (58.8)	244 (56.7)
At risk of overweight	16 (9.2)	51 (21.3)	67 (15.6)
Obese	7 (4.0)	18 (7.5)	25 (6.0)
Overweight and obese	23 (13.2)	69 (28.8)*	92 (21.6)
Height-for-age z score category (HAZ)	n = 59	n = 83	n = 142
Severely stunted	18 (10.3)*	10 (4.2)	28 (6.8)
Stunted	41 (23.6)	73 (30.4)	114 (27.5)
Normal	115 (66.1)	157 (65.4)	273 (65.7)
Waist circumference (percentile)#	n = 175	n = 240	n = 415
< 10	32 (18.3)	29 (12.1)	61 (14.7)
10–24.9	43 (24.6)	35 (14.6)	78 (18.8)
25–49.9	43 (24.6)	81 (33.8)	124 (29.9)
50–74.9	35 (20.0)	51 (21.3)	86 (20.7)
75–89.9	18 (10.3)	35 (14.6)	53 (12.8)
≥ 90	4 (2.3)	9 (3.8)	13 (3.1)

*, Statistically significant difference;
#, Percentiles based on American cut-off points.[17]

Waist circumference was also normal in most of the children, with only 68 (15.9%) of the children being above the 75th percentile of the ethnic-specific cut-off points. Although not statistically significant, more girls (n = 44; 18.4%) than boys (n = 22; 12.6%) had a waist circumference above the 75th percentile.

Table 3 shows the association between BMI-for-age and height-for-age with regard to different sociodemographic and economic indices. Because of the under-representation of other racial groups, associations between BMI and height-for-age could not be established with regard to race and home language.

The prevalence of wasting was significantly higher in children of skilled parents than those of graduate parents (n = 31; 20.5% and n = 10; 9.0%, respectively) (p = 0.01). Significantly more children of graduate parents (n = 9; 8.1%) were overweight/obese than those of skilled parents (n = 6; 4.0%) (p = 0.004). Considering overall SES based on parents' level of education and parents' occupation, children classified as being of medium SES (n = 42; 20.6%) were significantly more wasted than those of low (n = 11; 10.5%) and high SES (n = 11; 10.5%) (p = 0.03). A significant association could not be made between overall SES and overweight/obesity in these children.

Only five children of parents with specialist occupations and three of those with parents with graduate occupations were either stunted or severely stunted. The difference in the prevalence of severe stunting was significant between unskilled (n = 12; 9.0%) and graduate (n = 3; 2.7%) parents' children (p = 0.03). Despite the fact that there was no significant association between weight and parental level of education, the children whose parents had matric as their highest level of education (n = 12; 10.1%) were significantly

TABLE 3: Body mass index-for-age and height-for-age comparisons according to socioeconomic indicators of children 13–15 years of age.

Demographics	Body mass index-for-age (BAZ)					Height-for-age (HAZ)	
	Underweight n (%)	At risk n (%)	Normal weight n (%)	At risk n (%)	Overweight/ obese n (%)	Stunted n (%)	At risk n (%)
Race							
Black	13 (3.9)	53 (15.7)	199 (58.9)	52 (15.4)	21 (6.2)	27 (8.0)	103 (30.5)
Coloured	1 (4.8)	1 (4.8)	16 (76.2)	3 (14.3)	0 (0)	1 (4.8)	6 (28.6)
Indian	0 (0)	0 (0)	1 (100)	0 (0)	0 (0)	0 (0)	0 (0)
White	0 (0)	10 (19.2)	26 (50.0)	12 (23.1)	4 (7.7)	0 (0)	5 (9.6)
Other (Chinese)	0 (0)	0 (0)	2 (100)	0 (0)	0 (0)	0 (0)	0 (0)
Home language							
Afrikaans	1 (1.6)	9 (14.1)	40 (62.5)	10 (15.6)	4 (6.3)	1 (1.6)	11 (17.2)
English	0 (0)	3 (20.0)	7 (46.7)	5 (33.3)	0 (0)	0 (0)	2 (13.3)
Sesotho	2 (1.2)	22 (12.9)	106 (62.0)	30 (17.5)	11 (6.4)	18 (10.5)	53 (31.0)
Setswana	8 (8.0)	24 (24.0)	45 (45.0)	18 (18.0)	5 (5.0)	8 (8.0)	34 (34.0)
isiXhosa	3 (4.9)	5 (8.2)	44 (72.1)	4 (6.6)	5 (8.2)	1 (1.6)	14 (23.0)
Chinese	0 (0)	1 (33.3)	2 (66.7)	0 (0)	0 (0)	0 (0)	0 (0)
Parents' occupation							
Unskilled	5 (3.7)	19 (14.2)	79 (58.9)	21 (15.7)	10 (7.5)	12 (9.0)*	41 (30.6)
Skilled	7 (4.6)	31 (20.5)*	89 (58.9)	18 (11.9)	6 (4.0)	13 (8.6)	45 (29.8)
Graduate	2 (1.8)	10 (9.0)	65 (58.6)	25 (22.5)	9 (8.1)*	3 (2.7)	23 (20.7)
Specialist	0 (0)	4 (22.2)	11 (61.1)	3 (16.7)	0 (0)	0 (0)	5 (27.8)
Parents' level of education							
Post-Matric	2 (4.3)	4 (8.5)	29 (61.7)	6 (12.8)	6 (12.8)	3 (6.4)	14 (29.8)
Matric	6 (5.0)	20 (16.8)*	71 (59.7)	16 (13.5)	6 (5.0)	12 (10.1)*	44 (36.9)
High school	5 (4.2)	24 (20.2)	65 (54.6)	20 (16.8)	5 (4.2)	8 (6.7)	30 (25.2)
Primary school	1 (0.8)	16 (12.4)	79 (61.2)	25 (19.4)	8 (6.2)	5 (3.9)	26 (20.2)
Socioeconomic status							
Low	5 (4.8)	11 (10.5)*	65 (61.9)	16 (15.2)	8 (7.6)	9 (8.6)	33 (31.4)*
Medium	8 (3.9)	42 (20.6)	113 (55.4)	32 (15.7)	9 (4.4)	16 (7.8)	62 (30.4)*
High	1 (0.9)	11 (10.5)*	66 (62.9)	19 (18.1)	8 (7.6)	3 (2.9)	19 (18.1)

*, Statistically significant difference

TABLE 4: Logistic regression predicting nutritional status in children 13–15 years of age.

Variable	Indicator	Odds ratio	95% CI	p-value
Parental education (high school and upwards)	Overweight	0.373	0.148–1.071	0.0397*
Male gender	Underweight	2.776	1.673–4.674	0.0001*
High socioeconomic status	Underweight	0.475	0.252–0.852	0.0145*
Graduate and specialist occupations	Stunting	0.496	0.307–0.786	0.0031*

*, Statistically significant

more severely stunted than those whose parents had primary school (n = 5; 3.9%) as their highest level of education (p = 0.003). Furthermore, children of low SES (n = 33; 31.4%) and medium SES (n = 62; 30.4%) were significantly more stunted than children of high SES (n = 19; 18.1%) (p = 0.03 and 0.02, respectively).

On logistic regression (Table 4), the odds of being underweight were higher in boys and less likely in children with a medium to high SES. Children whose parents had a level of education of high school, matric and post-matric were more likely to be overweight. Additionally, children whose parents had graduate or specialist occupations were less likely to be stunted.

Discussion

The current study was the first of its kind to be carried out in the Free State Province of South Africa to investigate factors associated with adolescents' nutritional status. The study was conducted in Bloemfontein, an urban area of the province consisting largely of built-up areas and informal settlements. Consequently, most of the children lived in brick houses (89.7%) and had access to water and sanitation facilities (87.5%). McVeigh, Norris and DeWet[21] obtained similar results with their sample of children living in Johannesburg, South Africa. In their study, 88% of the children lived in brick houses, 95% and 94% of these households had a television set and refrigerator, respectively, whilst only 39% owned a microwave.[21] The fact that our study was based in an urban area also meant that a high percentage of the children had storage and cooking facilities, such as fridges, stoves and microwave ovens, available in their homes.

Using the WHO classification for BMI-for-age, the prevalence of overweight and obesity (> + 2 SD) was relatively low (6%). However, the number of children classified as being at risk for overweight was higher (15.6%). The coexistence of undernutrition in these children, as indicated by the high number of wasted (< -2 SD) and severely wasted children (< -3 SD) (18.3% combined), confirms the double burden of over- and undernutrition common in developing countries.[13,22] Almost a third (27.5%) of the children in this study were stunted, whilst 6% were severely stunted. These figures emphasise the fact that even though there is an observed increase in the prevalence of overweight and obesity, the problem of undernutrition continues to affect South African children.[23] The high prevalence of wasting and stunting can also be seen as a reflection of the high levels of underdevelopment typical of the Free State Province[16,24] and food poverty experienced by most South African families.[25]

Similar to other South African studies,[16,24,26] the prevalence of overweight and obesity in our study was higher amongst girls than boys, even though these studies used different methods of interpreting nutrition status. Furthermore, as confirmed by logistic regression, wasting and stunting occurred more amongst boys than girls. These differences in nutritional status as a result of gender can possibly be ascribed to earlier sexual maturation in girls, which influences body fat[26,27] or possibly to the fact that the boys in this study might have been physically more active than the girls, as reported elsewhere.[28]

The association between waist circumference and BMI in our study was statistically significant. Only a small percentage of the children (15.9%) had a waist circumference above the 75th percentile, compared with 27.9% of the children in a Mexican study.[29] In children where waist circumference was above the suggested cut-off point, the risk of metabolic complications is increased. Adolescents with a waist circumference above the 90th percentile have been shown to have higher concentrations of low density lipoprotein (LDL) cholesterol, triglycerides and insulin, as well as lower concentrations of high density lipoprotein (HDL),[20,30] increasing their risk of developing chronic diseases of lifestyle in later years.

SES has been established as a predictor of nutritional status in several studies.[13,26,31] Pathways through which SES may be associated with nutritional status include income, education and occupation.[3] In developed countries, lower SES has been found to be a strong predictor of obesity,[13,32] whilst a high SES status in developing countries is associated with an increased risk for obesity.[31,33] The current study failed to find any significant linear association between the prevalence of obesity and overall SES.

Significantly more children whose parents had graduate occupations were overweight/obese and tended to be less wasted than children whose parents were skilled labourers. The THUSA BANA study,[16] conducted in the North-West Province of South Africa, also compared children's weight status with their parents' occupation. They found that children whose parents were employed as domestic or contract workers (unskilled) were less inclined to be overweight/ obese than children whose parents had professional or business occupations (graduate and specialists).[16] This could possibly be attributed to more money being available to spend on food in these households than in the domestic or contract workers' households. In contrast to this current study, Ekelund et al.[34] established an inverse association between the parents' education level and BMI in the girls in their study in Stockholm.

Whilst no associations could be established with overweight and obesity and SES, stunting and underweight presented a different picture. The odds of being underweight were

low in children with a medium to high SES and the odds of being stunted were low in children whose parents had graduate or specialist occupations. Stunting in the children was associated with being from a low SES group, having a parent who had completed secondary education and having a parent who had an occupation categorised as unskilled. These results confirm the fact that household food insecurity, low parental education and low levels of employment are amongst the main determinants of stunted growth.[35] Education and employment typically translate into opportunities to earn money and therefore secure adequate food for the family. Furthermore, a low level of education may predict a deficiency in nutritional knowledge and thereby affect children's nutritional status.[3]

Although race has been noted as a predictor of nutritional status in some studies, no such association could be made in our study, mainly because of the under-representation of race groups other than black people (81.7%) and white people (12.5%). The THUSA BANA study found that the prevalence of obesity was twice as high in white children compared with the other racial groups.[16] Mamabolo et al.[36] also reported that white primary school children had a higher body weight than their black counterparts. Nationally, Indian children (25.3%) were more overweight than the white (23.4%) and black (16.6%) children.[24] It is important to note, however, that in all these studies, a limited number of white children were included and the data may not be representative of the total population.

Recommendations

Policies on the prevention of under- and overnutrition in children and adolescents need to be planned and supported in order to address the double burden of malnutrition in South Africa.

Because of the ambiguity relating to sociodemographic factors and their effect on nutritional status, researchers and/or programme planners need to conduct in-depth assessments of possible factors leading to under- or overnutrition in their targeted intervention communities prior to commencement of the programme.

Conclusion

The effect of sociodemographic factors on the prevalence of under- and overnutrition remains important when effective intervention programmes have to be planned. However, limited literature is available on sociodemographic factors in South Africa and its influence on adolescent nutritional status. This study aimed to contribute to the literature by focusing on the Free State Province in South Africa, which is somewhat neglected with regard to research in this specific area. A coexistence of under- and overnutrition was found in this study population, which is typical of developing countries. Male gender and the parents' occupation and level of education were indicated as determinants of nutritional status.

Acknowledgements

The authors would like to thank Dr Daleen Struwig, medical writer, Faculty of Health Sciences, University of the Free State, for technical and editorial preparation of the manuscript.

Competing interests

The authors declare that they have no financial or personal relationship(s) that may have inappropriately influenced them in writing this article.

Authors' contributions

L.N.M.M. (University of the Free State) designed and conducted the research, analysed the data, wrote and approved the manuscript and takes primary responsibility for the final content. M.S-S. (University of the Free State) designed and conducted the research and approved the manuscript. C.M.W. (University of the Free State) designed the research, wrote and approved the manuscript. S.H.K. (North-West University) designed the research and approved the manuscript. M.N. (University of the Free State) analysed the data and approved the manuscript.

References

1. Rennie KL, Johnson L, Jebb SA. Behavioural determinants of obesity. Best Pract Res Clin Endocrinol Metab. 2005;19(3):343–358. http://dx.doi.org/10.1016/j.beem.2005.04.003. PMID 16150379.

2. Subramanian SV, Perkins JM, Khan KT. Do burdens of underweight and overweight coexist among lower socioeconomic groups in India? Am J Clin Nutr. 2009;90(2):369–376. http://dx.doi.org/10.3945/ajcn.2009.27487. PMID 19515733.

3. Kimani-Murage EW, Kahn K, Pettifor JM, et al. The prevalence of stunting, overweight and obesity, and metabolic risk in rural South African children. BMC Public Health. 2010;10:158. http://dx.doi.org/10.1186/1471-2458-10-158. PMID 20338024.

4. Black RE, Allen LH, Bhutta ZA, et al. Maternal and child undernutrition: Global and regional exposures and health consequences. Lancet. 2008;371(9608):243–260. http://dx.doi.org/10.1016/S0140-6736(07)61690-0. PMID 18207566.

5. Abegunde DO, Mathers CD, Adam T, et al. The burden and costs of chronic diseases in low-income and middle-income countries. Lancet. 2007;370(9603):1929–1938. http://dx.doi.org/10.1016/S0140-6736(07)61696-1. PMID 18063029.

6. Lopez AD, Mathers CD, Ezzati M, et al. Global burden of disease and risk factors. New York: Oxford University Press; 2006.

7. Victora CG, Adair L, Fall C, et al. Maternal and child malnutrition: Consequences for adult health and human capital. Lancet. 2008;371(9609):340–357. http://dx.doi.org/10.1016/S0140-6736(07)61692-4. PMID 18206323.

8. Reilly JJ. Descriptive epidemiology and health consequences of childhood obesity. Best Pract Res Clin Endocrinol Metab. 2005;19(3):327–341. http://dx.doi.org/10.1016/j.beem.2005.04.002. PMID 16150378.

9. Li Y, Yang X, Zhai F, et al. Childhood obesity and its health consequence in China. Obes Rev. 2008;9(Suppl 1):82–86. http://dx.doi.org/10.1111/j.1467-789X.2007.00444.x. PMID 18307705.

10. Steyn NP. Nutrition and chronic diseases of lifestyle in South Africa. In: Steyn K, Fourie J, Temple N, editors. Chronic Diseases of Lifestyle in South Africa since 1995–2005. Tygerberg, South Africa: Medical Research Council Chronic Diseases of Lifestyle Unit; p. 33–47 [document on the Internet]. c2006 [cited 2014 Jul 24]. Available from: http://www.mrc.ac.za/chronic/cdlchapter4.pdf

11. Janssen I, Boyce WF, Simpson K, et al. Influence of individual- and area-level measures of socioeconomic status on obesity, unhealthy eating, and physical inactivity in Canadian adolescents. Am J Clin Nutr. 2006;83(1):139–145. PMID 16400062.

12. Phipps SA, Burton PS, Osberg LS, et al. Poverty and the extent of child obesity in Canada, Norway and the United States. Obes Rev. 2006;7(1):5–12. http://dx.doi.org/10.1111/j.1467-789X.2006.00217.x. PMID 16436098.

13. Deckelbaum RJ, Williams CL. Childhood obesity: The health issue. Obes Res. 2001;9(S11):239S–243S. http://dx.doi.org/10.1038/oby.2001.125. PMID 11707548.

14. Frühbeck G. Overnutrition. In: Gibney MJ, Elia M, Ljungquist O, et al., editors. Nutrition Society Textbook Series: Clinical nutrition. Oxford: Blackwell Publishing, 2005; pp. 30–61.

15. Armstrong ME, Lambert MI, Sharwood KA, et al. Obesity and overweight in South African primary school children – the Health of the Nation Study. S Afr Med J. 2006;96(5):439–444. PMID 16751921.

16. Kruger R, Kruger HS, MacIntyre UE. The determinants of overweight and obesity among 10- to15- year-old schoolchildren in the North West Province, South Africa – the THUSA BANA (Transition and Health during Urbanisation of South Africans; BANA, children) study. Publ Health Nutr. 2006;9(3):351–358. PMID 16684387.

17. Lee RD, Nieman DC. Nutritional Assessment. 3rd ed. Boston: McGraw Hill; 2003.

18. World Health Organization. WHO child growth standards: Methods and development. Length/height-for-age, weight-for-age, weight-for-length, weight-for-height and body mass index-for-age. Geneva: WHO; 2006.

19. Genovesi S, Antolini L, Giussani M, et al. Usefulness of waist circumference for identification of childhood hypertension. J Hypertens. 2008;26(8):1563–1570. http://dx.doi.org/10.1097/HJH.0b013e328302842b. PMID 18622233.

20. Fernández JR, Redden DT, Pietrobelli A, et al. Waist circumference percentiles in nationally representative samples of African-American, European-American, and Mexican-American children and adolescents. J Pediatr. 2004;145(4):439–444. http://dx.doi.org/10.1016/j.jpeds.2004.06.044. PMID 15480363.

21. McVeigh JA, Norris SA, De Wet T. The relationship between socio-economic status and physical activity patterns in South African children. Acta Paediatr. 2004;93(7):982–988. http://dx.doi.org/10.1111/j.1651-2227.2004.tb02699.x. PMID 15303817.

22. Prentice AM. The emerging epidemic of obesity in developing countries. Int J Epidemiol. 2006;35(1):93–99. PMID 16326822.

23. Gericke GJ, Labadarios DL. A measure of hunger. In: National food consumption survey: fortification baseline. Stellenbosch: Department of Health, 2007; pp. 255–257.

24. Medical Research Council. Umthente uhlaba usamila: the 2nd South African national youth risk behaviour survey [document on the Internet]. c2008 [cited 2010 Oct 16]. Available from: http://www.mrc.ac.za/healthpromotion/yrbs_2008_final_report.pdf

25. Rose D, Charlton KE. Prevalence of household food poverty in South Africa: Results from a large, nationally representative survey. Publ Health Nutr. 2002;5(3):383–389. http://dx.doi.org/10.1079/PHN2001320. PMID 12003648.

26. Wang Y. Cross-national comparison of childhood obesity: The epidemic and the relationship between obesity and socioeconomic status. Int J Epidemiol. 2001;30(5):1129–1136. http://dx.doi.org/10.1093/ije/30.5.1129. PMID 11689534.

27. Lobstein T, Baur L, Uauy R. 2004. Obesity in children and young people: A crisis in public health. Obes Rev. 2004;5(Suppl 1):4–85. http://dx.doi.org/10.1111/j.1467-789X.2004.00133.x. PMID 15096099.

28. Meko NML. Associations between the determinants of overweight and obesity in children aged 13–15 years in Bloemfontein, in the Free State province. Doctoral thesis. Bloemfontein: Faculty of Health Sciences, University of the Free State; 2010.

29. Halley-Castillo E, Borges G, Talavera JO, et al. Body mass index and the prevalence of metabolic syndrome among children and adolescents in two Mexican populations. J Adolesc Health. 2007;40(6):521–526. PMID 17531758.

30. McCarthy HD, Ellis SM, Cole TJ. Central overweight and obesity in British youth aged 11–16 years: Cross-sectional surveys of waist circumference. BMJ. 2003;326(7390):624–626. http://dx.doi.org/10.1136/bmj.326.7390.624. PMID 12234.

31. Pérez-Cueto A, Almanza M, Kolsteren PW. Female gender and wealth are associated to overweight among adolescents in La Paz, Bolivia. Eur J Clin Nutr. 2005;59(1):82–87. http://dx.doi.org/10.1038/sj.ejcn.1602040. PMID 15305181.

32. Kleiser C, Rosario AS, Mensink GBM, et al. Potential determinants of obesity among children and adolescents in Germany: Results from the cross-sectional KiGGS study. BMC Public Health. 2009;9:46. http://dx.doi.org/10.1186/1471-2458-9-46. PMID 19187531.

33. Poskitt EM. Tackling childhood obesity: Diet, physical activity or lifestyle change? Acta Paediatr. 2005;94(4):396–398. http://dx.doi.org/10.1080/08035250510026733. PMID 16092449.

34. Ekelund U, Neovius M, Linné Y, et al. Associations between physical activity and fat mass in adolescents: the Stockholm Weight Development Study. Am J Clin Nutr. 2005;81(2):355–360. PMID 15699221.

35. Monteiro CA, Benicio MHD, Conde WL, et al. Narrowing socioeconomic inequality in child stunting: the Brazilian experience, 1974–2007. Bull World Health Organ. 2010;88:305–311. http://dx.doi.org/10.2471/BLT.09.069195. PMID 20431795.

36. Mamabolo RL, Kruger HS, Lennox A, et al. 2007. Habitual physical activity and body composition of black township adolescents residing in the North West Province, South Africa. Pub Health Nutr. 2007;10(10):1047–1056. http://dx.doi.org/10.1017/S1368980007668724. PMID 17381956.

Permissions

All chapters in this book were first published in PHCFM, by AOSIS Publishing; hereby published with permission under the Creative Commons Attribution License or equivalent. Every chapter published in this book has been scrutinized by our experts. Their significance has been extensively debated. The topics covered herein carry significant findings which will fuel the growth of the discipline. They may even be implemented as practical applications or may be referred to as a beginning point for another development.

The contributors of this book come from diverse backgrounds, making this book a truly international effort. This book will bring forth new frontiers with its revolutionizing research information and detailed analysis of the nascent developments around the world.

We would like to thank all the contributing authors for lending their expertise to make the book truly unique. They have played a crucial role in the development of this book. Without their invaluable contributions this book wouldn't have been possible. They have made vital efforts to compile up to date information on the varied aspects of this subject to make this book a valuable addition to the collection of many professionals and students.

This book was conceptualized with the vision of imparting up-to-date information and advanced data in this field. To ensure the same, a matchless editorial board was set up. Every individual on the board went through rigorous rounds of assessment to prove their worth. After which they invested a large part of their time researching and compiling the most relevant data for our readers.

The editorial board has been involved in producing this book since its inception. They have spent rigorous hours researching and exploring the diverse topics which have resulted in the successful publishing of this book. They have passed on their knowledge of decades through this book. To expedite this challenging task, the publisher supported the team at every step. A small team of assistant editors was also appointed to further simplify the editing procedure and attain best results for the readers.

Apart from the editorial board, the designing team has also invested a significant amount of their time in understanding the subject and creating the most relevant covers. They scrutinized every image to scout for the most suitable representation of the subject and create an appropriate cover for the book.

The publishing team has been an ardent support to the editorial, designing and production team. Their endless efforts to recruit the best for this project, has resulted in the accomplishment of this book. They are a veteran in the field of academics and their pool of knowledge is as vast as their experience in printing. Their expertise and guidance has proved useful at every step. Their uncompromising quality standards have made this book an exceptional effort. Their encouragement from time to time has been an inspiration for everyone.

The publisher and the editorial board hope that this book will prove to be a valuable piece of knowledge for researchers, students, practitioners and scholars across the globe.

List of Contributors

Tenna Ephrem
Oromia Regional Health Bureau, Addis Ababa, Ethiopia

Bezatu Mengiste and Frehiwot Mesfin
College of Health and Medical Sciences, Haramaya University, Ethiopia

Wanzahun Godana
College of Medicine and Health Sciences, Arba Minch University, Ethiopia

Modjadji M. Maake
Department of Public Health, School of Health Sciences, University of Limpopo, South Africa

Olalekan A. Oduntan
Department of Optometry, School of Health Sciences, University of Kwazulu-Natal, South Africa

Ronel Roos, Hellen Myezwa and Helena van Aswegen
Department of Physiotherapy, University of the Witwatersrand, South Africa

Katijah Khoza-Shangase and Shannon Harbinson
Faculty of Humanities, Department of Audiology, University of the Witwatersrand, South Africa

Zelra Malan and Bob Mash
Family Medicine and Primary Care, Stellenbosch University, South Africa

Katherine Everett-Murphy
Chronic Diseases Initiative in Africa (CDIA), Faculty of Health Sciences, University of Cape Town, South Africa

Ayodeji M. Adebayo and Michael C. Asuzu
Department of Preventive Medicine and Primary Care, College of Medicine, University of Ibadan, Ibadan

Radiance M. Ogundipe and Robert Mash
Division of Family Medicine and Primary Care, Faculty of Medicine and Health Sciences, Stellenbosch University, Tygerberg, South Africa

Ntambwe Malangu and Omotayo D. Adebanjo
Department of Epidemiology & Biostatistics, University of Limpopo, Medunsa Campus, South Africa

Gershom Chongwe and Charles Michelo
University of Zambia, School of Medicine, Department of Public Health, Zambia

Nathan Kapata
Ministry of Health, National TB/Leprosy Control Program, Zambia

Mwendaweli Maboshe and Olusegun Babaniyi
World Health Organization Country Office, Zambia

Rory du Plessis
Department of Visual Arts, University of Pretoria, South Africa

Andrew Ross and Laura Campbell
Department of Family Medicine, University of KwaZulu-Natal, South Africa

Gavin MacGregor
Umthombo Youth Development Foundation, South Africa

Asafa R. Adedeji, John Tumbo and Indiran Govender
Department of Family Medicine and Primary Health Care, Sefako Makgatho Health Sciences University, South Africa

Joseph N. Ikwegbue, Andrew Ross and Harbor Ogbonnaya
Department of Family Medicine, University of KwaZulu-Natal, South Africa

Amon Siveregi and Phatisizwe Dlamini
Mankayane Government Hospital, Swaziland

Lilian Dudley
Division of Community Health, Department of Interdisciplinary Health Sciences, Stellenbosch University, South Africa

Courage Makumucha
Institute of Development Management, Mbabane, Swaziland

Sihle Moyo
Hlatikhulu Government Hospital, Swaziland

Sibongiseni Bhembe
Piggs Peak Government Hospital, Swaziland

Martin Bac and Jannie Hugo
Faculty of Health Sciences, Department of Family Medicine, University of Pretoria, South Africa

Anne-Marie Bergh and Mama E. Etsane
MRC Unit for Maternal and Infant Health Care Strategies, Faculty of Health Sciences, University of Pretoria, South Africa

Abigail Dreyer, Audrey Gibbs, Scott Smalley and Motlatso Mlambo
Centre for Rural Health, Department of Family Medicine, Faculty of Health Sciences, University of the Witwatersrand, South Africa

Himani Pandya
Centre for Rural Health, Department of Family Medicine, Faculty of Health Sciences, University of the Witwatersrand, South Africa
Faculty of Health Sciences, Department of Paediatrics and Child Health, Division of Community Paediatrics, University of the Witwatersrand, South Africa

Evans Chinkoyo
Faculty of Medicine and Health Sciences, Department of Interdisciplinary Health Sciences, Division of Family Medicine and Primary Care, University of Stellenbosch, South Africa
Chipata Level 1 Hospital, Lusaka, Zambia

Michael Pather
Faculty of Medicine and Health Sciences, Department of Interdisciplinary Health Sciences, Division of Family Medicine and Primary Care, University of Stellenbosch, South Africa

Thembisile M. Chauke and Hendry van der Heever
Department of Public Health, University of Limpopo, Medunsa Campus, South Africa

Muhammad E. Hoque
Graduate School of Business and Leadership, University of KwaZulu-Natal, Westville Campus, South Africa

David P. van Velden
Department of Pathology, Faculty of Medicine and Health Sciences, Department of Pathology, Stellenbosch University, South Africa

Helmuth Reuter
Winelands Medical Research Centre, South Africa

Martin Kidd
Centre for Statistical Consultation, Department of Statistics and Actuarial Sciences, Stellenbosch University, South Africa

F. Otto Müller
Clinical Trials and Drug Development Consultant, George, South Africa

Johan Schoevers
Division of Family Medicine and Primary Health Care, Faculty of Health Sciences, Stellenbosch University, South Africa
Family Physician, Mossel Bay subdistrict, Western Cape Department of Health, South Africa

Louis Jenkins
Division of Family Medicine and Primary Health Care, Faculty of Health Sciences, Stellenbosch University, South Africa
George Provincial Hospital, Eden District, Western Cape Department of Health, South Africa

Graham Bresick, Abdul-Rauf Sayed, Cynthia le Grange, Susheela Bhagwan and Nayna Manga
Faculty of Health Sciences, University of Cape Town, South Africa

Zamir A. Gilani
Department of Family Medicine, Prince Mshiyeni Memorial Hospital, South Africa

Kantharuben Naidoo and Andrew Ross
Department of Family Medicine, University of KwaZulu-Natal, South Africa

Robin E. Dyers
Division of Community Health, Faculty of Medicine and Health Sciences, Department of Interdisciplinary Health Sciences, Stellenbosch University, South Africa
Health Programmes, Western Cape Government: Health, South Africa

Robert Mash
Division of Family Medicine and Primary Care, Faculty of Medicine and Health Sciences, Department of Interdisciplinary Health Sciences, Stellenbosch University, South Africa

Tracey Naledi
Health Programmes, Western Cape Government: Health, South Africa

Khathutshelo P. Mashige, Olalekan A. Oduntan and Rekha Hansraj
Discipline of Optometry, School of Health Sciences, University of KwaZulu-Natal, South Africa

Vivien Essel
Public Health Registrar, University of Cape Town, South Africa
Western Cape Provincial Health Services, South Africa

Unita van Vuuren
Chronic Disease Management, Western Cape Provincial Health Services, South Africa

Angela De Sa, Katie Murie, Mosedi Namane and Elma de Vries
Family Physician, University of Cape Town, South Africa
Western Cape Metro District Health Services, South Africa

Srini Govender and Arina Schlemmer
Western Cape Metro District Health Services, South Africa
Family Physician, Stellenbosch University, South Africa

Colette Gunst
Cape Winelands District Health Services, Western Cape Government: Health, South Africa

Andrew Boulle
Western Cape Provincial Health Services, South Africa
Public Health Specialist, University of Cape Town, South Africa

Phillip Mubanga and Wilhelm J. Steinberg
Faculty of Health Sciences, Department of Family Medicine, University of the Free State, South Africa

Francois C. Van Rooyen
Faculty of Health Department Sciences, Department of Biostatistics, University of the Free State, South Africa

Chandra R. Makanjee
Faculty of Health Sciences, Department of Radiography, University of Pretoria, South Africa

Anne-Marie Bergh
MRC Unit for Maternal and Infant Health Care Strategies, Faculty of Health Sciences, University of Pretoria, South Africa

Willem A. Hoffmann
Department of Biomedical Sciences, Tshwane University of Technology, South Africa

Zelra Malan and Bob Mash
Family Medicine and Primary Care, Stellenbosch University, South Africa

Katherine Everett-Murphy
Chronic Diseases Initiative in Africa (CDIA), Faculty of Health Sciences, University of Cape Town, South Africa

Elsje Scheffler and Surona Visagie
Centre for Rehabilitation Studies, Stellenbosch University, South Africa
Psychology Department, Stellenbosch University, South Africa

Marguerite Schneider
Psychology Department, Stellenbosch University, South Africa
Centre for Public Mental Health, Department of Psychiatry and Mental Health, University of Cape Town, South Africa

Ian Couper
Centre for Rural Health, Faculty of Health Sciences, University of the Witwatersrand, South Africa

Oladele V. Adeniyi, Parimalane Yogeswaran and Benjamin Longo-Mbenza
Department of Family Medicine, Faculty of Health Sciences, Walter Sisulu University, Mthatha, South Africa

Graham Wright
Centre for Health Informatics Research and Development (CHIRAD), University of Fort Hare, South Africa

Lucia N. M. Meko, Marthinette Slabber-Stretch and Corinna M. Walsh
Nutrition and Dietetics, University of the Free State, South Africa

Salome H. Kruger
School of Physiology and Nutrition, North-West University, Potchefstroom Campus, South Africa

Mariette Nel
Biostatistics, Faculty of Health Sciences, University of the Free State, South Africa